Health Policy and Advanced Practice Nursing

Kelly A. Goudreau, PhD, RN, ACNS-BC, FAAN, is the Associate Director Patient Care Services/Nurse Executive at the Veterans Affairs Southern Oregon Rehabilitation Center and Clinics (VA SORCC). Dr. Goudreau has administrative responsibility for a number of patient care services such as Audiology, Chaplain, Nutrition and Food Services, Radiology, Laboratory, Infirmary Nursing Staff, Infection Control, Infusion Center, Occupational Health, Sleep Lab, Wound Care, Home-Based Primary Care, Home Telehealth, and Sterile Processing Services. She has been working at local, regional, and national levels in the development of policy that has a specific impact on advanced practice registered nurses (APRNs) as a member of the Joint Dialogue Group that created the APRN Consensus Paper. As a champion for APRNs (Clinical Nurse Specialists in particular) and originally completing her generic baccalaureate nursing program in Canada, she sees the health policy implications from an international perspective. She is a past president of the National Association of Clinical Nurse Specialists and is an Associate Editor of *Clinical Nurse Specialist: The Journal for Advanced Nursing Practice.*

Mary C. Smolenski, EdD, MS, FNP, FAANP, is a consultant and family nurse practitioner with a career path that spans the health care field in a variety of areas such as nurse practitioner education, government contracting, the military, primary care, independent practice, and associations with an emphasis on certification and accreditation. She is a retired Air Force Reserve Colonel flight nurse and a Fellow of the American Association of Nurse Practitioners. She served as Director of Certification Services at the American Nurses Credentialing Center (ANCC) for 11 years in which she devoted a significant portion of her role to advanced practice issues. She was a member of the APRN Consensus Process Work Group during the development of the APRN Consensus Paper. She was active on several accreditation nonprofit boards and has presented and published on certification, competency, advanced practice nursing, and on-line portfolios. Her initial work on portfolios while at ANCC paved the way for specialty nursing recognition process through on-line portfolios.

Health Policy and Advanced Practice Nursing

Impact and Implications

EDITORS
Kelly A. Goudreau, PhD, RN, ACNS-BC, FAAN
Mary C. Smolenski, EdD, MS, FNP, FAANP

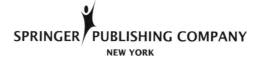

SPRINGER PUBLISHING COMPANY

NEW YORK

Springer Publishing Company, LLC
11 West 42nd Street
New York, NY 10036
www.springerpub.com

Acquisitions Editor: Margaret Zuccarini
Composition: Exeter Premedia Services Private Ltd.

ISBN: 978-0-8261-6942-6
e-book ISBN: 978-0-8261-6943-3

13 14 15 16 17 / 5 4 3 2 1

The author and the publisher of this Work have made every effort to use sources believed to be reliable to provide information that is accurate and compatible with the standards generally accepted at the time of publication. The author and publisher shall not be liable for any special, consequential, or exemplary damages resulting, in whole or in part, from the readers' use of, or reliance on, the information contained in this book. The publisher has no responsibility for the persistence or accuracy of URLs for external or third-party Internet websites referred to in this publication and does not guarantee that any content on such websites is, or will remain, accurate or appropriate.

Library of Congress Cataloging-in-Publication Data
Health policy and advanced practice nursing : impact and implications / editors, Kelly A. Goudreau, Mary C. Smolenski.
        p. ; cm.
    Includes bibliographical references and index.
    ISBN 978-0-8261-6942-6—ISBN 978-0-8261-6943-3 (e-book)
  I. Goudreau, Kelly A., editor of compilation.   II. Smolenski, Mary C. (Mary Catherine),
    1950– editor of compilation.
    [DNLM: 1. Advanced Practice Nursing—United States.   2. Health Policy—United States.
    WY 128]
    RT89
    362.17′3—dc23
                                                                                        2013041334

Printed in the United States of America by Gasch Printing.

This book is dedicated to APRNs everywhere. The hardest part of becoming the best that you can be, is to incorporate the global perspective and consider the implications of health policy to your practice. It is our sincere hope that this text will assist you to begin the journey regardless of where you are in your career. As a new or developing APRN, welcome. As an existing APRN in mid-career, welcome. As an APRN at the end of your career … it is about time you joined the battle! All joking aside, the need for APRNs to become engaged in the dialogue has never been more important than it is right now. We are pleased to be able to dedicate this perspective on health policy to all of you so that you can engage in discussion, dialogue, and discourse about the future of APRNs everywhere around the globe.

Contents

Contributors   *xi*
Foreword   Loretta C. Ford, RN, EdD, PNP, FAAN, FAANP   *xv*
Preface   *xvii*
Acknowledgments   *xix*

UNIT I: INTRODUCTION TO HEALTH POLICY FROM AN ADVANCED PRACTICE PERSPECTIVE

1. Prolific Policy: Implications for Advanced Practice Registered Nurses   *3*
   Melissa Stewart

2. Turning Health Policy Into Practice: Implications for Advanced Practice Registered Nurses   *13*
   James L. Harris

3. Johnson & Johnson Campaign for Nursing's Future: An Impetus for Change   *23*
   Mary C. Smolenski

4. Policy Implications for Optimizing Advanced Practice Registered Nurse Use Nationally   *29*
   Robin P. Newhouse, Jonathan P. Weiner, Julie Stanik-Hutt, Kathleen M. White, Meg Johantgen, Don Steinwachs, George Zangaro, Jillian Aldebron, and Eric B. Bass

5. The IOM Report: The Future of Nursing   *41*
   Liana Orsolini

6. Implications for Practice: The Consensus Model for Advanced Practice Registered Nurse Regulation   *57*
   Kelly A. Goudreau

7. The Coalition for Patients' Rights—A Coalition That Advocates for Scope of Practice Issues   *67*
   Melinda Ray and Maureen Shekleton

8. The Future of Nursing: Campaign for Action   *75*
   Susan Hassmiller, Susan Reinhard, and Andrea Brassard

UNIT II: IMPLICATIONS OF HEALTH CARE REFORM AND FINANCE ON ADVANCED PRACTICE REGISTERED NURSE PRACTICE

9. **The Patient Protection and Affordable Care Act**   *87*
    Jan Towers

10. **AARP Initiatives**   *95*
    Andrea Brassard and Susan Reinhard

11. **A Million Hearts® Initiative**   *103*
    Liana Orsolini and Mary C. Smolenski

12. **Joining Forces: Taking Action to Serve America's Military Families—A White House Initiative**   *121*
    Cathy Rick

13. **Effective State-Level Advanced Practice Registered Nursing Leadership in Health Policy**   *135*
    Christine Filipovich

14. **Funding of Advanced Practice Registered Nurse Education and Residency Programs**   *145*
    Suzanne Miyamoto

15. **Interface of Policy and Practice in Psychiatric Mental Health Nursing: Anticipating Challenges and Opportunities of Health Care Reform**   *163*
    Kathleen R. Delaney and Andrea N. Kwasky

UNIT III: HEALTH POLICY AND SPECIAL POPULATIONS

16. **The Aging Population**   *185*
    Pat Kappas-Larsen

17. **The Certified Nurse Midwife in Advanced Nursing Practice**   *197*
    Janelle Komorowski

18. **Health Policy Implications for Advanced Practice Registered Nurses Related to End-of-Life Care**   *215*
    Judy Lentz

19. **Health Policy Implications for Advanced Practice Registered Nurses Related to Oncology Care**   *235*
    Cynthia Abarado, Kelly Brassil, Garry Brydges, and Joyce E. Dains

UNIT IV: HEALTH POLICY AND ITS IMPACT ON ADVANCED PRACTICE REGISTERED NURSE-DRIVEN QUALITY

20. **Policy Implications for Advanced Practice Registered Nurses: Quality and Safety**   *253*
    Mary Jean Schuman

21. **Moving Toward Accountable Care: A Policy Framework to Transform Health Care Delivery and Reimbursement**   *273*
    Susan M. Kendig

22. **A Systemic Approach to Containing Health Care Spending** *287*
Ezekiel Emanuel, Neera Tanden, Stuart Altman, Scott Armstrong, Donald Berwick,
François de Brantes, Maura Calsyn, Michael Chernew, John Colmers, David Cutler,
Tom Daschle, Paul Egerman, Bob Kocher, Arnold Milstein, Emily Oshima Lee,
John D. Podesta, Uwe Reinhardt, Meredith Rosenthal, Joshua Sharfstein,
Stephen Shortell, Andrew Stern, Peter R. Orszag, and Topher Spiro

UNIT V: EFFECTS OF THE SHIFTING SANDS OF POLICY ON NURSING ORGANIZATIONS

23. **The Effects of Shifting Sands of Health Policy on Advanced Practice Nursing Organizations** *297*
Anita Finkelman

24. **The American Nurses Association** *311*
Cindy Balkstra and Andrea Brassard

25. **State Implementation of the APRN Consensus Model** *323*
Tracy Klein

26. **Advanced Practice Registered Nursing: The Global Perspective** *337*
Judith Shamian and Moriah Ellen

27. **Credentialing Across the Globe: Approaches and Applications** *349*
Frances Hughes and Catherine Coates

UNIT VI: WHAT DOES THE FUTURE HOLD FOR ADVANCED PRACTICE REGISTERED NURSE PRACTICE AND HEALTH CARE POLICY

28. **Health Policy for Advanced Practice Registered Nurses: An International Perspective** *361*
Madrean M. Schober

29. **The Future for Nurse Practitioners** *373*
Jan Towers

30. **What the Future Holds for Clinical Nurse Specialist Practice and Health Policy** *379*
Rachel Moody

31. **Health Policy and Special Needs Populations: Advanced Nursing Practice in Low-Income Countries** *393*
Patricia L. Riley, Jessica M. Gross, Carey F. McCarthy, Andre R. Verani,
and Alexandra Zuber

32. **Health Care Policy and Certified Registered Nurse Anesthetists: Past, Present, and Future** *417*
Christine S. Zambricki

Index *443*

Contributors

Cynthia Abarado, DNP, MSN, APRN, GNP-BC   Advanced Practice Registered Nurse, MD Anderson Cancer Center, Houston, TX

Jillian Aldebron, JD   Independent Consultant, Baltimore, MD

Stuart Altman, PhD   Brandeis University, Waltham, MA

Scott Armstrong, MBA   Group Health Cooperative, Seattle, WA

Eric B. Bass, MPH, MD   The Johns Hopkins University, School of Medicine, Baltimore, MD

Cindy Balkstra, MS, RN, ACNS-BC   First Vice President, ANA and Case Manager, United Hospice, Dahlonega, GA

Donald Berwick, MD, MPP   Center for American Progress, Washington, DC, and Harvard Medical School, Boston, MA

Andrea Brassard, PhD, MPH, FNP-C, FAANP   Former Senior Strategic Policy Advisor, Center to Champion Nursing, AARP, Current Senior Policy Fellow, ANA, Washington, DC

Kelly J. Brassil, BASW, MSN, ACNS-BC, AOCNS   Associate Director Nursing Programs, MD Anderson Cancer Center, Houston, TX

Garry J. Brydges, CRNA, DNP, ACNP-BC   Certified Registered Nurse Anesthetist, MD Anderson Cancer Center, Houston, TX

Maura Calsyn, JD   Center for American Progress, Washington, DC

Michael Chernew, PhD   Harvard Medical School, Boston, MA

Catherine Coates, BA   Senior Advisor, Office of Mental Health, Ministry of Health, Blemhem, NZ

John Colmers, MPH   Johns Hopkins Medicine, Baltimore, MD

David Cutler, PhD   Center for American Progress, Washington, DC, and Harvard University, Cambridge, MA

Joyce E. Dains, DrPH, JD, RN, FNP-BC, DPNAP, FAANP   Associate Professor, the Department of Nursing, University of Texas, MD Anderson Cancert Center, Houston, TX

François de Brantes, MBA   Health Care Incentives Improvement Institute, Newtown, CT

Tom Daschle, BA   Center for American Progress, Washington, DC, and DLA Piper, Washington, DC

Kathleen R. Delaney, PhD, RN   Professor of Nursing and Graduate Nursing Education Project Director, Rush University, Chicago, IL

Paul Egerman, BS   Co-founder, IDX and eScription, Inc., Needham, MA

Moriah Ellen, PhD, MBA   McMaster University, Toronto, Ontario, Canada

Ezekiel Emanuel, MD, PhD   Center for American Progress, Washington, DC, and University of Pennsylvania, Philadelphia, PA

Christine Filipovich, MSN, RN   Executive Assistant, Office of Quality Assurance, Pennsylvania Department of Health, Harrisburg, PA

Anita Finkelman, MSN, RN   Faculty, Bouve College of Health Sciences and School of Nursing, Northeastern University, Boston, MA

Kelly A. Goudreau, PhD, RN, ACNS-BC, FAAN   Associate Director Patient Care Services/Nurse Executive, VA Southern Oregon Rehabilitation Center and Clinics, White City, OR

Jessica M. Gross, ANP-BC, MPH   Health Systems Strengthening (The Task Force for Global Health), Consultant, Centers for Disease Control and Prevention, Nairobi, Kenya

James L. Harris, DSN, RN, CNS, CNL, FAAN   Acting Chief Nurse, Veterans Affairs, Washington, DC

Susan Hassmiller, PhD, RN, FAAN   Senior Advisor for Nursing, Director, Future of Nursing: Campaign for Action, Robert Wood Johnson Foundation, Princeton, NJ

Frances Hughes, RN, DNurs, ONZM   Visiting Professor, University of Sydney, Sydney, Australia

Meg Johantgen, PhD, RN   University of Maryland, Baltimore, MD

Pat Kappas-Larsen, DNP, APN-C, FAAN   Independent Consultant, Hastings, MN

Susan Kendig, JD, MSN, WHNP-BC, FAANP   Teaching Professor and WHNP Emphasis Area Coordinator, College of Nursing, University of Missouri-St. Louis, St Louis, MO

Tracy Klein, PhD, FNP, ARNP, FAANP, FAAN   Assistant Professor, School of Nursing, Washington State University Vancouver, WA

Bob Kocher, MD   Venrock, Palo Alto, CA, and Brookings Institution, Washington, DC

Janelle Komorowski, CNM, MS   Nurse-Midwife, Women First, Loveland, CO

Andrea N. Kwasky, DNP, PMHCNS-BC, PMHNP-BC   Family Psychiatric/Mental Health Nurse Practitioner, University of Detroit Mercy, McAuley School of Nursing, Detroit, MI

Emily Oshima Lee, MA   Center for American Progress, Washington, DC

Judy Lentz, RN, MSN   Retired CEO, Hospice and Palliative Nurses Association, Pittsburgh, PA

Carey F. McCarthy, PhD, RN   Human Resources for Health Advisor, Centers for Disease Control and Prevention, Atlanta, GA

Arnold Milstein, MD, MPH   Stanford University School of Medicine, Stanford, CA

Suzanne Miyamoto, PhD, RN   Director of Government Affairs, American Association of Colleges of Nursing, Washington, DC

Rachel Moody, MS, CNS, RN   Immediate Past President, National Association of Clinical Nurse Specialists, Harrisburgh, PA

Robin P. Newhouse, PhD, RN, NEA-BC, FAAN   University of Maryland, Baltimore, MD

Liana Orsolini, PhD, RN, ANEF, FAAN   Care Delivery and Advanced Practice System Consultant, Bon Secours Health System, Inc., Center for Clinical Excellence and Innovation, Marriottsville, MD

Peter R. Orszag, PhD   Citigroup and the Council on Foreign Relations, New York, NY

John D. Podesta, JD   Center for American Progress, Washington, DC

Melinda Ray, MSN, RN   Executive Director, National Association of Clinical Nurse Specialists, Pittsburgh, PA

Susan Reinhard, PhD, RN, FAAN   Senior VP and Director, AARP Public Policy Institute, Chief Strategist, Center to Champion Nursing, Washington, DC

Uwe Reinhardt, PhD   Princeton University, Princeton, NJ

Cathy Rick, RN PhD (H), NEA-BC, FAAN, FACHE   Chief Nurse, Veterans Affairs, Washington, DC

Patricia L. Riley, CNM, MPH, FACNM   Senior Nurse Midwife, Maternal and Child Health Branch, Centers for Disease Control and Prevention, Atlanta, GA

Meredith Rosenthal, PhD   Harvard School of Public Health, Boston, MA

Madrean M. Schober, PhD, MSN, BGS, ANP, FAANP President, Schober Consulting, International Healthcare Consultants, Indianapolis, IN

Mary Jean Schuman, DNP, MBA, RN, CPNP, FAAN Assistant Professor of Nursing, The George Washington University School of Nursing, Washington, DC

Judith Shamian, RN, PhD, LLD, LLD (Hon), D.Sci (Hon), FAAN President, International Council of Nurses, Geneva, Switzerland

Joshua Sharfstein, MD Department of Health and Mental Hygiene, State of Maryland, Baltimore, MD

Maureen Shekleton, PhD, RN Owner, Shekleton LLC, Chicago, IL

Stephen Shortell, PhD, MPH, MBA University of California, Berkeley, School of Public Health, Berkeley, CA

Mary C. Smolenski, EdD, MS, FNP, FAANP Consultant, Lakewood Ranch, FL

Topher Spiro, JD Center for American Progress, Washington, DC

Julie Stanik-Hutt, PhD, ACNP, CCNS, FAAN The Johns Hopkins University, School of Nursing, Baltimore, MD

Don Steinwachs, PhD The Johns Hopkins University, School of Public Health, Baltimore, MD

Andrew Stern, BA Center for American Progress, Washington, DC, and Columbia University, New York, NY

Melissa Stewart, DNP, RN, CPE Assistant Professor, Our Lady of the Lake College, St. Francisville, LA

Neera Tanden, JD Center for American Progress, Washington, DC

Jan Towers, PhD, NP-C, CRNP, FAANP, FAAN Senior Policy Advisor, American Association of Nurse Practitioners, Washington, DC

Andre R. Verani, JD, MPH Public Health Policy Analyst, Division of Global HIV/AIDS, Center for Global Health, Centers for Disease Control and Prevention, Atlanta, GA

Jonathan P. Weiner, DrPH The Johns Hopkins University, School of Public Health, Baltimore, MD

Kathleen M. White, PhD, RN, NEA-BC, FAAN The Johns Hopkins University, School of Nursing, Baltimore, MD

Christine S. Zambricki, DNAP, CRNA, FAAN Former Senior Director, Federal Affairs Strategies, American Association of Nurse Anesthetists, Washington, DC

George Zangaro, PhD, RN The Catholic University of America, School of Nursing, Washington, DC

Alexandra Zuber, MPP Human Resources for Health Advisor, Health Systems and Human Resources Team, Centers for Disease Control and Prevention, Atlanta, GA

Foreword

As this nation, finally after 100 years of political strife, adopts a national health policy and embraces universal health care, the opportunities and options for advanced practice nurses could not be more politically, socially, and economically timely and opportunistic. One of the most hopeful trends in the new health care legislation, the Patient Protection and Affordable Care Act (PPACA) is a perfect match for nursing because of its transformation of the current sick care system to a bona fide "health care system." With the term Patient Protection, which is often ignored in reports, indicates that the PPACA has at its core, prevention and health promotion to achieve optimal population health. Since Florence Nightingale's leadership in creating a healthy environment in which healing can take place, nursing has had at its caring core prevention and health promotion to preserve and protect the health of individuals and populations. Not that this has been recognized, reported, respected, or rewarded among colleagues or the public media. In this world of high-tech medicine, public attention is focused on the dramatic, esoteric, and unique procedures that help a few unfortunate patients. Granted much can be learned from these marvels, but application to the larger populations is in question. However, achieving this monumental effort to reorient this humongous health care sector with all its social, economic, and political woes, legislative stalemates, and professional territorial battles would not be easy. But a crisis is an opportunity for change and *now* is nursing's time to jump into the fray.

Internally, unifying our nursing forces and resources across a diversely educated populace is the first hurdle. Externally, we must remove artificial barriers to changes in state practice laws, address the competition among a host of nursing organizations, settle disagreements on the political strategies, and do whatever is called for to form a united front. All this will require a well-organized, well-funded, fast-moving national campaign—one that not only unifies nursing and nursing organizations, but also cultivates new partners outside the traditional health professionals, such as other stakeholders, consumer groups, industries and corporations, and faith-based and public service agencies. It is a huge undertaking, but there are a number of signs on the horizon to encourage us. Politically, we must stop requesting changes in state practice laws, one task at a legislative session. Nursing, and in particular APRNs, must seek full statutory authorization and autonomy to practice to the full extent of the practitioner's preparation. We must gain our freedom to practice *now*.

The timeliness of the Institute of Medicine's *The Future of Nursing*, the *Consensus Report on Licensure, Accreditation, Credentialing and Education*, and many other recently published documents (*The Governors' Report*, Florida watchdog tax group, etc.) offer monumental support for nurses everywhere and, in particular, nursing leaders especially APRNs to move quickly and decisively to achieve the goals of addressing the nation's problems of access, quality, and affordability in health care. Perhaps most importantly, it is an opportunity for nurses to re-orient a medically disease-focused sick care system to a true *health* system with prevention at the core of the services. Knowledge is power. Gaining a better understanding of the political landscape and its impact on nursing and the APRN practice environment, by learning through textbooks such as this and then through active involvement at any level in the political process itself, can only strengthen nursing and its influence on health policy. Nursing leaders and nurses everywhere must not miss the opportunities that this new enabling environment in health care offers to innovate, invent, imagine, and inspire. Our patients deserve this, the nation needs it, and *now* is the time!

Loretta C. Ford, RN, EdD, PNP, FAAN, FAANP
Dean and Professor Emerita
School of Nursing
University of Rochester

Preface

The original concept for this book was to bring into discussion the many events, campaigns, initiatives, documents, and legislative efforts that have laid the groundwork for change and have impacted advanced practice registered nurse (APRN) practice in today's world. As a book written by APRNs from an APRN perspective, it was also intended to identify the implications that these changes might have for current and future practice, and get APRNs thinking about them and involved in creating conditions that will improve patient outcomes. Many books give you an outside-in view of events. This book is to give you an inside-out view, placing you right in the middle of things, helping you to see the importance of understanding the basics of health policy development, and recognizing that each person can play a part in the process.

Health policy is not something that most APRNs or APRN faculty can hold near and dear to their hearts. Political events of the past few years along with current-day partisanship have unfortunately turned more people off to the political process than enamored them to it. Discomfort with the health policy process can be viewed in the same way that research used to be viewed. Everyone realized that research was important and necessary, it seemed to be a little complex and scary, and it got a mention and some cursory attention in curricula with the hope that someone else would take care of it. Well, that has certainly changed over the past few decades with the influence of graduate education, the advent of evidence-based practice, and the need to have data-supporting practice in order to initiate changes. Everyone is much more concerned about research-based evidence, patient safety, and quality.

Health policy has taken on that same persona as research once had and more APRNs and consumers in general have taken up their banners for specific causes. The world has become a smaller place and with the influence of television and social media, initiating interest in change has never been easier. Action is the harder task. Whereas some advanced practice groups such as certified registered nurse anesthetists (CRNAs) have been thrown into the political arena to defend their practice and reimbursement, others are only beginning to see the need for involvement. This book hopefully points out numerous areas where APRNs are already taking action to create better practice environments and conditions, how they can work to define positive change for their patients/clients, and how they can have an impact on the health of communities and the nation through the health policy process.

It is our hope that this book will show you, the reader, how health policy has and will affect your practice as an APRN, regardless of role. This "boots on the ground" perspective is intended to show you a global point of view on how nurses in advanced practice are presently making a difference and how you too can make a difference. Join the dialogue, speak your concerns, and become engaged. Learn from your predecessors and take up the challenge … the world is yours.

Kelly A. Goudreau
Mary C. Smolenski

Acknowledgments

Many thanks are in order as this book comes to fruition. First of all, many thanks to Margaret Zuccarini, Publisher at Springer Publishing Company, for her question, "Hey, Kelly ... do you have any ideas for a new book?" Thanks to the team at Springer who assisted in pulling together all the bits and pieces and made this book a reality.

A special thanks to the contributors to this book. In every book, there is a story and this one has been interesting with life events that happened and are happening (aging parents, deaths, births, new jobs, moving, being overwhelmed and overcommitted, and retiring). The product of the contributors' labors is within these pages for you to digest and learn from the lessons lived.

Finally, many thanks to those who put work into the chapters not only as authors, but as editors and supporters of the authors. Your expertise is valued beyond all.

Thank you all for assisting us in the development and completion of this text. May it guide you well in your learning.

INTRODUCTION TO HEALTH POLICY FROM AN ADVANCED PRACTICE PERSPECTIVE

Prolific Policy: Implications for Advanced Practice Registered Nurses

Melissa Stewart

True health care reform cannot happen in Washington. It has to happen in our kitchens, in our homes, in our communities.

—Mehmet Oz

Policy can serve as a vehicle for movement or progress in practice. Policy can open doors for opportunity and provide methodology for systematic solidarity in action. Unfortunately, many health care practitioners allow policy to happen around them but not through them. To truly be an effective advocate, policy must become a tool used to sharpen our practice to meet the needs of our consumers. Tomajan (2012) defined advocacy as "work on the behalf of self and/or others to raise awareness of a concern and to promote solutions to the issues. Advocacy often requires working through formal, decision-making bodies to achieve desired outcomes."

Milstead (2013) defined policy as "A purposeful, general plan of action, which includes authoritative guidelines, that is developed to respond to a problem. The plan directs human behavior toward specific goals." Policy statements detail values and guidelines to provide precise direction. Actions in the legislative arena at every level, local, state, and federal, directly impact the practice arena, and what occurs in the practice arena in turn impacts legislative action. In order to support the profession and provide for those entrusted to our care, it is essential that advanced practice nurses assume advocacy roles and strengthen their leadership skills in order to become policy leaders. Nursing leaders need a basic platform of understanding, both in advocacy and policy, to combine resources to accomplish identified goals. Advanced practice nurses must recognize that policy is an integral part of everyday professional nursing practice.

OUR RIGHT TO PROMOTE WELL-BEING

We the people of the United States, in order to form a more perfect union, establish justice, insure domestic tranquility, provide for the common defense, promote the general welfare, and secure the blessings of liberty to ourselves and our posterity, do ordain and establish this Constitution for the United States of America.

The authors of the preamble to the Constitution called for union of Americans to create optimal conditions for the safety and well-being of America's citizens. This sacred document established a priority to promote welfare among American citizens. Government action toward this directive is derived through policy. Prudent, pragmatic approaches are designed through policy to yield optimal results.

As practitioners, policy often surfaces as regulatory mandates or organizational improvements. Personally and professionally, policy surrounds us daily. From the protection of patient confidentiality to the code used to charge a payer, policy is deeply embedded in our everyday life. The power to influence policy through the political arena is a right of every American. Legislative representatives are servants of the voters who empower them with their political appointment. The right to vote and contact political figures is often an underutilized resource. Although one may choose to label self as not being politically active, they cannot escape the consequences acquiesced from the political arena.

To many health care professionals, policy is just not appealing enough to hold the providers' attention. The tedious nature of policy is how regulatory changes can sneak in and make chaos out of a once highly functional practice. Legal terms in law, ambiguous terminology in regulations, and robotic language in organizational policy can serve to disengage health care providers. Unfortunately, the perceived pleonasm of policy can deter the health care practitioners who need to understand and implement the directives in practice. According to Anderson (2011), there are five stages of policy making (Table 1.1).

Stage 1 is policy agenda. In stage 1, the focus is on problems that receive attention of public officials. In policy formulation, stage 2, concentration is on the development of courses of action, acceptable and proposed, for dealing with a public problem. Stage 3 is policy adoption when support for a specific proposal is procured so the policy can be legitimized. Policy implementation is the focus of stage 4; this is where the administrative machinery of government begins to apply the policy. Finally, in stage 5, policy evaluation, policy is evaluated for effectiveness, barriers, and consequences. Table 1.2 compares the five stages of policy making with the nursing process.

Policy is born out of need for communal actions. The need may be identified within an organization to achieve optimal performance from employees, or because of market changes or new legislation passed. Socially, policy is developed to help maintain a civility among populations. Common drivers that influence policy are social and environmental factors, voters, professional organizations, and advocacy groups (Figure 1.1). Irrespective of the reason for the policy, once created individuals are affected by policy.

TABLE 1.1 Stages of Policy Development

Stage 1 Policy agenda	Assessment
Stage 2 Policy formulation	Diagnosis
Stage 3 Policy adoption	Plan
Stage 4 Policy implementation	Implement
Stage 5 Policy evaluation	Evaluate

TABLE 1.2 Five Stages of Policy Making Compared With the Nursing Process

STAGE 1 POLICY AGENDA	STAGE 2 POLICY FORMULATION	STAGE 3 POLICY ADOPTION	STAGE 4 POLICY IMPLEMENTATION	STAGE 5 POLICY EVALUATION
Those problems that receive the serious attention of public officials	Development of pertinent and acceptable proposed courses of action for dealing with a public problem	Development of support for a specific proposal so a policy can be legitimized or authorized	Application of the policy by the government's administrative machinery	Efforts by the government to determine whether the policy was effective and why or why not

Social and environmental factors include newsworthy topics such as unemployment, illegal aliens, and the stock market crash. The stock market influences companies' revenue, which in turn impacts employment. The crash of the stock market caused a decrease in capital for companies that translated into layoffs and downsizing. With the loss of employment comes the loss of benefits such as health care benefits. The Affordable Care Act was framed as a way to provide health care coverage for the unemployed and illegal aliens. From bill to law, the Affordable Care Act has ignited political astuteness from political influencers.

It is imperative that health care professionals understand the political process. Health care providers, either (or both?) individually, or through professional organizations or advocacy groups, directly influence local, state, and national policy on a regular basis. Professional organizations and advocacy groups through the weight of their votes impact policy. Because the legislative and executive branches of government comprise elected officials, votes and organized groups of voters carry strong lobbying influence when dealing with these two political arms.

Within professional organizations, such as the American Association of Nurse Practitioners and the American Nurses Association, member-created resolutions help to push an issue up to the state and national level for organizational support. In the past, a house of delegates would vote on resolutions to help the direction for national organizational boards. The new trend is to have various specialty committees work together to offer expert support. The Institute of Medicine (IOM) often holds round-tables for specific health care issues as a way to provide direction and influence to members, legislators, and other significant parties.

Knowledge of where to introduce proposed policy can determine success or failure. Through the three branches of government, that is, legislative, judicial, and

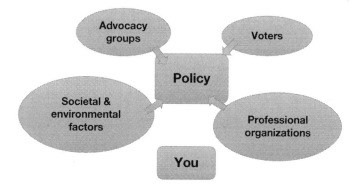

FIGURE 1.1 Drivers of Policy.

executive, policy is created, implemented, and enforced. The legislative branch, the House of Representatives and the Senate, creates law. The executive branch, which consists of the president federally, at the state level the governor, and at the city level the mayor, implements law. The judicial branch, courts and regulatory agencies, enforces law. To be effective when advocating for law, point of access is critical.

Appropriate point of access for impact is contingent on what a provider is trying to accomplish, because this will determine where personal or professional influence should be introduced. For example, if a bill is in the House, which may limit the practice of the advanced practice registered nurse (APRN), the practitioner may want to contact legislators and attend committee meetings about the bill. Whereas if the bill has passed into law and the provider wants to ensure the law is interpreted into practice appropriately the APRN would want to connect with the executive branch's assigned government entity tasked with implementing the new law. Government entities often tasked with implementing health care laws are the Centers for Medicare and Medicaid Services (CMS), or the State Department of Health and Human Services. Finally, the APRN accesses the judicial arm of government through reporting illegal activity or serving as an expert witness to safeguard intent of the law. Each state's Board of Nursing serves as a judicial arm of government protecting the state's citizens from negligence and/or error of practitioners. Knowing when and where to access can help the health care provider to maximize their influential potential (Figure 1.2).

In the process of developing law, a bill has to go through several stages of debate, revision, and voting before it sees the light of day. A proposal from a member of Congress, either the Senate or the House of Representatives, proposes an idea for a new law or an idea to alter a law that already exists. After the proposal is submitted, it then becomes the proposing official's job to get the proposal written into a bill. Once the bill is created, it must be submitted to one of the two houses of Congress, the Senate or the House of Representatives. The bill is then assigned to a particular committee that deals with the subject of the proposed law. It is the assigned committee's job to debate the value of the law, including its necessity to be passed, and the pros versus the cons. If the bill is favorably passed by the committee it then goes in front of the entire House or the Senate for debate. It is similar to the debate that occurred within the committee but now the whole branch of Congress debates the merits and implications of the proposed bill. Once a bill has met with the approval of one of the branches of Congress, it then moves to the other branch to go through the same process. Throughout the journey in Congress, the bill is modified in an effort to be passed by the general consensus. Once the bill is passed by both branches of

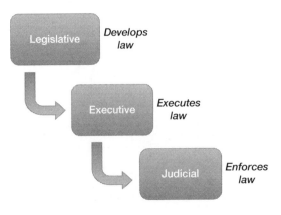

FIGURE 1.2 Point of Access for Maximum Influence.

Congress, it goes to a conference committee to get the modifications added to the original bill figured out. After the bill has been revised, both houses of Congress vote on it. Finally, the bill is submitted to the president of the United States, who has the power to either put the law into effect or veto it. Even if the president decides to veto the bill, the legislative branch can vote to overrule his decision. If two thirds of the representatives vote to overrule it, the bill becomes a law anyway.

It is not uncommon, and probably most likely, that organizations and/or lobbyists of special interest groups will try to have as much impact on the early stages of this process, as the idea is being proposed, accepted, and written up as a bill. Getting in on the ground floor of a proposal submission and following it allows for maximum input and to ensure that there is clarity in terminology. It also helps to craft components of the bill with the best interests of the particular group. Most, if not all of the initial bills, are written by House or Senate staffers, who research elements of the proposal and work on draft after draft until it is ready for committee assignment. The work continues throughout the whole process, because as outlined previously, the bill can be modified, changed, and possibly lose the impact that was originally intended. Knowing where the bill is in the process, what committee it is assigned to and who is on that committee, and contacting legislators and committee members with facts and data to support (or rebuke) the bill are important steps that any APRN can take.

POLICY SHIFT TOWARD ILLNESS PREVENTION

As the 21st century unfolds, a new paradigm in health care begins to emerge with the implementation of the Affordable Care Act. The expansion of health care deliverables, coupled with the movement in health maintenance through prevention services, presents new challenges to address. Redefining providers' scope of practice, adjusting to result-oriented payment structures, and establishing new delivery realms such as transitions in care are just a few of the issues that must be addressed to successfully move forward (CMS, 2011a, 2011b).

The present prevention/wellness movement in health care has always held a presence in our delivery system, especially in the practice of nursing. Nursing theorists such as Florence Nightingale, Dorothea Orem, Betty Neuman, and Nora Pender, are just a few who include wellness through prevention as a construct in their theories (Figure 1.3). Although healing related to insult or injury has historically been the crux of health care, the 21st century is focused on personal sustainability through health prevention. With the ever-growing shortage of primary care physicians, frontline access providers are becoming less and less available to the public. In an attempt to address the frontline provider crisis, which has traditionally been a physician,

THEORIST	THEORY
Florence Nightingale	Environmental Theory
Dorothea Orem	Self-Care Deficit
Betty Neuman	Systems Theory
Nora Pender	Health Promotion Model

FIGURE 1.3 Nursing Theorists With a Prevention Focus.

APRNs and in particular nurse practitioners (NPs) are assuming this role to meet the public access crisis.

SCOPE OF PRACTICE

Although APRNs are meeting the need of the consumer they are still limited by reimbursement and collaboration agreements. Even though APRNs are delivering the same level of care in many cases as is rendered by a generalist physician, they are not reimbursed 100% of the treatment billing codes like their physician colleagues. Instead, APRNs are reimbursed at the rate of only 85% of the code allotment. Payer discrimination between APRNs and physicians only serves to fiscally limit investment in their practices. The harnessing of APRNs through collaboration agreement mandates between APRNs and physicians further attempts to publicly restrict the independent role of the APRN. To maximize the role of APRNs, the legislatively created scope of practice in each state will need to remove these independent practice barriers. The issues of payment and collaborative agreements are regulatory mandates that are hindering the progression of APRNs as they attempt to maximize their practice autonomy. Understanding these issues and having a knowledge of the legislative system can assist in removing the barriers of practice maximization.

RESULTS-ORIENTED PAYMENT

Result-oriented reimbursement for health care services was derived from the exponentially rising costs of care with a perception of an ever decreasing quality of care outcomes. Health care services in our present delivery system continue to have large mounting costs while consumers experience lower quality in care delivered than that of other industrialized countries as evidenced in comparable preventable mortality, number of uninsured, and care system efficiency scores (Davis, Schoen, & Stremikis, 2010). It is estimated that by year 2019, health care spending will comprise 20% of the U.S. gross national product (Alonso-Zaldivar, 2010). The United States also pays far more per capita than any other nation when compared with other industrialized nations (Organization for Economic Co-operative Development, 2011). Hospital care consumes the largest and growing section of the U.S. health care system. According to Millman Medical Index (2012), inpatient and outpatient services now represent 32% and 18% of the U.S. health care budget, respectively. Mergers and acquisitions are taking place as health care reform unfolds with insurers, for-profit companies, and private equity firms entering into the health care delivery market (Caramenico, 2012). Despite hopes for savings through the efficiency of size, these unions of companies and investors have been associated with rising health care costs and a system-wide decrease in patient satisfaction (Berenson, Ginsburg, Christianson, & Yee, 2012; Office of Attorney General Martha Coakley, 2010).

According to National Public Radio, the Robert Wood Johnson Foundation, and the Harvard School of Public Health (2012), a recent survey of U.S. residents with illness found that 73% felt that the cost of health care was a very serious problem and 45% felt that quality was a very serious problem. The survey found that the United States has a below-average life expectancy rate and an above-average infant mortality rate (Organization for Economic Co-operative Development, 2011). Quality in care continues to be a growing concern in health care as two recent studies have found that approximately one in seven hospitalized patients experience an adverse event (Landrigan et al., 2010; Office of Inspector General [OIG], 2010), with 44% to 66% of these events found to be preventable. Unfortunately, more than not, hospital administration may not even be aware that these events have occurred. As noted in the OIG report, only 14% of events that cause harm to patients are captured by hospital tracking systems (OIG, 2012). Downey and colleagues (Downey, Hernandez-Boussard, Banka, & Morton, 2012) examined the Agency for Healthcare Research and Quality (AHRQ) patient safety indicators between the years 1988 and 2007, and found little overall change in that time frame. This lack of progress in safety is a poor response to the IOM's publication of the 1999 report, which estimated that almost 100,000 patients die each year from medical errors (IOM, 2000). Another reflection of the quality of care seen in today's health care system can be observed in health care-acquired infections (HAIs), which inflict 1.7 million hospitalized patients each year (Klevens et al., 2007), or approximately 1 in 20 patients. HAIs afflict the U.S. health care system at a cost of $35.7 to $45.0 billion each year (Scott, 2009), resulting in 100,000 deaths and untold disability (Klevens et al., 2007). According to a recent survey, 8% of hospitalized patients report getting an HAI (National Public Radio, Robert Wood Johnson Foundation, & Harvard School of Public Health, 2012). The health care system continues to face many challenges in quality of care coupled with elevating costs, which is evident in the slow progress toward reducing adverse events. In response, the CMS through the Patient Protection and Affordable Care Act (PPACA), along with some private insurance companies, are trying to implement financial incentives that will reward quality care while (at the same time) penalizing care that does not meet quality standards.

Fiscal transparency is a type of health care value-based purchasing incentive (Woodward, 2012). Transparency of measures allows consumers and referrers to make choices between different hospitals and providers based on quality and performance, and cost of services. There are approximately 27 states and the District of Columbia that publicly report HAIs (Frieden, 2010). Provider data on hospital-acquired conditions (HACs), process measures, and patient satisfaction surveys are accessible for public viewing online through Hospital Compare (CMS, n.d.). Beyond referrals and the individual consumer, use of the reporting of quality measures can be a factor in a provider negotiation of insurance contracts and third-party payers. Transparency in value-based purchasing can impact a provider's revenues.

To address the gross disparity between cost and outcomes in care, the PPACA directed the CMS to initiate a value-based purchasing system to financially incentivize quality in health care and lower societal health care costs. At present, in the shift toward outcomes-oriented reimbursement, there are two categories for financial incentives. The first category penalizes payment for the care rendered to an individual patient who acquires an HAC. The second category penalizes or rewards the entire fee for all services and patients who are treated at a facility. The incentive that is selected depends on whether a facility's reimbursement is a payment for individual (line item) services or a bundled payment. Unfortunately, the PPACA provides only a framework for change. A proactive stance in health policy formulation is needed that is based on the best information available.

APRNs must engage in the national redesign and construction of health care under a quality care/wellness delivery paradigm. The literature strongly supports the cost effectiveness of NPs as well as strong quality in care delivery and outcomes of other APRN roles such as clinical nurse specialists (CNSs) (Blackmore et al., 2013; Clavelle, 2012; National Nursing Centers Consortium, n.d.; Schiff, 2012). As the nation moves to redefine health care and apply fiscal incentives, it is a nursing duty to ensure patients receive optimal care for a reasonable fee. It is imperative that advanced practice nurses such as APRNs lead nursing in their political efforts to move health care toward a more patient-centric delivery model.

NEW DELIVERY MODELS

As the nation's health care system revolutionizes its way into a new paradigm of health delivery, policy will need perpetual refurbishment. New areas of health care delivery will unfold such as the newly reimbursable transitions in care, which originated from CMS's ninth Scope of Work's (SOW) Care Transitions pilot. CMS's care transitions pilot was framed around Mary Naylor and Erik Coleman's work in transitioning the patient from an acute level of care to home, where self or caregiver deliver personal care. The focus of both Naylor and Coleman's work is to decrease patient readmissions in chronic care patients by injecting a health care provider's presence into the transitional time frame, which is usually 30 to 45 days postdischarge.

CMS's pilot focused on decreasing the readmission rate of Medicare patients with one or more of five diagnoses—chronic obstructive pulmonary disease, congestive heart failure, myocardial infarction, diabetes, and pneumonia. Both Naylor and Coleman used a coaching model for patient intervention. Naylor's model utilized an APRN to do home visits, whereas Coleman's model used a registered nurse who did home visits and telephonic coaching. Selected quality improvement organizations (QIOs) were awarded contracts to participate in the care transitions pilot. The QIOs were charged with forging a working relationship with established hospitals for pilot patients. Once recruited, patients were to be enrolled into the QIO's coaching program. Naylor's and Coleman's work helped to inaugurate basic face-to-face and telephonic communication between hired health care providers and patients.

Of the pilot contracts awarded, one QIO found that they were able to make some impact in decreasing readmissions but not as profound as they wanted. This QIO chose to delve deeper in the communication between patient and provider by implementing the Medagogy© Model and Understanding Personal Perspectives Instrument© in their coaching program (Stewart, 2012). Then the pilot was able to decrease the enrolled population's inherited 18% readmission rate down to 3% (Griggs, 2011). The marked improvement yielded from their improved patient education efforts and patient engagement led to CMS's acknowledging their work as the nation's most innovative pilot in 2011. Because of the success of the pilot, CMS has created two billing codes that physicians, physician assistants, nurse midwives, CNSs, and NPs can bill under to receive reimbursement for their care transitions work (CMS, 2013). This serves as one example of how nursing, through the work of Naylor, Coleman, and Stewart, made an impact on a policy change at CMS that has improved the bottom line for both patients and providers.

CONCLUSION

Policy making, as it relates to health care during the first part of the 21st century, has been at an all-time record high. Although it is generally agreed that health care is overregulated, much of the policy that is sought at this time regards dramatic change in the status quo, to include breaking down traditional provider definitions and creating what would almost appear to be new hybrids of medical professionals. As attempts are made to curtail and control spending, one of the fundamental questions proposed is what constitutes "good" health care, which generates the next question—What role/who is qualified to provide it? A resounding call has been made to utilize APRNs as primary care providers in the face of the projected shortage of approximately 45,000 primary care physicians expected in the next decade (AARP, 2013). Unfortunately, at present, only 16 states allow APRNs to practice autonomously and without oversight. The vast majority of states require limitations to practice, most prominently the requirement that a collaborating practice physician must be contracted in order for any form of health care provision at the APRN level to occur. And despite having data that the quality of care provided by APRNs is commensurate to that of physicians, many managed care organizations do not credential APRNs as primary care providers. This limits the ability to be reimbursed by insurance companies.

Of particular need within the APRN and nursing community at large is to acknowledge, embrace, and embark on participating in the political action process so necessary for these times. The intent of the development of laws in the United States was citizen freedom to create and implement action through regulation for the good of all citizens. The process was meant to represent the population of the country and directly address the needs of the citizens. The initiation and support of legislation is a fundamental right of our birth as Americans; however, it is a laborious process in our whirlwind existence that is unfortunately far too often seen as the responsibility of others. As nurses, we must step up and drive policy—it is in the best interest of all.

REFERENCES

AARP. (2013). *Nurse practitioners: The answer to the doctor shortage*. Retrieved from http://blog.aarp.org/2013/03/29/nurse-practitioners-the-answer-to-the-doctor-shortage

Alonso-Zaldivar, R. (2010). *Gov't: Spending to rise under health care overhaul*. Associated Press. Retrieved from http://www.washingtontimes.com/news/2010/sep/9/govt-spending-to-rise-under-health-care-overhaul

American Academy of Nurse Practitioners (AANP). (2012). *Reimbursement: Medicare update*. Retrieved from http://www.aanp.org/practice/reimbursement/68-articles/326-medicare-update

Anderson, J. E. (2011). *Public policymaking* (7th ed.). Boston, MA: Wadsworth.

Berenson, R. A., Ginsburg, P. B., Christianson, J. B., & Yee, T. (2012). The growing power of some providers to win steep payment increases from insurers suggests policy remedies may be needed. *Health Affairs, 31*, 973–981.

Blackmore, C. C., Edwards, J. W., Searles, C., Wechter, D., Mecklenburg, R., & Kaplan, G. S. (2013). Nurse practitioner-staffed clinic at Virginia Mason improves care and lowers costs for women with benign breast conditions. *Health Affairs, 32*(1), 20–26.

Caramenico, A. (2012, March 8). Hospital groups grow with insurer, private equity partners. *Fierce Health Care*. Retrieved from http://www.fiercehealthcare.com/story/hospital-groups-grow-insurer-private-equity-partners/2012-03-08

Centers for Medicare and Medicaid Services (CMS). (2011a). Medicare program; Hospital inpatient value-based purchasing program. Final rule. *Federal Register, 76*(88), 26490–26547.

CMS. (2011b). *CMS issues final rule for first year of hospital value-based purchasing program. Fact sheets.* Retrieved from http://www.cms.gov/apps/media/press/factsheet.asp?Counter=3947

CMS. (2013). *Frequently asked questions about billing medicare for transitional care management services.* Retrieved from http://www.cms.gov/Medicare/Medicare-Fee-for-Service-Payment/PhysicianFeeSched/Downloads/FAQ-TCMS.pdf

CMS. (n.d.). *Hospital compare*. Retrieved from http://www.hospitalcompare.hhs.gov

Clavelle, J. T. (2012). Implementing Institute of Medicine Future of Nursing recommendations: A model for transforming nurse practitioner privileges. *Journal of Nursing Administration, 42*(9), 404–407.

Davis, K., Schoen, C., & Stremikis, K. (2010, June). *Mirror, mirror on the wall: How the performance of the U.S. health care system compares internationally, 2010 update*. New York, The Commonwealth Fund.

Downey, J. R., Hernandez-Boussard, T., Banka, G., & Morton, J. M. (2012). Is patient safety improving? National trends in patient safety indicators: 1998–2007. *Health Services Research, 47*(1), 414–430.

Frieden, T. R. (2010). Maximizing infection prevention in the next decade: Defining the unacceptable. *Infection Control Hospital Epidemiology, 31*(Suppl 1), S1–S3.

Griggs, T. (2011, October). Communication key to patient education. *Louisiana Medical News*, 4–5.

Institute of Medicine (IOM). (2000). *To err is human, building a safer health environment.* Washington, DC: National Academy of Science Press (actually paper says Nov 1999 but copyright is 2000 by NAS).

Klevens, R. M., Edwards, J. R., Richards, C. I., Jr., Horan, T. C., Gaynes, R. P., Pollock, D. A., & Cardo, D. M. (2007). Estimating health care-associated infections and deaths in U.S. hospitals, 2002. *Public Health Reports, 122*(2), 160–166.

Landrigan, C. P., Parry, G. J., Bones, C. B., Hackbarth, A. D., Goldmann, D. A., & Sharek, P. J. (2010). Temporal trends in rates of patient harm resulting from medical care. *New England Journal of Medicine, 363*(22), 2124–2134.

Millman Medical Index. (2012). *Healthcare costs for American families in 2012 exceed $20,000 for the first time.* Retrieved from http://www.publications.milliman.com/periodicals/mmi/pdfs/milliman-medical-index-2012.pdf

Milstead, J. A. (2013). *Health policy and politics: A nurse's guide* (4th ed.). New York, NY: Jones and Barlett.

National Nursing Centers Consortium. (n.d.). *The cost effectiveness of nurse practitioner care.* Retrieved from http://www.nncc.us/site/images/pdf/cost-effectiveness_npcare.pdf

National Public Radio, Robert Wood Johnson Foundation, & Harvard School of Public Health. (2012, May). *Sick in America poll: Chartpack.* Retrieved from http://www.rwjf.org/files/downloads/Cost_Quality%20Summary%20Final20120518.pdf

Office of Attorney General Martha Coakley. (2010, March 16). *Examination of health care cost trends and cost drivers.* Retrieved from http://www.mass.gov/ago/docs/healthcare/final-report-w-cover-appendices-glossary.pdf

Office of Inspector General (OIG). (2010). *Adverse events in hospitals: National incidence among Medicare beneficiaries* (OEI-06-09-00090). Washington, DC: Department of Health and Human Services.

OIG. (2012). *Hospital incident reporting systems do not capture most patient harm* (OEI-06-09-00091). Washington, DC: Department of Health and Human Services.

Organization for Economic Co-operative Development. (2011). *OECD factbook 2011: Economic, environmental and social statistics.* Paris, France: OECD Publishing.

Schiff, M. (2012). *The role of nurse practitioners in meeting increasing demand for primary care.* Retrieved from http://www.nga.org/cms/home/nga-center-for-best-practices/center-publications/page-health-publications/col2-content/main-content-list/the-role-of-nurse-practitioners.htm

Scott, R. D. (2009). *The direct medical costs of healthcare-associated infection in U.S. hospitals and the benefits of prevention.* Atlanta, GA: Centers for Disease Control and Prevention.

Stewart, M. (2012). *Practical patient literacy: The Medagogy model.* New York, NY: McGraw-Hill.

Tomajan, K. (2012, January 31). Advocating for nurses and nursing. *OJIN: The Online Journal of Issues in Nursing, 17*(1), Manuscript 4.

Woodward, N. H. (2012). Seeking transparency: More employers are providing pricing and quality information to help employees make smarter health care purchasing decisions. *HRMagazine, 57*(9), 39–42. Society for Human Resource Management (republished by High Beam Research).

CHAPTER 2

Turning Health Policy Into Practice: Implications for Advanced Practice Registered Nurses

James L. Harris

Escalating health care costs continue. Approximately 15% of the gross domestic product is spent nationally on health care with projections to increase by 20% on or before 2050 (Congressional Budget Office, 2009). Although there has been rapid growth in biomedical advances and knowledge generation over the past decade, care providers, consumers, and stakeholders remain concerned about the quality, safety, and efficiency of clinical care. Care access coupled with quality and safety concerns is closely aligned with cost containment (Ridenour & Trautman, 2009).

The ongoing debate about health care reform and how to finance escalating costs is an opportunity for advanced practice registered nurses (APRNs) to engage in policy formation that can shape and influence advanced nursing practice. Policy formation is an overarching process, and the complexities associated with health policy can be even more complex and multidimensional as individuals from various public and private sectors are involved. This complexity requires numerous checks and balances as different strategies are formulated. Although there are a number of definitions of health policy, Block's (2004, p. 7) definition, "the collection of authoritative decisions made within government that pertains to health and the pursuit of health" is foundational for the estimated 241,000 APRNs in practice, and similarly those who engage in policy development and lobbying activities that have practice, education, and research implications.

BACKGROUND

The evolution of advanced practice nursing has been influenced by many factors such as advances in care, finances, consumer demands, evolving health care reform legislation, and regulatory stands to cite a few (Furlong & Smith, 2005). In particular, three converging factors are drivers of APRN demand to include (a) increased demands among an aging American population, (b) enhanced access made possible by Patient Care Action, and (c) the Institute of Medicine's (IOM) report calling for less restrictive scope of practice (Clabo et al., 2012). What paradoxically seems inevitable is actually a result of multiple years of activity culminating in policies that will continuously influence APRN practice and affect all populations across the life span (Kronenfeld, 2002).

Numerous authors have written about the various levels, components, and processes associated with health policy development (Block, 2004; Fawcett & Russell, 2001; Hinshaw, 1988). For example, Block (2004) identified six stages of public policy making to include setting the agenda, formulating the policy, adopting the policy, implementing the policy, assessing the policy impact, and modifying the policy as indicated. As health policy is formed, consideration should be given to all levels to include health care agencies—state, national, and international interests (Hinshaw & O'Grady, 2011).

So one may pose the question, how do APRNs fit into the processes associated with health policy development? In order to respond to this question, one should first consider four developmental components when developing health policy: (a) policy process—government sets public policy to include formation, implementation, and evaluation; (b) policy reform—changes in programs that may positively or negatively affect practices such as priority reform, financial structures, and the regulatory environment that affect institutions and organizations; (c) policy environment—areas where the process occurs such as government, public, and/or media; and (d) policy makers—the primary stakeholders and participants within the policy environment. Therefore, APRNs fit into the health policy development through the following actions and activities: (a) policy process—systematically reviewing identified issue(s) and developing dialogue based upon the best available evidence; (b) policy reform—remaining informed and involved in lobbying activities, polls, and meetings; (c) policy environment—remaining visible, articulating position, and disseminating information to stakeholders; and (d) policy makers—demonstrating the value of nurses' contributions to the group and providing credible evidence to support positions. An incremental approach is advisable whereby APRNs can start with current and publicly charged issues that have impacts on health and health services such as community development, social determinants of health, and financing activities.

CONCEPTUAL FOUNDATION

The conceptual foundation for this chapter is based on a model of nursing and specifically health policy by Fawcett and Russell (2001). Fawcett and Russell's (2001) model "was designed to extend the substantive knowledge of health policy within the discipline of nursing" (p. 108). Ten underlying philosophic assumptions underpin the model, but most notable to this discussion are those specific to public policies, organizational policies, and professional policies. "Public policies are those that are developed by nations, states, cities, and towns. The health policies promulgated by public entities typically have a broad impact on individuals, groups, communities, and health care organizations. Organizational policies are developed by health care institutions, such as hospitals, clinics, and home health agencies, to guide practice of a particular institution. Professional policies are standards or guidelines developed by discipline-specific and multidisciplinary associations to provide direction for those individuals and groups who work for or with the associations" (Russell & Fawcett, 2005, p. 320). For the purposes of this chapter, the American Nurses Association (ANA), the National Organization of Nurse Practitioner Faculties

(NONPF), the National Association of Clinical Nurse Specialists, and the American Association of Colleges of Nursing are examples of professional policy-making organizations to be used to guide discussion and related content. Regardless whether it is public, organizational, or professional policies, health care services, personnel, and expenditures are interrelated as related to nursing and health policy.

The model by Russell and Fawcett (2005) consists of four increasingly broad and interacting levels that encompass the concepts of the nursing metaparadigm (human beings, environment, and nursing) posed by Fawcett (2005). The levels are not hierarchical, but are rather increasingly broad as nursing and health policies advance to health care systems. Level 1 emphasizes health policy by focusing on quality relative to the efficacy of nursing practice on the outcomes of individuals, families, groups, and communities. Level 2 focuses on health policy related to quality and cost associated with the effectiveness and efficiency of nursing practice and the health care delivery subsystems created by providers on outcomes of individuals, families, groups, and communities. Level 3 highlights health policy associated with access by focusing on societal demands for equity of access to effective nursing practice, efficient nursing delivery systems, and equity of costs and care delivery burdens distribution. Level 4 stresses health policy links to quality, cost, and access in relation to social and economic quality and cost-effective services, and health-related resources.

Much dialogue has ensued as to how the model should be used for policy analysis and evaluation. Although there are differing beliefs, the model can be a valuable resource when designing advanced nursing practice learning opportunities and delivering care to individuals, families, groups, and communities. Moreover, the model can also guide policy analysis and evaluation aligned with access, quality, cost, efficiency, and effectiveness. For purposes of this chapter, the utility of the model is applicable to APRN practice evaluation.

APPLICATION OF HEALTH POLICY TO APRNs

APRNs are in pivotal roles to continuously advance nursing practice, education, policy, and the spread of best available evidence. The historical opportunity with health care reform further highlights how APRNs can use policy to leverage widespread social change, especially public policy (Ridenour & Trautman, 2009). This supports the aforementioned conceptual discussion and how the value of health policy priorities shape and influence the welfare of others and development of implementation of organizational policies.

The impact of APRN practice on health care costs, quality, safety, efficiency, and effectiveness cannot be understated or underestimated. The definitive actions and interventions by APRNs who are linked to individual, family, group, and community needs have never been more profound than today, especially in an era of diminishing resources, manpower, and escalating chronic illnesses. Whether addressing discrepancies in access, prevention and health maintenance, chronic disease management, or workforce education and development, APRNs are a powerful force that influences policy makers and engages numerous stakeholders in advancing health policy. In an epoch of information technology and knowledge expansion, APRNs can use advanced knowledge and skill sets of health informatics to engage in comparative analysis of evidentiary interventions and delivery systems that ultimately shape policies in today's constantly changing health care environment.

The myriad of opportunities for APRNs to optimize influence on health care and workforce needs can be more effective when evidence guides actions and there is consistent engagement in policy development. For example, in primary care, APRNs improve access for underserved populations. With the advent of policy reducing the number of medical resident hours, APRNs became an immediate part of the solution (Christmas et al., 2005). The convenience of seeking care has expanded through the use of APRNs in retail clinics and the proliferation of advances in telehealth (Hansen-Turton, Ryan, Miller, Counts, & Nash, 2007; Newhouse et al., 2012). As an integrated workforce, opportunities are abundant for APRNs to advance patient-centered care and drive policy, which will allow innovative models of care that bring value to recipients across the life span.

As APRNs continue to fill faculty positions in academia, developing the provider workforce for the next decade requires practice, technology and information, policy, and systems leadership competencies to name a few (National CNS Competency Task Force, 2010; NONPF, 2007, 2009) and is in support of the IOM (2011) recommendations. For the purposes of this chapter, APRNs must be able to demonstrate the six policy competencies posed by the National Task Force on Quality Nurse Practitioner Education (2012). For example, two of the six competencies include understanding of the specifics for the interdependence of policy and practice, and analyzing the implications of health policy across disciplines. Similarly, the nine clinical nurse specialist core competencies and behaviors associated with the sphere of influence and the nurse characteristics must be demonstrated (National CNS Competency Task Force, 2010). For example, the systems leadership competency (ability to manage change and engage others to influence clinical practice and political processes within and across multiple systems) is imperative as health policy is turned into APRN practice.

EVALUATION CONCEPTS

Numerous outcomes data are continuously collected in health care systems. Although data collection systems and outcomes management vary between systems, both inform public, organization, and professional policies. As data are collected and analyzed, approaches to evidence-based care drive policy revision and change. Polit and Beck (2008) support the notion that data stimulate discussions about practice improvement, policy change, validity of evidence-based practices, what groups are at risk for adverse outcomes, and the most pressing priorities. Outcomes measurement linked to quality, cost effectiveness, and value-based care is foundational to advancing APRN practice and complementary policy formation and change.

Although a myriad of issues and variation in care exists in the United States, patient, family, and community engagement are increasingly identified as a primary component in achieving a high-quality, affordable health system (National Quality Forum, 2012). Metrics that align with measuring all provider, such as APRN, impacts in an integrated workforce are fundamental to the overarching goal of meeting needs and moving from single provider, discipline-specific care delivery (Pawlson et al., 2011). The preparation of APRNs allows for individual and group choice in care provision. Care outcomes can subsequently be compared among providers and lead to any policy changes needed to enhance quality, safe, and value-based care. Policy change will be guided by outcomes that benefit consumers and communities. As the number of APRNs increase to meet the escalating care demands, active involvement in policy is an imperative for quality. Crafting metrics that amplify efficiency and provider incentives for good care can underpin reimbursement policies that maximize payment for APRN services beyond current rates. Improving workforce data in regard to APRN practice must be included in national databases and will serve as the basis for health care and workforce policy (Newhouse et al., 2012).

The rapid pace of health care change and engagement of the patient at the center of care delivery will continue to require data that will shape policy and generate viable solutions that culminate in evaluating the effectiveness of APRN care delivery. The capacity to use outcomes data and collection systems require APRNs to be knowledgeable of these and policy in order to increase the development of effective policies that will shape practice, education, and inquiry in succeeding decades. Being consistent in message, communicating a shared perspective, being visible and innovative, and tailoring activities to identified needs will offer many prospects to evaluate APRN outcomes (Ridenour & Trautman, 2009).

DISCUSSION

"The national landscape surrounding advanced practice nursing roles is undergoing significant change. A perfect storm of forces presents a unique window of opportunity for APRNs to realize their full potential" (Clabo et al., 2012, p. 1). Advances in technology, science, and practice innovation have resulted in people living longer and presenting with multiple care needs. The APRN community and educators are in a unique position to be the catalyst for policy development that will shape the preparation of future advanced practice nurses who will ultimately function as licensed independent practitioners. Regulation of APRNs varies widely among the 50 states, thus generating mobility barriers that can subsequently limit access to care and the underutilization of skill sets that differentiate advanced and generalist registered nursing practice (Lugo, O'Grady, Hodnicki, & Hanson, 2007; National Council of State Boards of Nursing [NCSBN] et al., 2006; Pearson, 2010). Mobility and access barriers potentiate the creation of roadblocks toward achievement of the nation's goals for safe, efficient, and cost-effective care to all citizens (Lugo et al., 2007; Safriet, 2002).

Multiple issues and barriers related to education, scope of practice, reimbursement, and prescriptive authority are all embedded in policy and regulatory languages that make it difficult for APRN practice potential and contributions to be realized across the nation. Equally, issues are compounded when collaborative relationships with other regulated disciplines are limited, if not absent. Unquestionably, the issues have significant relevance to advanced nursing practice today and in the future as policies are revised and developed (Hamric, Spross, & Hanson, 2009). This is further rationale for the involvement of APRNs in health policy development that will ultimately impact practice and address the needs of all consumers of care.

For the purposes of this chapter, three issues and potential barriers are further discussed that have significance as public, organizational, and professional policies are developed and implemented. The three issues include (a) education, (b) scope of practice, and (c) reimbursement.

The majority of APRN education is designed and accomplished using a model developed almost a half-century ago where students were involved in siloed clinical learning situations using volunteer preceptors to provide the direct supervision. This education often disregards the growing number of collaborative interprofessional educational opportunities where students learn with and from other disciplines (Culliton & Russell, 2010; Interprofessional Education Collaborative, 2011; IOM, 2011). As Tanner (2012) challenged, "We are approaching a crisis in both the cost of clinical education and the insufficient supply of suitable clinical sites if we continue to use the traditional approach to clinical education" (p. 419). To remedy this situation, changes in educational policy are requisite to success where collaboration between academia and practice across all health professions designs, tests, and implements new models of clinical education. The questions are therefore posed as

to, should there be a specific number of clinical hours for each course, the number of clinical simulation hours used, and how and by whom should precepting occur? Practicing APRNs, educators, interprofessional colleagues, and preceptors can guide this historical journey and craft policy that will contribute to meeting the care needs among various cohorts of consumers in order to meet the impending care demands.

Ongoing challenges remain in overcoming the limits imposed on the sole authority in scope to practice. Several states possess sole authority from state boards of nursing; whereas other states possess joint authority with other professional boards (Hamric et al., 2009). The landmark recommendations by the IOM (2011) are a starting point calling for nurses to practice to the full extent of preparation. These calls for changes create opportunities directed at policy involvement that will ultimately result in the best care possible—a timely and responsive patient-centric opportunity.

Although the title, APRN, is a value-based asset, the challenge of equitable reimbursement remains as an impending issue that requires action. Policy makers must continuously be educated about the contribution of APRNs in order to address the debate of equal pay for equal service. The care provided by APRNs cannot be viewed as inferior to that of physicians. But the impending and imposing questions remain—will the education requirement of a doctoral degree for the APRN and recognition of the APRN as a licensed independent practitioner resolve the reimbursement inequity?

Turning health policy into practice has many implications for APRN practice beyond the current decade. The landscape of APRN practice is changing as a result of the rapid pace of impending health needs of the population. The changes imposed by health care reform, cost containment, and mandates for safe and quality care that are patient-centric have become impending requisite actions for active engagement. The time is now for APRNs to become active players in shaping health policy that will guide practice and prove themselves as safe and cost-effective providers to society and move forward as professionals who are entrusted as future providers for a healthy America.

ETHICAL CONSIDERATIONS

Ethical considerations are moral principles governing behavior with integrity, honesty, and opportunities for advocacy. The ANA Code of Ethics is guidelines available to nurses in practice guiding the conduct of actions in accordance with primary values and standards of the profession (ANA, 2008). The practice of APRNs is central to individual, family, and community needs. According to Kjervik and Brous (2010), APRNs have expanded the standards of care beyond the generalist nursing care. With expanded knowledge and skills, APRNs must understand the obligations and rights associated with advanced practice nursing and roles in advancing health policy that are directed at ethical protection of society. Many ethical situations present daily in practice environments and may not have the same outcomes. Gray areas exist where there is no specific answer. The APRN must function as an advocate for the patient, family, community, and peer practice. Building consensus among the APRN community can support ethical considerations that must strengthen high-quality, safe, and affordable care.

The nursing and ethical pedagogy for APRNs allows options to utilize knowledge and skills when becoming policy advocates for patients, families, and communities. Evidence-based knowledge is a powerful tool for change and building interprofessional strength that will guide ethical policies and ethical decision making.

As pioneers for change, policy development, and ultimately ethical care, APRNs rely on the knowledge and skills gained through education, practice, and collaboration. As entrusted providers of care, the role of the APRN in ethical policy development engagement will continue to direct the use of available resources that culminate in quality, safe, and efficient care delivery.

HEALTH POLICY AND APRN PRACTICE IMPLICATIONS

- Convey how health policy shapes the meeting of emerging needs of Americans.
- Motivate and educate others to shift priorities in order to guide policy that will shape APRN practice currently and in the future.
- Illustrate the skills, expertise, and dedication of APRNs to meet emerging needs and to strengthen the nation's communities.
- Outline the importance of involving APRNs in developing and implementing health policies and core competencies that result in measurable outcomes.
- Create awareness for policy change, interprofessional learning, and skill development directed at quality, safe, and efficient care delivery.

DISCUSSION QUESTIONS

1. How does policy shape current and future APRN practice?
2. Considering the current and impending health care reform mandates, how can a policy framework assist the APRN to become involved in turning health policy into practice?
3. What are the impending needs necessary to reform APRN practice, educational preparation, and reimbursement in order to provide quality, safe, and cost-effective care?
4. What is the relation of policy formation and implementation to APRN practice in addressing ethical issues?
5. What are additional issues that should be considered in turning health policy into APRN practice?

SYNTHESIS AND CLINICAL APPLICATION EXERCISES

1. Conduct a focus group of APRNs and educators to gain an understanding of the impact of policy development on future APRN preparation.
2. Conduct a focus group of providers and consumers of care to gain an understanding of the impact of APRN practice.
3. Interview a policy maker to discuss the advantage(s) of turning health policy into practice for APRNs.
4. Interview an elected professional organization member to identify the advantage of APRN involvement in health policy.
5. Develop ways to disseminate practices that support policies that guide APRN activities.
6. Review the literature and generate a priority list of policy formulation and implementation factors affecting current and future APRN practice.
7. Identify ways to expand evidence that will benefit all citizens and differentiate generalist and advanced practice nursing.

REFERENCES

American Nurses Association (ANA). (2008). *Code of ethics for nurses with interpretive statements*. Silver Spring, MD: Author.

Block, L. E. (2004). Health policy: What it is and how it works. In C. Harrington & C. L. Estes (Eds.), *Health policy: Crisis and reform in the U.S. health care delivery system* (4th ed., pp. 4–14). Sudbury, MA: Jones & Bartlett.

Clabo, L. L., Giddens, J., Jeffries, P., McQuade-Jones, B., Morton, P., & Ryan, S. (2012). A perfect storm: A window of opportunity for revolution in nurse practitioner education. *Journal of Nursing Education, 51*, 539–541.

Christmas, A. B., Reynolds, J., Hodges, S., Frankline, G. A., Millier, F. B., Richardson, J. D., & Rodrigquez, J. L. (2005). Physician extenders impact trauma systems. *Journal of Trauma: Injury, Infection & Critical Care, 58*, 917–920.

Congressional Budget Office (CBO). (2009, March 1). *Health*. Retrieved from http://www.cbo.gov /publications/collections/health.cfm

Culliton, B. J., & Russell, S. (Eds.). (2010). *Who will provide primary care and how will they be trained* [Conference proceedings]? Durham, NC: Josiah Macy, Jr., Foundation.

Fawcett, J. (2005). *Contemporary nursing knowledge: Analysis and evaluation of nursing models and theories* (2nd ed.). Philadelphia, PA: F. A. Davis.

Fawcett, J., & Russell, G. (2001). A conceptual model of nursing and health policy. *Policy, Politics & Nursing Practice, 2*(2), 108–116.

Furlong, E., & Smith, R. (2005). Advanced nursing practice: Policy, education and role development. *Journal of Clinical Nursing, 14*(9), 1059–1066.

Hamric, A. B., Spross, J. A., & Hanson, C. M. (2009). *Advanced practice nursing: An integrated approach* (4th ed.). St. Louis, MO: Elsevier.

Hansen-Turton, T., Ryan, S., Miller, K., Counts, M., & Nash, D. B. (2007). Convenient care clinics: The future of accessible health care. *Disease Management, 10*, 61–73.

Hinshaw, A. S. (1988). Using research to shape policy. *Nursing Outlook, 36*(1), 21–24.

Hinshaw, A. S., & O'Grady, P. A. (Eds.). (2011). *Shaping health policy through nursing research*. New York, NY: Springer Publishing Company.

Institute of Medicine (IOM). (2011). *The future of nursing: Leading change, advancing health*. Washington, DC: National Academies Press.

Interprofessional Education Collaborative. (2011). *Team-building competencies: Building a shared foundation for education and clinical practice* [Conference proceedings]. Durham, NC: Josiah Macy, Jr., Foundation.

Kjervik, D., & Brous, E. A. (2010). *Law and ethics for advanced practice nursing*. New York, NY: Springer Publishing Company.

Kronenfeld, J. J. (2002). *Health care policy: Issues and trends*. Westport, CT: Praeger.

Lugo, N. R., O'Grady, E., Hodnicki, D., & Hanson, C. (2007). Ranking state NP regulation: Practice environment and consumer healthcare choice. *American Journal of Nurse Practitioners, 11*, 8–24.

National CNS Competency Task Force. (2010). *Clinical nurse specialist core competencies: Executive summary 2006–2008*. Philadelphia, PA: National Association of Clinical Nurse Specialists.

National Council of State Boards of Nursing (NCSBN), Association of Social Work Boards, Federation of State Board of Physical Therapy, Federation of State Medical Boards, National Association of Boards of Pharmacy, & National Board of Certification of Occupational Therapy (Eds.). (2006). *Changes in healthcare professions' scope of practice: Legislative considerations*. Chicago, IL: NCSBN.

National Task Force on Quality Nurse Practitioner Education. (2012). *Criteria for evaluation of nurse practitioner programs*. Washington, DC: National Organization of Nurse Practitioners Faculties.

National Organization of Nurse Practitioners Faculties (NONPF). (2007, 2009). *The APRN consensus process*. Washington, DC: Author.

National Quality Forum. (2012). *Patient reported outcomes (PROs) in performance measurement*. Draft report for comment. Washington, DC: Author.

Newhouse, R. P., Weiner, J. P., Stanki-Hutt, J., White, K. M., Johantgen, M., Steinwachs, D., … Bass, E. B. (2012). Policy implications for optimizing advanced practice registered use nationally. *Policy, Politics, & Nursing Practice, 13*(2), 81–89.

Pawlson, L. G., Bagley, B., Barr, M., Sevilla, X., Torda, T., & Scholle, S. (2011). *Patient-centered medical home: From vision to reality.* Retrieved from http://pcpcc.net/content/pcmh-vision-reality

Pearson, L. J. (2010). The Pearson Report. *American Journal for Nurse Practitioners, 14*(2). Retrieved from http://www.webnpolinie.com

Polit, D. F., & Beck, C. T. (2008). *Nursing research: Generating and assessing evidence for nursing practice.* Philadelphia, PA: Lippincott Williams & Wilkins.

Ridenour, N., & Trautman, D. (2009). A primer for nursing on advancing health reform policy. *Journal of Professional Nursing, 25*(6), 358–362.

Russell, G. E., & Fawcett, J. (2005). The conceptual model for nursing and health policy revisited. *Policy, Politics & Nursing Practice, 6*(4), 319–326.

Safriet, B. (2002). Closing the gap between can and may in healthcare providers' scope of practice: A primer for policymakers. *Yale Journal of Regulation, 19,* 301–334.

Tanner, C. A. (2012). Reflections—On leaving the JNE editorship. *Journal of Nursing Education, 51,* 419–420.

CHAPTER 3

Johnson & Johnson Campaign for Nursing's Future: An Impetus for Change

Mary C. Smolenski

Corporate America has had an impact on nursing, and one company that has helped to change the face of nursing in a positive way is Johnson & Johnson (J&J). J&J is an international company developed by three brothers (Robert Wood Johnson, James Wood Johnson, and Edward Mead Johnson) in 1886 and from its beginning has a record of helping communities and populations to solve health care and public health problems. From producing one of the first commercial "First-Aid Kits" and manuals, introducing the first commercially produced sanitary pads—a breakthrough for women's health—and mass producing dental floss to provide better dental care, to donating products and cash for disaster relief in 1900 starting a long tradition, J&J has been innovative and involved. This company continued to branch out developing maternity/family planning products, baby products such as baby powder and shampoo, the Band-Aid, various surgical items, and the list goes on and on. The company, started by the three brothers over 125 years ago, has grown into a worldwide partnership of over 250 companies in 57 countries. There are products, projects, and efforts in the areas of consumer health, medical devices and diagnostics, and pharmaceuticals touching every facet of health and global community and helping to solve problems with a goal of making the world a better place to live.

The company's credo, written by Robert Wood Johnson in 1943, remains unchanged today and attests to the fact that J&J is committed to and has a responsibility to the doctors, nurses, patients, communities, and the world we live in. J&J's progressive and future-oriented set of values began some 70 plus years ago long before the terminology "corporate social responsibility" came into vogue. The credo outlines J&J's responsibilities to health care providers, recipients of health care, J&J employees, local and worldwide communities, and the J&J stockholders. A portion is quoted below:

> We are responsible to the communities in which we live and work and the world community as well. We must be good citizens—support good works and charities and bear our fair share of taxes. We must encourage civic improvement and better health and education. We must maintain in good order the property we are privileged to use, protecting the environment and natural resources.
>
> *J&J Credo (1943)*

This dedication and corporate responsibility contributes to, if it is not the reason for, its survival as one of only a handful of companies that has weathered the world's changes over the last 125-year period.

When James Lenehan, a former Vice Chairman of J&J, made the rounds on one of his routine executive business reviews in 2001, over 12 years ago, he was asking one major question—"What's going on in health care and what do we need to focus on?"

One of the recurring comments he received was about the nursing shortage and the impact it might have on health care. Lenehan, whose mother was a nurse, knew well how nurses can and do impact health. Nursing shortages have been a cyclical problem. Numerous factors contributed to the shortage in the early 2000s. The nursing population at the time had an average age in the late 40s and nurse educators were also quickly reaching the retirement age. Few young people, typically women, were entering the profession, especially because many more lucrative professions were open to women, unlike decades ago. Men did not typically enter nursing because it was considered as a profession for women. Along with the decreased numbers was an increased need for nurses and other caregivers because of the aging population and extended life span. Lenehan asked himself if J&J could make an impact on this problem. The rest is history.

The J&J *Campaign for Nursing's Future* was initiated over 10 years ago in February 2002, as a multiyear, 50 million dollar national campaign with its major goals to enhance the nursing profession's image, to recruit nurses and nursing faculty, and to improve retention in the profession. J&J formed alliances with nursing organizations, schools, hospitals, and other health care organizations already involved in their own efforts to improve nursing's image. Initial efforts also focused on how to increase the number of students entering nursing as a profession at both regional and community levels by helping raise monies for grants and scholarships in nursing. Even nursing camps for elementary and high-school students were supported.

The "Dare to Care" television commercials, which were aimed at potential new nurses, were born and launched nationwide. Nursing has long been the most trusted profession by consumers and the campaign helped to increase that awareness and get others asking questions. But over time as awareness increased and efforts around the United States focused more on how to get more individuals to enter the nursing profession, the campaign broadened its view. It was time to emphasize not only that nurses "care" about patients, but also to focus on what nurses "do" for patients (Andrea Higham, personal communication, August 16, 2012). The campaign expanded its reach to develop an appreciation for the acute skills and knowledge base held by nurses in the variety of areas they work. It started to look at the technical and diagnostic expertise of nurses along with the many specialties they enter. This broader emphasis also looked at the advanced practice areas open to nurses, once again educating consumers to the variety of roles that nursing professionals are educated for and the level of skills they bring to the health care arena. Primary health care and who would be providing this type of care in the future were a new question that J&J wanted to impact and advanced practice nurses make a key contribution to the solution.

With the numbers of nurses starting to slowly increase in the early 21st century as a result of the coordinated efforts of many groups, it also became clear that numbers could not continue to increase if there was no one to educate these aspiring "nurses to be," mentor them, provide leadership for them, and find ways to fund their education. J&J reached out and developed multiple partnerships with major nursing organizations to focus more directly on these specific problems.

in their own countries rather than leave for the United States, Britain, or Canada. Working with the Caribbean nursing leaders and government, an initiative called the Year of the Caribbean Nurse was born. "In many ways, [the campaign] understood that there was an issue of connecting need, people and resources in ways that have never been done before," Salmon said. "The campaign set the table for nursing around the world, not just the United States."

More recently, Auerbach and colleagues (Auerbach, Staiger, Meunch, & Buerhaus, 2013) published about the nursing workforce and the amazing turnaround in the number of nurse graduates. Between 2002 and 2010, the number of graduates went from 74,000 to 157,000, more than doubling, with many of these being baccalaureate grads. Nearly 5% of first-year college students in 2010 claimed nursing as their probable major, the highest level since the 1960s. Initially, there was a surge of 30-somethings returning to the workforce in nursing, attending associate degree programs. This helped to increase nurse graduate numbers. But then the idea of viewing nursing as a career hit the 20-year-olds. Commitment to a career in nursing frequently leads to future education and advancement, a desire to become involved and be more independent in the workplace, all a good sign for the future of advanced practice nursing. Data from AACN Enrollments and Graduations depicting APRNs 2002–2011 (see Table 14.3; Miyamoto, 2013) show that in Master's programs alone, the number of advanced practice nurses enrolled, except for clinical nurse specialists (CNSs), increased from 2002 to 2011: nurse practitioners (NPs) 2002—16,675 and 2011—43,475, more than doubling; certified nurse midwives (CNMs) 2002—677 and 2011—1,272, almost double; and certified registered nurse anesthetists (CRNAs) 2002—2,198 and 2011—3,614. CNSs have remained above 3,000 enrollment but went from 3,730 in 2002 to 3,139 in 2011. This could be due in part to the Consensus Model and its potential impact on advanced practice authority for CNSs. This model reflects a role (NP, CNS, CNM, or CRNA) and population focus (family, pediatrics, etc.) for legal authority, and the CNS model has generally always been a "specialty or system focus" (rehab, pulmonary, cardiac, etc.), which may decrease the desirability of CNS programs from an advanced practice standpoint.

The authors state that this phenomenon of large increases in nursing graduates is caused by a confluence of factors. The J&J *Campaign*, initiated in 2002, is identified as a major private sector effort focusing on the nursing shortage affecting these results. The *Campaign* with its multifocused, responsive approach to solving the shortage has made a significant impact on the nursing workforce and ultimately on patient care. The *Campaign* "continues to inform the country about the importance of the nursing profession, promote a positive image of that profession, and entice a new generation of men and women into nursing careers" (p. 1471). Adding to the *Campaign*'s efforts was the initiation of health workforce centers in over three dozen states that complemented the efforts. The national growing interest and attractiveness of nursing, in conjunction with the recession, increased health care spending and jobs, and a dynamic response from the nursing education system have paved the way for a strong foundation in the nursing workforce for the coming years. Reinforcement will be necessary however and sustainment is not fail-proof, as nursing shortages are cyclical, learning from past history. More important reasons to sustain the growth in the nursing workforce now is the massive aging population and the changes in health care reform seeking to provide health care for all.

The *Campaign* continues to evolve and Higham says that there is no end date in sight. The impact of the *Campaign* on policies within communities, cities, states, organizations, and probably even federal policy is evident when reviewing the 10 years plus history and the changes over the last decade. The shape and focus of the message are tailored to meet the need. As health care focuses on primary care and community, away from acute hospital settings, J&J has modified its emphasis. As the emphasis on prevention, holistic care, and care coordination grow and the improved care of chronic health conditions become more a key focus of health care reform, the nursing model and advanced practice nurses are at the forefront of care in helping to make changes and provide quality "health" care. And J&J has helped to lead the way just as their credo of 1943 says "We are responsible to the communities in which we live and work and the world community as well. We must be good citizens—support good works...."

REFERENCES

Auerbach, D. I., Buerhaus, P. I., & Staiger, D. O. (2011). Registered nurse supply grows faster than projected amid surge in new entrants ages 23 to 26. *Health Affairs, 30*(12), 2286–2292.

Auerbach, D. I., Staiger, D. O., Meunch, U., & Buerhaus, P. I. (2013, April 18). The nursing workforce in an era of health care reform. *New England Journal of Medicine, 368*, 1470–1472.

J&J Credo. (1943). Retrieved from http://www.jnj.com/about-jnj/jnj-credo

Miyamoto, S. (2013, April 3). APRN Enrollments and Graduations 2002–2011 extracted from AACN Enrollments and Graduation data, submitted by Susan Miyamoto, AACN.

Stringer, H. (2012, November 12). *Johnson & Johnson Campaign for Nursing's Future turns 10* [quote from Beverly Malone]. Retrieved from http://news.nurse.com/article/20121112/HL01/311120008

Policy Implications for Optimizing Advanced Practice Registered Nurse Use Nationally*

*Robin P. Newhouse, Jonathan P. Weiner, Julie Stanik-Hutt,
Kathleen M. White, Meg Johantgen, Don Steinwachs, George Zangaro,
Jillian Aldebron, and Eric B. Bass*

Advanced practice registered nurses (APRNs) (nurse practitioners [NPs], certified nurse midwives [CNMs], certified registered nurse anesthetists [CRNAs], and clinical nurse specialists [CNSs]) are crucial providers of care that have not been used to their full potential in the health care delivery system. An estimated 240,460 APRNs are currently practicing in environments where they exercise a high degree of professional autonomy in the delivery of care to millions of patients annually (Health Resources and Services Administration, 2004). Our systematic review of nearly two decades of research conclusively found that care delivered by APRNs and care delivered by physicians (alone or in teams without an APRN) produce equivalent patient outcomes (Johantgen et al., 2012; Newhouse et al., 2011).

Table 4.1 provides the key findings of our review, including the frequency of studies reviewed, research designs, and level of evidence (high, moderate, or low). These studies measured discrete patient outcomes and compared care delivered by APRNs (both on their own and as part of teams) to care delivered by other providers (mainly physicians) practicing without APRNs. The review summarizes the significance as reported by the authors. A patient outcome was included in the summary if it was measured in at least three studies. A total of 28 patient outcomes derived from 69 studies (20 randomized controlled trials and 49 observational) were aggregated on this basis. A high level of evidence was considered present if there were at least two experimental studies of high quality or three high-quality observational studies that supported the outcome.

These findings offer a firm evidentiary basis for supporting an enhanced role for APRNs in the health care workforce consistent with the breadth and depth of

*From *Policy, Politics, & Nursing Practice* (2012), 12, 81–89, Sage.

TABLE 4.1 Key Findings of a Systematic Review of APRN Outcomes, Number of Studies, Randomized Controlled Trials, and Level of Evidence

	NUMBER OF STUDIES (*N* OF RCTs)	LEVEL OF EVIDENCE
Nurse practitioner (NP) outcomes are similar to physician groups for the following:		
Patient satisfaction with provider/care	6 (4 RCT)	High
Self-report of perceived health status	7 (5 RCT)	High
Functional status	10 (6 RCT)	High
Blood glucose	5 (5 RCT)	High
Blood pressure	4 (4 RCT)	High
Emergency department visits	5 (3 RCT)	High
Hospitalization	11 (3 RCT)	High
Mortality	8 (1 RCT)	High
Length of stay	16 (2 RCT)	Moderate
Duration of ventilation	3 (0 RCT)	Low
NP patient outcomes are better than physician groups for:		
Management of serum lipids	3 (3 RCT)	High
Certified nurse midwife (CNM) outcomes are similar to physicians for:		
Apgar scores	11 (1 RCT)	High
Low birth weight	8 (1 RCT)	High
CNM care compared with physicians has proportionally fewer:		
Cesarean sections	15 (1 RCT)	High
Epidurals	10 (0 RCT)	Moderate
Labor augmentations	9 (1 RCT)	High
Episiotomies	8 (1 RCT)	High
Labor inductions	9 (0 RCT)	Moderate
Vaginal operative deliveries	8 (1 RCT)	High
Labor analgesia use	6 (1 RCT)	High
Perineal lacerations	5 (1 RCT)	High
CNM care compared with physicians is comparable or proportionally better outcomes:		
Vaginal birth after cesarean	5 (0 RCT)	Moderate
Neonatal intensive care unit (NICU) admission	5 (0 RCT)	Moderate
Breastfeeding	3 (0 RCT)	Moderate
Clinical nurse specialists (CNS) group outcomes compared with non-CNS groups:		
Inpatient length of stay comparable or lower	7 (2 RCT)	High
Inpatient costs comparable or lower	4 (2 RCT)	High
Complications comparable or lower	3 (1 RCT)	Moderate
Satisfaction comparable	3 (2 RCT)	High

Source: Newhouse et al. (2011).

their education and training. As we move away from silos to embrace integrated models of health care delivery in which professionals collaborate across disciplinary boundaries to produce new, more effective methods of care, the success of these efforts will depend in large part on the ability of each practitioner to maximize its contribution as a member of the team (Choi & Pak, 2007; Committee on the Robert Wood Johnson Foundation Initiative on the Future of Nursing, at the Institute of Medicine, 2011).

THE CASE FOR EXPANDED ROLES FOR APRNs

Over the years, APRNs have assumed an increasingly prominent place in the health care system, in particular, stepping in to fill certain provider shortages. In some measure, these shortages have been driven by employment trends as fewer physicians opt to practice alone or with only a single physician partner—a drop from 40.7% in 1996–1997 to 32.5% in 2004–2005 (Liebhaber & Grossman, 2007). It is especially noteworthy that APRNs have long been relied on to provide care for the most vulnerable (e.g., elderly and disabled), minority populations, and those living in inner-city and rural areas (Lewandowski & Adamle, 2009).

This is evident in federally qualified health centers (FQHCs), which increase access to primary care services in areas where resources are constrained. FQHCs provide primary care for all ages including dental, mental health, and substance abuse services (Rural Assistance Center, 2011). A team-based approach to primary care uses varied nonphysician providers. In 2010, 9,100 physicians and 5,800 NPs, physician assistants (PAs), or CNMs provided essential primary and preventive care in FQHCs (Medpac, 2011). Many jurisdictions already permit NPs to deliver care as independent providers (Christian, Dower, & O'Neil, 2007). Twenty-two states allow totally autonomous NP practice (NCSBN, 2012). Seventeen accord NPs full prescriptive authority (NCSBN, 2012): Alaska, Arizona, Colorado, District of Columbia, Hawaii, Idaho, Iowa, Maine, Maryland, Montana, New Hampshire, New Mexico, Oregon, Rhode Island, Utah, Washington, and Wyoming (NCSBN, 2012). Twenty-seven jurisdictions condition NP practice on a "collaborative agreement" of some type (NCSBN, 2012). In reality, this usually means that NPs autonomously perform comprehensive health assessments (history and physical examinations) and medical diagnoses, but are required to have a written agreement of collaboration with a physician to do so. The physician does not oversee the work or sign off on charts and may not even be located at the same practice site.

Still, APRNs on the whole remain an underutilized resource with the demonstrable potential to do more for special populations and others. Expanding APRNs' scope of practice to take full advantage of their educational preparation could go far toward alleviating the growing strain on our primary care physician workforce exerted by the combined pressures of demography and expanded insurance coverage under the Patient Protection and Affordable Care Act (ACA). There are also practice model arguments for enhancing the role of APRNs. Nursing skills complement those of physicians in the case of chronically ill patients.

The "medical home" model for serving patients with chronic illness, for example, envisions 24/7 provider access—something that is not likely achievable unless there is a team. Yet, most descriptions of the medical home refer to physician-directed care. For example, the Patient-Centered Primary Care Collaborative endorses access to care based on "an ongoing relationship with a personal physician trained to provide first contact, continuous, and comprehensive care" who "leads a team of individuals at the practice level who collectively take responsibility for the ongoing care of patients" (Pawlson et al., 2011). That said, a growing number of states (e.g., Maryland, Pennsylvania, Colorado) have allowed APRNs to function as primary care providers, some even permitting nurse-led medical homes. This movement has prompted the National Committee for Quality Assurance (NCQA), Utilization Review Accreditation Commission (URAC), and the Joint Commission to include nurse-led primary care practices in their patient-centered medical home recognition and accreditation programs, and to replace the term "physician" with "clinician" in their relevant materials to accommodate NPs and physician assistants (PAs) (Joint Commission, 2011; NCQA, 2011). Federal legislation that incorporates NPs as providers who are responsible and accountable for care has been introduced, representing a further positive step.

Emerging trends of physician visits in the home (house calls) and the incorporation of medical care into residential settings also make the case for integrated teams in which each profession, including APRNs, contributes its unique range of competencies in a collaborative model of care (Bookbinder et al., 2011; Deitrik et al., 2011; Landers, Gunn, & Stange, 2009; Naylor et al., 1999; Ornstein, Smith, Foer, Lopez-Cantor, & Soriano, 2011). Complex and chronic diseases are best managed by a team with diverse expertise sufficient to meet a patient's multiple needs (Interprofessional Education Collaborative Expert Panel, 2011; Shih et al., 2008).

OPPORTUNITIES FOR OPTIMIZING APRN USE

There are a number of ways that APRNs are meeting present health care workforce needs but could be used more effectively to address these and future needs. Table 4.2 summarizes key areas in which APRNs can have a potential role in addressing workforce needs.

Primary Care

Evidence suggests that we need to rethink how to deliver primary care. Over the past decade there has been an inexorable decrease in the number of American medical students going into primary care residency training programs (Jeffe, Whelan, & Andriole, 2010). The critical shortage of primary care physicians that was identified before passage of health care reform will be further exacerbated by the mandates of the new law (Dodoo et al., 2005). The number of primary care physicians grew just 1.2% to 90 per 100,000 people from 1995 to 2005. By comparison, the number of primary care NPs rose 9.4% to 28 per 100,000 people over the same period (Steinwald, 2008). APRNs have already been deployed to improve access where primary care physicians are in short supply, such as rural settings and among underserved urban populations. Sixty-eight percent of NPs practice in primary care (American Academy of Nurse Practitioners, 2010). Rather than relying on physicians alone to satisfy the primary care needs of the general population, using APRNs (and PAs, among others) would stretch the workforce and improve access.

Medical Resident Care

When medical resident work hours were reduced because excessively long hours were found to compromise patient safety, NPs immediately became part of the workforce solution (Christmas et al., 2005; Lundberg, Wali, Thomas, & Cope, 2006; Molitor-Kirsch, Thompson, & Milonovich, 2005; Resnick, Todd, Mullen, & Morris,

TABLE 4.2 Potential Role of APRNs in Addressing Workforce Needs

Primary care shortages	Provide a pool of primary care providers capable of alleviating the shortage of primary care physicians in certain areas
Supplement medical resident care	Replace residents and fellows who are practicing fewer hours due to graduate medical education reform
Provide care for vulnerable populations	Expand access to care in rural or inner-city areas. Promote public health/population-based initiatives including prenatal/infant mortality improvement programs
Disease and chronic care management and medical homes	Improve chronic care management and medical home expansion to improve quality of life, reduce complications and readmissions
TeleHealth	Support consumer-based e-health/technology supported care models, including remote patient monitoring
Access/convenient care	Provide care through retail clinics and other models of community-based care

2006). This substitution was based on emerging evidence that APRN care was not only safe, but also substitutable for most resident care (Brown & Grimes, 1995; Horrocks, Anderson, & Salisbury, 2002; Laurant et al., 2005). The success of this solution can and should be extended to other settings that are still struggling to meet the resident hour restrictions.

Serving Vulnerable Populations

APRNs often care for the nation's uninsured and vulnerable populations. As we expand coverage for the uninsured, APRNs can have a greater role in providing primary care (NPs and CNMs), pregnancy care and delivery (CNMs), chronic disease management (NPs and CNSs), and anesthesia care (CRNA). Eighteen percent of NPs (American Academy of Nurse Practitioners, 2010) practice in rural areas where distances to access care are great and practitioners sparse. CNMs attend a substantial portion of births in the nation's most rural states (American College of Nurse-Midwives [ACNM], 2012). CRNAs are the sole anesthesia providers in 85% of rural hospitals (Pine, Holt, & Lou, 2003).

APRNs have long demonstrated their value as central actors in innovative care delivery models that address shortages of both primary and specialty care for underserved population groups. Eliminating barriers that restrict the scope of their practice would enable them to be still more effective in this area of persistent and growing need.

Disease Management and Chronic Care

APRNs can optimize health in the delivery of primary care and disease management of patients with chronic illnesses. Examples include management of patients with diabetes (Lenz, Mundinger, Hopkins, Lin, & Smolowitz, 2002) and heart failure (Naylor et al., 2004). These two chronic diseases as a primary diagnosis alone account for more than 1.54 million hospital discharges in 2010 generating charges of more than U.S. $52 billion (HCUPnet, 2010). Based on our systematic review, in comparisons of teams with and without APRNs, NPs and CNSs are effective at reducing readmissions, improving adherence to evidence-based care, and reducing hospital length of stay when patients are admitted. APRNs used to their full potential can have a profound effect on the efficiency and cost of care in the chronic care population.

Medical Homes

As medical homes and other types of coordinated programs (both primary care and specialized "principal care" for persons with a "dominant condition") become major features of the health care infrastructure, it will be essential that collaborative teams with the right "skill mix" are defined and used. The inclusion of APRNs providing care to the full extent of their competencies and skills is a crucial component. The medical home should determine the best way to use APRNs—and, indeed, all other types of qualified health care providers—to attain the best outcomes for patients.

Telehealth and HIT

As use of health information technology (HIT) spreads, including remote patient monitoring and the use of personal health record/consumer-centric e-health self-care, there will be an increased need for appropriate practitioners to provide professional support from a "distance." Patients with chronic illnesses, such as heart failure, benefit by telehealth care accessed in the home. APRNs, with their expertise in patient communication and education, can for example, assess a patient's progress in nutrition, weight management, or adherence to medications to identify and treat symptoms before they develop to a level that requires hospitalization. This opportunity for expanded use of APRNs will be applicable in a variety of settings and practices, but especially for patients isolated by geography, age, or disability who have difficulty accessing specialty or chronic care services.

Retail Clinics

Consumers' increasing desire for ready access to care on their own terms is a trend not likely to go away. Demand for user-friendly health care has propelled the convenient care (a.k.a. "retail clinic") movement (Hansen-Turton, Ryan, Miller, Counts, & Nash, 2007). There are more than 1,200 retail clinics operating nationwide, and their number is expected to reach 3,400 by 2014 (Herrick, 2010). NPs are generally the providers of care in retail clinics (Mehrotra et al., 2009). For three commonly treated acute conditions (otitis media, pharyngitis, and urinary tract infections), costs at retail clinics are lower and quality of care is similar to that in physicians' offices and urgent care centers (Mehrotra et al., 2009; Weinick, Pollack, Fisher, Gillen, & Mehrotra, 2010). Setting-based outcomes were compared for the selected conditions because they are commonly managed in all ambulatory care settings. Results also indicate that antibiotic prescribing patterns and provision of preventive services were similar across care settings (Mehrotra et al., 2009). Patient satisfaction with the care they receive at retail clinics is high (Weinick et al., 2010). Given the popularity of care provided by NPs in these clinics, it is likely that NPs will continue to be found well suited to meet patients' needs and improve care access by practicing in these and other primary care settings.

APRNs IN AN INTEGRATED WORKFORCE: CHALLENGES AND SOLUTIONS

As the Institute of Medicine (IOM) recommended in its landmark report, Crossing the Quality Chasm, the nation needs to move away from single providers and single disciplines working as islands unto themselves (Committee on Quality of Health Care in America, Institute of Medicine, 2001). Members of well-supported, integrated teams need to have authority and accountability to maximize the contributions of each practitioner toward system goals that benefit the patient and society.

- Patient-centered care based on patient need in integrated care model
- Outcome-driven policy to allow innovative models of care to bring value to consumer and community
- Focus on quality gaps for priority population, quality metrics, and support for interdisciplinary care
- Avoid professional protectionism in expanding systems of care
- Educate an interprofessional workforce
- Reform provider reimbursement to maximize efficiency and quality
- Improve workforce data to evaluate outcomes and inform policy

FIGURE 4.1 Integrated Workforce Challenges and Solutions.

In an integrated workforce, APRNs will have differing roles and relationships with primary care and specialty physicians. There will be models of care in which APRNs work directly with specialty physicians (e.g., endocrinologists managing patients with diabetes) and/or with primary care physicians (who will have patients with a wide variety of acute and chronic conditions, and an increasing number of patients having multiple chronic conditions). Primary care physicians will refer patients to APRNs with expertise in managing chronic care populations. APRNs will refer to specialists for specific patient conditions, or to primary care physicians for complex symptom management. The role of an APRN is likely to vary according to whether the team involves family physicians, general internists, or medical specialists. How physicians organize their practice will also vary depending on the roles that APRNs play.

Once the issue of comparability between APRN care and that delivered by physicians is set aside in favor of an integrated team concept, disciplines can focus on the overarching goals (Pawlson et al., 2011). Some of the issues and challenges that must be confronted to develop an integrated workforce include development of patient-centered integrated teams, supporting outcome-driven policy, building a shared health care vision to reduce quality gaps, avoiding professional protectionism, educating an interprofessional workforce, reforming reimbursement, and improving workforce data collection (see Figure 4.1).

Integrated Teams

Patient-centered care should be driven by patient need. Rather than framing assessments of care quality in terms of that delivered by provider type "A" versus provider type "B," we propose a more productive policy framework that focuses on an integrated care model in which the providers assume responsibility for care based on the needs of the patient. The right provider may be an APRN, physician, or APRN-physician team that could include an array of other professionals as well. NPs (and CNMs and CRNAs depending on the care needed) are well prepared and legally authorized to provide many of the same services now provided by physicians. A patient's choice of provider in an integrated team context should not be impeded by unnecessary barriers. Patients should be able to decide who they want to see for their annual exam or who they prefer to monitor and manage their blood pressure as an outpatient, as long as it is within the provider's legally authorized scope of practice based on their education and experience.

Outcome-Driven Policy

Policy should be guided by outcomes, value, and consumer and community benefit, rather than taking a provider-centric perspective. Our systematic review of the evidence revealed that there are many opportunities for APRNs to contribute as "substitutes," "alternatives," "complements," or "extenders" to the care provided by physicians.

Focus on Quality Gaps

The 2011 National Healthcare Quality Report indicates that quality of care in the United States has had uneven improvements and is lagging in making care safer, promoting healthy living, and disparities related to race, ethnicity, and socioeconomic status and access (Agency for Healthcare Research and Quality, 2012). An expanded APRN workforce can have a positive influence in all three. In addition, quality metrics should refocus on the continuum of care instead of episodic care (Christian et al., 2007; Committee on Redesigning Health Insurance Performance Measures, Payment, and Performance Improvement Programs, Board on Health Care Services, Institute of Medicine, 2006). Refocusing on patient outcomes across all providers and teams of providers is a first step in implementing a comprehensive metric of quality. There should be priority funding for interdisciplinary studies that include practitioners (APRNs, physicians, etc.) in the development of protocols that are patient centric. Measures of integrated care across the continuum of care need to be developed and tested in different settings and populations. Consensus should be established on the important outcomes of quality.

Avoid Professional Protectionism

As others have suggested, we need to avoid workforce policy that is unduly influenced by professional protectionism and instead base policy decisions on individual and community welfare and system performance (Phillips, Harper, Wakefield, Green, & Fryer, 2002). Public and private policy should sustain such goals. The American College of Physicians recently issued statements supporting incorporation of NPs into health care teams (American College of Physicians, 2009). Such policy positions open the door to discourse among multiple parties, with the goal of creating optimal systems of care. To create these optimal systems, regulatory barriers for APRN practice will need to be eliminated.

Educate an Interprofessional Workforce

Future health care workforce policy must reject practice "silos." Likewise, university and clinical settings need to incorporate collaboration across professions as part of their education process. Core competencies of this interprofessional education are teamwork, evidence-based practice, quality improvement, informatics, and patient-centered care (Committee on the Health Professions Education Summit, 2003; Interprofessional Education Collaborative Expert Panel, 2011). Continuing education, which is often conducted in an interprofessional environment, can be used effectively to foster collaboration and improve care quality (Hager, Russell, & Fletcher, 2008). We must continue to invest in and test model systems of interprofessional education, continuing education, safety, and quality monitoring.

There will be many barriers to providing interprofessional education, not the least of which are incompatible curriculum schedules. Furthermore, professional schools will need to negotiate how workload will be distributed for faculty and how each school will be reimbursed for student tuition. Interprofessional faculty will need to consider options where no best practices or evidence exists to guide decisions. For example, they will need to evaluate how important is it for medical students and nursing students to be together for learning activities. Is it sufficient to have medical students learning from nursing faculty, and nursing students learning from medical faculty?

Within nursing, progress could be gained by fostering common definitions and scope of practice for APRNs. State policy should adopt licensing requirements that reflect standard definitions for APRNs, with concomitant licensing requirements (APRN Consensus Work Group & the National Council of State Boards of Nursing APRN Advisory Committee, 2008).

Reform Provider Reimbursement

We need to design reimbursement systems that maximize efficiency and provide appropriate incentives for good care and good workforce policy. This includes structuring payment models that support the use of interdisciplinary teams and, as appropriate, independent APRN practice. Medicare and Medicaid reimbursement for NP services historically has been lower than reimbursement for physician services. Payments by private payers vary widely (Chapman, Wides, & Spetz, 2010), and reimbursement to physicians for APRN visits are billed under "incident services," further obscuring the actual scope and extent of APRNs' contribution to care (Chapman et al., 2010). These incident services are delivered by APRNs in physician practices (or where there is a common employer). Under some circumstances, they may be billed as services "incident to" those of a physician, in which case they are paid at 100%.

Changes in reimbursement policy could provide an incentive to better use APRNs in primary care (Chapman et al., 2010). The American College of Nurse-Midwives worked from 1988 when CNMs were first recognized under Medicare to secure passage of legislation providing for equitable reimbursement at 100% of the Part B fee schedule for midwifery services. Such a provision was finally incorporated in the ACA, and went into effect on January 1, 2011 (American College of Nurse-Midwives [ACNM], 2010).

Improve Workforce Data

Data collection related to provider practice must improve. This will be key to setting future health care workforce policy. Provider categories for APRNs should be included among the data collected by federal databases, and the databases made available for research so that the distribution and practice contributions of APRNs can be better assessed. Currently, important public and private data collection efforts such as the National Ambulatory Medical Care Survey, the Center Studying Health Systems Change surveys, and the Area Resource File (which is the basis for health professional shortage area identifications) do not collect sufficiently granular data on APRNs.

CONCLUSION

Many critical workforce gaps will have major implications for the health care delivery system and, ultimately, the health of the U.S. population. Present challenges and recent evidence support the premise that health care reform should embrace APRNs to the full extent of their knowledge, skills, and competencies, and that these highly trained nurses represent one very important solution for addressing workforce needs over the coming decades. Indeed, the IOM has strongly recommended elimination of regulatory barriers to APRN practice, in particular singling out restrictive physician-nurse practitioner collaborative agreements for needlessly reducing access to primary care (Committee on the Robert Wood Johnson Foundation Initiative on the Future of Nursing, at the Institute of Medicine, 2011).

APRNs must be fully integrated into emerging models of care that foster collaboration among health care providers from appropriate disciplines to meet the patient's health care needs. This team approach does not mean that professional disciplines merge boundaries in a transdisciplinary way, but rather that each discipline contributes in a unique way to achieve a shared goal in the care of the patient. APRNs will not be able to function effectively in teams unless the legal, regulatory, and reimbursement barriers to their practice are eliminated (Cronenwett & Dzau, 2010).

As we proceed to transform our health care system over the coming decades, it is essential that workforce policy assessment, planning, and investment be guided by scientific evidence on staffing approaches that offer the greatest value to patients and communities. This, rather than provider-centric politics or parochialism, should serve as framework and guideposts. Accordingly, we have grounded our recommendations on just such evidence, derived from decades of comparative effectiveness research. We offer them here in the hope and expectation that they will move the national workforce policy discourse in a similar direction.

REFERENCES

Advanced Practice Registered Nurses (APRN) Consensus Work Group & the National Council of State Boards of Nursing APRN Advisory Committee. (2008). *Consensus model for APRN regulation: Licensure, accreditation, certification & education.* Retrieved from https://www.ncsbn.org/APRN Joint_/Dia_report_May_08.pdf

Agency for Healthcare Research and Quality. (2012, March). *National Healthcare Quality Report 2011.* Rockville, MD: U.S. Department of Health and Human Services, Agency for Healthcare Research and Quality. Retrieved from http://www.ahrq.gov/qual/qrdr11.htm

American Academy of Nurse Practitioners. (2010). *Nurse practitioner facts.* Retrieved from http://www.aanp.org/images/documents/research/2010-11_NPFacts.pdf

American College of Nurse-Midwives (ACNM). (2010). *Equitable reimbursement.* Retrieved from http://www.midwife.org/EquitableReimbursement

American College of Nurse-Midwives (ACNM). (2012). *Where midwives work.* Retrieved from http://www.midwife.org/ACNM/files/ACNMLibraryData/UPLOADFILENAME/000000000277/Where%20Midwives%20Work%20June2012.pdf

American College of Physicians. (2009). *Nurse practitioners in primary care* (Policy monograph). Retrieved from http://www.acponline.org/advocacy/where_we_stand/policy/np_pc.pdf

Bookbinder, M., Glajchen, M., McHugh, M., Higgins, P., Budis, J., Solomon, N., ... Portenoy, R. K. (2011). Nurse practitioner-based models of specialist palliative care at home: Sustainability and evaluation of feasibility. *Journal of Pain Symptom Management, 4*(1), 25–34.

Brown, S. A., & Grimes, D. E. (1995). A meta-analysis of nurse practitioners and nurse midwives in primary care. *Nursing Research, 44,* 332–339.

Chapman, S., Wides, C., & Spetz, J. (2010). Payment regulations for advanced practice nurses: Implications for primary care. *Policy, Politics & Nursing Practice, 11,* 89–98.

Choi, B. C., & Pak, A. W. (2007). Multidisciplinarity, interdisciplinarity, and transdisciplinarity in health research, services, education and policy: 2. Promotors, barriers, and strategies of enhancement. *Clinical and Investigative Medicine, 30,* E224–E232.

Christian, S., Dower, C., & O'Neil, E. (2007). *Chart overview of nurse practitioner scopes of practice in the United States.* San Francisco: Center for the Health Professions, University of California. Retrieved from http://www.acnpweb.org/files/public/UCSF_Chart_2007.pdf

Christmas, A. B., Reynolds, J., Hodges, S., Franklin, G. A., Miller, F. B., Richardson, J. D., & Rodriguez, J. L. (2005). Physician extenders impact trauma systems. *Journal of Trauma: Injury, Infection & Critical Care, 58,* 917–920.

Committee on Quality of Health Care in America, Institute of Medicine. (2001). *Crossing the quality chasm: A new health system for the 21st century.* Washington, DC: National Academy Press.

Committee on Redesigning Health Insurance Performance Measures, Payment, and Performance Improvement Programs, Board on Health Care Services, Institute of Medicine (IOM). (2006). *Performance measurement: Accelerating improvement.* Washington, DC: National Academies Press.

Committee on the Health Professions Education Summit. (2003). *Health professions education: A bridge to quality.* Washington, DC: National Academy of Sciences.

Committee on the Robert Wood Johnson Foundation Initiative on the Future of Nursing, at the Institute of Medicine. (2011). *The future of nursing: Leading change, advancing health.* Washington, DC: National Academies Press.

Cronenwett, L., & Dzau, V. (2010). Who will provide primary care and how will they be trained? In B. Culliton & S. Russell (Eds.), *Proceedings of a conference sponsored by the Josiah Macy Jr. Foundation, 2010.* Durham, NC: Josiah Macy Jr. Foundation. Retrieved from http://www.josiahmacy foundation.org

Deitrik, L., Rockwell, E., Gratz, N., Davidson, C., Lukas, L., Stevens, D., & Sikora, B. (2011). Delivering specialized palliative care in the community: A new role for nurse practitioners. *Advances in Nursing Science, 34*(4), E23–E36.

Dodoo, M. S., Phillips, R. L. J., Green, L. A., Ruddy, G., McCann, J. L., & Klein, L. (2005). Excess, shortage, or sufficient physician workforce: How could we know? *American Academy of Family Physicians, 72,* 1670.

Hager, M., Russell, S., & Fletcher, S. W. (Eds.). (2008). Continuing education in the health professions: Improving health care through lifelong learning. *Proceedings from a conference sponsored by the Josiah Macy Jr. Foundation.* New York, NY: Josiah Macy Jr. Foundation. Retrieved from http://www .josiahmacyfoundation.org

Hansen-Turton, T., Ryan, S., Miller, K., Counts, M., & Nash, D. B. (2007). Convenient care clinics: The future of accessible health care. *Disease Management, 10,* 61–73.

HCUPnet. (2010). *National statistics on all stays, specific diagnoses 2010.* Retrieved from http://hcupnet .ahrq.gov

Health Resources and Services Administration. (2004). *The registered nurse population. Findings from the March 2004 national sample survey of registered nurses.* Retrieved from http://bhpr.hrsa.gov/health workforce/rnsurveys/rnsurvey2004.pdf

Herrick, D. (2010). *Retail clinics: Convenient and affordable care* (Brief Analysis No. 686). Washington, DC: National Center for Policy Analysis.

Horrocks, S., Anderson, E., & Salisbury, C. (2002). Systematic review of whether nurse practitioners working in primary care can provide equivalent care to doctors. *British Medical Journal, 324*(7341), 819–823.

Interprofessional Education Collaborative Expert Panel. (2011). *Core competencies for interprofessional collaborative practice: Report of an expert panel.* Washington, DC: Interprofessional Education Collaborative. Retrieved from http://www.aacn.nche.edu/Education/pdf/IPECReport.pdf

Jeffe, D. B., Whelan, A. J., & Andriole, D. A. (2010). Primary care specialty choices of United States medical graduates, 1997–2006. *Academic Medicine: Journal of the Association of American Medical Colleges, 85,* 947–958.

Johantgen, M., Fountain, L., Zangaro, G., Newhouse, R., Stanik-Hutt, J., & White, K. (2012). Comparison of labor and delivery care provided by certified nurse-midwives and physicians: A systematic review, 1990 to 2008. *Women's Health Issues, 22*(1), e73–e81.

Joint Commission. (2011). *Approved standards & EPs with scoring for the joint commission primary care medical home option.* Retrieved from http://www.jointcommission.org/assets/1/18/PCMH_Standard _EPs_Scoring_20110718.pdf

Landers, S., Gunn, P., & Stange, K. (2009). An emerging model of primary care for older adults: The house call-home care practice. *Care Management Journals, 10,* 110–114.

Laurant, M., Reeves, D., Hermens, R., Braspenning, J., Grol, R., & Sibbald, B. (2005). Substitution of doctors by nurses in primary care. *Cochrane Database of Systematic Reviews.* doi: 10.1002/14651858 .CD001271.pub2

Lenz, E. R., Mundinger, M. O., Hopkins, S. C., Lin, S. X., & Smolowitz, J. L. (2002). Diabetes care processes and outcomes in patients treated by nurse practitioners or physicians. *Diabetes Educator, 28,* 590–598.

Lewandowski, W., & Adamle, K. (2009). Substantive areas of clinical nurse specialist practice: A comprehensive review of the literature. *Clinical Nurse Specialist, 23*(2), 73–90.

Liebhaber, A., & Grossman, J. (2007). *Physicians moving to mid-size, single-specialty practice* (Tracking report #18). Washington, DC: Center for Studying Health System Change. Retrieved from http://hschange.org/CONTENT/941/#top

Lundberg, S., Wali, S., Thomas, P., & Cope, D. (2006). Attaining resident duty hours compliance: The acute care nurse practitioners program at Olive View-UCLA medical center. *Academic Medicine, 81,* 1021–1025.

Medpac. (2011). *Report to the Congress: Medicare and the health care delivery system.* Retrieved from http://www.medpac.gov/chapters/Jun11_Ch06.pdf

Mehrotra, A., Liu, H., Adams, J. L., Wang, M. C., Lave, J. R., Thygeson, N. M., & McGlynn, E. A. (2009). Comparing costs and quality of care at retail clinics with that of other medical settings for 3 common illnesses. *Annals of Internal Medicine, 757,* 321–328.

Molitor-Kirsch, S., Thompson, L., & Milonovich, L. (2005). The changing face of critical care medicine: Nurse practitioners in the pediatric intensive care unit. *AACN Clinical Issues, 16*(2), 172–177.

National Committee for Quality Assurance (NCQA). (2011). *Standards and guidelines for NCQA's patient centered medical home (PCMH) 2011.* Washington, DC: Author.

National Council of State Boards of Nursing (NCSBN). (2012). NCSBN's APRN campaign for consensus: State progress toward uniformity. Retrieved from https://www.ncsbn.org/2567.htm

Naylor, M. D., Brooten, D. A., Campbell, R. L., Jacobsen, B., Mezey, M., Pauly, M., & Schwartz, J. (1999). Comprehensive discharge planning and home follow-up of hospitalized elders: A randomized, controlled trial. *Journal of the American Medical Association, 281,* 613–670.

Naylor, M. D., Brooten, D. A., Campbell, R. L., Maislin, G., McCauley, K. M., & Schwartz, J. S. (2004). Transitional care of older adults hospitalized with heart failure: A randomized, controlled trial. *Journal of the American Geriatrics Society, 52,* 675–684.

Newhouse, R., Stanik-Hutt, J., White, K., Johantgen, M., Bass, E. B., Zangaro, G., … Weiner, J. P. (2011). Advanced practice nurse outcomes 1990–2008: A systematic review. *Nursing Economics, 29,* 230–250.

Ornstein, K., Smith, K., Foer, D., Lopez-Cantor, M., & Soriano, T. (2011). To the hospital and back home again: A nurse practitioner-based transitional care program for hospitalized, homebound people. *Journal of the American Geriatrics Society, 59,* 544–551.

Pawlson, L. G., Bagley, B., Barr, M., Sevilla, X., Torda, T., & Scholle, S. (2011). *Patient-centered medical home: From vision to reality.* Retrieved from http://pcpcc.net/content/pcmh-vision-reality

Phillips, R. L., Jr., Harper, D. C., Wakefield, M., Green, L. A., & Fryer, G. E., Jr. (2002). Can nurse practitioners and physicians beat parochialism into plowshares? *Health Affairs, 21*(5), 133–142.

Pine, M., Holt, K. D., & Lou, Y. B. (2003). Surgical mortality and type of anesthesia provider. *AANA Journal, 71*(2), 109–116.

Resnick, A. S., Todd, B. A., Mullen, J. L., & Morris, J. B. (2006). How do surgical residents and non-physician practitioners play together in the sandbox? *Current Surgery, 63*(2), 155–164.

Rural Assistance Center. (2011). *FQHC frequently asked questions.* Retrieved from http://www.raconline.org/topics/clinics/fqhcfaq.php

Shih, A., Davis, K., Schoebaum, S., Gauthier, A., Nuzum, R., & McCarthy, D. (2008). *Organizing the US health care delivery system for high performance.* New York, NY: Commonwealth Fund. Retrieved from http://www.commonwealthfund.org/usr_doc/Shih_organizingushltcaredeliverysys_1155.pdf

Steinwald, A. B. (2008, February 12). *Primary care professionals: Recent supply trends, projections, and valuation of services. Testimony before the committee on health, education, labor and pensions, U.S. Senate* (GAO-08-472T). Washington, DC: Government Accountability Office.

Weinick, R. M., Pollack, C. E., Fisher, M. P., Gillen, E. M., & Mehrotra, A. (2010). *Policy implications of the use of retail clinics* (No. TR-810-DHHS). Santa Monica, CA: RAND Corporation.

CHAPTER 5

The IOM Report: The Future of Nursing

Liana Orsolini

No one predicted this report would go viral. Since its release, "The Future of Nursing: Leading Change, Advancing Health" has been the most widely read report released by the Institute of Medicine (IOM) (2010) and is associated with a grassroots effort that has spread to 49 states and the District of Columbia to implement its recommendations. As of this writing, Alaska is making plans to officially join the Future of Nursing's Campaign for Action. The report's inception came about because Robert Wood Johnson Foundation (RWJF) partnered with the IOM to study how to best transform the nursing profession to effectively function in a future of health care delivery redesign and be a part of the solution to increasing access to health care for millions more Americans. During the IOM's work, committee members were cognizant that if the Patient Protection and Affordable Care Act, also known as the ACA, became law, 30 million more Americans would have access to health care but millions more illegal immigrants would remain without affordable coverage. This report was never meant to aggrandize nursing but rather to significantly increase access to health care and to serve as a blueprint for nursing for how to accomplish this.

BACKGROUND INFORMATION

Let us start with the RWJF. Who are they and why are they so interested in nursing's future? Robert Wood Johnson II of Johnson & Johnson started the foundation in 1972 (RWJF, 2013a). The mission of the foundation is to improve public health and it spends over 350 million dollars a year on grants to accomplish this (RWJF, 2013b). The RWJF views public health as increasing access to and improving the quality of health care, improving health, reducing health disparities, stemming the obesity epidemic, increasing prevention effectiveness, reducing the rising cost of health care, and creating leaders who are change agents in the community and in government. When the RWJF realized that the status quo was not sustainable and that sickness prevention would have to be incentivized, they turned to the potential of the nursing workforce for solutions. There are no other health care professional groups that are over 3 million strong, 2.6 million of which are actively working in the health care industry (Health Resources and Services Administration [HRSA], 2010). Nursing was a sleeping giant.

Why did RWJF approach the IOM? Founded in 1970, the IOM is part of the National Academy of Sciences and studies issues around health and health care. The National Academy of Sciences is a bit older than the IOM as it was established under Lincoln's presidency. The IOM is often sanctioned by Congress, a federal agency such as the National Institutes of Health, or an other division within the Department of Health and Human Services (DHHS) to undertake a study with recommendations (IOM, 2013a). Sometimes, the IOM is privately funded to hold a study such as the Future of Nursing report. The IOM is held to section 15 of the Federal Advisory Committee Act, which means that most of its committee work and process is transparent to the public when a report contains recommendations aimed at a government entity (IOM, 2013b). Each IOM committee has stakeholders from many different disciplines as well as content experts. Committee makeup goes through a national public vetting process and its final reports go through a more structured vetting process with key stakeholders who are not committee members. The IOM is a trusted, nonbiased entity that holds their reports to high scientific rigor; they must be evidence-based and strive to have consensus-based recommendations. When one wants stakeholders who hold multiple perspectives to take a report seriously, many turn to the IOM.

RWJF needed a process for the Future of Nursing report that would ensure credibility, transparency, and an established vetting process to ensure a diversity of stakeholders and that report recommendations were evidence-based. Although these methods of operations were well in place at the IOM, RWJF needed the IOM to implement some changes to their methods that would not affect the credibility of their process. These changes were unprecedented for the IOM and included allowing RWJF to provide just-in-time research support by an external group of experts, providing a Study Director from outside the IOM (Susan Hassmiller, Senior Advisor for Nursing for RWJF), and providing communications staff (Hassmiller, personal communication, March 9, 2013). The Study Director's, Susan Hassmiller, PhD, RN, FAAN, role was to not only serve as a symbolic message that RWJF sanctioned this study, but also provided crucial continuity between the report recommendations and their implementation through the Campaign for Action. The research team implemented needed data analysis to fill gaps the committee members discovered as they poured through evidence. RWJF also funded outside consultations (invited papers) for important topics committee members discovered few publications about. The communication team blogged and tweeted, helping to keep the public cognizant of the three open public forums on Nursing Education, Care in the Community, and Acute Care held throughout the country, and kept the committee members cognizant about any new evidence that was newly published in peer-reviewed journals or findings reported by the RWJF research team. They also blogged and tweeted the unveiling of the report that was met with much fanfare including a mention in the *New York Times* (Chen, 2010). It is important to note that although social media were applied throughout the IOM process, the core of the process was adhered to, and internal discussions and construction of recommendations were strictly confidential at all times.

THE REPORT

The Future of Nursing: Leading Change, Advancing Health committee's charge included reconceptualizing nursing practice with the knowledge that (a) 78 million baby boomers were rapidly reaching retirement age knowing that a significant number of nurses fit into this category; (b) Americans were living with a higher number of chronic conditions; (c) a third of children were now either overweight or obese; (d) if the ACA passed about 30 million more Americans would have access to primary and preventive services; and (e) there was already an acute shortage of primary care practitioners. The committee assumed that health care delivery was going to change; they were already seeing a movement away from fee-for-service to Accountable Care Organizations and to other models of care where those with chronic conditions were being managed by interprofessional teams who received bundled payments for services. The complexity of care needed for patients was rising while the cost of care was increasing at a proportion far beyond the rate of inflation. Future nurses would have to be prepared for a new way of doing business, whereas nurses in practice would have to be retooled with new competencies. Although no one could predict when we would completely eliminate the fee-for-service payment structure, many were, and still remain certain that this is inevitable. A little known fact of the ACA is that if the Center for Medicare and Medicaid Innovation (CMMI) collects enough evidence to support a new payment structure, which incentivizes health, through large enough pilot and regional grant-funded projects, the Secretary of Health from the Department of Health and Human Services can scale payment reform nationally without the need for legislation (CMMI, 2013). It is only a matter of time before CMMI collects enough data to support such a move and there are already 500 hospitals participating in their new bundled payment demonstration project (Forbes, 2013). The committee was also given the task to expand the ranks of nursing faculty because they knew that thousands of qualified undergraduate and graduate nursing students were turned away each year (and still are as of this writing) due to faculty shortages. The committee was also asked to examine solutions to health care delivery and health professional education in preparation for future changes; in essence, they were given the leadership baton for writing an action plan for how to utilize the profession of nursing to get America where it needed to go.

COMMITTEE'S VISION

The Committee envisions a future system that makes quality care accessible to the diverse populations of the United States, intentionally promotes wellness and disease prevention, reliably improves health outcomes, and provides compassionate care across the life span. In this envisioned future, primary care and prevention are central drivers of the health care system. Interprofessional collaboration and coordination are the norm. Payment for health care services rewards value, not volume of services, and quality care is provided at a price that is affordable for both individuals and society. The rate of growth of health expenditures slows. In all these areas, the health care system consistently demonstrates that it is responsive to individuals' needs and desires through the delivery of patient-centered care.

IOM (2010, p. 2)

Many different stakeholders served on the committee. Donna Shalala, former Secretary of Health for the Department of Health and Human Services under the Clinton administration was the chair, whereas Linda Burnes Bolton, a nurse executive, served as the vice chair. Six members were registered nurses (Liana Orsolini-Hain; Michael Bleich; Jennie Chin Hansen; Rosa Gonzalez-Guarda; Anjli Aurora Hinman; Linda Burnes Bolton [Vice Chair]), whereas 12 came from diverse backgrounds in business, medicine, health policy, consumer advocacy, academia, health care, philanthropy, political science, medical insurance, and economics. This level of diversity increased the credibility and integrity of the report; hence it was taken more seriously by nonnurses such as physicians because there were physicians on the committee. Lawmakers and the Department of Health and Human Services also took the report seriously. It was a dream team.

The report consists of four key messages, eight major recommendations, and 42 subrecommendations. It named 31 actors: actors are entities that are directed to carry out the recommendations. Examples of actors named include those from the national level such as Congress, the Health Resources and Services Administration (HRSA), the Department of Labor to those at the local level such as frontline nurses and health care organizations. Included in the subrecommendations are strategies for how the actors are to go about implementing the recommendations. For example, recommendation 2, "Expand opportunities for nurses to lead and diffuse collaborative improvement efforts," names the actors: private funders (usually philanthropic organizations), public funders (government), health care organizations (hospitals, clinics, and insurance companies), nursing education programs, and nursing associations. The actors are urged to provide more opportunities for nurses to lead when collaborating with others to conduct research and improve the quality of health practice environments. This level of specificity embedded within each of the subrecommendations makes it a "blueprint" for how to enact these changes.

KEY MESSAGES OF THE REPORT

1. Nurses should practice to the full extent of their education and training.
2. Nurses should achieve higher levels of education and training through an improved education system that promotes seamless academic progression.
3. Nurses should be full partners, with physicians and other health professionals, in redesigning health care in the United States.
4. Effective workforce planning and policy making require better data collection and an improved information infrastructure.

IOM (2010, p. 4)

The first key message is often mistaken to refer solely to advanced practice nurses. *All* nurses should practice to the full extent of their education and training. It is shocking, however, how few states allow advanced practice nurses to practice independently of a physician whether it is in running a nurse-managed clinic, assessing patients, prescribing medications, or delivering anesthesia and treatments for chronic pain. Since the report was released in October of 2010, a total of 21 states, the District of Columbia (DC), and one U.S. territory have laws that allow nurse practitioners (NPs) to practice and prescribe independently from a physician. This is an increase from 16 states in 2010 (National Council of State Boards of Nursing [NCSBN], 2013a). Certified registered nurse anesthetists (CRNAs) can both practice and prescribe independently in only 14 states, DC, and one U.S. territory, whereas clinical nurse midwives (CNMs) can both practice and prescribe independently in only 17 states, DC, and one U.S. territory. Clinical nurse specialists (CNSs) fare the worst with only 11 states, DC, and one U.S. territory allowing both independent practice and prescribing. The committee saw the value of the care millions of nurses could deliver if only allowed to work at their full capacity. This would probably exponentially increase access to health care and hopefully, significantly reduce health disparities. This key message could lead to achieving a little more social justice for those without access to a primary care provider. This would be a difficult key message for others to accept and, sure enough, it became the most controversial key message pulling along with it recommendation 1, "Remove scope-of-practice barriers." Nurses and supportive stakeholders would have to battle professional territorialism and fear.

The second key message, "Nurses should achieve higher levels of education and training through an improved education system that promotes seamless academic progression," called for a better educated nursing workforce but stopped short of demanding that the baccalaureate degree be the entry level into nursing practice. This key message disappointed many academic nurses because they had been advocating for the baccalaureate in nursing degree (BSN) as the entry requirement for nurses to sit for their state board licensing exam since at least the mid-1960s (Orsolini-Hain & Waters, 2009). Why did not this landmark report call for the BSN as entry level into practice? It seemed the perfect opportunity, especially after the Carnegie Foundation for the Advancement of Teaching's national nursing education study, "Educating Nurses: A Call for Radical Transformation," not only called for the BSN as entry into practice but also recommended that all nurses get a master's degree within 10 years of initial licensure (Benner, Sutphen, Leonard, & Day, 2010).

The evidence the IOM had available at the time of this report was mixed. Although some studies showed a difference in outcomes for nurses with at least a BSN degree (Aiken, Clarke, Cheung, Sloane, & Silber, 2003; Estabrooks, Midodzi, Cummings, Ricker, & Giovannetti, 2005; Tourangeau et al., 2006) others did not (Sales et al., 2008), and instead linked outcomes with level of experience (Blegen, Vaughn, & Goode, 2001). So if the evidence was mixed and the IOM did not have enough research findings to support such a key message or recommendation why did the report call for a better educated nursing workforce? There were several reasons for this. Of the 850,000 nurses reaching retirement age, a significant number of them were nursing educators. One of two main reasons nursing programs have been turning away thousands of qualified students each year from nursing schools is due to shortages of faculty. All knew we were heading toward a retirement cliff in nursing, but especially so with nursing faculty. Aging and retiring nursing faculty desperately needed to be replaced. Most of the nursing faculties have a master's degree if they are teaching at the community college, and community colleges educate about 60% of our undergraduate nursing workforce. At least 50% of faculties in BSN programs have a PhD or other doctoral level degree and most faculties who teach in graduate programs have a doctoral level degree because they conduct clinical nursing and other research. Some committee members were wondering if we could even replace the number of nursing researchers needed to continue the level of National Institute of Health funded nursing research. To replace the number of retiring nurses seemed a daunting task with the worsening nursing faculty shortage; in addition, more advanced practice nurses were needed to provide access to care for at least 30 million more Americans after the ACA passed. Although the master's degree has been the required entry point into advanced practice nursing for many years now there is a strong national movement to require the doctorate of nursing practice (American Association of Colleges of Nursing [AACN], 2004), which would require even more faculties who could teach at the doctoral level. We would also need to retool the current nursing workforce for the inevitable changes in health care delivery, which would require more continuing education. Finally, because of the rising complexity of patients and the rising need for chronic care management, we would need a better educated nursing workforce with higher-level competencies to deliver more preventive and population health services.

The third key message, "Nurses should be full partners, with physicians and other health professionals, in redesigning health care in the United States," was the second most controversial statement in the report. This key message ties into recommendation 2, which states, "Expand opportunities for nurses to lead and diffuse collaborative improvement efforts." When an IOM report states that nurses should "lead," many physicians get very nervous. The American Medical Association was anxious about this key message and recommendation and publicly stated so at the convening in Washington, DC, to unveil the report at a public forum in 2010. The only way Virginia's Action Coalition could get buy-in legislation to increase the independence for its advanced practice nurses was to agree that physicians would always lead the patient care team and that physicians could now "collaborate" with six NPs instead of four (HB 346, 2012).

With a growing national movement toward interprofessional health education and practice, the IOM's Global Forum on Innovations in Health Professional Education sponsored Lloyd Michener, MD, Director, Duke Center for Community Research in North Carolina at their meeting in November 2012 who showcased how medical homes using NPs and other health professionals collaborate in interprofessional teams (Michener, 2012). They used a patient-centered approach: the health professional who could best help the patient's problem became the designated "leader" for that patient in that situation. Dr. Michener stated, "'Lead' isn't quite the right term, as it suggests that individuals are either leading or following, as opposed to a sense of shared, coordinated leadership with clear roles, well coordinated around the needs of the patient(s). If the primary need is for social services, the 'lead' is likely a social worker; if mental health, might be a psychologist" (Michener, personal communication, November 4, 2012). Leadership was fluid and contextual. When professional egos do not get in the way, this approach can work well. In addition, Duke University recently partnered with Johnson & Johnson to offer a nurse leadership fellowship program to teach leadership competencies to APRNs necessary to successfully lead nurse-managed health clinics (NMHCs) and to "act on behalf of patients to address needs within the larger health care system" (Duke University, 2013). How can nurses and how should nurses lead on a national level so they can make a significant impact to improve the health of the nation? The obvious answer is to not wait to be asked to lead; just lead. Examples of this on a national scale are evident in three areas: (a) the sweeping movement in the Action Coalitions; (b) the proliferation of NMHCs; and (c) the Million Hearts Initiative.

The RWJF approached AARP and AARP Foundation's Center to Champion Nursing in America to create a nationwide grassroots effort to implement the recommendations of the IOM report. This national phenomenon in nursing is creating a new national awareness in leaders among several stakeholder groups about nurses' goals to do what needs to be done to make a dent in improving access to health care and to improve health for millions more people living in America. The Action Coalition movement has reached the awareness of politicians on the Hill, the White House, and leaders in the Administration such as in the Department of Health and Human Services. There are nurses throughout the Hill and in the Administration who work in health policy that are very interested in the potential of the nursing workforce to help implement the ACA and to make implementation of the ACA sustainable. For example, Marilyn Tavenner is only the second nurse ever to lead the Centers for Medicare and Medicaid Services (CMS). Mary Wakefield, a PhD prepared registered nurse, is the administrator of HRSA, an agency that is key to developing the health professional workforce. They both understand the potential of nurses who act to the full extent of their education and training.

NMHCs are proliferating. These clinics are run by advanced practice nurses and are staffed by a variety of health professional practitioners who work together in teams. They provide primary care and preventive services to communities traditionally underserved who remain vulnerable to chronic illness. They are usually associated with an institution such as a college, university, department or school of nursing, a federally qualified health center, a nonprofit foundation, or some other group (National Nursing Centers Consortium [NNCC], 2013). Federally qualified health centers (FQHCs) are community-based centers that provide comprehensive primary care services to populations, which have traditionally had significantly less health care than average Americans (HRSA, 2013).

SERVICES PROVIDED BY NMHCS

1. Promotion and maintenance of health
2. Prevention of illness and disability
3. Basic care during acute and chronic phases of illness
4. Guidance and counseling of individuals and families
5. Referral to other health care providers and community resources when appropriate
6. Nurse-midwifery services

HRSA (2012)

In 2010, when the IOM released the Future of Nursing report, there were at least 200 NMHCs in 37 states with an estimated two million patient encounters per year (Kovner & Walani, 2010). About 60% of these patients were either uninsured or had Medicaid. According to Jamie Ware, the Policy Director of the NNCC as of October 2012, there were about 500 nurse-managed primary care clinics, preventive care clinics, birthing centers, and school-based health centers across the country that NNCC can track (Ware, personal communication, November 1, 2012). It is difficult to track all these centers because they use different funding sources.

The Million Hearts Initiative, which will be discussed in more detail in another chapter, is a CMS and Centers for Disease Control led national effort to prevent one million heart attacks and strokes by 2017 (www.millionhearts.hhs.gov/index.html). Advanced practice nurses led by national nurse leaders are taking the challenge of lowering blood pressure in hypertensive patients without asking permission to join their interprofessional peers. Instead, advanced practice nurses are asking their interprofessional peers to join them in efforts to improve the health of the nation and are even being asked to lead in this effort due to this initiative. Most health professionals are beginning to realize that they need to work together instead of in separate silos to make a difference in eliminating health disparities and to significantly improve health, which is the ultimate goal of increasing access to health care.

The fourth key message of the IOM Future of Nursing report, "Effective workforce planning and policy making require better data collection and an improved information infrastructure," reflects the lack of ability for the report committee to predict how many and which types of nurses we need to prepare for the future, and in which geographic areas do shortages exist. The committee did not know where advanced practice nurses practice geographically and what type of practices they were working in. At the time of the report's formation, the committee did not know how quickly health service delivery redesign was going to occur, even if the ACA was going to pass, or if it did pass, whether President Obama would be re-elected for a second term in office. The committee did not know how quickly CMS would be able to eliminate a fee-for-service system, which provides incentives for volume of care versus a system of regional health-bundled payments that would provide hospitals incentives to keep their beds empty by incentivizing health. If this happened, the committee speculated that hospitals would surely turn into big intensive care units with operating rooms and an emergency room. Hospitals would require fewer beds and regions would require more community-based clinics. Telehealth would expand because care teams would be able to see more patients virtually at home. These changes would require academic institutions to change the way they educate the health professional workforce. Health care professionals would have to learn new competencies for caring for people in their own environments versus in the hospital. In addition, new competencies would be needed to work in inter- and transprofessional teams. Examples of interprofessional colleagues are registered nurses, advanced practice nurses, registered dieticians, physical therapists, pharmacists, and physicians, whereas examples of transprofessional colleagues include certified nurse assistants, health coaches, and community workers. There were too many variables and uncertainty for the IOM report committee to list the number and types of registered nurses that Americans needed for the future.

RECOMMENDATIONS OF THE REPORT

1. Remove scope-of-practice barriers
2. Expand opportunities for nurses to lead and diffuse collaborative improvements efforts
3. Implement nurse residency programs
4. Increase the proportion of nurses with a baccalaureate degree to 80% by 2020
5. Double the number of nurses with a doctorate by 2020
6. Ensure that nurses engage in life-long learning
7. Prepare and enable nurses to lead change to advance health
8. Build an infrastructure for the collection and analysis of interprofessional health care workforce data

IOM (2010, pp. 9–15)

In addition to the four key messages, the Future of Nursing report has eight recommendations. The first recommendation, "Remove scope-of-practice barriers," is necessary in order for nurses to practice to the full extent of their education and training. As stated earlier in this chapter, the Center to Champion Nursing in America, through its Action Coalitions, is working toward increasing the independence of all advanced practice nurses through state legislation. Whereas the Action Coalitions work to remove scope of practice barriers at the state level, the Federal Trade Commission (FTC) is working to prevent physician run monopolies that squeeze out advanced nursing practice. Directed by the Senate Commerce Committee, the FTC is reviewing all state practice laws and regulations to see if any of these preclude nurses from working to the full extent of their education and training. They are asking several state legislatures such as those in Texas, West Virginia, Missouri, Louisiana, and other states to remove "unduly restrictive regulations … to amend them to allow advanced practice registered nurses to provide care to patients in all circumstances in which they are qualified to do so" (FTC, 2013). Subrecommendations in the report also asked CMS to change regulations to permit more direct reimbursement to advanced practice nurses for services rendered independently of a physician. For example, the Physician Fee Schedule Rule was revised in 2012 to include stronger language to enable CRNAs to get direct Medicare reimbursement for chronic care management to include related care such as all the diagnostic and interventional measures for monitoring, placement of medication, and treatment (CMS, 2013). Health policy scholars in CMS and throughout DHHS realize that this is likely to reduce the cost of health care and improve access.

The second recommendation, "Expand opportunities for nurses to lead and diffuse collaborative improvement efforts," was not only a call for a variety of organizations to invite registered nurses to lead in redesigning and improving health practice environments but it was also a call to these nurses to seek out these types of leadership roles. There are few nurses and fewer nurse leaders in health policy arenas. These areas are hard to break into mid-career because many high-level positions in the Administration require that one starts from a low-paid position in order to get hired into an agency. Many mid-career nurses cannot afford to remain in a low-level position until they have worked their way up into a position of higher influence. It is the same for elected officials who are nurses, and it usually takes most many years of local and regional public service before being elected to be a state or federal legislator. Although there are many physicians in leadership in public health arenas and there are many physicians and lawyers in Congress and in the Administration, there are few nurses whose voices are heard. Conversely, although most hospitals and employers of registered nurses have a chief nursing officer, there are few nurses on their boards. In 2011, the percentage of registered nurses on hospital boards was only 6% whereas 20% were physicians (Hassmiller & Combs, 2012). Even more dismal, the percentage of nurses on boards of nonprofit hospitals was a mere 2% in 2010 (Totten, 2010). To help ensure a higher number of registered nurses in boardrooms, leadership training should include competencies needed to serve on governing boards. In addition, more health policy leadership strategies such as offering dual degrees for advanced practice nurses are needed. Many schools of medicine offer a Medical Doctor *and* Master's in Public Health dual degree program. Advanced practice nurses can also minor in health care or public health administration. More nurses need to work in the Administration in agencies such as CMS, the Agency for Healthcare Research and Quality (AHRQ), Institutes at the National Institutes of Health besides National Institute of Nursing Research, and the Immediate Office of the Secretary of Health in DHHS.

Recommendation 3 states that we should "implement nurse residency programs." Nurse residency programs are also known as transition-to-practice programs and include transition to new practice areas, not solely to new nursing practice. For example, a nurse who wishes to move to intensive care from medical surgical hospital practice should have a transition-to-practice residency. New graduate-registered nurses should have transition-to-practice programs that last longer than an orientation of new employees program. Nurses entering advanced practice should have a transition-to-practice program. Although the National Council of State Boards of Nursing is conducting a study of patient health outcomes linked to transition-to-practice programs for new graduate nurses in three states there is a need for research in this area for experienced nurses transitioning to new practice areas and for new advanced practice nurses (NCSBN, 2013b). Funding for these residencies may be perceived as a challenge by employers of registered nurses and advanced practice nurses. Increased retention of nurses will likely pay for these programs because orienting even experienced nurses takes thousands of dollars in these care environments that must be compliant with much regulation.

Recommendation 4, "Increase the proportion of nurses with a baccalaureate degree to 80% by 2020," and recommendation 5, "Double the number of nurses with a doctorate by 2020," tie in with the second key message that nurses should "achieve higher levels of education." The report speaks extensively about making it seamless for nurses to continue with their education whether they are continuing students or have been in practice for years. Seamless refers to processes in place that go beyond the ease of good articulation agreements between community college and university nursing programs. Seamless means without barriers or roadblocks (Orsolini-Hain & Waters, 2009). Many studies have shown that deterrents to returning to school for a more advanced degree in nursing are redundant curricula, needing to be on site too often during working hours, lack of flexibility with courses, and many others (Kovner, Brewer, Katigbak, Djukic, & Fatehi, 2012; Orsolini-Hain, 2008). Being seamless address all these issues, not just admission into a BSN or higher-level nursing program. In order to achieve recommendation 4, 778,879 nurses or about one-third of the workforce will need to earn a BSN by 2020; to achieve recommendation 5, 21,000 more nurses will need to earn a doctoral level degree (Kovner et al., 2012). This seems unlikely when nursing schools continue to turn away thousands of qualified applicants yearly in both undergraduate and graduate programs because of faculty and/or clinical site shortages. The AACN's survey data show that of 75,587 qualified applications who were turned away to all professional nursing programs, 14,354 qualified applications were turned away from graduate programs in 2011 (AACN, 2012). We may achieve the goal of recommendation 5, however, because many nurses are returning to school to earn their doctor of nursing practice (DNP). The DNP has become more attractive to nurses than a PhD in nursing such that as of 2011 there are double the enrollments in DNP programs as in research-focused doctorates (AACN, 2013). This demand for DNP programs has encouraged their growth. Since 2004, the number of DNP programs grew from 20 to 217 whereas the number of research-focused doctoral programs grew from 103 to only 126 (AACN, 2013).

Recommendations 4 and 5 are critical to facilitate nursing's success in interdisciplinary health professional practices of the future. The paradigm of nursing blindly following physician's orders is becoming prehistoric as accountability and engagement into higher levels of frontline leadership requires a more active role in the health care team. Better educated nurses will be taken more seriously and are likely to acquire more credibility as they increase interactions with other health professionals whose entry into their practice requires graduate degrees. If your advanced practice nursing program does not require interprofessional health education learning experiences you are not being prepared for future practice. All health professionals, even advanced practice nurses and not solely physicians, are being called to practice together. Emerging evidence shows that it is more effective to practice together instead of alone, especially to reduce blood pressure in complex patients (Centers for Disease Control and Prevention [CDC], 2012). Even if allowed to practice independently, advanced practice nurses work with physicians and psychiatrists, social workers, pharmacists, physical therapists, and a myriad of others in care teams.

Recommendation 6, "Ensure that nurses engage in life-long learning," speaks to staying competent to give safe and culturally appropriate care in a changing environment and in changing health care delivery systems. It is not enough to get a more advanced degree in nursing; one must continually strive to stay up to date with constantly emerging evidence, for improvement of skills for chronic care management, and for effective population preventive health measures. Care is becoming more complex as we are urged by legislatures, the Administration, employers, and health insurers to lower health care costs while improving care safety and effectiveness. The Institute for Healthcare Improvement (IHI), a nonprofit organization, which believes everyone should receive the best health care possible developed the Triple Aim framework. The three aims are to (a) improve the quality of care that should increase patient satisfaction; (b) improve the health of populations; and (c) reduce the cost of health care (IHI, 2013). These aims must happen simultaneously by everyone in the business of health care for this approach to make a difference. We can no longer afford *not* to operate by the triple aim framework. For access to health care for all in America to be sustainable, we must reduce the expenditures of health care down from 17% of the gross national product that is projected to rise to even higher levels (CMS, 2012).

One of the best ways to ensure that all nurses engage in life-long learning is for employers of nurses to form strong collaborative partnerships. These partnerships can bring nursing academia and health care organizations together to combine strengths to provide residency programs, continuing education to retool the current workforce, seamless education pathways that lead to more advanced degrees, and process improvements. These partnerships can work together to transition interprofessional education of health professionals into new ways of doing interprofessional practices. The literature on models of these new collaboratives is expanding. These collaboratives have the potential to help nursing faculty stay current in the nursing field as they can lead to joint appointments and exposure to health care organizations' quality and safety committees. Conversely, these collaboratives can strengthen undergraduate and graduate nursing curricula because health care organization leaders can be exposed to nursing program curriculum committees and serve on nursing program advisory boards. Perhaps, we will begin to see nursing educators on health care boards of directors.

Recommendation 7, "Prepare and enable nurses to lead change to advance health," ties to keynote message 3, "Nurses should be full partners, with physicians and other health professionals, in redesigning health care in the United States," and with the title of the report itself "Leading Change, Advancing Health." In order to implement this recommendation, nurses need to be leaders at the national level and not solely at regional and local levels. Nurses need to think beyond their own practice environments and start to care about the health of communities and populations. Nurses have to care about social justice and feel the need to reduce health disparities by reducing or eliminating social determinants that reduce health. These social determinants include poverty, social structures, lack of resources to improve health literacy, substance abuse, tobacco use, unsafe physical living environments, social environments that encourage racial discrimination, reduced or no physical access to health preventive and primary care services, and a myriad of others that lead to health inequities (CDC, 2013). Nurses have to start caring beyond their single patient encounters and work on what really matters on improving health if they are seriously determined to improve the health of this nation.

Advanced practice nursing students can prepare for leadership roles by taking as many courses in leadership, health policy, health administration, and economics as possible while in school. Advanced practice nurses can lead by joining their national organizations and by getting involved. Most advanced practice nursing organizations are headquartered or have an office in Washington, DC, which gives them access to legislators and to agencies in DHHS such as Medicare and Medicaid. It is critical that APRNs stay abreast of Medicare and Medicaid regulations because future proposed rules and legislation may eliminate direct reimbursement or limit independent practice. Limiting direct reimbursement to APRNs and limiting their scope of practice will certainly decrease access to care, especially to the already disenfranchised. Some advanced practice organizations are working on getting state insurance exchanges mandated by the ACA to recognize nurse led health clinics as "essential community providers" that allow direct reimbursement by Medicare and Medicaid insurance contractors (NNCC, 2011). Advanced practice nurses can engage in life-long learning by taking executive leadership courses and training through their professional and other organizations. They can step up to the plate and run a clinic or medical center and even run for public office.

The last recommendation, 8, states, "Build an infrastructure for the collection and analysis of interprofessional health care workforce data." We could not have leveraged 200 million dollars in graduate nursing education monies had we not shown a shortage in primary care providers in the United States. We need these data and these data need to be uniform across states. The Forum of State Nursing Workforce Centers has developed three minimum datasets that each state should collect as frequently as is affordable in order to continue monitoring the makeup of the nursing workforce. The three datasets include nurse supply, nurse demand, and level of nurse education (Forum of State Nursing Workforce Centers, 2013). This national effort to standardize states' collection of data about the nursing workforce is especially important because HRSA is no longer able to fund conducting the National Sample Survey of Nursing in the near future that they have been previously conducting every 4 years since 1977. Although it is unlikely Congress will appropriate money for the ACA's mandated National Health Care Workforce Commission, IOM recommendations are still calling for it. The IOM's recent report, "Geographic Adjustment in Medicare Payment Phase II: Implications for Access, Quality, and Efficiency," calls for the Workforce Commission as one of six recommendations in order to propose evidence-based actionable items regarding professional health workforce distribution, supply, and to allow APRNs to practice at the full extent of their education and training (IOM, 2012).

DIVERSITY AND THE IOM REPORT

Many nurses criticized the IOM Future of Nursing report because they perceived that it did not do enough to increase the diversity of the nursing workforce. If one reads the Future of Nursing report cover to cover the reader will notice that increasing the diversity in the nursing workforce is a thread throughout the chapters. The report calls for bringing and educating more people from diverse ethnic backgrounds, including men, into the profession of nursing. Nurses should racially, ethnically, and by gender reflect the population in the United States; all nurses must have or gain the competency of providing culturally competent care and that concern over diversity must be integrated into all levels of nursing practice. Diversity is so integral to the Campaign for Action (2013) in order to fully implement the Future of Nursing recommendations that the Campaign unveiled its Diversity Steering Committee to work on implementing a national diversity action plan and is giving technical assistance to state Action Coalitions on diversity strategies.

Members on the Diversity Steering Committee represent the following national nursing organizations: National Black Nurses Association, National Association of Hispanic Nurses, American Assembly for Men in Nursing, Asian American/Pacific Islander Nurses Association, Philippine Nurses Association, and National Alaska Native American Indian Nurses Association. Why was diversity in nursing such a

> ### MISSION OF THE CAMPAIGN FOR ACTION DIVERSITY STEERING COMMITTEE
>
> To narrow the health care disparities gap, to support the importance of a diverse workforce, and to help prepare the discipline of nursing to care for an increasingly diverse population, the Future of Nursing: Campaign for Action's Diversity Steering Committee is organized to ensure that all Americans, regardless of race, religion, creed, ethnicity, gender, sexual orientation, or any aspect of identity will have access to high quality, patient-centered care in a health system where nurses contribute as essential partners in achieving success.
>
> *Campaign for Action (2013)*

concern to the IOM Future of Nursing committee and continues to be a concern to the Campaign for Action? By 2042, the U.S. Census Bureau predicts that minority groups will make up 54% of our population (U.S. Census Bureau, 2012). By 2042, although the non-Hispanic White population will be the largest single group, no single ethnic group will be the majority. Contrast this to the racial makeup of nurses in 2008 that remains predominantly White and female (HRSA, 2010). Although about 85% of registered nurses in the U.S. are White, only 5.5% are Asian, 5.4% are Black, 3.6% are Hispanic, and Alaska Native and American Native Indian are combined at less than 1%. It is widely believed that a more diverse nursing workforce will give more culturally competent care. An executive summary published by the Commonwealth Fund reports that this racial discordance in professional health care has serious consequences. The degree of continued racial disparities in health care is the fruit of this gross mismatch of mostly White practitioners to non-White patients and populations. It is naïve to think that the color of skin is solely the issue. As many White health professionals come from a background that facilitated them to go to medical or nursing school they likely lead mostly middle to upper-middle class lives. They do not have the kind of cultural insight that comes with living in poverty where life is completely different than being White and middle class in America. White, middle-class health professionals constantly make assumptions about their racially and ethnically non-White patients such as they can afford to fill their prescriptions, they have access to transportation, and they can afford to buy nonsubsidized fruits and vegetables. Several studies link racial concordance with better patient satisfaction and better health outcomes (Cooper & Powe, 2004).

CONCLUSION

The Future of Nursing report has put a strong spotlight onto the nursing profession. This report is essentially challenging the profession of nursing to commit to mobilize for changes that will make a difference in people's health and in their quality of life. Would not it be more meaningful for nurses if interventions could make lasting health changes in patients' lives rather than solely relief from a single acute illness event? Nurses must take to heart the rest of the American Nurses Association (ANA) definition of nursing which is to advocate for the health of families, communities, and populations (ANA, 2010). The IOM's Future of Nursing report is not only telling nurses they are capable of increasing the health of Americans but also that they must care enough to return to school and to lead in these efforts.

DISCUSSION QUESTIONS

1. How could the push for increased interprofessional health practice change the current practice of APRNs?
2. How can health coaches and community workers affect the practice of APRNs?
3. Is a transition to practice residency really necessary for APRNs, especially since research shows good health outcomes of APRNs who never had such a residency?
4. Are there any practice barriers in your state and if so what are they and what does this mean for your practice?
5. Do APRNs really need a DNP? Why or why not?

ANALYSIS AND SYNTHESIS EXERCISES

1. Interview leaders in your state or district's Action Coalition and analyze the extent to which your state has implemented any or all of the eight recommendations of the Future of Nursing report.
2. Interview an APRN who works in a NMHC about their practice in relation to the eight recommendations of the Future of Nursing report. Ask them their concerns about the health of the community in which they serve and what their ideas are to promote the health of their community.
3. Find an APRN who is racially/ethnically not White or not female and ask them what (if any) the barriers were for them to become an APRN.

CLINICAL APPLICATION CONSIDERATIONS

1. APRNs will have to learn ways of increasing interprofessional practice, especially if their state allows independent practice.
2. APRNs will increasingly be asked to extend their practices by engaging in transprofessional teams such as including community health workers.
3. APRNs will increasingly work with registered nurses in increasingly complex care environments.
4. APRNs will increasingly use Telehealth to manage patients with chronic illness.
5. APRNs will increase their engagement in population/preventive health measures.

REFERENCES

Aiken, L. H., Clarke, S. P., Cheung, R. B., Sloane, D. M., & Silber, J. H. (2003). Educational levels of hospital nurses and surgical patient mortality. *Journal of the American Medical Association, 290*(12), 1617–1623.

American Association of Colleges of Nursing (AACN). (2004). *AACN position statement on the practice doctorate in nursing.* Retrieved from http://www.aacn.nche.edu/publications/position/DNP positionstatement.pdf

AACN. (2012). *New AACN data show an enrollment surge in baccalaureate and graduate programs amid calls for more highly educated nurses.* Retrieved from http://www.aacn.nche.edu/news/articles /2012/enrollment-data

AACN. (2013). *DNP fact sheet.* Retrieved from http://www.aacn.nche.edu/media-relations/fact-sheets /dnp

American Nurses Association (ANA). (2010). *Nursing's social policy statement: The essence of the profession* (3rd ed.). Silver Spring, MD: Author.

Benner, P., Sutphen, M., Leonard, V., & Day, L. (2010). *Educating nurses: A call for radical transformation.* San Francisco, CA: Jossey-Bass.

Blegen, M. A., Vaughn, T. E., & Goode, C. J. (2001). Nurse experience and education: Effect on quality of care. *Journal of Nursing Administration, 31*(1), 33–39.

Campaign for Action. (2013). *Diversity steering committee: Supporting efforts to build a diverse workforce ready to care for an increasingly diverse population.* Retrieved from http://www.campaignforaction.org/whos-involved/diversity-steering-committee

Centers for Disease Control and Prevention (CDC). (2012). *Task force recommends team-based care for improving blood pressure control.* Retrieved from http://www.cdc.gov/media/releases/2012/p0515_bp_control.html

CDC. (2013). *Social determinants of health.* Retrieved from http://www.cdc.gov/socialdeterminants/Definitions.html

Center for Medicare and Medicaid Innovation (CMMI). (2013). *About the CMS innovation center.* Retrieved from http://www.innovation.cms.gov/about/index.html

Centers for Medicare and Medicaid Services (CMS). (2012). *National health expenditures projections 2010–2012.* Retrieved from http://www.cms.gov/Research-Statistics-Data-and-Systems/Statistics-Trends-and-Reports/NationalHealthExpendData/Downloads/proj2010.pdf

CMS. (2013). *Physician fee schedule.* Retrieved from http://www.cms.gov/Medicare/Medicare-Fee-for-Service-Payment/PhysicianFeeSched/index.html?redirect=/PhysicianFeeSched

Chen, P. W. (2010, November 18). Nurses' role in the future of health care. *New York Times.* Retrieved from http://www.nytimes.com/2010/11/18/health/views/18chen.html?_r=0

Cooper, L. A., & Powe, N. R. (2004). *Disparities in patient experiences, health care processes, and outcomes: The role of patient–provider racial, ethnic, and language concordance.* Retrieved from http://www.commonwealthfund.org/programs/minority/cooper_raceconcordance_753.pdf

Duke University. (2013). *Nurse leadership program.* Retrieved from http://www://duke-jjnurseleadership.duhs.duke.edu

Estabrooks, C. A., Midodzi, W. K., Cummings, G. C., Ricker, K. L., & Giovannetti, P. (2005). The impact of hospital nursing characteristics on 30-day mortality. *Nursing Research, 54*(2), 74–84.

Federal Trade Commission (FTC). (2013). *Protecting America's consumers.* Retrieved from http://www.ftc.gov

Forbes. (2013). *Though Obama care pays less, providers flock to 'bundled' Medicare payments.* Retrieved from http://www.forbes.com/sites/brucejapsen/2013/02/01/though-obamacare-pays-less-medical-providers-flock-to-bundled-medicare-payments/

Forum of State Nursing Workforce Centers. (2013). *National nursing workforce minimum data sets.* Retrieved from http://www.nursingworkforcecenters.org/minimumdatasets.aspx

Hassmiller, S., & Combs, J. (2012). Nurse leaders in the boardroom: A fitting choice. *Journal of Healthcare Management, 57*(1), 8–11.

HB 346. (2012). *Nurse practitioners; practice as part of patient care teams that includes a physician.* Retrieved from http://lis.virginia.gov/cgi-bin/legp604.exe?121+sum+HB346

Health Resources and Services Administration (HRSA). (2010). *The registered nurse population: Initial findings from the 2008 National Sample Survey of Registered Nurses.* U.S. Department of Health and Human Services. Retrieved from http://www.bhpr.hrsa.gov/healthworkforce/rnsurveys/rnsurveyinitial2008.pdf

HRSA. (2012). *Affordable Care Act nurse managed health clinics: Frequently asked questions.* U.S. Department of Health and Human Services. Retrieved from http://www.bhpr.hrsa.gov/grants/nursemangfaq.pdf

HRSA. (2013). *What is a health center?* U.S. Department of Health and Human Services. Retrieved from http://www.bphc.hrsa.gov/about

Institute for Healthcare Improvement (IHI). (2013). *IHI triple aim initiative.* Retrieved from http://www.ihi.org/offerings/Initiatives/TripleAim/Pages/default.aspx

Institute of Medicine (IOM). (2010). *The future of nursing: Leading change, advancing health.* Retrieved from http://www.iom.edu/Reports/2010/The-Future-of-Nursing-Leading-Change-Advancing-Health.aspx

IOM. (2012). *Geographic adjustment in Medicare payment—phase II: Implications for access, quality, and efficiency.* Retrieved from http://www.iom.edu/Reports/2012/Geographic-Adjustment-in-Medicare-Payment-Phase-II.aspx

IOM. (2013a). *About the IOM.* Retrieved from http://www.iom.edu/About-IOM.aspx

IOM. (2013b). *Federal Advisory Committee Act*. Retrieved from http://www.iom.edu/About-IOM/Study -Process/FACA.aspx

Kovner, C. T., Brewer, C., Katigbak, C., Djukic, M., & Fatehi, F. (2012). Charting the course for nurses' achievement of higher education levels. *Journal of Professional Nursing, 28*(6), 333–343.

Kovner, C., & Walani, S. (2010). *Nurse managed health centers*. Retrieved from http://www.thefuture ofnursing.org/sites/default/files/Research%20Brief-%20Nurse%20Managed%20Health%20 Centers.pdf

Michener, L. (2012, November). *Durham and Duke: A story of one community's journey towards health and what it has meant for practice and training*. Paper presented at the Institute of Medicine Global Forum on Innovation in Health Professional Education, Washington, DC.

National Council of State Boards of Nursing (NCSBN). (2013a). *APRN maps*. Retrieved from http:// www.ncsbn.org/index.htm

NCSBN. (2013b). *Nurse exchange comments—Transition to practice*. Retrieved from http://www.ncsbn .org/363.htm

National Nursing Centers Consortium (NNCC). (2011). *Nurse exchange comments—Transition to practice*. Retrieved from http://www.nncc.us/site/images/pdf/nnccexchangecommentssubmitted _september.pdf

NNCC. (2013). *Nurse-managed health clinics: Increasing health care workforce capacity and access to care*. Retrieved from http://www.nncc.us/site/images/pdf/nmhc_general_fact_sheet_2012.pdf

Orsolini-Hain, L. M. (2008). *An interpretive phenomenological study on the influences on associate degree prepared nurses to return to school to earn a higher degree in nursing* (Doctoral dissertation, University of California). Retrieved from ProQuest (3324576).

Orsolini-Hain, L., & Waters, V. (2009). Education evolution: A historical perspective of associate degree nursing. *Journal of Nursing Education, 48*(5), 266–271.

Robert Wood Johnson Foundation (RWJF). (2013a). *About RWJF—Our history*. Retrieved from http:// www.rwjf.org/en/about-rwjf/our-mission/our-history.html

RWJF. (2013b). *Grants*. Retrieved from http://www.rwjf.org/en/grants.html#q/maptype/grants

Sales, A., Sharp, N., Li, Y. F., Lowy, E., Greiner, G., Liu, C. F., … Needleman, J. (2008). The association between nursing factors and patient mortality in the Veterans Health Administration: The view from the nursing unit level. *Medical Care, 46*(9), 938–945.

Totten, M. K. (2010, May/June). Nurses on healthcare boards: A smart and logical move to make. *Healthcare Executive Magazine*. Retrieved from http://www.bestonboard.org/website/pdf/MJ10 _GovInsights_reprint.pdf

Tourangeau, A. E., Doran, D. M., McGillis-Hall, L., O'Brian-Pallus, L., Pringles, D., Tu, J. V., & Cranley, L. A. (2006). Impact of hospital nursing care on 30-day mortality for acute medical patients. *Journal of Advanced Nursing, 57*(1), 32–44.

U.S. Census Bureau. (2012). *U.S. Census Bureau projections show a slower growing, older, more diverse nation a half century from now*. Retrieved from http://www.census.gov/newsroom/releases/archives /population/cb12-243.html

Implications for Practice: The Consensus Model for Advanced Practice Registered Nurse Regulation

Kelly A. Goudreau

The Consensus Model by APRN Consensus Work Group and National Council of State Boards of Nursing APRN Advisory Committee (2008) is an historic document that will have implications for practice for all four of the identified Advanced Practice Registered Nurse (APRN) roles (Clinical Nurse Specialist [CNS], Nurse Practitioner [NP], Certified Nurse Midwife [CNM], and Certified Registered Nurse Anesthetist [CRNA]) for many years to come. The effects of the statements made in that document were felt immediately upon its release in July 2008 and continue to be felt across the four roles in numerous ways and in all states. Other chapters in this text define the specific implications of the Consensus Model as the document has come to be known. This chapter provides a brief history of how the document was created, explores how it is being applied today to APRN practice, evaluates the outcomes of the document to date, and identifies how and why APRNs continue to need to be engaged in the discussions relative to the implementation of the Consensus Model.

BRIEF HISTORICAL BACKGROUND

The landscape of advanced practice nursing has been a confusing patchwork quilt of differing definitions for scope of practice, expectations of autonomy, prescriptive authority, and educational preparation. Prior to the Consensus Model (APRN Consensus Work Group and National Council of State Boards of Nursing APRN Advisory Committee, 2008), each state had to work with their legislative body to affirm the existence of APRNs and define the functionality of each of the roles. The Consensus Model (APRN Consensus Work Group and National Council of State Boards of Nursing APRN Advisory Committee, 2008) was created through a difficult and sometimes laborious process that took approximately 4 years of discussion between 23 nursing organizations and the National Council of State Boards of Nursing (NCSBN).

The chaos that is regulation of advanced practice nursing has been recognized for a long time. As roles were added in the 1980s (NP) and the clear delineation between nursing practice and medical practice became blurred, there was increasing resistance from medical practitioners in a variety of states. That resistance took the form of negotiated limits on the function and autonomy of nurses in advanced roles. Those limits were different in each state and, therefore, there were multiple models for regulation of advanced practice nurses. In an effort to bring some order to the national chaos that was advanced practice regulation, the NCSBN adopted a position paper on the licensure of advanced practice nursing in 1993 that included model language for legislation and a template for state-level administrative rules (Stanley, 2009). Unfortunately, the work performed in the position paper had little effect and the confusion and chaos in state-by-state rules and regulation of advanced practice nurses continued. Areas of concern were lack of uniformity in how an APRN was defined, inability to cross state lines and provide care of a consistent nature, and a clear definition of a specialty or subspecialty and how one was educated to provide specialized care. Each state was doing what they could to try to make the APRN language work in concert with the legislative understanding of the roles and how they could impact quality, safety, and access to care for constituents.

In 2004, in a continuing effort to more clearly define the advanced practice role and provide guidance to the state member constituents, the NCSBN APRN Advisory Panel—essentially a special interest group of the NCSBN focused on APRN regulatory issues nationally—began work on a draft APRN vision paper. This document was being created simultaneously with another document that was being created by the APRN Consensus Work Group, which had been convened in response to concerns from the American Nurses Association (ANA), the National Organization of Nurse Practitioner Faculties (NONPF), and the American Association of Colleges of Nursing (AACN). The APRN Consensus Work Group had also been working on a document since 2004 in parallel to the NCSBN but unaware of the work that was being carried out by the NCSBN APRN Advisory Panel.

The APRN Advisory Panel completed a draft of their paper and disseminated it in 2006 to a broad audience including multiple nursing organizations that were engaged in the APRN Consensus Work Group process. Response was immediate and not favorable. Although created in a parallel process there were significant differences from the document that was nearing completion in the APRN Consensus Work Group.

Rather than continue on parallel pathways, it was determined that APRNs would be better served by a consensus among the various organizations. In order to achieve that consensus, there needed to be significant dialogue to explore the similarities and differences between the NCSBN draft document and the APRN Consensus Work Group draft document. In order to do that work, seven representatives were selected from the NCSBN APRN Panel and the APRN Consensus Work Group to represent equally the content of the documents and discuss how best to ensure that the content was at least complementary and not contradictory if two documents were to be maintained. The decision was that there could not be differing documents in an already chaotic environment. There needed to be consistency in the recommendations in order to guide the work of states as they wrestled with how best to categorize and ensure the ongoing access to advanced practice nurses. This smaller group of 14 nurses became known as the APRN Joint Dialogue Group and began meeting in early 2007.

The work of the APRN Joint Dialogue group progressed for another year. The group took on a specific aim of "doing no harm" to any APRN group in order to better the lot of another, and also determined that the group must listen to each concern voiced and determine a collective and consensus response. In that year, each area of the two papers was examined, openly discussed in regards to implications, and a decision was made to combine the documents and come forward with a single consensus paper that could guide the regulation of APRN practice across the country. The final document, *The Consensus Model for APRN Regulation: Licensure, Accreditation, Certification and Education* (APRN Consensus Work Group & National Council of State Boards of Nursing APRN Advisory Committee, 2008) was released to nursing and regulatory organizations in July 2008.

The "Consensus Model," as it has come to be known, has generated much discussion among the four APRN roles as the implications of the statements in it have been dissected and analyzed in the effort to implement the recommendations. The document was also used in part as an element of the document created by the Institute of Medicine (IOM) (2010), further validating its impact on the APRN roles.

APPLICATION TO APRN PRACTICE

Since the release of the Consensus Model in 2008 there has been much work accomplished in each of the four areas of licensure, accreditation, certification, and education (LACE). The work of reducing the chaos and standardizing the expectations for APRNs across the United States has begun and is well under way. The stated goal of full implementation of the model by 2015 is fast approaching, however, and there continues to be a significant amount of work still left to complete. Each of the organizations that represent the four areas of LACE has work to do. This work includes considerations in licensure, accreditation processes for educational programs, certification, and changes to the core educational process for each of the four roles involved. Each of the roles has been impacted differently. An analysis of the impact to each of the areas reveals much about the intrinsic philosophic approach taken in the foundation of each of the roles.

Licensure

The nature of the comprehensive change this agreement is generating is clearly evident when one looks at the issues arising from the proposed changes in licensure across the country. The Consensus Model is intended to provide standardization of licensure, accreditation, certification, and education in nursing. Licensure is the only one of those elements that is not truly controlled by nursing. The laws that become the licensure regulations in each state are developed as an outcome of the political process in that state. As such, the rules are different in each and every state. It is a monumental undertaking to change the laws governing nursing in each state. The Consensus Model calls for some consistent rules to apply to all four of the advanced practice roles.

These requirements may seem simple on the surface but when attempting to implement them consistently across the nation for four advanced practice roles, the issues become complex. Difficulty arises when the state board of nursing in the various states must open the state practice act in order to have the language modified to meet the above requirements. Opening the state practice act allows for any interested stakeholder to voice their concerns with one or more sections of the existing law and any proposed changes. Great opposition has been raised by physician groups in particular in relation to prescriptive authority or supervised/collaborative practice.

FOUNDATIONAL REQUIREMENTS FOR LICENSURE

Boards of nursing will:

1. license APRNs in the categories of CRNA, CNM, CNS, or Certified NP within a specific population focus;
2. be solely responsible for licensing APRNs;
3. only license graduates of accredited graduate programs that prepare graduates with the APRN core, role and population competencies;
4. require successful completion of a national certification examination that assesses APRN core, role and population competencies for APRN licensure;
5. not issue a temporary license;
6. only license an APRN when education and certification are congruent;
7. license APRNs as independent practitioners with no regulatory requirements for collaboration, direction or supervision;
8. allow for mutual recognition of advanced practice registered nursing through the APRN Compact;
9. have at least one APRN representative position on the board and utilize an APRN advisory committee that includes representatives of all four APRN roles; and
10. institute a grandfathering clause that will exempt those APRNs already practicing in the state from new eligibility requirements.

APRN Consensus Work Group and National Council of State Boards of Nursing
APRN Advisory Committee (2008, pp. 14–15)

Another issue is the one surrounding licensure of existing APRNs when no prior recognition for them existed under the old rules or regulations. Many issues are arising for those individuals who may have been carrying the name of one or more of the groups of APRNs without the appropriate education or certification to match.

The NCSBN has been actively engaged in the discussion from the outset of the Joint Dialogue Group and has developed some tools that can be used by nurses with an interest in the current discussion related to where their state is presently as measured against the Consensus Model language and whether or not their state or neighboring states are proposing changes to the laws and subsequently the rules and regulations surrounding licensure of APRNs. Look to the NCSBN webpage located at www.ncsbn.org/2567.htm for a synopsis of all states and territories and where they are in reaching the goal of compliance with the Consensus Model.

Accreditation

The Consensus Model outlined expectations for the accrediting bodies as well as the licensure, certification, and education entities. Those changes were defined as follows.

The accrediting bodies, inclusive of the Accreditation Commission for Education in Nursing, Inc. (ACEN), formerly known as the National League for Nursing Accreditation Commission (NLNAC), the Commission on Collegiate Nursing Education (CCNE), the Accreditation Commission for Midwifery Education (ACME), and the Council on Accreditation of Nurse Anesthesia Educational Programs (COA) have all undergone some changes as a result of the implementation of the Consensus Model. The major changes have occurred as a reflection of the requirement that

Accreditors will:

1. be responsible for evaluating APRN education programs including graduate degree granting and postgraduate certificate programs;
2. through their established accreditation standards and process, assess APRN education programs in light of the APRN core, role core, and population core competencies;
3. assess developing APRN education programs and tracks by reviewing them using established accreditation standards and granting preapproval, preaccreditation, or accreditation prior to student enrollment;
4. include an APRN on the visiting team when an APRN program/track is being reviewed; and
5. monitor APRN educational programs throughout the accreditation period by reviewing them using established accreditation standards and processes.

APRN Consensus Work Group and National Council of State Boards of Nursing
APRN Advisory Committee (2008, p. 15)

APRN programs are evaluated in relation to the role and population foci. This is new territory for many of the accrediting agencies, let alone the shift in thought process that must occur at the educational level for the four roles.

In addition, two of the accrediting agencies had never considered preaccreditation review of programs. Both the ACEN and the CCNE needed to shift their perspectives and realign their accreditation standards to meet this requirement. The preaccreditation process was in use by the ACME and COA prior to the Joint Dialogue discussions and is intended to ensure that educational programs in the role meet the outcome standards and expectations prior to final accreditation. Previously, the preaccreditation assessment of programs was conducted only by the nurse anesthetists and midwifery program accrediting agencies. This standardization was called for during the LACE discussions and is intended to provide counsel, strength, and consistency to both the CNS and NP educational programs in addition to the nurse anesthetist and midwifery programs.

The inclusion of an APRN on the team when programs are being evaluated is a work in process. At present, there may be an NP on the team, or a CNS and they are then responsible for reviewing both the NP and CNS tracks when they themselves may not be as knowledgeable as they could be for the alternative role. For the CNM and CRNA programs, there is no question that there will be an appropriate APRN on the team as the program review is specific to the role. This is an area that continues to need refinement as time nears for the full implementation of the Consensus Model.

All of the accrediting agencies for higher education programs are overseen by the Department of Education (2013) through a process of review and evaluation of the standards set by each of the accrediting agencies. As per the Department of Education website, "The goal of accreditation is to ensure that education provided by institutions of higher education meet acceptable levels of quality" (Department of Education, 2013). The Department of Education relies on review of all educational accrediting agencies by the National Advisory Committee on Institutional Quality and Integrity (NACIQI), a politically appointed board of 18 individuals who are nominated in equal numbers by each party. The members are identified by peers and reviewed for political appointment to the committee. Criteria for selection include expertise in educational matters and a proclivity for integrity and objectivity. All four of the nursing accrediting bodies have been reviewed by the NACIQI and are approved to accredit nursing programs in higher education. In order to maintain their ability to accredit programs, they must meet or exceed the standards articulated by the Department of Education and reviewed by the NACIQI.

Certification

CRNAs and CNMs already determined many years ago that they needed certification as an entry to practice element prior to the Consensus Model discussions and subsequent to its implementation. CRNAs and CNMs developed certification as an adjunct to their educational process and an outgrowth of the professional expectations for competency-based assessments of skill. NPs, too, were using certification as an entry to practice assessment of competency prior to practice in most states. CNSs however were not. Until the discussions at the Joint Dialogue Group table, the CNS leadership had maintained the perception that certification was a mark of excellence rather than an element to assess competence for entry to practice. Therefore most, if not all, CNS certification examinations had a requirement for 2 to 3 years of practice as an element of eligibility to sit for the examination. This major paradigm shift has created great difficulty in the transition period for the CNSs. The conceptual framework for CNSs was based on some core elements of competency that span all of the specialty foci but each CNS was flexible enough to move fluidly within and between populations based on the specialty content of their practice. For example, a CNS who specialized in diabetes or pulmonary could move between populations in acute, community, or age brackets. Their specialty was foremost in their practice. Within a regulatory model, however, which calls for standardization in order to protect the public, there is little tolerance of unique perspectives, regardless of the need. CNSs have had to reframe their entire construct of certification and ultimately of the core educational framework.

All four of the roles needed to look at the certification examinations they were offering and refine them to meet the criteria of the new model. Specifically, the primary change for the roles has been to align in the format of role and population foci. As mentioned previously, CNSs did not focus on a single population as described in the Consensus Model. The population foci in the model include six primary groupings: adult gerontology, pediatrics, gender-specific, psychiatric, family/individual across the life span, and neonatal.

CNSs moved across these population foci depending on their specialty focus. Primary certification for CNSs has been in the specialty role, so moving to a population foci has meant a complete shift in how the CNS certification examinations are written. The NPs have also had to shift somewhat. Although the population foci fit much better with the NP perspective, there has been some drift as CNSs have been nonexistent in many areas yet the specialty need has continued so they too moved into a specialty focus in many instances. The realignment of both the NP and the CNS examinations has been a disruptive innovation for both groups. The CNMs can fit into multiple categories as well, which has opened up their perspective on caring for individual women and their partners through young, middle, and old adulthood as well as the neonate. Nurse anesthetists have, like CNSs, moved fluidly across the populations because of their specialty approach to care. It is still unclear how the certification examinations will change over time for each of the roles but changes are pending in all four roles and will be fully implemented by 2015 per the timeline outlined in the Consensus Model.

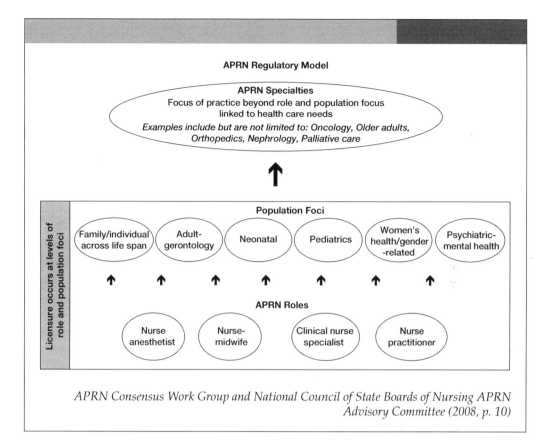

APRN Consensus Work Group and National Council of State Boards of Nursing APRN Advisory Committee (2008, p. 10)

Education

Again the need for change has varied among the four APRN roles and the Consensus Model language has impacted one or two more than the others. Primary elements of the needs in education are outlined below as defined in the Consensus Model.

FOUNDATIONAL REQUIREMENTS FOR EDUCATION

APRN education programs/tracks leading to APRN licensure, including graduate degree granting and postgraduate certificate programs will:

1. follow established educational standards and ensure attainment of the APRN core, role core, and population core competencies;
2. be accredited by a nursing accrediting organization that is recognized by the U.S. Department of Education (USDE) and/or the Council for Higher Education Accreditation (CHEA);
3. be preapproved, preaccredited, or accredited prior to the acceptance of students, including all developing APRN education programs and tracks;
4. ensure that graduates of the program are eligible for national certification and state licensure; and
5. ensure that official documentation (e.g., transcript) specifies the role and population focus of the graduate.

APRN Consensus Work Group and National Council of State Boards of Nursing APRN Advisory Committee (2008, p. 16)

In addition, there were changes to the curriculum expectations for the four roles. Some of the changes experienced by the CRNAs, CNMs, and CNSs have been the inclusion of three separate courses on pathophysiology, physical and health assessment, and pharmacology, commonly referred to as the "three Ps." The course content may have been present for all three of the roles in the curriculum but not necessarily pulled out in three separate and distinct courses as defined in AACN (1998) as it had been for the NP programs since the implementation of the NONPF agreement on core competencies and outcome expectations in the "Task Force Criteria" document first published in 1990 and updated most recently in 2012. The CNM and CRNA curricula have been established for a very long time and are based on demonstrated competency in tasks and skills and repetitive application of same. The CNS, however, has seen many changes in licensure (simple recognition as an APRN role in some states), accreditation (incorporation of the core competency documents into accreditation standards is still pending), certification (transition from recognition of expert specialty focus to entry to practice population focused examinations), and education (establishment of core competencies through a consensus process and refocusing to a population rather than specialty) (Goudreau, 2009; National Association of Clinical Nurse Specialists, 2012). All of these are significant paradigm shifts for any role but ones that will pay dividends in the end.

The changes have been substantial for all four of the roles. Some of the roles have had the backbone and infrastructure in place for most of the needed implementation (CRNA and CNM), some have had old battles to fight in state legislatures regarding independent practice and prescriptive authority (NP), and some have had to build again essentially from the ground up in defining consistent curriculum expectations and outcomes (CNS) but the changes are occurring and are doing so in a timely manner so as to meet the expectations for a 2015 implementation.

EVALUATION OF THE CONSENSUS MODEL

The evaluation of the Consensus Model will take many years. The work was carried out over a period of 4 years and took much discussion, collaboration, and assessment of the principle of doing no harm to any of the four advanced practice roles. It also took a lot of dialogue to determine the definition of APRN versus nurses who practice at an advanced level. When looking at the discussions in the remainder of this text this definition may seem arbitrary and lacking in substance but it is the definition of terminology that will help to clearly define the boundaries of APRN practice. When the next generation of APRNs looks back on the work done in the early 2000s will they look at it with appreciation of the work done or disdain for the barriers that were put in place for APRN practice? It is hard to tell at this point. There are many gains for the APRN roles but also many losses for the values of the past and the intent of the roles when they were first created. All things must evolve. This is the evolution or the revolution of APRN practice in the 21st century in the United States. Perhaps, it will reach out to other countries and impact the consideration of outcomes of APRN definitions and practice in other countries. Also, it will be used as an exemplar of what not to do or will clearly define the pitfalls that need to be avoided. Only time will tell.

THE CONSENSUS MODEL AS HEALTH POLICY

The Consensus Model for APRN regulation is the epitome of health policy that will have a direct impact on the practice of advanced practice nurses across the United States. It will also influence the outcomes of similar discussions around the world as other countries consider their need for expansion of the APRN role. The role of the leaders in APRN practice in the United States was significant and took 4 years to bring to consensus. This document will provide guidance for the development of health policies specific to the recognition and implementation of the APRN role in each and every state in the union.

Although the work of the leaders is complete at this time, the words are now being taken and put to task in new documents that are being created in each state. It is truly up to the APRNs in each state, region, or county to speak up as to their specific needs that can support the patients they see and the access to health care in their community. Only by speaking with a singular voice about the impact of APRN care can the legislators hear about the impact and possibilities of APRN practice.

Now, it is your turn to work on the issues. Raise your voice and address your legislator(s). Let them know what you need in order to practice to the full scope of your license as defined by the IOM (2010). Identify health policies that need to be generated as a result of this landmark consensus document and work for a brighter future for all APRNs and their patients.

CONCLUSION

The Consensus Model was a work of collaboration, integration, focused energy, and a will to define clearly for now and the future what an APRN is and should be able to do. The consensus around the elements of regulation was a landmark and groundbreaking. To have more than 40 nursing organizations agree in principle to elements that provide the foundation for licensure, accreditation, certification, and education of advanced practice nurses across the country took tremendous work from all involved. The key element of not wanting to do any harm to any of the four groups was upheld by all. The right to self-determination of the roles was also upheld and respected and the members around the discussion table stopped and listened to the needs of each group as issues of concern were raised. It was not a perfect process and although there are many issues that have been raised for a variety of the roles, it is at least and at last a place to start. The recognition of the four roles and provision of definitions for each has set an expectation and a standard that will be discussed and perhaps emulated internationally. Time will tell.

It is the sincere hope of this author that the work that was performed will stand the test of time and will endure so that changes can be made at all levels of policy across the United States. Only through sweeping changes such as proposed in the Consensus Model can there be clear understanding of the importance, role, and implications for APRNs everywhere. On to the future now that we have the past more clearly defined.

DISCUSSION QUESTIONS

1. Identify one change in your state that has already occurred or is in process as a result of the Consensus Model implementation.
2. Discuss how the Consensus Model has impacted your role as an APRN. Has it been positive or negative? Has the Consensus Model created or removed barriers for your APRN role?
3. Identify how the Consensus Model has changed certification of APRNs in your role or population focus.
4. Identify how the Consensus Model has changed your educational program. Have there been curriculum changes that have occurred over the last 2 to 5 years? How has that change impacted your education specifically?

SYNTHESIS EXERCISES

1. Go to the website for your state legislature and/or your state board of nursing and look for legislation that is being proposed. Determine if the legislative change being proposed is in relation to the changes required by the Consensus Model. If related to the Consensus Model plan to attend the hearings in the committee where the legislation was created or is being heard. Identify how your voice should be heard on the issue and prepare written testimony for presentation to the committee for their consideration.

2. Is there a rule or regulation that simply does not make sense in your state? Example could include the inability of APRNs to sign state orders for life-sustaining treatment, death certificates, or orders for physical therapy for patients who need it. Does the rule or regulation impact your practice directly? Consider approaching a legislator to educate them about the situation and propose new legislation that would address the issue.

REFERENCES

American Association of Colleges of Nursing (AACN). (1998). *Essentials of Master's education for advanced practice nursing.* Washington, DC: Author.

APRN Consensus Work Group & National Council of State Boards of Nursing APRN Advisory Committee. (2008, April). *Consensus model for APRN regulation: Licensure, accreditation, certification & education.* Retrieved from http://www.aacn.nche.edu

Department of Education. (2013, March 12). *Accreditation standards and criteria.* Retrieved from http://www2.ed.gov/admins/finaid/accred/accreditation_pg13.html

Goudreau, K. A. (2009). What clinical nurse specialists need to know about the Consensus Model for Advanced Practice Registered Nurse Regulation. *Clinical Nurse Specialist, 23*(2), 50–51.

Institute of Medicine (IOM). (2010). *Future of nursing: Leading change, advancing health.* Author. Retrieved from http://www.iom.edu/Reports/2010/The-Future-of-Nursing-Leading-Change-Advancing-Health.aspx

National Association of Clinical Nurse Specialists. (2012). *Statement on the APRN Consensus Model Implementation.* Author. Retrieved from http://www.nacns.org/docs/PR-ConsensusModel120313.pdf

Stanley, J. M. (2009). Reaching consensus on a regulatory model: What does this mean for APRNs? *Journal for Nurse Practitioners, 5*(2), 99–104.

CHAPTER 7

The Coalition for Patients' Rights— A Coalition That Advocates for Scope of Practice Issues

Melinda Ray and Maureen Shekleton

The cost of health care has been an issue in the United States for decades. It has been a growing concern for individuals, businesses, and government over the last decade (The Henry J. Kaiser Family Foundation, 2012, p. 1). The portion of gross domestic product (GDP) that is attributed to health care has increased from 7.2% in 1970 to 17.9% in 2009 and 2010. The trend of health care spending outpacing the national GDP has occurred since the 1960s. Further analysis shows that health care costs per capita have grown an average 2.4 percentage points above GDP since 1970 (The Henry J. Kaiser Family Foundation, 2012, p. 1).

The Centers for Medicare and Medicaid Services (CMS) identified that the United States spent over $2.6 trillion on health care in 2010. This translates to approximately $8,160 per U.S. resident and 17.6% of the GDP. In order to appreciate the growth in these costs, in 1970, health spending accounted for $75 billion or $356 per resident and was 7.2% of GDP (The Henry J. Kaiser Family Foundation, 2012, p. 1). These numbers alone do not make the case for health care reform, but they do illustrate the importance of the United States facing this trend and implementing efforts to decrease the rate of cost increases. Important goals of health care reform include promoting access to care while reducing the cost of health care services and maintaining quality patient care.

One mechanism to achieve cost reductions in health care services is the full utilization of a wide range of licensed, qualified health care professionals. Although this seems like a straightforward, logical approach, its implementation is actually hindered by years of tradition in the provision of health care in the United States. Full utilization of a wide range of licensed health care providers creates competition between these health care professionals and traditional health care providers such as medical physicians, osteopathic physicians, and dentists. A response to this scenario has been the evolution of two coalitions—the Coalition for Patients' Rights (CPR) (www.patientsrightscoalition.org) and the American Medical Association's (AMA) Scope of Practice Partnership (SOPP).

One of the key strategies in moving issues forward at the federal, state, and local levels is coalition building. Coalitions are established around a common mission or purpose, and the members agree to work together to move this mission forward. Often that translates into legislation, regulation, and/or media coverage on the issue. The coalition typically elects or appoints leadership that guides the group in their work. Coalition members, typically associations, organizations and/or businesses, and other stakeholders, pool their resources and work together on the issues of concern. The CPR is an excellent example of a long-standing and effective multidisciplinary coalition.

The demands of the patient in the evolving reformed health care system are juxtaposed against the history of health care professionals in care delivery. Traditional, medically driven care is being challenged to accept the entry of qualified advanced practice registered nurses (APRNs), physician assistants (PAs), and other health care professionals who are legally qualified to provide specific health care services. This need for change has generated a strident response from organized medicine that has organized a coalition of medical physician membership organizations called the SOPP. The SOPP was formed in 2006 to challenge what physicians and osteopaths describe as "inappropriate scope of practice expansions, such as those that are not commensurate with a nonphysician provider group's education and training" (American Osteopathic Association [AOA], 2013). The stated goals of the SOPP were to protect patient safety by supporting the "team" approach to medical care. They are advocating for the physician-led, team-based medical model, which they maintain ensures that professionals with complete medical education and training are adequately involved in patient care (AOA, 2013).

Although many SOPP member organizations note that they value the contributions of nonphysician clinicians to the health care delivery system, there is a continued theme that expansion of their authority to provide services to patients should not happen without medical and osteopathic physician oversight.

The CPR was formed in response to this coalition of medical physician organizations and years of interprofessional rivalry between organized medicine/osteopathy and other health care professional groups. The CPR member organizations represent (but are not limited to) nursing, physical therapy, occupational therapy, psychology, family therapy, chiropractic physicians, naturopathic physicians, nutrition specialists, speech and hearing therapists, and foot and ankle surgeons. In the past, if one of the physician/osteopathic organizations made an effort to oppose a scope of practice issue for another health care provider group, that provider group would organize a targeted coalition and mount a response. The CPR has grown out of these ongoing challenges by professional medicine and optimizes the voice of a number and variety of health care provider organizations. It is rather unique to have such a large number of varied health care groups work together on scope of practice issues.

The CPR consists of approximately 35 health care professional membership organizations. The CPR website notes there are "… a variety of licensed health care professionals who provide a diverse array of safe, effective, and affordable health care services to millions of patients each year. These competent, well-prepared health care professionals complete years of education in their respective specialties, and have long been recognized at the federal and state levels as qualified and essential contributors to the U.S. health system" (CPR, 2011a).

One of the strengths of the CPR is the wide variety of health care providers that are members. This broad-based composition allows the CPR to generate a strong support from many different fronts when needed. When asked what is the most significant contribution the CPR has made to the protection and enhancement of scope of practice of health care professionals other than MDs and DOs, Maureen Shekleton, PhD, RN, FAAN, who was the Professional Relations Specialist for the American Association of Nurse Anesthetists, the organization that serves as the co-chair of CPR stated, "providing a unified, multidisciplinary voice for over 3 million health care professionals to support their ability to practice to the fullest extent of their preparation so that patients are allowed a choice of quality cost-effective providers through whom they can access care...." (CPR, 2011b).

CPR ACTIVITIES

The purpose of a coalition is to bring together an alliance of parties and/or groups for joint action. The CPR has worked to take a proactive approach to the issues that are of concern to its members. One important effort is in the public relations arena. Early in the formation of the coalition, members recognized the importance of having a unified communication strategy that was designed to promote the role of CPR member organizations in health care. The coalition has generated a series of press releases that articulate the added value of its members to the health care system. The CPR has also published a brochure that serves as a resource for members and the public. This brochure was developed to introduce health care professionals and consumers to the coalition. It is available as a hard-copy brochure and a downloadable one-page version that can be found on the coalition's website (CPR, 2011a).

As most scope of practice issues are dealt with at the state level, CPR has most recently been focused on efforts to support and assist state coalitions. The CPR members have access to a state issues-focused tool kit that they can use to support their state advocacy efforts. In addition, the CPR members have access to conference calls where members update each other on state activities. This update has the impact of allowing organizations to support each other's efforts in the states.

Dr. Shekleton identified one of the challenges the coalition faces is engaging and empowering the local affiliates of the national organizations because the actual scope battles occur at the state level. A new and exciting effort of the coalition is a State-Based Coalition (SBC) Program for state/regional organizations, branches, and representatives of the national CPR organizations. The purpose of these state-based coalitions is to enable a coordinated, proactive response by stakeholders to scope of practice developments at the state level, particularly attacks by the SOPP through state and local medical societies. The SBC Program works to facilitate networking and information sharing at the state level between CPR organizations and the creation of state-based CPR coalitions that reflect the national membership of the CPR. One excellent resource that is available on the coalition website (www.patientsrightscoalition.org) is a virtual training session on how to build state-level coalitions that will have an impact. Some of the topics covered in this webinar include background information on the coalition: the role a coalition can play in addressing scope of practice issues on the state level and an overview of tools that are available to support coalition development in your state (CPR, 2011b).

THE SCOPE OF PRACTICE PARTNERSHIP

Between individual health care professionals of different disciplines who provide care together, there is a positive and supportive relationship between the individual medical and/or osteopathic physicians and other collegial professionals who are represented by the CPR member organizations. Unfortunately, these expert medical clinicians may not have a voice within their professional societies and associations. As a result, there is, at times, a wide gap between what many practitioners experience at the bedside and what is articulated by the medical and osteopathic association on the national policy front. Health care economics and the passage of health care reform have provided many new opportunities for all categories of health care professionals to work in new, innovative integrated health care delivery models of care. As state and federal entities have worked to find solutions to health care professional shortages and reduce medical costs, the use of all qualified health care providers has become more of a norm for best practices. Although at times this may require a modification in the state's scope of practice for a specific professional group, most often, it is a matter of regulatory and/or legislative changes at the state or federal level to allow these qualified professionals to work within their current scope of practice to provide better care to their patients.

The CPR seeks to counter efforts by professional medicine/osteopathy and specifically the efforts of the AMA's (SOPP) initiative that is designed to limit patients' choice of health practitioners. The SOPP efforts are extensive and have been artfully framed as patient protections.

According to a presentation given by Michael D. Maves, MD, MBA, chief executive officer and executive vice president, AMA, on February 18 and 19, 2010, in Geneva, Switzerland, at the World Health Professions Conference on Regulation, the membership included 49 state medical associations and the District of Columbia, 14 national medical associations, the AMA, and the AOA (and AOA's 20 state associations) (Maves, 2010). Their stated interests included state and federal regulation and legislation related to the scope of practice of a variety of non-MD/DO health care providers. Some of the health care groups SOPP has specifically targeted include, but are not limited to, podiatrists, optometrists, nurse anesthetists, nurse practitioners, nurse midwives, psychologists, audiologists, physical therapists, chiropractors, and naturopathic physicians (Maves, 2010). Limited information is publicly available concerning the goals and planned activities of SOPP. According to the AMA website, information on the SOPP can be accessed via the AMA website's members-only site.

The presentation given by Dr. Maves identified three major initiatives to curtail the scope of practice of other members of the health care provider team. The first is strategically called the "Truth in Advertising Campaign" (AMA, 2013). This campaign highlights the SOPP's concern with the use of the title "doctor" by nonmedical providers. If an individual has an earned doctorate in a discipline such as psychology or nursing, they would require these individuals to forgo the use of their earned title and require them to identify their type of professional licensure and training. This initiative seeks to require nonmedical providers to include the full designation in their title, such as doctorate in psychology or doctorate in nursing. In an article detailing the efforts of Reps. John Sullivan (R. OK.) and David Scott (D. GA.)'s legislation—The Healthcare Truth and Transparency Act (H.R. 452 introduced January 21, 2011)—it was noted that the goals of these efforts are to clarify title misrepresentation and minimize patient confusion about who is providing medical care (Krupa, 2011). The rhetoric used in this initiative is phrased in terms of patient protections but essentially serves to limit patient choice of health care providers. This legislation failed in the 112th Congress but variations of this legislation have been seen in a number of different states.

Two other initiatives are part of the SOPP's efforts—the AMA Scope of Practice Data Series and the AMA GeoMapping Initiative. The AMA Scope of Practice Data

Series provides the AMA's analysis of the preparation and scope of practice of 10 provider groups (AMA, 2013). A number of CPR member organizations made efforts to proactively work with AMA to provide accurate information regarding their respective practitioner roles. Despite these efforts, the final products in the AMA Scope of Practice Data Series were disappointing to the CPR organizations whose members were targeted including nurse practitioners and nurse anesthetists as well as physical therapists, podiatrists, audiologists, naturopaths, and psychologists. In response to the AMA Scope of Practice Data Series, the coalition publicly requested that it be withdrawn. The CPR's recommendation to withdraw the SOPP Data Series modules was based on many concerns, including those related to conflict of interest, inaccuracies, restricting patient access, and redundancies. The CPR maintains that there is a fundamental conflict of interest for one professional group to define the scope of practice of another (CPR, 2010). According to the CPR website, it is not reasonable for medical physicians to purport that they are seeking to protect patients when (a) there is no credible evidence to suggest that preventing patients from choosing their health care professional would, in any way, improve patient care; and (b) the economic interests of MDs and DOs are intertwined with scope of practice issues. These efforts amount to protecting "turf," and the needs of patients are lost in the discussion (CPR, 2010).

In addition to this concern, the SOPP Data Series has been criticized as being "rife" with inaccuracies and misstatements about the training, education, and accreditation of health care professionals other than MDs/DOs. In spite of these statements, the AMA continues to support and disseminate the Scope of Practice Data Series as advocacy documents (AMA, 2013).

The third publicly identified initiative of the SOPP is the AMA GeoMapping Initiative. This project attempts to map the practice areas of different providers on a state-by-state level. In a 2012 advocacy summary, the AMA spoke about their GeoMapping Initiative, "The AMA GeoMapping Initiative compares the practice locations of physician specialists and nonphysicians to demonstrate that, despite the claims of lack of access, health care professionals tend to practice in the same, large urban areas" (AMA, 2010). The power of these maps lies in how they are interpreted. Many health care providers, because of restrictions in direct payment policies, must be associated to an employer in order to be reimbursed.

The CPR has been quite busy anticipating and responding to these assaults to scope of practice. This is a strong coalition that is likely to continue to grow and work to represent the concerns of health care professionals. When asked what has made CPR such a long-lasting and effective coalition, Dr. Shekleton identified that the reasons go beyond mere opposition to the SOPP efforts. "I believe that the coalition members have come to the realization that the problems each discipline faces are similar to those faced by others—in other words, they see each as more alike than different. Also the reason we initially came together (to counter the SOPP) is not the reason we stay together—our focus has expanded to consumer education about the abilities of health care professionals other than MDs and DOs and engaging our state affiliates in coalition building" (Shekleton, 2012).

IMPLICATIONS FOR THE APRN

APRNs must actively engage in local, state, and national issues that impact their practice. There are many public policy implications to APRNs working to practice to the full extent of their scope of practice. It is critical that APRNs work to articulate and take action in concert with their colleagues on public policy issues that have an impact on patients, their family, health care providers, systems, the community, and on local, state, and federal public policy levels. In order to stay on top of these issues, APRNs should maintain memberships in their professional associations. Often, APRNs gravitate to single memberships in organizations that provide solid clinical and practice support to their members. These memberships are important; but in order to be professionally engaged in scope of practice issues, APRNs should also consider membership in the state nurses association and their APRN membership organizations. APRNs should seek out opportunities to be engaged on the state and local level through coalitions and state association chapters that will focus colleague efforts on key issues of importance to the APRNs in the state.

Beyond this basic level of engagement, APRNs can work on their personal policy advocacy skills. Often membership associations offer training sessions and lobby days on the state and federal level. These sessions are excellent ways to begin to refine your skills in these areas.

Coalitions form around issues of mutual interest for individuals and associations. With the advent of health care reform and the efforts to fully utilize all health care providers to the full extent of their scope of practice, the tensions with the professional medical associations are expected to continue. As with many policy issues, evaluation is not a clear-cut process. Success can, at times, be defined as passage or failure of passage of specific legislation. More often, success can be seen in more subtle results, such as legislative delay tactics, budget implications that sideline a policy discussion, and/or negotiated bill language that solves a smaller percent of the concerns a group has with specific legislation.

APRN ENGAGEMENT

Scope of practice, the core issues around which the CPR coalition is formed, requires a high level of APRN engagement for change to be realized. It is essential to see personal political activity as part of your professional role. Scope of practice issues are largely fought and won on the state level. Therefore, the APRN has the opportunity to invest time in building relationships with colleague APRNs and policy makers to make change over a period of time. Being engaged and active on the local and state level allows individual APRNs to work together with each other to achieve public policy success. Although it is important that all nurses support APRNs operating under their full scope of practice, the APRN is uniquely qualified to speak to the needs of the health care system and their patients and families.

It is challenging to always measure the success of public policy issues. It is a clear success when a bill is passed or fails; but success can also be the development of a strong, well-functioning coalition, or long-term engagement of APRNs. All national competencies mention the importance of public policy awareness and engagement. An individual APRN can feel amazingly empowered when they are able to serve as a resource for their legislators and/or testify to the state legislature or even on the national level. Once an APRN gets involved in public policy issues, they often are motivated to stay involved. The ability to represent the concerns of the profession and the needs of the patients and families the APRNs serve helps the individual APRN to achieve a new aspect of their professional identity. It often motivates these individuals to stay involved and pursue other legislative and regulatory issues of concern.

DISCUSSION QUESTIONS

1. Consider the impact of rising health care costs and the implementation of health care reform in the United States. With this in mind, discuss the advantages for payers to include a wide range of health care providers to their clients.
2. Identify how an APRN working at their full scope of practice can contribute to decreased health care costs.
3. Identify and discuss the advantages of working in a coalition to represent the public policy concerns of a given issue. What could be some disadvantages to working within a coalition to advance a public policy issue and how might they be resolved? Examine the arguments presented by the American Medical Association in their Scope of Practice Partnership and identify how these positions would limit the scope of practice of other licensed health care providers.

SYNTHESIS EXERCISES

1. Divide into two groups with each group selecting a position to defend. One group will represent the American Medical Association's Scope of Practice Partnership and the other will represent the CPR. Each group should prepare key talking points for testimony that represents their position on a scope of practice issue. Some scope of practice issues the groups might consider: expansion of prescriptive authority (Schedule III medications) for APRNs; ordering of x-rays by APRNs; ordering of home health care services for patients by nurse practitioners and clinical nurse specialists; and use of fluoroscopy and interventional pain management by CRNAs.
2. Review the Truth and Transparency legislation found at www.thomas.gov/. Develop a factsheet in opposition to this legislation from the APRN perspective.

REFERENCES

American Medical Association (AMA). (2010). *Advocacy update: AMA GeoMapping initiative provides powerful scope of practice snapshot* (p. 5). Retrieved from http://www.phlebology.org/20100119_Advocacy_Update.pdf

AMA. (2013). *Truth in advertising*. Retrieved from http://www.ama-assn.org//ama/pub/advocacy/state-advocacy-arc/state-advocacy-campaigns/truth-in-advertising.page

American Osteopathic Association (AOA). (2013). *Scope of practice partnership*. Retrieved from http://www.osteopathic.org/inside-aoa/advocacy/state-government-affairs/scope-of-practice-partnership/Pages/default.aspx

Coalition for Patients' Rights (CPR). (2010). *CPR responds to AMA scope of practice modules*. Retrieved from http://www.patientsrightscoalition.org/Advocacy-and-Legislation/AMA-Initiatives/Response-to-AMA-Scope-of-Practice-Modules.aspx

CPR. (2011a). *Protecting health care quality, access and choice of providers*. Retrieved from http://www.patientsrightscoalition.org/default.aspx

CPR. (2011b). *State-Based Coalition (SBC) Program*. Retrieved from http://www.patientsrightscoalition.org/Advocacy-and-Legislation/State-Coalition.aspx

Krupa, C. (2011). Credential disclosure sought by bill. *Amednews.com*. Retrieved from http://www
.ama-assn.org/amednews/2011/02/07/prl20207.htm

Maves, M. (2010). *Scope of practice in the United States*. Proceedings from the World Health Professions
Conference on Regulation, Geneva, Switzerland. Retrieved from http://www.whpa.org
/whpcr2010/presentations/Michael%20Maves%20WHPCR2010.pdf

The Henry J. Kaiser Family Foundation. (2012). *Health care costs: A primer* (pp. 2–5). Retrieved from
http://kff.org/health-costs/report/health-care-costs-a-primer

CHAPTER 8

The Future of Nursing: Campaign for Action

Susan Hassmiller, Susan Reinhard, and Andrea Brassard

BACKGROUND: THE ROBERT WOOD JOHNSON FOUNDATION

The mission of the Robert Wood Johnson Foundation (RWJF) is to improve the health and health care of all Americans. Expanding access to primary care has been an RWJF focus since its beginning, 40 years ago. Ahead of its time in 1973, RWJF envisioned the promise of advanced practice registered nurses as primary care providers. Four regional demonstration projects in Alabama, California, Tennessee, and rural New England educated nurses to become family nurse practitioners or certified nurse midwives. A few years later, this demonstration project transitioned to the Nurse Faculty Fellowship Program, which funded master's level nurse practitioner programs within schools of nursing between 1975 and 1982. To further increase access to primary care, RWJF created the School Health Services Program, which funded nurse practitioner-managed school health services between 1977 and 1984. This early RWJF funding was the impetus for federal funding for advanced practice registered nurses (APRNs) education (Charting Nursing's Future, 2013).

In addition to funding APRN education, RWJF funded a sentinel research study on outcomes of nurse practitioner services provided by the Columbia University School of Nursing's nurse practitioner-run primary care practice. Mundinger and her colleagues (Mundinger et al., 2000) in their groundbreaking article reported that outcomes of nurse practitioner care—patient satisfaction, service utilization, and health status—were comparable with care provided by physicians.

Strengthening the profession of nursing has been an RWJF priority for many years as evidenced by more than $583 million in grants since 1972 to improve nursing education and practice and more than $350 million in just the last 10 years alone (see Figure 8.1). Programs such as the RWJF Executive Nurse Fellows and Nurse Faculty Scholars contribute capacity-building efforts to an up and coming generation of nurse leaders. Other programs such as the Interdisciplinary Nurse Quality Research Initiative and the Quality, Transforming Care at the Bedside, and Safety in Nursing Education demonstrate the link between nursing care and high-quality patient outcomes. This chapter will focus on the *Future of Nursing: Campaign for*

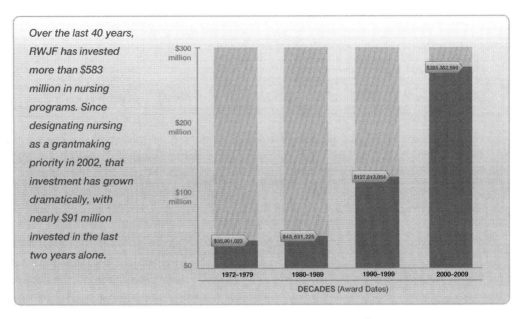

FIGURE 8.1 RWJF Investments in Nursing Surpass $583 Million.

Source: The Robert Wood Johnson Foundation.

Action, beginning with a brief description of the RWJF funded Center to Champion Nursing in America (CCNA) and the Institute of Medicine (IOM) (2011) report *The Future of Nursing: Leading Change, Advancing Health.*

The CCNA was launched in 2007 as an initiative of RWJF, AARP, and the AARP Foundation with a mission to ensure that every American has access to a highly skilled nurse, when and where they need one (see Chapter 10 on AARP Initiatives).

In 2008, RWJF approached the IOM to propose a partnership between the two organizations to respond to the need to transform the nursing profession to become partners and leaders in improving health care. The resulting collaboration became the RWJF Initiative on the Future of Nursing at the IOM, with Susan Hassmiller serving as the Study Director. The stipulation that an RWJF employee serve in this capacity was unprecedented for the IOM and served as a statement of the importance of this report for RWJF (see Chapter 5 on the IOM report by Liana Orsolini).

CAMPAIGN FOR ACTION

The Future of Nursing: Leading Change, Advancing Health was released on October 5, 2010. The *Campaign for Action* launched shortly thereafter at the "National Summit on Advancing Health through Nursing" on December 1, 2010. The *Campaign for Action* is a national initiative to guide implementation of the recommendations of the IOM report. Five pilot state Action Coalitions were announced at the National Summit: California, Mississippi, Michigan, New Jersey, and New York. Action Coalitions are the driving force of the campaign at the local and state levels, forming a strong, connected grassroots network of diverse stakeholders working to transform health care through nursing. Each Action Coalition has nurse and non-nurse ("nurse champion") leaders. Examples of organizations that are represented by nonnurse leaders include AARP state offices, state workforce centers, state hospital associations, and large health insurers. *Campaign for Action* work on removing barriers to APRN practice and care is supported through AARP (see Chapter 10 AARP initiatives).

First-Year Progress: "Visibility"

By the end of the first year, Action Coalitions were operational in 36 states. In March 2011, the following 10 states joined ("Wave II"): Colorado, Florida, Idaho, Illinois, Indiana, Louisiana, New Mexico, Utah, Virginia, and Washington. In October 2011, 21 more states joined ("Wave III"): Arkansas, Delaware, Georgia, Hawaii, Kansas, Kentucky, Maryland, Massachusetts, Minnesota, Missouri, Montana, Nebraska, North Carolina, Ohio, Pennsylvania, Rhode Island, South Carolina, Texas, West Virginia, Wisconsin, and Wyoming.

At the national level, the *Campaign for Action* has sparked widespread support. National organizations have publicly supported the report and its key messages, such as the American Red Cross, the Healthcare Information and Management Systems Society, the National Association of Hispanic Nurses, the National Association of Public Hospitals and Health Systems, the National Medical Association, and the World Health Organization. On the state level, more than 150 events were held related to the *Campaign for Action*, such as statewide strategic planning sessions, stakeholder presentations, launch events, and Action Coalitions webinars. *Campaign for Action* spokespeople presented at more than 120 venues in more than 21 states.

Second-Year Progress: "Infrastructure Building and Advancing Education Progression"

By the end of the second year, 48 states had Action Coalitions. Twelve more Action Coalitions were announced in March 2013 ("Wave IV"): Alabama, Arizona, Connecticut, Iowa, Maine, Nevada, New Hampshire, North Dakota, Oklahoma, South Dakota, Tennessee, and Vermont. Action Coalition liaisons from the CCNA provided technical assistance to assist each state with developing infrastructure, setting priorities, recruiting key stakeholders, and documenting progress. The IOM

FUTURE OF NURSING COMPAIGN FOR ACTION

Area of Focus

- Leadership
- Practice and Care
- Education
- Interprofessional Collaboration
- Diversity

Adapted from Future of Nursing®, Campaign for Action (2010).

report recommendations were conceptualized as pillars to provide an infrastructure for organizing the *Campaign for Action* work: leadership, practice and care, education, interprofessional collaboration, and diversity.

The goal of "Advancing Education Progression" was targeted as the main focus for year 2 activities. To build the infrastructure for advancing education progression, the *Campaign* created a state- and national-level network of nursing leaders and stakeholders to accelerate progress on goals to increase the education level of nurses. The *Campaign for Action* highlighted four promising models of nursing education progression including expanding accelerated Associate Degree in Nursing (ADN) to Master of Science in Nursing (MSN) programs. The accelerated ADN to MSN model can help prepare all four categories of APRNs. Regional meetings of 30 to 40 state nursing education leaders were held in each of the four regions such as the Southeast (December 2011), West (February 2012), Midwest (April 2012), and Northeast (May 2012) to engage the Action Coalitions in this work. Following the regional meetings, *Campaign for Action* nurse experts facilitated regional webinars to help the Action Coalitions to develop and implement action plans to advance education progression in their states. To accelerate education progression, RWJF provided funding through the Academic Progression in Nursing (APIN) program to nine Action Coalitions (California, Hawaii, Massachusetts, Montana, New Mexico, New York, North Carolina, Texas, and Washington). The American Organization of Nurse Executives serves as the National Program Office for this grant, as a representative of the Tri-Council of Nursing.

The *Campaign for Action*'s second year focus on academic progression is at the core of nursing leadership and advancing nursing practice. The *Campaign for Action* is built on decades of work by nursing organizations and leaders in education as well as the other pillar focus areas. For example, the APIN program recognizes the efforts of the Tri-Council for Nursing, an alliance between the American Association of Colleges of Nursing, the American Nurses Association, the American Organization of Nurse Executives, and the National League for Nursing. The Tri-Council's statement on the Educational Advancement of Registered Nurses released in May 2010 echoes many of the recommendations outlined in the IOM report.

Year Three: "Strategic Activation"

As the *Campaign for Action* moves into its third year, it builds on progress from years 1 and 2 by moving forward with strategic activation. With the District of Columbia joining the *Campaign for Action* in mid-January 2013, the grassroots network of Action Coalitions now includes 51 coalitions.

A *Campaign for Action* website was launched in September 2012 providing a national hub of information about the *Campaign*, the 51 Action Coalitions, and an online community connecting the grassroots network and stakeholders nationwide. Designed to be forward thinking and interactive, the website is the *Campaign's* platform to reach new audiences and tell the story of how nurses are transforming health care across the country. The website allows for easy and timely access to resources, communications tools, and templates from the national campaign. Each Action Coalition has its own state page that includes contacts, news, state specific resources, and a progress report. Much of the state-to-state interaction is through the website's dynamic interactive community (www.campaignforaction.org).

To further the implementation of the IOM recommendations, RWJF is providing grants to up to 30 Action Coalitions through the State Implementation Program (SIP).

Grants of up to $150,000 are awarded to Action Coalitions to implement two priority recommendations of the IOM report. The SIP requires Action Coalitions to secure matching funds to sustain efforts over the long term. To date, there are 240 additional funders that are providing resources to Action Coalitions, leveraging over $5 million additional dollars to the campaign.

NATIONAL SUMMIT

From February 28 to March 1, 2013, Action Coalitions from 50 states and the District of Columbia convened in Washington, DC, to work on transformative strategies to accelerate on-the-ground momentum of the *Campaign for Action.* Risa Lavizzo-Mourey, MD, president and CEO of RWJF, kicked off the summit with a conversation about the Foundation's commitment to transforming health care through nursing. She called upon nurses as key partners to forward the Foundation's vision of a "culture of health" for all Americans. Action Coalition teams developed shared understandings of next steps and strategy, created plans for bold action, and identified ways to attract more diverse people to the work. Susan Hassmiller and Susan Reinhard, senior VP for public policy at AARP, unveiled five Campaign Imperatives that lay the groundwork to achieve and sustain meaningful results.

CAMPAIGN IMPERATIVES

I. Must move beyond *NURSING*.

II. Must deliver short term *RESULTS* in the next 18 months even as you develop long term plans.

III. Must have *COURAGE* to place the right *LEADERS* at the helm or remove weak, ineffective leaders.

IV. Must have *FUNDING* to sustain this work.

V. Must not ignore *DIVERSE* stakeholders critical to our success.

Reprinted with permission of AARP.

Importantly, they emphasized that unless Action Coalitions successfully engaged stakeholders other than nurses, they would not have the requisite power, influence, and resources to make the policy and culture changes needed to implement the IOM recommendations. Understanding that the *Campaign for Action* is about what is best for patients and communities is a core ingredient in aligning key stakeholders.

CAMPAIGN FOR ACTION CHALLENGES

The *Campaign for Action*'s greatest asset is also its greatest challenge. In order to immediately respond to and capitalize on the momentum of the IOM report, RWJF quickly organized a massive, multifaceted effort to transform the nursing profession in order to improve health and health care. In a very short time, the *Campaign for Action* mounted a vast field effort at the national and state levels to achieve that vision. With 50 states and the District of Columbia working to implement the IOM recommendations with policy makers and in health care facilities and communities, at colleges and universities, and in many other settings, the *Campaign for Action* must move beyond its focus on mobilization and shift to meaningful action. The *Campaign for Action* must sustain the changes being made; establish and maintain relationships that bring influence, resources, and funding; and measure outcomes in order to make course corrections and adjustments for the long term.

An ongoing challenge is to ensure that all relevant stakeholders are not only involved but also have a consequential way to engage—both nursing and nonnursing. For example, overcoming the opposition to implementing IOM recommendations surrounding education progression and practice and care is critical to success and involves engaging physicians and others in the health professions as well as community colleges and other educational institutions. Some of the opposition voiced from these groups has been reflected in the media in the past year ("State Directors Focus on Nursing Data," 2013) and in an American Academy of Family Physicians (2012) report.

Although nurses are at the heart of the *Campaign for Action*, there are still challenges to be overcome in engaging some of our own: students, public health nurses, staff nurses, and others. Siloes within the health professions have also made it difficult to engage our colleagues in other disciplines and in particular physicians. National physician professional organizations have presented a significant challenge to the *Campaign*, particularly in regards to progress on scope of practice issues. The *Campaign for Action* must continue to work on engaging with others in and outside of our profession to advance this work.

EVALUATION

In late 2011, TCC Group, a consulting firm with extensive experience evaluating coalitions, was engaged to conduct a formative evaluation of the *Campaign for Action*. The TCC's evaluation was designed to provide constant feedback to *Campaign for Action* stakeholders so that findings could inform decision making and improve the *Campaign*. This evaluation includes assessments of the collaboration between RWJF and CCNA as well as the *Campaign*'s relationship with stakeholders such as the Champion Nursing Coalition and Champion Nursing Council. In addition, site visits to eight state Action Coalitions and the nine APIN projects, a survey of Action Coalitions, and a survey of RWJF alumni regarding their engagement in the *Campaign for Action* will also be conducted. Early learning from the evaluation includes:

1. Action Coalitions will likely need significant personalized assistance in fund development.
2. When Action Coalition structure includes a standalone workgroup dedicated to data, groups working on other *Campaign* pillars have been left without sufficient expertise in data. As a result of this realization, Action Coalitions have been dissolving their data workgroups and integrating team members into other workgroups.

3. Previous RWJF and CCNA efforts in the states have provided a foundation for the Action Coalitions, current work.

In addition to this formal external evaluation of the *Campaign for Action*, RWJF and CCNA have been observing and learning from the Action Coalitions since the *Campaign for Action*'s launch and throughout the visibility, infrastructure building, and strategic activation phases. Action Coalitions' quarterly reports capture descriptions of their work under each pillar, successes, and challenges, as well as requests for technical assistance that will facilitate their work toward implementing the IOM recommendations in their state. CCNA and RWJF have also administered operational and communication-focused surveys to determine what is working and where Action Coalitions would benefit from additional support. The observations of each Action Coalitions' dedicated liaison provide an additional lens through which progress is evaluated with an understanding of the states' unique context. As noted earlier (see *National Summit* section), Action Coalitions' capacity to move beyond nursing, deliver short-term results (next 18 months) as long-term plans are developed, place the right leaders at the helm, obtain funding to sustain work, and engage diverse stakeholders have been recognized by *Campaign for Action* leadership as essential elements for sustainability and success. Through observations, surveys, self-reports, and TCC's external evaluation, RWJF and CCNA will continue to identify key elements that will strengthen the *Campaign for Action* while also measuring progress toward implementing the IOM recommendations on a state level.

DASHBOARD INDICATORS

The IOM report recommendations serve as a foundation to fully realize nursing's potential (see Table 8.1). Successful implementation will lead to a transformed health care delivery system and improved patient care. Through extensive analysis, the *Campaign for Action*'s research team determined the best indicators to measure its progress on a national level. And just as sound evidence grounds the IOM's report recommendations, solid, reliable evidence will inform its progress. Yearly, the *Campaign for Action* will analyze established data sets to evaluate where we are gaining ground and areas that require additional emphasis.

FUTURE PLANS: WHAT WILL SUCCESS LOOK LIKE?

According to Risa Lavizzo-Mourey, *Campaign for Action* success would be implementation of the Future of Nursing report recommendations. Success "looks like people … across America practicing to the full extent of their training and education. It looks like a diverse nursing workforce that is really able to start with bachelor's degree and continue to grow and provide the kind of care that we know is going to evolve over our lifetimes and beyond. It looks like, frankly, a country that … has a culture of health" (http://www.rwjf.org/en/about-rwjf/newsroom/newsroom-content/2013/02/transforming-nursing-to-create-a--culture-of-health-.html).

Success will rely on good communication and continued evidence to support the messages that drive our action and movement toward a culture of health. Key messages have been developed so that Action Coalitions can communicate with nonnursing stakeholders such as hospital CEOs, physicians, and other audiences. Unified messages that help articulate the IOM recommendations in a way that resonates with diverse groups will expand the impact of the *Campaign for Action*. And

TABLE 8.1 Future of Nursing: Campaign for Action DASHBOARD Indicators and Data Sources

IOM RECOMMENDATION	INDICATOR	DATA SOURCE
Increase the proportion of nurses with a baccalaureate degree to 80% by 2020	Percentage of employed nurses with baccalaureate degree in nursing or higher degrees	American Community Survey
Double the number of nurses with a doctorate by 2020	Total fall enrollment in nursing doctorate programs	American Association of Colleges of Nursing
Advanced practice nurses to be able to practice to the full extent of their education and training	State progress in removing regulatory barriers to care by advanced practice registered nurses	National Council of State Boards of Nursing
Expand opportunities for nurses to lead and disseminate collaborative improvement efforts	Number of required clinical courses and/or activities at top nursing schools that include both RN students and other graduate health professional students	Top nursing schools (as determined by U.S. News and World Report rankings) that also have graduate-level health professional schools at their academic institutions. Course offerings and requirements include clinical and/or simulation experiences
Health care decision makers should ensure leadership positions are available to and filled by nurses	Percent of hospital boards with RN members	American Hospital Association Health Care Governance Survey and the National Governance Institute
Build infrastructure for collection and analysis of interprofessional health care workforce data	Number of recommended data items collected by the states	Forum of State Nursing Workforce Centers

continued visibility and promotion of the importance of the IOM recommendations in addressing health care challenges are paramount to creating this culture shift within the profession, within health care, and in the community.

The Future of Nursing: Leading Change, Advancing Health continues to be the most viewed report on the IOM website. The people viewing, buying, and printing this report are from 150 countries. With more than 1,200 mentions in major media and more than a quarter million impressions since its release, the report continues to be highly influential. It serves as an evidence base for supporting efforts toward transforming health and health care. This report has been covered or mentioned in national media such as *The New York Times*, *Wall Street Journal*, *Washington Post*, and *The Economist*.

The call from the *Campaign for Action* and the recommendations of the IOM report to transform health care through nursing have been echoed with support from several national reports. A recent report by the National Governors Association (2012) on December 20 states that "to better meet the nation's current and growing need for primary care providers, states may want to consider easing their scope of practice restrictions and modifying their reimbursement policies to encourage greater nurse practitioner involvement in the provision of primary care." The American Hospital Association (2013) released a model in January, which calls for increased interprofessional education and practice, with APRNs responsible for diagnosing and implementing the plan of care for patients and families in healthy communities. Action Coalition and national leaders have been able to utilize these reports as further evidence to support our messages at professional meetings and in communities.

We will also measure our success through our Campaign Imperatives. Engaging key stakeholders is a *Campaign for Action* imperative. The Champion Nursing Coalition

FUTURE OF NURSING™
Campaign for Action

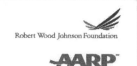
Robert Wood Johnson Foundation
AARP

2013 STRATEGIC ACTIVATION PRIORITIES

Our goal is to ensure that people get the care they need, when and where they need it. The Campaign for Action is working to improve health care through nursing.

> The Campaign for Action, *now in its third year, has previously focused on 1) broad awareness building among key health stakeholders around the Institute of Medicine future of nursing report; and 2) infrastructure building through the designation of volunteer Action Coalitions in all 50 states and the District of Columbia. In its third phase, the* Campaign *will focus on strategic action at the national and state levels, working to engage stakeholders and advance policy and program priorities.*

Education: **Prepare our nursing workforce for the future** by strengthening education and training. A more highly educated nursing workforce can lead system improvements and improve quality, accountability, and coordination of care. More nurses with bachelor and graduate degrees can manage challenges in an increasingly complex system, lead improvements, and prepare the next generation of nurses. We will:
- Leverage partnerships with community colleges and four year universities that enable nurses to achieve higher levels of education through an improved education system.

Leadership: We need to **prepare the next generation of nurses to address health care challenges** and position nurses to lead system change. As the primary coordinators of patient care, nurses must contribute their unique experience to decision making platforms. We will:
- Increase the number of nurses in leadership positions across all settings (practice, local, state, national and federal).
- Identify and share state based leadership programs that will prepare nurses to lead.

Practice and Care: **Expand access to care** by maximizing the use of nurses. Nurse practitioners, for example, provide an immediate and cost-effective solution to care delivery challenges caused by primary care provider shortages, an aging population, and patients with more chronic conditions. We will:
- Work with state and national stakeholders to increase consumers' access to care.

Diversity: Nursing needs to **reflect the changing demographics** of the U.S. population to meet workforce demands, provide culturally appropriate care, and address health disparities. Racial and ethnic minorities make up 30 percent of the population, but only 10 percent of nurses. Men represent 49% of the U.S. population but only 7% of nurses. We will:
- Develop state based diversity outreach initiatives that increase the diversity of the nursing workforce.

Interprofessional Collaboration: We must **improve quality and coordination of health care** by promoting a team-based approach to education and practice. We will:
- Identify and develop state based programs that encourage greater collaboration among all health professionals to significantly improve patient care.

Capacity Building: The *Campaign* will expand the capacity of all Action Coalitions to sustain their efforts over time. We will:
- Work with all Action Coalitions to develop strong strategic action plans that demonstrate a process for achieving goals, have measurable benchmarks, and are supported and sustained by outside financial resources.
- Urge all Action Coalitions to develop synergistic, long term partnerships with diverse stakeholders, including business, consumer, and other health professional organizations.

Communications and Outreach: The *Campaign* joins together a broad spectrum of groups including Action Coalitions, businesses, consumer organizations, and other health professionals each with a stake in transforming health care through nursing. *Campaign* supporters collaborate via the *Campaign for Action* online community and periodic convenings.

Please visit us at www.campaignforaction.org to learn more.

includes more than 50 diverse national organizations representing business, consumers, and health professional organizations. Health insurers such as Aetna, Cigna, and United Health Group are some of the largest employers of nurses, and have historically promoted nurses to leadership positions in their organizations. Through the *Campaign for Action*, health insurers have built awareness around nurse-led health plan programs that help their members and consumers. Another Champion Nursing Coalition member, the American Hospital Association, envisions a society of healthy communities, where all individuals reach their highest potential for health. More than 30 state hospital associations have joined Action Coalitions to advance nursing and health care.

Sustainable funding is a campaign imperative. As noted earlier, to date, 30 states report receiving external funding, which totals more than $5 million. These grants come from more than 240 institutions and 150 individuals.

The *Campaign for Action* offers an unprecedented opportunity for nurses to engage diverse health care stakeholders to improve health and health care through nursing. The nursing community is united as never before around the need to implement the IOM recommendations, and diverse stakeholders have pledged support for the *Campaign*. It is truly a historical time for nursing. To join this national effort, go to www.campaignforaction.org and sign up. Help shape the future of health care for all Americans.

DISCUSSION QUESTIONS

1. Describe your involvement in the *Campaign for Action*. If you are not currently involved, visit www.campaignforaction.org and your state webpage. Sign up for the online community.
2. Visit the Dashboard Indicators. What progress has been made nationally and in your state?
3. What else can the *Campaign* do to transform health and health care through nursing? To contribute toward creating a culture of health?
4. What role can students play in the *Campaign for Action*? What can the *Campaign for Action* do to engage students? Other stakeholders?
5. Discuss some activities that you might be able to lead to help advance the *Campaign* priorities.

REFERENCES

American Academy of Family Physicians. (2012). *Primary care for the 21st century: Ensuring a quality, physician-led team for every patient.* Retrieved from http://www.aafp.org/online/etc/medialib/aafp_org/documents/membership/nps/primary-care-21st-century/whitepaper.Par.0001.File.dat/AAFP-PCMHWhitePaper.pdf

American Hospital Association. (2013). *Workforce roles in a redesigned primary care model.* Retrieved from http://www.campaignforaction.org/sites/default/files/PCwhitepaper%20FINAL%20Jan102013.pdf

Charting Nursing's Future. (2013). *Celebrating a sustained commitment to improving health and health care: RWJF marks its 40th anniversary.* Retrieved from http://www.rwjf.org/content/dam/files/file-queue/CNF_January%202013__Issue%2019__FINAL.pdf

Institute of Medicine (IOM). (2011). *The future of nursing: Leading change, advancing health.* Washington, DC: National Academies Press (prepublication copy). Retrieved from http://www.nap.edu/catalog/12956.html

Mundinger, M. O., Kane, R. L., Lenz, E. R., Totten, A. M., Tsai, W. Y., Cleary, P. D., … Shelanski, M. L. (2000). Primary care outcomes in patients treated by nurse practitioners or physicians: A randomized trial. *Journal of the American Medical Association, 283*(1), 59–68.

National Governors Association. (2012). *The role of nurse practitioners in meeting increasing demand for primary care.* Retrieved from http://www.nga.org/cms/home/nga-center-for-best-practices/center-publications/page-health-publications/col2-content/main-content-list/the-role-of-nurse-practitioners.html

State directors focus on nursing data to support ADN. (2003, April 3). *Community College Times.* Retrieved from http://www.communitycollegetimes.com/Pages/Workforce-Development/State-directors-focus-on-nursing-data-to-make-case-for-ASN.aspx

IMPLICATIONS OF HEALTH CARE REFORM AND FINANCE ON ADVANCED PRACTICE REGISTERED NURSE PRACTICE

The Patient Protection and Affordable Care Act

Jan Towers

Improving and updating the health care system in the United States has been on the agenda of legislators, regulators, and other policy makers as well as health care providers for decades. Beginning with unsuccessful national health insurance proposals of Theodore Roosevelt and later with Franklin Roosevelt's more successful social reforms, it has been continuously on the agenda of both Republicans and Democrats in the White House and Congress as well as many state legislatures to the present day (CMS, 2013).

The initiation of the Medicare and Medicaid Programs in 1965 was arguably the most significant step taken to assure the elderly and underserved of health care access and payment for care. As early as 1945, President Truman proposed the formation of these programs that were signed into law 20 years later by Lyndon Johnson. Although many attempts to improve upon these programs were initiated through the years, it was not until 2003 that the next piece of legislation to improve access to health care was signed into law. That was when the Medicare Modernization Act (MMA) that sought to improve outpatient care and payment for medications to eligible Medicare recipients was passed and signed by President George W. Bush.

In the intervening years, the need for health care reform was recognized by President Richard Nixon in the early and mid-1970s, when his proposed legislation (the Comprehensive Health Manpower Act and the Nurse Training Act) that initiated, among other things, federal funding for nurse practitioner education was passed and signed into law. At that time, he also proposed a "National Health Strategy" that included a fee for service or Health Maintenance Organization coverage for all citizens through their employer or special government programs. Likewise, President Gerald Ford signed into law the first health care privacy act and President Jimmy Carter, in anticipation of the implementation of national health insurance, consolidated various health care administration entities into what was first known as the Health Care Financing Administration (HCFA) and more recently as the Centers for Medicare and Medicaid (CMS).

Most of the health care reform proposals, however, were controversial. Both President Reagan and President Clinton encountered setbacks in proposals that slowed the progression of health care reform for close to 20 years. A bill was passed during the Reagan administration (the Medicare Catastrophic Coverage Act of 1988) that included catastrophic medical care coverage and prescription drug benefits that was subsequently repealed in the George H. W. Bush administration. Later, in the 1990s, although the Health Insurance Portability and Accountability Act that provided patients with privacy and insurance protection benefits was passed, a major health care reform bill providing for universal health care coverage to all Americans, proposed by President Clinton, disintegrated before votes could be taken because there was so much controversy over its provisions. Then in 2003, legislation that included drug benefits and preventive care benefits was passed under George W. Bush.

During those intervening years, nurse practitioners did become federally authorized providers first in the Federal Employees Health Insurance Program, then in rural and long-term care settings, and finally in the Medicare Program at large.

THE ACT

With the advent of the Obama administration, another attempt to initiate and pass health care reform legislation was undertaken. Bills were introduced in both the House and the Senate that would revise many costly and cumbersome provisions in Medicare and Medicaid law, provide increased access to health care by the nation's large uninsured population, and establish insurance processes to enhance access, protect patients, stimulate increases in the primary care workforce, and implement the provision of primary care services such as health promotion and disease prevention. Creating legislation that would lead to cost-effective care and bend the spiraling cost curve for health care soon became a contentious and convoluted process. As the contentiousness increased, mainly along party lines, the ability to reach agreement in the House and Senate decreased. Added to the confusion was the death of one of the lead Senators in the Democratic-led proposal for this legislation, which initially included provisions for a publicly funded universal health care program. In the end, a somewhat watered-down proposal was passed and signed into law. The bill was called the Patient Protection and Affordable Care Act (PPACA) of 2010.

Provisions in the Act were constructed so that they were not required to be implemented immediately. Instead, their implementation would be phased in over several years, in order to allow time for insurance carriers, providers, hospitals, and government agencies such as state governments to prepare for the new or revised provisions included in the legislation.

Patient protection provisions such as banning preexisting condition clauses in insurance contracts that prevent patients from obtaining later coverage for those conditions began immediately after passage of the bill in 2010. Those provisions were immediately implemented for children and 6 months later for adults. Similar approaches were taken regarding provisions that limited the practice of setting caps on coverage that would subsequently prohibit patients from obtaining needed health care services.

Provisions that protected patient choice of provider and payment nondiscrimination toward providers were to be implemented as the new requirements were implemented. These provisions protect the right of patients to keep or choose the health care provider they desire to see and prohibit health care insurers providing new insurance to patients to discriminate against a class of providers such as nurse practitioners. Other provisions, such as increasing Medicare payment for medical care including prescriptions to close gaps (commonly referred to as the doughnut hole) created by the 2003 MMA payment schemes, were designed to gradually go into effect over a 10-year period. The 2003 "doughnut hole" legislation provided payment for prescriptions of Medicare patients up to a certain level, then the patient was responsible for payment beyond that level until costs reached what was considered to be catastrophic, at which time payment would again be initiated for prescription costs that exceeded that threshold (prior to the 2003 legislation, Medicare did not cover prescriptions for medications). The PPACA provision continues to pay for prescriptions as legislated in 2003, and gradually raises the first level threshold until it meets the second or "catastrophic level" by the year 2010, thus eliminating the "doughnut hole" for payment for prescriptions initiated in 2003.

Other provisions such as the implementation of universal coverage and Medicaid expansion were delayed to allow regulations to be developed and methodologies for implementation put in place. These delayed provisions were the most controversial pieces of the legislation and led to drastic attempts by its opponents to remove the provisions. Initially, the House of Representatives voted to repeal the entire bill. However, the Senate rejected that proposal and the president had announced that such a piece of legislation would be vetoed by his office. This was followed by attempts to challenge the constitutionality of the legislation in the courts and further attempts to repeal or block appropriations for some of the provisions in the statute.

As the challenges moved through the courts, implementation of many of the provisions moved forward according to the required schedule set in the legislation. It was not until the spring of 2012 that the Supreme Court agreed to hear the case against the constitutionality of the new legislation. The questions the Court considered included whether the Supreme Court could actually hear the case prior to implementation of the legislation, whether the universal coverage mandate was constitutional, whether expansion of Medicaid (basically a state-controlled entity) was constitutional, and whether pieces of the proposed legislation could be determined unconstitutional without declaring the entire bill unconstitutional (severability).

The conclusion was that the Court determined they could hear the bill, despite the fact that not all parts had been implemented; that the universal health provision was constitutional; and that the federal government could not require the states to implement the expanded Medicaid coverage in the bill. The rest of the statute remained untouched (567 U.S., 2012). Although the road had been opened for implementation of the new legislation, opponents of the legislation determined that they would keep this bill from being implemented by blocking implementation through other means. The House (with a Republican majority) has voted twice to repeal the entire new statute, but the measure will not be taken up in the Senate that has a Democratic majority. Likewise, measures have been successfully introduced to repeal sections of the bill in the House; again these are not being addressed by the Senate, thus stopping their progress, and steps are being taken in proposed appropriations legislation to block the funding of many of the measures within the statute that require funding in order to implement them. Although expansion of Medicaid may suffer some setbacks, depending on whether the states opt to cover the additional populations/groups authorized federally to receive Medicaid, the steps to initiate all of the provisions of the bill continued to move forward. As of this writing, updated information is maintained at the following websites: www.kff.org or www .whitehouse.gov/healthreform.

NURSE PRACTITIONERS AND THE PPACA

Through the years, beginning in the late 1980s, nurse practitioners made progress with every reform bill that was passed. The Patient Protection Affordable Care bill was no exception. In the well-known presence of the need for primary care providers, nurse practitioners were identified as a significant part of the resolution of the health care crisis. At the time this legislation was passed, there were greater than 155,000 nurse practitioners. More than 88% of them were prepared as primary care providers and approximately 70% were practicing in primary care settings (American Association of Nurse Practitioners [AANP], 2013).

For the first time, legislation was predominantly provider neutral and "clinicians," rather than "physicians," were identified as providers throughout the statute. In addition, nurse practitioners and clinical nurse specialists were recognized as primary care providers throughout the legislation, and deemed eligible for primary care incentive payments that were previously limited to primary care physicians. Although the PPACA addresses all clinicians, nurse practitioners and clinical nurse specialists, rather than all advanced practice registered nurses (APRNs), are most affected by this legislation because of their recognition as primary care providers.

In the area of strengthening the health care workforce, Title VIII funding for the nursing workforce that includes appropriations for APRN education programs and traineeships, faculty loan repayment, and grants to nurse-managed clinics was reauthorized. In addition, payment to nurse-managed clinics and fellowships for family nurse practitioners in federally qualified health centers was authorized, though not immediately funded. What was immediately funded was a Graduate Nurse Education (GNE) demonstration that provided funding for clinical preparation through a competitive bidding process to five APRN programs to increase the number of APRN graduates prepared to practice in community-based primary care. The participants are Rush University, Chicago, IL; Duke University, Durham, NC; Hospitals of the University of Pennsylvania, Philadelphia, PA (consortia); Memorial Medical Center, Houston, TX (consortia); and Scottsdale Medical Center, Scottsdale, AZ (consortia).

Other significant programs within this legislation afforded opportunities for APRNs to obtain funding or participate in innovative programs focusing on the delivery of primary care services. A CMS innovation (Center for Medicare and Medicaid Innovation [CMMI]) was created to allow CMS to experiment and implement programs more efficiently than currently allowed. Prior to its development, successful demonstrations had to be reapproved by Congress if the programs were to be continued. Of particular importance to nurse practitioners is that CMMI innovations were not limited to physicians and hospitals. Although the first rounds of the funding cycle were dedicated to large established practices, later funding cycles included more innovative projects that incorporated APRNs and allowed for smaller practices to compete.

Among the most prominent innovations included in this legislation were the formation of insurance exchanges for individuals not covered by existing government or third-party insurance programs, the formation of a Medicare primary care accountable care organization pilot called Shared Savings, an emphasis placed on the utilization of medical home standards in a variety of government payment innovations, the development of a medical home for homebound patients, the development of programs that reimburse for transitional care of patients being discharged from hospitals, and funding for the coordination of complex patient care. All of these programs have potential for APRN involvement and leadership. As the rules for implementation of these programs are developed, it will be important for APRNs to be recognized as eligible providers within the programs and for them to assert themselves and their practices by becoming involved in the programs.

INSURANCE EXCHANGES AND MEDICAL HOMES

Currently, the regulations for the development of insurance exchanges allow APRNs to become providers within the systems being developed. However, because there is no mandate, APRNs will need to be vigilant within their states in order to become involved in the development and implementation of these programs. This means they must be at the table, acquainted with the state's insurance commissioners, involved in associated task forces and committees, and involved with the insurance carriers associated with the programs. Likewise, it will be important for APRNs to be vigilant, as state regulations are developed, to be sure that practices are recognized as medical homes within those regulations and regulations for other state-controlled programs affecting health care. Currently, nurse practitioner practices are recognized by Medical Home certifiers and may receive recognition from the recognized national certification programs. The principles of the Medical Home Practice have been the centerpiece for nurse practitioner practice from the beginning: holistic patient-centered care, with an emphasis on access, quality, and safety (AANP, 2012).

ACCOUNTABLE CARE ORGANIZATIONS

In this legislation, nurse practitioners are recognized as Accountable Care Organization (ACO) providers. However, last-minute changes in the Shared Savings provision for Medicare patients have determined for that program that the only eligible beneficiaries will be patients of primary care physicians. In this instance, changes continue to be needed in the statute that will allow patients of nurse practitioners to be beneficiaries in this program. Although this provision disincentivizes APRNs in the Shared Savings Program, it does not prevent them from becoming members of other ACOs or forming ACOs of their own.

The Shared Savings Program is a pilot Medicare primary care ACO, designed for primary care practices within the Medicare system. Practices will participate in shared savings activities that include the performance of a predetermined set of quality indicators and reported cost savings by practices of physicians performing primary care services to Medicare patients. The statute is in place as of this writing; however, it requires a change to allow patients of APRNs to become beneficiaries in the program. It is unclear how this will impact APRNs and their patients in the long run as it, like numerous aspects of the PPACA, is still evolving,

TRANSITIONAL CARE AND CARE COORDINATION AND MEDICAID EXPANSION

As in other areas, studies have already demonstrated that advanced practice nurses are particularly skilled in implementing transitional care and coordinating care for patients both in public and commercial insurance plans. Transitional care speaks to the care of patients postdischarge (usually 30 days) from hospitals and other health care institutions usually at home and in primary care practices; care coordination refers to the activities all professional nurses have been prepared to provide, which involves the maintenance of patient-centered continuity of care and communication among health care providers, families, other community resources, and the patient that provide for and maintain the health and welfare of patients in our communities. The goal of both transitional care and care coordination is to sustain maximal functioning outside the health care institution and keep the patients from being admitted or readmitted with the same problem or some sequelae. Involvement in the development of these programs at the community level and involvement with the reimbursement planning at the policy level are musts for advanced practice nurses. Likewise, the expansion of Medicaid coverage will necessitate the continued authorization of advanced practice nurses as full participants in the health care systems, if the projected increased numbers of patients are to receive primary care services.

HEALTH PROMOTION/DISEASE PREVENTION

The legislation has continued to emphasize the importance of health promotion and disease prevention through the expansion of payment for health promotion, disease prevention services, and the development of programs that APRNs are particularly prepared to deliver. It will be important for APRNs to seek out opportunities to utilize this authorization in the provision of the care upon which advanced practice nurse education is built.

OBSTACLES/BARRIERS

One of the unfortunate aspects of the passage of legislation such as this has been the opposition of some power brokers in the country's health care system. Of particular significance to APRNs is organized medicine's opposition to changes in the care models that are being authorized. This has created particular challenges to APRNs, who have the potential to increase the quantity and quality of health care services to both public and private patients throughout the country.

Likewise, the presence of other statutory barriers to practice that are grounded in obsolete laws will continue to interfere with the ability of APRNs to fully implement the opportunities provided in this piece of legislation until they are changed. The need for all advanced practice nurses to function at their full scope of preparation and for obsolete barriers related to physician oversight and Medicare Conditions of Participation to be removed continues to exist at this writing.

CONCLUSION

As with all legislation, the statutory provisions in this legislation have their limitations, but similar to health care reform legislation in the past, they provide significantly increased opportunities for advanced practice nurses to practice to the full extent of their education and licensure. It will be important for APRNs to take advantage of the opportunities provided in the PPACA, to seize the moment once again to demonstrate their worth and expertise in meeting the health care needs of the nation and to continue to use their influence to make changes in the country's health care system that will improve the health and welfare of its citizens.

DISCUSSION QUESTIONS

1. What do you think an APRN should/can do to assist with the implementation of the PPACA?
2. How should the PPACA affect your patient's health?
3. Identify two provisions of the PPACA that would help the patients of APRNs.
4. Identify two provisions of the PPACA that would help APRNs in their practices. Give examples.

REFERENCES

American Association of Nurse Practitioners (AANP). (2012). *Survey results national database.* Austin, TX: Author.

AANP. (2013). *Nurse practitioners in primary care.* Austin, TX: Author. Retrieved from http://www.aanp.org/publications/position-statements-papers

Centers for Medicare and Medicaid (CMS). (2013). *Tracing the history of CMS programs: From President Theodore Roosevelt to President George W. Bush.* Retrieved from http://www.cms.gov/About-CMS/Agency-Information/History/downloads/presidentcmsmilestones.pdf

U.S. House of Representatives Office of Legislative Council. (2010). *Patient Protection and Affordable Care Act* (as amended through May 1, 2010, including *Patient Protection and Affordable Care Act health-related portions of the Health Care and Education Reconciliation Act of 2010*). Washington, DC: U.S. Government Printing Office.

567 U.S. (2012). Opinion of Roberts, C.J. Supreme Court of the United States Nos. 11-393, 11-398, and 11-400. National federation of Independent Business, et al., Petitioners vs. Kathleen Sebelius, Secretary of Health and Human Services, et al., Department of Health and Human Services, et al., Petitioners vs. Florida et al. Petitioners, Florida et al. vs. Department of Health and Human Services et al. On Writs of Certiorari to the United States Court of Appeals for the Eleventh Circuit.

CHAPTER 10

AARP Initiatives

Andrea Brassard and Susan Reinhard

WHAT IS AARP?

Established in 1958, and formerly known as the American Association of Retired Persons, AARP, now its official name, is the nation's leading membership organization for people aged 50 and over. This is a nonprofit, nonpartisan membership organization with a membership of more than 37 million, and is dedicated to enhancing the quality of life for all, nationally and globally, and leading positive social change by providing information, advocacy, and service to its members and the public. AARP's founder, Dr. Ethel Percy Andrus, was a high-school principal in Los Angeles when she retired at the age of 60 to take care of her mother. Her mother recovered and Dr. Andrus volunteered with the California Retired Teachers Association and led its committee for retired teachers' welfare. Learning that many retired educators had no health insurance and inadequate pensions, Dr. Andrus testified before the California legislature. Her efforts resulted in the formation of the National Retired Teachers Association in 1947 that advocated for educators throughout the United States. Dr. Andrus developed benefits and programs such as group health insurance for older persons and a discount mail order pharmacy service. These programs were so popular that thousands of persons asked the association to open its membership for noneducators and, in 1958, AARP was founded. In 1999, its name was changed to the four-letter acronym AARP because the membership is open to persons of age 50 years and above, with almost half of the current membership continuing to work. The National Retired Teachers Association continues as a division of AARP.

AARP is a nonprofit, nonpartisan organization that helps people of age 50 years and above have independence, choice, and control in ways that are beneficial to them and society as a whole. AARP does not endorse candidates for public office or make contributions to either political campaigns or candidates. The AARP Foundation is an affiliated charity that provides security, protection, and empowerment to older persons in need with support from thousands of volunteers, donors, and sponsors. AARP has staffed offices in all 50 states, the District of Columbia, Puerto Rico, and the U.S. Virgin Islands.

Located within AARP is the prestigious Public Policy Institute (PPI), staffed by approximately 40 researchers and issue experts who inform public debate on critical issues. PPI conducts policy research and analysis, and convenes leading policy experts for discussion of national and state policy issues. This PPI's research and analysis informs AARP's national policy efforts aimed at improving economic security, health care and quality of life, and advocacy work by AARP state offices. These research findings are shared throughout the national policy-making community, such as other researchers, advocacy organizations, legislative and executive branch officials, and the media.

CENTER TO CHAMPION NURSING IN AMERICA

Launched in December 2007, the Center to Champion Nursing in America (CCNA) is a joint initiative of the Robert Wood Johnson Foundation (RWJF), AARP, and the AARP Foundation. CCNA's chief strategist is Dr. Susan Reinhard, who is a Senior Vice President of AARP's PPI. CCNA's vision is that all Americans will have access to a highly skilled nurse when and where they need one.

In its first 2 years, CCNA focused primarily on building nursing education capacity through state teams and two national invitation only summits. The first summit was held in June 2008. Eighteen state teams of diverse stakeholders such as representatives from nursing education, employers, state nursing workforce centers, government agencies, and AARP state offices developed action plans to increase nursing education enrollment in their states. In preparation for the summit, RWJF, CCNA, and the U.S. Department of Labor, Employment, and Training Administration commissioned a white paper, "Blowing Open the Bottleneck: Designing New Approaches to Increase Nurse Education Capacity" (www.rwjf .org/content/rwjf/en/research-publications/find-rwjf-research/2008/05/blowing -open-the-bottleneck.html). Four approaches to effective solutions were outlined as follows: (a) create strategic partnerships to align and leverage stakeholder resources; (b) increase nurse faculty capacity and diversity; (c) redesign nurse education—for example, use simulation technology, redesign clinical education, and create dedicated educational units; and (d) capitalize on the role played by government and accrediting organizations in nurse education.

CCNA's initial goals were to (a) strengthen our nation's educational pathways to prepare the nursing workforce of the future; (b) increase the number and diversity of nurses entering and remaining in the profession; (c) remove barriers that limit nurses' ability to provide the health care consumers need; and (d) enhance the influence of nurses in high levels of health care, policy, business, and community decision making. In December 2008, CCNA founded the Champion Nursing Coalition, whose member organizations such as Aetna, Families USA, and Verizon represent the voices of consumers, purchasers, and providers of health care. The Champion Nursing Coalition is raising awareness of the roles of nurses in increasing access to primary care, transitional care, and chronic care management in a reformed health care delivery system. CCNA also convened the Champion Nursing Council, an advisory group made up of national nursing organizations. In 2009, 12 additional state teams were added to focus on increasing education capacity in the states. The 30 multistakeholder teams included representatives from multiple AARP state offices. CCNA provided advocacy training and communications support to stakeholders to help them communicate more effectively with policy makers and private-sector leaders. Several AARP state offices contacted CCNA advocacy staff about scope of practice limitations for advanced practice registered nurses (APRNs) in their states.

In response to this advocacy work, the AARP Policy Book was amended with input from CCNA to increase access to APRN practice and care.

AARP POLICY BOOK 2010 REVISION

In the spring of 2010, the Health Chapter in the AARP Policy Book was amended to include all four APRN categories in its "Professional Schools and Licensing" section and in the Policy Book glossary (below). The new language called for states to "amend current nursing and, where applicable, medical licensing laws to allow nurses, APRNs and allied health professionals to perform duties for which they have been educated, and certified..." An additional bullet was added that "current state nurse practice acts and accompanying rules should be interpreted and/or amended where necessary to allow APRNs to fully and independently practice as defined by their education and certification" (AARP, 2013).

GLOSSARY

Advanced practice registered nurses (APRNs):

Nurses who receive advanced clinical preparation (generally a master's degree and/ or post-master's certificate, although the Doctor of Nursing Practice degree is increasingly being granted). Specific titles and credentials vary by state approval processes, formal recognition, and scope of practice as well as by board certification. APRNs fall into four broad categories: nurse practitioner, clinical nurse specialist, nurse anesthetist, and nurse midwife.

CCNA FOCUS EVOLVES TO IMPLEMENT THE RECOMMENDATIONS OF THE IOM REPORT

In October 2010, the Institute of Medicine (IOM) released *The Future of Nursing: Leading Change, Advancing Health*, a thorough examination of how nurses' roles, responsibilities, and education should change to meet the needs of an aging, increasingly diverse population, and to respond to a complex, evolving health care system. The four key messages and eight major recommendations (below) in the report focus on the critical intersection between the health needs of patients across the life span and the readiness of the nursing workforce. These recommendations are intended to support efforts to improve health care for all Americans by enhancing nurses' contributions to the delivery of care.

KEY MESSAGES

- Nurses should practice to the full extent of their education and training.
- Nurses should achieve higher levels of education and training through an improved education system that promotes seamless academic progression.
- Nurses should be full partners, with physicians and other health care professionals, in redesigning health care in the United States.
- Effective workforce planning and policy making require better data collection and an improved information infrastructure.

REPORT RECOMMENDATIONS

1. Remove scope-of-practice barriers.
2. Expand opportunities for nurses to lead and diffuse collaborative improvement efforts.
3. Implement nurse residency programs.
4. Increase the proportion of nurses with a baccalaureate degree to 80% by 2020.
5. Double the number of nurses with a doctorate by 2020.
6. Ensure that nurses engage in life-long learning.
7. Prepare and enable nurses to lead change to advance health.
8. Build an infrastructure for the collection and analysis of interprofessional health care workforce data.

CAMPAIGN FOR ACTION

The Future of Nursing: Campaign for Action is a national initiative to guide implementation of the recommendations in *The Future of Nursing: Leading Change, Advancing Health*, a landmark IOM (2011) report. The campaign envisions a health care system where all Americans have access to high-quality care, with nurses contributing to the full extent of their capabilities. It is coordinated through the CCNA, an initiative of AARP, the AARP Foundation, and the RWJF.

The campaign includes 50 states plus DC Action Coalitions and a wide range of health care providers, consumer advocates, policy makers, and business, academic, and philanthropic leaders. Many of the Action Coalitions evolved from CCNA's state teams.

The *Campaign for Action* is working to implement all eight recommendations of *The Future of Nursing: Leading Change, Advancing Health.* Any work performed by CCNA staff that relates to advocacy or lobbying is funded by AARP, because RWJF grant funds cannot be used to fund lobbying or political campaign activities. CCNA tracks legislative and regulatory activity pertaining to all eight recommendations. Advocacy efforts in areas such as advancing nursing education are funded by AARP. To date, of the eight recommendations, advocacy work has largely focused on removing scope of practice barriers for APRNs at both the federal and state levels.

RECOMMENDATION NO. 1: REMOVE SCOPE-OF-PRACTICE BARRIERS

To fully realize nurses' potential contribution to a patient-centered, seamless, transformed health care system, the *Campaign for Action* is leading efforts to modernize outdated policies (public and private), change state and federal laws and regulations, and remove cultural and organizational barriers. The *Campaign for Action* is implementing a learning collaborative to help states to achieve success; engaging national stakeholder partners in state, federal, and private sector efforts; and engaging stakeholders to ensure inclusion of nurses practicing in all sectors.

As described above, advocacy work around Recommendation No. 1 is funded through AARP's portion of the *Campaign for Action*. AARP has a consumer focus—the goal is to increase access to care by removing barriers to APRN practice. CCNA's placement within the PPI of AARP provides an opportunity to offer research and analysis to inform the consumer-focused health policy advocacy agenda of AARP.

AARP'S PPI PUBLICATIONS

To date the PPI of AARP has published two papers that align with the first recommendation of *The Future of Nursing: Leading Change, Advancing Health*. The first of these papers is titled "Removing Barriers to Advanced Practice Registered Nurse Care: Hospital Privileges" (Brassard & Smolenski, 2011). This article discusses barriers to hospital privileges and expands on the IOM report recommendations that APRNs be eligible for hospital clinical privileges, admitting privileges, and hospital medical staff membership and also be permitted to perform hospital admission assessments—documenting medical histories and performing physical examinations.

The second paper that aligns with the IOM report is "Removing Barriers to Advanced Practice Registered Nurse Care: Home Health and Hospice Services" (Brassard, 2012). This paper expands on the IOM report recommendations that APRNs be allowed to certify patients for Medicare payment of home health and hospice services and shows how removing this barrier would benefit consumers, physicians, and the health care system. Allowing APRNs to certify home health and hospice services can potentially decrease costs, expedite treatment by eliminating the need for physician sign-off, and allow patient-centered health care teams to practice more efficiently.

GRADUATE NURSE EDUCATION DEMONSTRATION PROGRAM

True to the CCNA vision to ensure that Americans have the highly skilled nurses needed to provide affordable, quality health care, now and in the future, AARP continues to advocate for state and national funding for nursing education. AARP advocates for funding to advance education progression in nursing and to increase the supply of RNs, APRNs, and nursing faculty.

AARP advocated for the Graduate Nurse Education (GNE) Demonstration Program, which is an important part of the 2010 Affordable Care Act (ACA). ACA set aside $200 million over 4 years to test the idea of providing Medicare funding for GNE to fund hospitals to train more APRNs. Selected hospitals are partnering with accredited schools of nursing and nonhospital community-based care settings to expand clinical education within and beyond the hospital setting. Consumers, nurses, and health care groups issued a collective cheer when the selected institutions—the Hospital of the University of Pennsylvania, Duke University Hospital, Scottsdale Healthcare Medical Center, Rush University Medical Center, and Memorial Hermann-Texas Medical Center Hospital—were announced in July 2012.

The GNE Demonstration Program will enable the selected graduate nursing programs to expand access to clinical training sites—especially in community-based clinics, which are ideal for educating APRNs and other primary care providers. AARP is supporting and monitoring GNE implementation. If the demonstration program is deemed as a success, it could prompt Medicare to change its current nursing education payment policies and create a permanent funding stream to boost graduate nursing education nationwide.

AARP EYE ON NURSING

AARP advocacy and lobbying activities that are related to nursing are posted on the "Eye on Nursing" and can be found at www.aarp.org/politics-society/advocacy /info-05-2010/eye_on_nursing.html (AARP's website). This webpage includes links to letters submitted by AARP national and state offices supporting legislation and revised federal regulations.

AARP members are watching for policy solutions and legislation that would fully realize nurses' potential contribution to a patient-centered, transformed health care system in the following areas:

Removing Barriers to Practice: Modernize outdated policies (public and private) and change state and federal laws and regulations to allow nurses to practice to the full extent of their education and training.

Patient-Centered Transformed Health Care System: Advances and contributions to the research, advocacy, and communications strategies through the national network of professional and health care-related stakeholders.

Advancing Nursing Education: Federal and state policies to increase the educational level of nurses through an improved education system that promotes seamless academic progression.

Nurses Leading Change and Advancing Health: Federal and state policy making bodies include nurses on advisory committees, commissions, and boards.

ONGOING AARP INITIATIVES

As previously described, CCNA is a strategic initiative within AARP's PPI. Another PPI strategic initiative aims to improve the capacity of nurses and social workers to meet the needs of family caregivers. This initiative is made possible by the John A. Hartford Foundation and the Jacob & Valeria Langeloth Foundation through AARP Foundation. Organizations supporting this effort include the Family Caregiver Alliance, the National Association of Social Workers, U.S. Administration on Aging, the Lewin Group, the Hilltop Institute, Nurses Improving Care to Health System Elders (NICHE), and the American Journal of Nursing.

In addition to these national strategic initiatives, PPI's work is organized into four teams—Consumer and State Affairs, Economics, Independent Living and Long-Term Care, and Health. PPI's Health Team works on policy related to a range of issues that impact APRN practice and care such as the Medicare and Medicaid Programs, improvement of health insurance coverage at the state and national level, the cost and appropriate use of prescription drugs, healthy behaviors, racial and ethnic disparities in care, and care delivery and coordination. APRNs are also interested in policy issues addressed by PPI's Independent Living/Long-Term Care Team such as expanding consumer access and choice, improving home and community-based services, and supporting family caregivers.

As our health care system continues to evolve, APRNs can look to AARP for ongoing research and policy initiatives that are relevant to APRN practice and care.

DISCUSSION QUESTIONS

1. Review the two AARP's PPI publications that refer to Recommendation No. 1 of the IOM report. How do these barriers impact your current or future practice? What other barriers to APRN practice and care impact consumers?
2. How does the GNE Demonstration Program impact your school's current or future APRN programs?

REFERENCES

AARP. (2013). *The Policy Book: AARP Public Policies, 2013–2014* (Chapter 7, p. 145). Washington, DC: Author.

Brassard, A. (2012, July). *Removing barriers to advanced practice registered nurse care: Home health and hospice services*. AARP Public Policy Institute, Insight on the Issues 66. Retrieved from http://www.aarp.org/health/medicare-insurance/info-07-2012/removing-barriers-to-advanced-practice-registered-nurse-care-home-health-hospice-AARP-ppi-health.html

Brassard, A., & Smolenski, M. (2011, September). *Removing barriers to advanced practice registered nurse care: Hospital privileges*. AARP Public Policy Institute, Insight on the Issues 55. Retrieved from http://www.aarp.org/health/doctors-hospitals/info-10-2011/Removing-Barriers-to-Advanced-Practice-Registered-Nurse-Care-Hospital-Privileges.html

Institute of Medicine (IOM). (2011). *The future of nursing: Leading change, advancing health.* Washington, DC: National Academies Press.

CHAPTER 11

A Million Hearts® Initiative

Liana Orsolini and Mary C. Smolenski

The Institute of Medicine's (IOM) future of nursing report's seventh recommendation calls everyone to "prepare and enable nurses to lead change to advance health" (2010, p. 43) and the American Nurses Association (ANA) Social Policy Statement's definition of nursing includes advocating for "...the care of individuals, families, communities and populations" (2010, p. 10). Both these documents call for nurses to improve the health of communities and populations, an imperative nursing has mostly ignored. Advanced practice registered nurses (APRNs) have opportunities to improve the health of communities and populations through public–private partnerships and through involvement with federal programs.

Federal efforts to improve health are certainly not new but have gathered momentum with the start of the U.S. Department of Health and Human Services (USDHHS) launch of Healthy People in 2000 (National Center for Health Statistics [NCHS], 2001). Unlike Healthy People 2020 (USDHHS, 2010), which covers a myriad of health topics from access to health services to improving the visual health of the nation, the Million Hearts® Initiative zeroes in on one Healthy People 2020 goal of improving cardiovascular health by preventing one million heart attacks and strokes by 2017 (HealthyPeople, 2020; USDHHS, 2013a).

A Million Hearts is a national initiative begun in 2011 by the Centers for Disease Control and Prevention (CDC) director Dr. Tom Frieden and former Administrator of the Centers for Medicare and Medicaid Services (CMS), Donald M. Berwick, under the Department of Health and Human Services. This initiative not only works to align existing efforts but is also creating new programs to improve heart health and to help Americans live longer, more productive lives. The CDC and CMS, co-agency leaders of A Million Hearts, are working alongside other federal agencies and private and public sector organizations to institutionalize effective cardiovascular disease prevention (CVD) strategies within communities. Community strategies include targeting smoking, artificial trans fat, and sodium consumption, whereas clinical strategies include targeting appropriate aspirin use, blood pressure control, cholesterol control, and smoking cessation (ABCS). Clinical strategies also include improving health information technology (HIT) and innovative care models to meet national goals. Federal agencies involved in Million Hearts include the Administration for

Community Living, National Institutes of Health (NIH), the Agency for Healthcare Research and Quality, the Food and Drug Administration (FDA), the Health Resources and Services Administration (HRSA), the Substance Abuse and Mental Health Services Administration, the Office of the National Coordinator, and the Veterans Administration. Among the many private-sector partners are the American Academy of Nursing, American Heart Association (AHA)/American Stroke Association, American Association of Nurse Practitioners (AANP), American Association of Colleges of Nursing, ANA, Association of Public Health Nurses, Preventive Cardiovascular Nurses Association (PCNA), and a nurse-managed clinic, Lewis and Clark Family Health Clinic. Dr. Janet Wright, an accomplished cardiologist who served as a Senior Vice President for Science and Quality at the American College of Cardiology, is the Executive Director of the Million Hearts Initiative. Under her leadership, many national nursing organizations have been asked and are still being asked to partner with Million Hearts. According to Dr. Wright, if this initiative is to be successful it will take a comprehensive interprofessional and transdisciplinary effort across multiple types of stakeholder organizations (Wright, personal communication, May 9, 2013).

The private-sector initiatives include a variety of efforts. The AHA pledges to help monitor progress of the initiative's goals and provide consumers with access to their heart health management tools, including Heart 360, My Life Check, and the Heart Attack Risk Calculator. Walgreens, with more than 26,000 health care providers, supports the Million Hearts initiative's prevention goal by providing blood pressure testing at no charge in consultation with a Walgreens pharmacist or with a Take Care Clinic Nurse Practitioner. The ANA has committed to continue their work to advocate for tobacco-free lives, whereas the AANP pledged to identify and share best practices and research regarding the prevention of heart disease and stroke. The PCNA is including Million Hearts in their clinical tools designed to educate health care providers, promote Million Hearts across multiple social media platforms, and will work to include Million Hearts as a supporter of PCNA's Summary of National Guidelines for CVD. The American Academy of Nursing is developing a white paper on nurse-led best practices and policy recommendations on the ABCS and plans to disseminate their results widely.

Why should APRNs be interested in the Million Hearts Initiative? Heart disease causes one in every four deaths or about 600,000 deaths per year in the United States, which costs about $110 billion each year for coronary disease alone in treatment costs and in loss of productivity (CDC, 2013a). While 81 million Americans are affected by some form of cardiovascular disease (Lloyd-Jones et al., 2010), this number is expected to increase as 75% of the U.S. population over 20 years of age are either overweight, obese, or extremely obese (CDC, 2012a) and one in every three children are overweight or obese (AHA, 2013). Strokes are also a leading killer taking 130,000 American lives each year (Kochanek, Xu, Murphy, Miniño, & Kung, 2011). If one adds up *all* deaths each year from heart attacks, strokes, and related vascular diseases, we are confronted with 800,000 deaths per year with accompanying staggering costs of $300 billion a year or $1 of every $6 spent for direct medical costs (CDC, 2011a) and an additional $161.5 billion worth in lost productivity (CDC, 2011b). Although the CDC (2013) Division for Heart Disease and Stroke Prevention began the National Heart Disease and Stroke Prevention Program in 1998, which is now in 41 states and in the District of Columbia, heart disease and stroke continue to increase. A likely cause of cardiovascular disease is that one in every three or 68 million Americans have high blood pressure and 20% of these, or about 14 million people, do not know they have it and less than half of those with high blood pressure have it controlled

(CDC, 2013b). Self-reported hypertension rose by almost 10% from 2005 to 2009 and the data continue to show racial and geographic disparities (CDC, 2013c). In addition, another 30% of Americans have pre-hypertension (CDC, 2013d). When documenting the extent of the problem of CVD and the lack of evidence-based treatment patients receive, Frieden and Berwick (2011) draw our attention to the chasm between clinical guidelines and practice as follows:

> Currently, less than half of people with ischemic heart disease take daily aspirin or another antiplatelet agent; less than half with hypertension have it adequately controlled; only a third with hyperlipidemia have adequate treatment; and less than a quarter of smokers who try to quit get counseling or medications.
>
> *Frieden and Berwick (2011)*

Clearly, cardiovascular disease in the United States is not well managed and this should have the attention of APRNs if nursing is to lead advancing the health of the nation. APRNs care for significant amounts of the U.S. population (ANA, 2011) and have an enormous capacity to bring blood pressure and other controllable risk factors under control (AAN, 2014). Data from the American Academy of Nurse Practitioners (now called the AANP) sample surveys from 2009 and 2010 indicate that 89% of the over 155,000 nurse practitioners (NPs) are prepared in primary care and 87% see patients covered by Medicare. Over 75% of them provide primary care to patients seeing from 10 to 25 patients daily, a majority of which are between the ages of 66 and 85. Of the 5.6% prepared as acute care NPs, the majority see patients over 60 years of age with multisystem disease in acute or critical care settings. Over 97% of NPs prescribe medications and of all the prescriptions written, two of the top three drugs prescribed are antihypertensives and dyslipidemics (AANP, 2010). NP-managed clinics have shown excellent outcomes for managing high blood pressure (Wright, Romboli, DiTulio, Wogen, & Belletti, 2011). Furthermore, nurse-managed health clinics are proliferating (Ware, personal communication, October 1, 2012) and are operating in at least 37 states with an estimated two million patient encounters per year, mostly for Medicaid recipients and for the uninsured (Kovner & Walani, 2010). More NPs work in rural areas and in other remote areas than any other primary care practitioner (Robert Wood Johnson Foundation [RWJF], 2012). Dr. McMenamin (2013), a Senior Policy Analyst for the ANA, analyzed Medicare data and discovered that APRNs served more than 30% of Medicare fee-for-service beneficiaries across the United States. Through nurse-managed health clinics, APRNs and registered nurses can lead the nation in improving blood pressure control and other controllable risk factors that contribute to heart attack and strokes. Figure 11.1 shows what all health professionals are asked to do by taking the Million Hearts Pledge.

Although prevention of illness and injury is a desirable proposition, it is difficult to sustain because success usually means the absence of a condition. Results are intangible and may take months or even years to realize. Patients often give up on strategies and methods because results seem slow, unreachable, or out of sight. Most effects and benefits of prevention have been shown in retrospective or highly controlled longitudinal studies. In a world where people are conditioned to expect instant feedback and immediate results, prevention efforts need to create incentives for both practitioners and patients alike. Integrating population health measures into primary care is a natural strategy for APRNs who actually have been leading the way in this arena for many years (Health Affairs, 2013). NPs and other APRNs are a natural fit to "lead change and advance health" through the Million Hearts Initiative.

By taking the pledge, as a health care provider, you commit to:

TREAT high blood pressure and cholesterol in your patients.

TREAT appropriate patients with aspirin.

ESTABLISH and **DISCUSS** with patients their specific goals for treatment and the most effective ways that they can help control their risk factors for heart disease and stroke.

COACH your patients to develop heart-healthy habits, such as regular exercise and a diet rich in fresh fruits and vegetables, and stress reduction techniques. Provide tools to show their progress and access to team members to help them succeed.

ASK your patients about their smoking status and provide cessation support and medication when appropriate.

ASK about barriers to medication adherence and help find solutions.

USE health information technology, such as electronic health records and decision support tools, to improve the delivery of care and control of the **ABCS.**

FIGURE 11.1 Million Hearts® Pledge.

Source: Available at: www.millionhearts.hhs.gov/providers.html

The Patient Protection and Affordable Care Act (ACA) created this opportunity by mandating prevention and quality care.

The ACA's Title III, Improving the Quality and Efficiency of Healthcare, Part II, National Strategy to Improve Health Care, mandates the first National Quality Strategy (NQS) (USDHHS, 2013b). The three aims of the NQS are given as follows:

1. Better Care: Improve the overall quality, by making health care more patient-centered, reliable, accessible, and safe.
2. Healthy People/Healthy Communities: Improve the health of the U.S. population by supporting proven interventions to address behavioral, social, and environmental determinants of health in addition to delivering higher-quality care.
3. Affordable Care: Reduce the cost of quality health care for individuals, families, employers, and government.

USDHHS (2011a)

The Million Hearts Initiative meets the National Quality Strategy's goal to "promote the most effective prevention and treatment practices for the leading causes of mortality, starting with cardiovascular disease" (USDHHS, 2012a). The Million Hearts Initiative has two main goals as follows:

1. Better Prevention Efforts by "empowering Americans to make healthy choices such as preventing tobacco use and reducing sodium and trans fat consumption," and

2. Better Treatment by, "improving care for people who do need treatment by encouraging a targeted focus on the ABCS," which includes **A**spirin as appropriate for people at risk, **B**lood pressure control, **C**holesterol management, and **S**moking cessation (ABCS).

CDC (2011c)

Strategies for prevention efforts aimed to improve the health of American lifestyles for preventing tobacco use and for reducing sodium and trans fat consumption rely on community engagement efforts. Let us begin by examining tobacco use in the United States.

Although tobacco use declined shortly after the 1998 Master Settlement Agreement that eliminated the use of advertising directed toward underage youth, the United States is currently quickly losing ground (USDHHS, 2012b). Tragically, nearly one in four high-school seniors smoke and most of these become adult smokers (USDHHS, 2012b). The success of big tobacco in the United States is evidenced by the figures that more than 600,000 middle-school students and three million high-school students smoke cigarettes. Also worrisome is that the number of middle school and high school students who have used e-cigarettes has recently doubled to equal almost 2 million and a growing number are trying e-cigarrettes without ever having tried a regular cigarette (CHC, 2013h). These numbers are expected to increase because while every day more than 1,200 people die due to smoking, at least two youth or young adults take their place. This means 2,400 young people begin smoking each day (USDHHS, 2012b). Certainly school nurses/practitioners and school-based health centers are key players in the prevention of tobacco product use and in smoking cessation in children and in youth. As of 2008, there were 73,697 registered nurses working as school nurses and nearly 2,000 school-based health centers (HRSA, 2010, 2013). School-based health centers routinely provide tobacco prevention services (National Assembly on School-Based Health Care, 2007–2008). In a study of 35 high schools, limited school nurse intervention using the 5As model (see Figure 11.2)

5As

- **Ask about smoking**
- **Advise smokers to stop**
- **Assess the smoker's willingness to stop**
- **Assist those smokers willing to stop**
- **Arrange follow-up**

5Rs

- Relevance (of quitting tobacco use)
- Risks (of continued tobacco use)
- Rewards (gained from quitting tobacco use)
- Roadblocks (to quitting)
- Repetition (repeat motivational interventions at each visit)

FIGURE 11.2 5As and 5Rs.

Source: The Tobacco Use and Dependence Clinical Practice Guideline Panel, Staff, and Consortium Representatives (2000).

resulted in successful short-term abstinence in adolescent boys (Pbert et al., 2011). More research needs to be conducted to determine if a longer intervention period will lead to sustained abstinence among all genders.

The incidence of tobacco use in adults in the United States remains problematic. The CDC (2013e) estimates that 45 million people or 19% of adults over 18 smoke cigarettes and that cigarette smoking accounts for over 440,000 deaths each year in the United States. Sadly, 70% of smokers wish to quit yet continue smoking (CDC, 2013f). The CDC is using the ACA's Prevention and Public Health Fund to finance its newest campaign against smoking. Most television viewers familiar with the CDC's "Tips from Former Smokers" campaign recognize Terrie, a middle-aged woman with a disfigured face and stoma, who tells her story of smoking that she started at the age of 13. The CDC television advertisements where Terrie and other former smokers tell their stories can be reviewed at: www.cdc .gov/tobacco/campaign/tips/resources /videos/terrie-videos.html#terrie-2. (Note: Terrie H. died September 16, 2013, at age 53.)

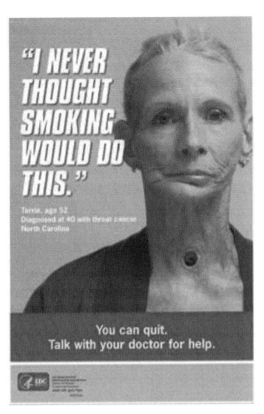

These ads caused the call volume to the CDC's 1-800-QUIT-NOW number to double and visits to the campaign website www.cdc.gov/tips increased more than fivefold (CDC, 2013f). Every APRN should follow the guidelines updated by USDHHS (2008). These guidelines list evidenced-based ways to facilitate successful tobacco use cessation in population-specific patients both willing and unwilling to quit at the time of visit with their health care practitioner. In an evidence review of over 8,000 articles from 1975, the 2008 updated guidelines stress that combining counseling and

Source: The Department of Health and Human Services, Centers for Disease Control Office on Smoking and Health.

medication are more effective than either alone. Also noteworthy is that the evidence to screen all patients for tobacco use at every visit to a primary care provider is an A level recommendation by the U.S. Preventive Services Task Force (USPSTF, 2013). Diet is another focus area for community prevention efforts of the Million Hearts Initiative.

With regard to hypertension, too much sodium intake increases the risk of developing high blood pressure (CDC, 2012b) and 90% of Americans eat more sodium than is recommended. Although the U.S. Dietary Guidelines recommend ingesting less than 2.3 g of sodium per day, Americans ingest an average of 3.3 g/day. Moreover, those at risk for cardiovascular disease such as African Americans, anyone older than 50, and those with high blood pressure, diabetes, or chronic kidney disease should ingest no more than 1,500 mg of sodium per day (U.S. Department of Agriculture & USDHHS, 2010). Although the IOM (2013) recommends further research on the effects of sodium on patient outcomes in population subgroups, there is much evidence to link a high sodium intake with cardiovascular disease. Most consumers are not aware that high amounts of sodium from the American diet come from surprising sources such as cottage cheese, raw chicken and pork injected with a sodium solution, bread, soup, and salsa. There are many resources for patients that APRNs can use to educate their patients about lowering their salt intake and salt intake's relationship to blood pressure. The NIH has a user-friendly guide for the public on how to lower their blood pressure by reducing salt consumption (NIH & National Heart, Lung and Blood Institute [NHLBI], 2013). This website has easy to read instructions on how to read food labels for sodium, quizzes to test knowledge of high sodium containing foods, and tips for smart shopping and meal preparation. The Preventive Cardiovascular Nurses Association (PCNA) has many downloadable resources as well as tools for health care providers at www.pcna.net/index.php. In addition to limiting salt intake or sodium, Americans must also limit their intake of trans fats.

The amount of publicity linking ingestion of trans fats to coronary heart disease (CHD) has led to a marked decrease in its consumption and in the reformulation of many foods to greatly decrease amounts of trans fat or completely eliminate it (CDC, 2012c). Despite this progress, Americans continue to consume 1.3 g of artificial trans fat or partially hydrogenated oils per day. Few realize that although an ingredient label states that there is 0 trans fat, manufacturers are allowed to add less than 0.5 g and remain within the law. As no trans fat is a good trans fat, patients should be told to avoid all products containing partially hydrogenated oils such as frozen pizza, microwave popcorn, ready-to-use-frostings, margarine, pies, cookies, coffee creamers, and fried foods. Many prepackaged foods and preprepared and fried foods still contain high amounts of trans fats. APRNs can encourage patients to read every label and cook for themselves as much as possible. Certainly, a nutritionist should be a part of the interprofessional team and should be available as a patient resource. Once an APRN determines that a patient needs treatment to prevent heart attacks and strokes, efforts are placed on the ABCS. A is for appropriate aspirin use. Appropriate aspirin use has been widely studied. The U.S. Preventive Services Task Force (USPSTF), a nongovernmental panel of interprofessional clinical experts and scientists, conducts evidence reviews on a large variety of primary care preventive health services and then publishes its recommendations. These recommendations are weighed according to the level of evidence. For instance, an A or B recommendation means there is high (A) or moderate (B) certainty that the preventive service should be offered to a targeted population, whereas a C recommendation means that the service should be used more selectively because the benefit is small (USPSTF, 2012). As of September 23, 2010, the ACA has mandated that the new insurance plans must cover all A and B preventive services recommended by the USPSTF at no cost sharing (Health Affairs, 2010). Figure 11.3 shows the USPSTF's recommendations for the use of aspirin to prevent cardiovascular disease. Note that the UPSTF is currently updating its recommendations on aspirin use.

The CDC analyzed data from the National Ambulatory Medical Care Survey and from the National Hospital Ambulatory Medical Care Survey representing a total of 198,042 patient visits among adults aged greater than or equal to 18 years in order to "estimate the prevalence of physician-prescribed aspirin and other antiplatelet medications" (George, Tong, Sonnenfeld, & Hong, 2012). Although prescribing increased from 32.8% in 2003 to 46.9% by 2008, this analysis concluded that prevalence of prescribing aspirin or other appropriate antiplatelet medications remains low for those in which prevention is recommended because of the presence of either ischemic vascular disease or presence of risk factors. Despite knowing which patients were already on an aspirin regimen and thus did not need their physician to prescribe it, or

- The USPSTF recommends the use of aspirin for men age 45 to 79 years when the potential benefit due to a reduction in myocardial infarctions outweighs the potential harm due to an increase in gastrointestinal hemorrhage.
  Grade: A recommendation

- The USPSTF recommends the use of aspirin for women age 55 to 79 years when the potential benefit of a reduction in ischemic strokes outweighs the potential harm of an increase in gastrointestinal hemorrhage.
  Grade: A recommendation

- The USPSTF concludes that the current evidence is insufficient to assess the balance of benefits and harms of aspirin for cardiovascular disease prevention in men and women 80 years or older.
  Grade: I statement

- The USPSTF recommends against the use of aspirin for stroke prevention in women younger than 55 years and for myocardial infarction prevention in men younger than 45 years.
  Grade: D recommendation

FIGURE 11.3 USPSTF Recommendations for Appropriate Aspirin Use.
Source: USPSTF (2009).

if aspirin use was contraindicated, the authors determined that a higher percentage of patients should be on aspirin prevention therapy. Appropriate aspirin therapy for the secondary prevention of cardiovascular disease is an integral part of the Million Hearts Initiative (Parekh, Galloway, Hong, & Wright, 2013). If APRNs followed the USPSTF guidelines, the gap in appropriate aspirin use can surely be narrowed.

B is for blood pressure control. Blood pressure control is challenging as evidenced by the millions of Americans who live with uncontrolled hypertension. The NIH and NHLBI published the seventh report of the Joint National Committee on Prevention, Detection, Evaluation, and Treatment of High Blood Pressure (JNC 7) in 2003 and is in the vetting process of the eighth report (NIH & NHLBI, 2004). The first step in effectively controlling hypertension is assessing for it correctly. The standard of care for in-office blood pressure measurement is to take the average of two readings 5 minutes apart with appropriate cuff size while the patient is sitting in a chair with both legs flat on the floor. An abnormal reading should be confirmed in the contralateral arm. Home blood pressure monitoring should be strongly encouraged for those with known or who are at high risk for hypertension. There is growing evidence to support home blood pressure monitoring over ambulatory blood pressure monitoring because patients' readings are closer to the readings taken by 24-hour ambulatory monitors, which eliminates falsely elevated readings from white coat syndrome (Pickering, Miller, Ogedegbe, Krakoff, Artinian, & Goff, 2008). With the plethora of technologically savvy health devices, there are blood pressure cuffs that plug into i-Phones, i-Pads, and other smart devices, collect blood pressure data, and can then transmit the data to clinicians. Electronic health records (EHR) can record the data and send an alert to the patient's clinician when the blood pressure becomes out of target range. Leslie L. Davis, PhD, RN, ANP-BC, published a useful tutorial for clinicians to use to implement home blood pressure monitoring for their patients (Davis, 2011). Dr. Davis is active in the Million Hearts Initiative and is a clinical assistant professor at the University of North Carolina at Chapel Hill in the School of Medicine, Division of Cardiology. Clearly, accurate and consistent blood pressure monitoring is necessary for diagnosing and controlling hypertension.

The algorithm for treating hypertension is seen in Figure 11.4. First-line measures include therapeutic lifestyle modifications. Therapeutic lifestyle modifications include weight loss, the Dietary Approaches to Stop Hypertension (DASH) eating plan, regular exercise, limited alcohol intake, and cessation of tobacco products. Heartening for both care practitioners and patients alike is that weight loss as little as 10 lb (4.5 kg) can reduce blood pressure significantly. The DASH diet includes eating many fruits and vegetables, choosing low-fat varieties of dairy products, choosing low-cholesterol protein sources, overall fat reduction intake to include reduced saturated fats and elimination of trans fat, and a reduced sodium intake. The overall diet should be rich in calcium and potassium. In addition, everyone should engage in aerobic physical activity for at least 30 minutes on most days.

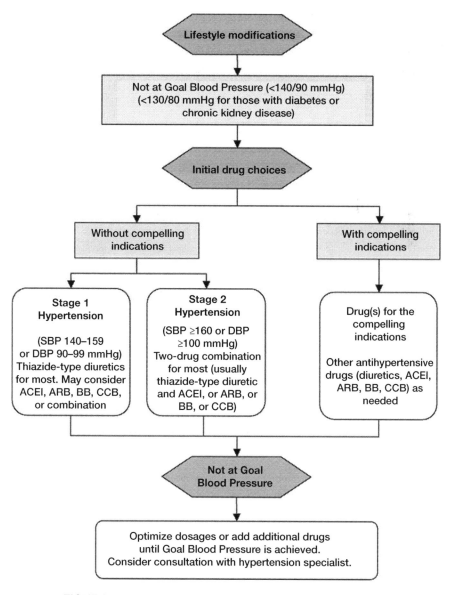

FIGURE 11.4. The JNC 7 Algorithm for Treating Hypertension.

Source: NIH and NHLBI (2004) (used with permission from USDHHS, NIH, & NHLBI).

If the patient is not successful with implementation of lifestyle modifications or progress is too slow or unsuccessful, then pharmacological therapy should be initiated. Most persons with hypertension will require more than one drug to bring their hypertension under adequate control. Some clinicians may begin therapy using a thiazide-diuretic alone or in combination with other classes of agents, especially if the patient is an African American, has diabetes, is obese, and/or has other cardiovascular chronic diseases. The JNC 7 includes goals and modifications of treatment for hypertension that vary for different categories of clinical complexity. The advantage of using multidrug therapy is to achieve greater blood pressure reduction at lower doses that creates fewer side-effects. The consideration to prescribe multiple medications should be balanced with the patient's ability to pay for multiple medications and their ability to adhere to taking multiple drugs, especially if they are needed to be taken more than once or twice a day. However, experiencing fewer side-effects will likely increase adherence. Also noteworthy for adherence considerations is that older diuretics and older beta-blockers dampen erectile function whereas many newer drugs do not (Manolis & Doumas, 2012). Some patients may be hesitant to speak about erectile dysfunction to their clinician so it behooves the clinician to consider erectile dysfunction when assessing causes of low medication adherence. Following the NIH and NHLBI guidelines for follow-up and monitoring of hypertensive patients is essential.

C is for cholesterol management. The NIH, NHLBI, and National Cholesterol Education Program (2002) published its Third Report of the Expert Panel on Detection, Evaluation, and Treatment of High Blood Cholesterol in Adults: Adult Treatment Panel III (ATP III). The guidelines stress that risk assessment is the first step to cholesterol management. In addition to assessing LDL and HDL cholesterol levels, high-risk factors such as tobacco use, genetic predisposition, age, hypertension, metabolic syndrome, and presence of CHD are taken into account. Presence of diabetes without CHD is considered to raise the risk bar considerably. Although some patients are candidates for therapeutic lifestyle changes alone, level of risk will direct clinicians to target lowering LDL cholesterol by adding medications to the treatment plan. While statins remain one of the classes of LDL-lowering agents recommended by the guidelines they are not without their side-effects. Side-effects such as myopathy or the perceived risk of side-effects has led to high levels of statin nonadherence (Harrison et al., 2013). The update of ATP III conducted in 2004 stressed that therapeutic lifestyle changes remain essential. Also reinforced is the treatment goal to lower LDL cholesterol, especially in high-risk patients, and diabetics remain classified as those whose risk is high. These recommendations are currently in review and will be updated again soon.

The S is for smoking cessation, which is already covered in this chapter. Although smoking cessation is critical for primary and secondary prevention of cardiovascular disease, it is also necessary to assess if the patient is using smokeless tobacco products. Nicotine, whether inhaled or absorbed through the mouth, causes vasoconstriction of blood vessels and rises in blood pressure. According to the American Lung Association, 3.3% of adults and 7.4% of high-school students use smokeless tobacco products. Appalling is that 2.6% of middle-school students use smokeless tobacco products as well (statistics available at: www.lung.org/stop-smoking/about-smoking/facts-figures/smokeless-tobacco-products.html#6). These numbers are likely to increase because tobacco companies are spending hundreds of millions of dollars promoting smokeless tobacco products.

HIT is an integral pillar of the Million Hearts Initiative. This technology includes the use of patient registries to identify gaps in CVD, use of multiple methods to track the progress of patients being treated for hypertension or hyperlipidemia, point-of-care risk assessment tools built into EHR to assist clinicians in identifying those at higher risk for disease, clinical decision support mechanisms through EHR systems to assist clinicians to deliver patient-specific care the first time and every time that the patient gets examined, and electronic reminders for consumers that assist them to develop and stick to new, healthier habits, which may include medication adherence (O'Brien, personal communication, March 3, 2011). Encouraging development of Applications or Apps for smart devices has also been a part of the Million Hearts Initiative. The winner of the 2012 Million Hearts Risk Check Challenge, sponsored by the Office of the National Coordinator, is the Marshfield Clinic Research Foundation in Wisconsin. Their Heart Health Mobile App is available in the Apple App Store or as a web-based version (www.hearthealthmobile. com) and is designed to reach those who may not know they are at risk for CHD. The App conducts a quick health risk assessment within an engaging user interface, motivates users to pursue learning their blood pressure and cholesterol values, and directs them to pharmacies in their own communities that offer affordable and convenient blood pressure and cholesterol screenings. Other App finalists include FLORNCE Healthy Heart Coach by mHealthCoach (www.mhealthcoach.com /flornce.html), Know Your Heart by XLBao Lab (www.appszoom.com/android _developer/xlbao-lab_fgrzh.html), HeartHealth Mobile also by Marshfield Clinic Research Foundation (www.hearthealthmobile.com/), HeartSpotter by Alexander Blair (www.heartspotters.com/index.php), and PharmaSmart Blood Pressure Tracker (www.pharma-smart.com). The Million Hearts website also has three App-like interfaces under their tool section to help consumers track and manage their heart health, determine 10-year risk of having a heart attack or dying from CHD, and learn the state of one's heart and about heart healthy behaviors (www.million hearts.hhs.gov/resources/tools.html). These and other innovations are increasing the reach of the Million Hearts Initiative.

A pleasant surprise of the Million Hearts Initiative has been its unintended consequences. This initiative's efforts have had an important positive impact on interagency collaboration within the Department of Health and Human Services, has resulted in the creation of many new private–public partnerships, especially for national nursing organizations, and has led to evidence discovery for interprofessional practice for the common goal of preventing and decreasing the harms of cardiovascular disease. The Community Preventive Services Task Force makes evidence-based reviews about interventions to promote public health and safety. Their members are appointed by the Director of the CDC. In an analysis of 80 studies, team-based care was significantly superior for lowering both systolic and diastolic pressure and improved outcomes for a greater proportion of patients with diabetes and hyperlipidemia than physicians practicing solo (CDC, 2013g). Teams consisted of a primary care provider and another health professional such as a nurse, pharmacist, social worker, dietician, and/or a community health worker. Teams with the greatest proportion of successful blood pressure control were those in which team members could change medications independently or with the approval of the primary care provider. Team member behaviors extended the work of the primary care provider by, "…providing support and sharing responsibility for hypertension care, such as medication management, patient follow-up, and helping the patient adhere to their blood pressure control plan, including monitoring blood pressure routinely, taking medications as prescribed, reducing sodium in the diet, and increasing physical activity (CDC, 2012d)." It is no coincidence that team-based care is a central pillar of the Million Hearts Initiative.

Another unintended consequence of the Million Hearts Initiative is that it is changing the paradigm of practice among the health professions. As discussed, there is a national "tipping point" push for interprofessional and transdisciplinary (includes direct care workers and others without advanced degrees) practice that involves the use of team-specific competencies (Frenk et al., 2010; Interprofessional Education Collaborative Expert Panel, 2011). This team approach to practice, which breaks institutionalized silos between the health professions, is creating higher quality care. Furthermore, through participation in the Million Hearts Initiative, these interprofessional teams and new public–private partnerships are creating more aggressive outreach to identify and begin early intervention of high blood pressure. Another paradigm change is the concept that "It takes a village to prevent and manage hypertension." Dentists, as well as optometrists and pharmacists, are taking blood pressures as a routine part of their intake process. Although the patient has always been the common element across providers of care, Million Hearts provides a more focused strategy and emphasizes the need for everyone to pay attention to the whole patient, whether they are having their eyes examined, getting their teeth cleaned, or having their medications evaluated at a regular checkup. Patients with high blood pressures or prehypertension will be referred to their primary care clinician for follow-up. As the ACA's reach and level of implementation widens, population health will become a greater focus of health professionals who were previously focused solely on their individual patients. There is great optimism that these unintended consequences and many other strategies will help the Million Hearts Initiative to meet its goals.

The Million Hearts Initiative has set both intervention target goals for clinical systems and target goals for the population as a whole to be reached by January of 2017. Table 11.1 shows baseline data from 2011 as well as the target goals.

In order to reach target goals, the Million Hearts Initiative has embedded reporting strategies such as quality measures such as the Physician Quality Reporting System (PQRS) for physicians and other eligible clinicians that supports the ABCS. This reporting system provides Medicare bonus payments or payment reduction for all eligible providers depending on their level of performance and patient outcomes. All APRNs are eligible to report PQRS measures (CMS, 2013a). Moreover, beginning in 2013, eligible health professionals who do not report quality measures will lose incentive payments and get less Medicare Part B reimbursement in a fee-for-service system (CMS, 2013b). Table 11.2 shows which PQRS measures align with which part of the ABCS. Another reporting strategy is that all community health centers funded by HRSA have to report their progress on the ABCS to track and improve their performance (USDHHS, 2011b).

In conclusion, APRNs can lead in improving the health of the nation by simply stepping up what they do really well, and that is blood pressure control and other means to prevent cardiovascular disease and its complications. There are so many opportunities for nurses to partner with the federal government and become a significant part of implementing the ACA in the area of population health than ever before through participation in the Million Hearts Initiative. Federal agencies as well as the White House have taken notice of the role APRNs can have in providing high-value primary care with integration of preventive services. For example, the American Academy of Nursing is producing a white paper on evidence-based best practices with policy recommendations to promote cardiovascular health and wellness based on the ABCS for individuals and populations to include nurse-led models of care. For more information about the Million Hearts Initiative and to access cardiovascular disease risk assessment tools, visit millionhearts.hhs.gov. Million Hearts is a trademark of the USDHHS.

TABLE 11.1 Million Hearts: Status and Targets for the ABCS

INTERVENTION	BASELINE (2011)	JANUARY 2017 TARGET FOR THE POPULATION AS A WHOLE	INTERVENTION TARGET FOR CLINICAL SYSTEMS OF CARE
Aspirin, for those at high risk	47%	65%	70%
Blood pressure control	46%	65%	70%
Cholesterol management	33%	65%	70%
Smoking cessation	23%	65%	70%
Smoking prevalence	19%	17%	
Sodium intake (average)	3.5 g/day	20% reduction	
Artificial trans fat consumption (average)	1% of calories/day	50% reduction	

Sources: Baseline: www.cdc.gov/mmwr/preview/mmwrhtml/mm6036a4.htm?s_cid=mm6036a4_w; 2017 goals of MH: www.millionhearts.hhs.gov/Docs/MH_Fact_Sheet.pdf; and Clinical target goals: www.cdc.gov/about /grand-rounds/archives/2012/pdfs/GR_MH_ALL_FINAL_Feb28.pdf

TABLE 11.2 PQRS Measures that Support the ABCS

ABCS	DOMAIN	MEASURES	2012 PHYSICIAN QUALITY REPORTING SYSTEM (PQRS)
A	Aspirin use	The percentage of patients aged 18 years and older with ischemic vascular disease will have documented use of aspirin or other antithrombotic therapy	#204
B	Blood pressure screening	The percentage of patients aged 18 years and older who are screened for high blood pressure (BP) and have a documented follow-up plan based on current BP readings	#317
	Blood pressure control	The percentage of patients aged 18–85 years who have a diagnosis of hypertension and whose BP was adequately controlled (<140/90) during the measurement year	#236
C	Cholesterol screening and control	The percentage of patients aged 20–79 years whose risk factors have been assessed and a fasting low-density lipoprotein (LDL). LDL test performed and their fasting LDL is at or below the recommended LDL goal after risk stratification	#316
	Cholesterol control–diabetes	The percentage of patients aged 18–75 years with diabetes mellitus who had their most recent LDL-C level in control	#2
	Cholesterol control–ischemic vascular disease	The percentage of patients aged 18 years and older with ischemic vascular disease who received at least one lipid profile within 12 months and who had their most recent LDL-C under control (<100 mg/dL)	#241
S	Smoking cessation	The percentage of patients aged 18 years and older who are screened for tobacco use one or more times within 24 months and received cessation counseling intervention(s) if identified as a tobacco user	#226

Source: Opportunities for Engagement in Million Hearts® (2012).

SCENARIO WITH QUESTIONS

Mrs. S, an African American obese female, has an appointment with you for a yearly physical that is mandated by her employer, a public metro agency where she works as a bus driver. You read on the electronic medical record that last year she weighed 275 lbs and that her height is 5′5″. She was borderline hypertensive and was encouraged to engage in lifestyle modifications. There is a history of adult onset diabetes and hypertension on her mother's side of the family and history of heart disease on her father's side of the family. You assess her on this visit and find that her resting blood pressure (average taken 5 minutes apart) is 150/95, pulse 85, and fasting blood sugar is 110. Her fasting cholesterol remains high with total cholesterol 275 mg/dL, LDL 180 mg/dL, HDL 30 mg/dL, and triglycerides 350 mg/dL. She reports that she drinks alcohol occasionally and is down to smoking 1 pack of cigarettes a day. She has no idea how many milligrams of sodium she consumes every day. She notices that she is getting more short of breath going up the stairs in her home.

1. Does Mrs. S need primary or secondary prevention measures to prevent heart attack and stroke?
2. What other physical and psychosocial information do you need to collect to come up with an appropriate treatment plan for Mrs. S?
3. How would you individualize the ABCS for Mrs. S?
4. Are there any referrals you would like to make and if so what are they?
5. How will you follow up with Mrs. S?

ACTIVITIES

1. Role play this scenario with one student playing Mrs. S and another student playing the APRN.
2. Write a sample office visit history and physical and treatment narrative. Practice the components of motivational interviewing using Mrs. S as the patient.

REFERENCES

American Academy of Nurses (AAN). (2014). *White paper: Evidence-based best practices and policy recommendations to promote cardiovascular health and wellness based on the ABCS for individuals and populations to include nurse-led models of care* [Manuscript in preparation].

American Academy of Nurse Practitioners (AANP). (2010). *2009–10 AANP national NP sample survey.* Retrieved from http://www.aanp.org/research/aanp-research

American Heart Association (AHA). (2013). *Overweight in children.* Retrieved from http://www.heart .org/HEARTORG/GettingHealthy/Overweight-in-Children_UCM_304054_Article.jsp

American Nurses Association (ANA). (2010). *Nursing's social policy statement: The essence of the profession.* Silver Spring, MD: Author.

ANA. (2011). *Advanced practice nursing: A new age in healthcare.* Retrieved from http://www.nursingworld .org/FunctionalMenuCategories/MediaResources/MediaBackgrounders/APRN-A-New-Age -in-Health-Care.pdf

Centers for Disease Control and Prevention (CDC). (2011a). *Most Americans with high blood pressure and high cholesterol at unnecessary risk for heart attack and stroke.* Retrieved from http://www.cdc.gov /media/releases/2011/p0201_vitalsigns.html

CDC. (2011b). *Rising health care costs are unsustainable.* Retrieved from http://www.cdc.gov/workplace healthpromotion/businesscase/reasons/rising.html

CDC. (2011c). *New Million Hearts tools announced by partners.* Retrieved from http://www.millionhearts .hhs.gov/docs/MH_Partners_Press_Release_11-3-2011.pdf

CDC. (2012a). *Prevalence of overweight, obesity, and extreme obesity among adults: United States, trends 1960–1962 through 2009–2010.* Retrieved from http://www.cdc.gov/nchs/data/hestat/obesity _adult_09_10/obesity_adult_09_10.pdf

CDC. (2012b). *CDC vital signs: Where's the sodium? There's too much in many common foods.* Retrieved from http://www.cdc.gov/vitalsigns/Sodium/index.html

CDC. (2012c). *Nutrition for everyone: Trans fat.* Retrieved from http://www.cdc.gov/nutrition/everyone /basics/fat/transfat.html

CDC. (2012d). *Task force recommends team-based care for improving blood pressure control.* Retrieved from http://www.cdc.gov/media/releases/2012/p0515_bp_control.html

CDC. (2013). *Division for Heart Disease and Stroke Prevention: CDC National Heart Disease and Stroke Prevention Program.* Retrieved from http://www.cdc.gov/dhdsp/programs/nhdsp_program

CDC. (2013a). *Heart disease facts.* Retrieved from http://www.cdc.gov/heartdisease/facts.htm

CDC. (2013b). *High blood pressure.* Retrieved from http://www.cdc.gov/bloodpressure

CDC. (2013c). Self-reported hypertension and use of antihypertensive medication among adults—United States, 2005–2009. *Morbidity and Mortality Weekly Report, 62*(13), 237–244. Retrieved from http:// www.cdc.gov/mmwr/preview/mmwrhtml/mm6213a2.htm?s_cid=mm6213a2_e

CDC. (2013d). *High blood pressure facts.* Retrieved from http://www.cdc.gov/bloodpressure/facts.htm

CDC. (2013e). *Adult cigarette smoking in the United States: Current estimate.* Retrieved from http://www .cdc.gov/tobacco/data_statistics/fact_sheets/adult_data/cig_smoking/index.htm

CDC. (2013f). *Education campaign returns with powerful stories to help Americans quit smoking.* Retrieved from http://www.cdc.gov/media/releases/2013/p0328_TIPS_campaign.html

CDC. (2013g). *Cardiovascular disease prevention: Team-based care to improve blood pressure control—Task force finding and rationale statement.* Retrieved from http://www.thecommunityguide.org/cvd /RRteambasedcare.html

CDC. (2013h). Notes from the field: Electronic cigarette use among middle and high school students—United States, 2011–2012. *Morbidity and Mortality Weekly Report (MMWR), September 6, 2013, 62*(35), 729–730. Retrieved from http://www.cdc.gov/mmwr/preview/mmwrhtml/mm6235a6 .htm

Centers for Medicare & Medicaid Services (CMS). (2013a). *Physician quality reporting system (PQRS): List of eligible professionals.* Retrieved from http://www.cms.gov/Medicare/Quality-Initiatives-Patient -Assessment-Instruments/PQRS/Downloads/PQRS_List-of-EligibleProfessionals_022813.pdf

CMS. (2013b). *Spotlight.* Retrieved from http://www.cms.gov/Medicare/Quality-Initiatives-Patient -Assessment-Instruments/PQRS/Spotlight.html

Davis, L. (2011). *How to implement home BP monitoring: The clinical advisor.* Retrieved from http://www .clinicaladvisor.com/how-to-implement-home-bp-monitoring/article/206808/1

Frenk, J., Chen, L., Bhutta, Z. A., Cohen, J., Crisp, N., Evans, T., ... Zurayk, H. (2010). Health professionals for a new century: Transforming education to strengthen health systems in an interdependent world. *Lancet, 376*(9756), 1923–1958.

Frieden, T. R., & Berwick, D. M. (2011). The "Million Hearts" initiative—Preventing heart attacks and strokes. *New England Journal of Medicine, 365,* e27. Retrieved from http://www.nejm.org/doi /full/10.1056/NEJMp1110421

George, M. G., Tong, X., Sonnenfeld, N., & Hong, Y. (2012). Recommended use of aspirin and other antiplatelet medications among adults—National ambulatory medical care survey and national hospital ambulatory medical care survey, United States, 2005–2008. *Morbidity and Mortality Weekly Report, 61*(2), 11–18. Retrieved from http://www.cdc.gov/mmwr/preview/mmwrhtml /su6102a3.htm

Harrison, T. N., Derose, S. F., Cheetham, T. C., Chiu, V., Vansomphone, S. S., Green, K., & Reynolds, K. (2013). Primary nonadherence to statin therapy: Patients' perceptions. *American Journal of Managed Care, 19*(4), e133-139.

Health Affairs. (2010). Health policy brief: Preventive services without cost sharing. *Health Affairs.* Retrieved from http://www.healthaffairs.org/healthpolicybriefs/brief.php?brief_id=37

Health Affairs. (2013). Health policy brief: Nurse practitioners and primary care. *Health Affairs.* Retrieved from http://www.healthaffairs.org/healthpolicybriefs/brief_pdfs/healthpolicybrief_92.pdf

Health Resources and Services Administration (HRSA). (2010). *The registered nurse population: Initial findings from the 2008 national sample survey of registered nurses.* Retrieved from http://bhpr.hrsa.gov /healthworkforce/rnsurveys/rnsurveyfinal.pdf

HRSA. (2013). *School-based health centers.* Retrieved from http://www.hrsa.gov/ourstories/school healthcenters

HealthyPeople. (2020). *Heart disease and stroke.* Retrieved from http://www.healthypeople.gov/2020 /topicsobjectives2020/overview.aspx?topicid=21#two

Institute of Medicine (IOM). (2010). *The future of nursing: Leading change, advancing health.* Washington, DC: National Academies Press. Retrieved from http://www.iom.edu/Reports/2010/The-Future-of -Nursing-Leading-Change-Advancing-Health.aspx

IOM. (2013). *Sodium intake in populations: Assessment of evidence.* Washington, DC: National Academies Press. Retrieved from http://www.iom.edu/Reports/2013/Sodium-Intake-in-Populations -Assessment-of-Evidence.aspx

Interprofessional Education Collaborative Expert Panel. (2011). *Core competencies for interprofessional collaborative practice: Report of an expert panel.* Washington, DC: Interprofessional Education Collaborative. Retrieved from http://www.aacn.nche.edu/education-resources/ipecreport.pdf

Kochanek, K. D., Xu, J. Q., Murphy, S. L., Miniño, A. M., & Kung, H. C. (2011). Deaths: Final data for 2009. *National Vital Statistics Reports, 60*(3). Retrieved from http://www.cdc.gov/nchs/data/nvsr /nvsr60/nvsr60_03.pdf

Kovner, C., & Walani, S. (2010). *Nurse managed health centers: Robert Wood Johnson Foundation Research Brief.* Retrieved from http://www.thefutureofnursing.org/sites/default/files/Research%20Brief-%20 Nurse%20Managed%20Health%20Centers.pdf

Lloyd-Jones, D., Adams, R. J., Brown, T. M., Carnethon, M., Dai, S., De Simone, G., ... Wylie-Rosett, J. (2010). Heart disease and stroke statistics—2010 update: A report from the American Heart Association. *Circulation, 121*(7), e46–e215. Retrieved from http://www.circ.ahajournals.org /content/121/7/e46.long

Manolis, A., & Doumas, M. (2012). Antihypertensive treatment and sexual dysfunction. *Current Hypertension Reports, 14*(4), 285–292.

McMenamin, P. (2013). *In 2011 in every state thousands of Medicare F-F-S beneficiaries were treated by an APRN.* American Nurses Association Nurse Space. Retrieved from http://www.ananursespace .org/BlogsMain/BlogViewer/?BlogKey=9632c2fa-6fc3-4a1b-93ad-343cd90058f1&ssopc=1

National Assembly on School-Based Health Care. (2007–2008). *School-based health centers: National census 2007–2008.* Retrieved from http://www.nasbhc.org/atf/cf/%7Bcd9949f2-2761-42fb-bc7a-cee 165c701d9%7D/NASBHC%202007-08%20CENSUS%20REPORT%20FINAL.PDF

National Center for Health Statistics (NCHS). (2001). *Healthy people 2000 final review.* Hyattsville, MD: Public Health Service. Retrieved from http://www.cdc.gov/nchs/data/hp2000/hp2k01.pdf

National Institutes of Health (NIH), & National Heart, Lung, and Blood Institute (NHLBI). (2004). *The seventh report of the joint national committee on prevention, detection, evaluation, and treatment of high blood pressure.* Retrieved from http://www.nhlbi.nih.gov/guidelines/hypertension/jnc7full.pdf

NIH & NHLBI (2013). *Your guide to lowering high blood pressure: Reduce salt and sodium in your diet.* Retrieved from http://www.nhlbi.nih.gov/hbp/prevent/sodium/sodium.htm

NIH, NHLBI, & National Cholesterol Education Program. (2002). *Detection, evaluation and treatment of high blood cholesterol in adults: Adult treatment panel III (ATP III).* Retrieved from http://www.nhlbi .nih.gov/guidelines/cholesterol/atp3full.pdf

Opportunities for Engagement in Million Hearts®. (2012). Retrieved from www.millionhearts.hhs.gov /docs/Field_Engagement_Opportunities.pdf

Parekh, A. K., Galloway, J. M., Hong, Y., & Wright, J. S. (2013). Aspirin in the secondary prevention of cardiovascular disease. *New England Journal of Medicine, 368*(3), 204–205.

Pbert, L., Druker, S., DiFranza, J. R., Gorak, D., Reed, G., Magner, R., ... Osganian, S. (2011). Effectiveness of a school nurse-delivered smoking-cessation intervention for adolescents. *Pediatrics, 128*(5), 926–936.

Pickering, T. G., Miller, N. H., Ogedegbe, G., Krakoff, L. R., Artinian, N. T., & Goff, D. (2008). Call to action on use and reimbursement for home blood pressure monitoring: A joint scientific statement from the American Heart Association, American Society of Hypertension, and Preventive Cardiovascular Nurses Association. *Hypertension, 52*, 10–29. Retrieved from http://hyper.aha journals.org/content/52/1/1.long

Robert Wood Johnson Foundation (RWJF). (2012). *Implementing the IOM future of nursing report—Part III: How nurses are solving some of primary care's most pressing challenges.* Retrieved from http:// www .rwjf.org/content/dam/files/file-queue/cnf20120810.pdf

The Tobacco Use and Dependence Clinical Practice Guideline Panel, Staff, and Consortium Representatives. (2000). A clinical practice guideline for treating tobacco use and dependence: A U.S. public health service report. *Journal of the American Medical Association, 283*(24), 3244–3254.

U.S. Department of Agriculture and the U.S. Department of Health and Human Services (USDHHS). (2010). *Dietary guidelines for Americans.* Retrieved from http://www.health.gov/dietaryguidelines /dga2010/dietaryguidelines2010.pdf

USDHHS. (2008). *Clinical practice guideline: Treating tobacco use and dependence—2008 update.* Retrieved from http://www.ahrq.gov/professionals/clinicians-providers/guidelines-recommendations /tobacco/clinicians/treating_tobacco_use08.pdf

USDHHS. (2010). *HealthyPeople 2020.* Office of Disease Prevention and Health Promotion. Retrieved from http://www.healthypeople.gov

USDHHS. (2011a). *Report to congress: National strategy for quality improvement in health care.* Retrieved from http://www.ahrq.gov/workingforquality/nqs/nqs2011annlrpt.pdf

USDHHS. (2011b). *New public–private sector initiative aims to prevent 1 million heart attacks and strokes in five years.* Retrieved from http://www.hhs.gov/news/press/2011pres/09/20110913a.html

USDHHS. (2012a). *Attachment to the annual progress report to congress national strategy for quality improvement in health care: Agency-specific quality strategic plans.* Retrieved from http://www.ahrq.gov /workingforquality/nqs/nqsplans.pdf

USDHHS. (2012b). *Preventing tobacco use among youth and young adults: A report of the Surgeon General.* Atlanta, GA: U.S. Department of Health and Human Services, Centers for Disease Control and Prevention, National Center for Chronic Disease Prevention and Health Promotion, Office on Smoking and Health. Retrieved from http://www.surgeongeneral.gov/library/reports/preventing -youth-tobacco-use/full-report.pdf

USDHHS. (2013a). *The million hearts initiative.* Retrieved from http://www.millionhearts.hhs.gov/index .html

USDHHS. (2013b). *The healthcare law and you: Read the law.* Retrieved from http://www.healthcare.gov /law/full/index.html

U.S. Preventive Services Task Force (USPSTF). (2009). *Aspirin for the prevention of cardiovascular disease.* Retrieved from http://www.uspreventiveservicestaskforce.org/uspstf/uspsasmi.htm

USPSTF. (2012). *Grade definitions.* Retrieved from http://www.uspreventiveservicestaskforce.org/uspstf /grades.htm

USPSTF. (2013). USPSTF A and B recommendations. Retrieved from http://www.uspreventive servicestaskforce.org/uspstf/uspsabrecs.htm

Wright, W. L., Romboli, J. E., DiTulio, M. A., Wogen, J., & Belletti, D. A. (2011). Hypertension treatment and control within an independent nurse practitioner setting. *American Journal of Managed Care, 17*(1), 58–65. Retrieved from http://www.ajmc.com/publications/issue/2011/2011-1-vol17-n1 /AJMC_2011jan_Wright_58to65/3

Joining Forces: Taking Action to Serve America's Military Families— A White House Initiative

Cathy Rick

> *Vision without action is merely a dream.*
> *Action without vision just passes the time.*
> *Vision with action can change the world.*
> —Joel Barker

The Joining Forces initiative was launched by First Lady Michelle Obama and Dr. Jill Biden in April 2010. This national initiative mobilizes all sectors of society to give service members, their families, and veterans the opportunities and support they have earned. According to Mrs. Obama and Dr. Biden, 1% of Americans may be fighting our wars, but we need 100% of Americans to be supporting our troops and their families. Mrs. Obama and Dr. Biden are asking Americans to get involved in any way they can. Representing only 1% of our population in the United States, our military willingly takes on the ultimate responsibility of protecting our entire nation. Missing small moments of each day that we often take for granted here at home, as well as irreplaceable milestones like birthdays, anniversaries, graduations, etc. with people they love, our service members make incredible sacrifices and put themselves in harm's way for the sake of us all. They do not make these sacrifices alone. When our troops are called to action, so are their families. In their unconditional support and care for those who are serving, military families show us what words such as "service," "strength," and "sacrifice" truly mean. They sustain the troops that are defending America, tend to our wounded warriors, and survive our fallen. Military families—spouses and children alike—remind us that with everything these families do to serve our country, in turn their nation has an obligation to serve them. The needs of our military families cannot be met solely in Washington, or by improving support provided by government alone. It is up to the other 99% to make sure that these families are receiving the respect and consideration they so deserve (www.whitehouse.gov/joiningforces).

BACKGROUND

Recognizing and supporting our nation's veterans dates back to the Civil War. First and foremost, it is the obligation of America's citizens to understand the primary needs of service members, their families, and veterans. Experiences related to preparing for combat, frequent uprooting of family, and vulnerability of engagement in war are encounters that impact day-to-day lives during and after separation from military service. Unless an individual is personally immersed in those experiences, it is a significant challenge to identify with or effectively support those who have served. The public sector (county, state, and federal) has dedicated specialized services to meet the needs of military service members, their families, and veterans. However, these specialized services do not have the capacity to meet the needs of all deserving their support. Thus, there is a need for all of our nation's citizens to become aware and better prepared to care for those who are currently serving or have served our country. Spelman and colleagues (Spelman, Hunt, Seal, & Burgo-Black, 2012) offer the following helpful insights. Since September 11, 2001, 2.4 million military personnel have deployed to Iraq and Afghanistan. As of May 2012, roughly 1.44 million separated from military service and approximately 772,000 of those veterans sought care at the Veterans' Health Administration (VHA) within the Department of Veterans Affairs (VA). Combat deployments impact the physical, psychological, and social health of veterans. Given that many veterans are receiving care from providers and practice settings other than the VHA, it is important that all community health care workers be familiar with the unique needs of this patient population, which include injuries associated with blast exposures such as mild traumatic brain injury (TBI), as well as a variety of mental health conditions such as post-traumatic stress disorder (PTSD).

There are many psychological stressors associated with combat deployment. These include anticipation of combat, combat and noncombatant-related psychological trauma, military sexual trauma, and separation from home and family. Psychosocial risks of combat include marital instability, unemployment/underemployment, financial decline, social isolation, and legal problems. In addition, recent evidence suggests a higher incidence of mental health diagnoses in spouses of veterans who have deployed, particularly if there has been prolonged deployment. Recent improvements in personal protective gear and battlefield emergency medical care has resulted in decreased mortality, yet increased morbidity in soldiers surviving their injuries.

Currently, many surviving soldiers face serious long-term consequences such as amputations, spinal cord injuries, and traumatic brain injuries. Common causes of TBI include blasts, bullets, shrapnel fragments, falls, or motor vehicle accidents. TBIs can range in severity from mild TBI (often used interchangeably with the term concussion) to severe TBI.

CONCEPTUAL FOUNDATION

Professional nursing practice considers conceptual frameworks or theories to be foundational guides for understanding the context of emerging needs. This section outlines a relevant theory that supports the work of the Joining Forces initiative. It is offered as a relevant background to those who develop specific strategies and action plans in support of service members, their families, and veterans.

Nurse clinicians, administrators, educators, and researchers would be well served by considering that health care that is based on the principles of partnerships for health and self-care would likely achieve the desired future state as outlined by the Joining Forces initiative. Although the specifics of how best to care for those who have served our country are vitally important, it is beyond the scope of this chapter to outline the detailed clinical skills or competencies to meet those needs. General concepts and strategies for developing partnerships to enhance the health and self-care management of military service members, their families, and veterans are described.

The Interagency Policy Committee, with the involvement of the National Economic Council, Office of the First Lady identified four areas to address the concerns and challenges of families of military service members, veterans, and those who have fallen (Figure 12.1). The White House Joining Forces initiative was

---

Four Priority Areas to Address Concerns and Challenges of Service Members, Families and Veterans

1. Enhance the well-being and psychological health of the military family
    a. By increasing behavioral health care services through prevention based alternatives and integrating community-based services;
    b. By building awareness among military families and communities that psychological fitness is as important as physical fitness;
    c. By protecting military service members and families from unfair financial practices and helping families enhance their financial readiness;
    d. By eliminating homelessness and promoting home security among veterans and military families; and
    e. By making our court systems more responsive to the unique needs of veterans and families.
2. Ensure excellence in military children's education and their development
    a. By improving the quality of the educational experience;
    b. By reducing negative impacts of frequent relocations and absences; and
    c. By encouraging the healthy development of military children.
3. Develop career and educational opportunities for military spouses
    a. By increasing opportunities for Federal careers;
    b. By increasing opportunities for private-sector careers;
    c. By increasing access to educational advancement;
    d. By reducing barriers to employment and services due to different State policies and standards; and
    e. By protecting the rights of service members and families.
4. Increase child care availability and quality for Armed Forces
    a. By enhancing child care resources within the Department of Defense and the Coast Guard.

This is an enduring effort. Each Cabinet secretary has pledged his or her individual commitment to this important task. Together as a team, we are committed to implementing our plans, assessing our results on a recurring basis with continued transparency, seeking constant feedback, and ensuring the Federal Government has the capacity to support and engage military families throughout their lives.

White House Report: Strengthening our Military Families: Meeting America's Commitment January 2011, Pages 2–3.

FIGURE 12.1 Four Priority Areas to Address Concerns and Challenges of Service Members, Families and Veterans.

launched to mobilize Americans to partner across multiple segments of society to become better prepared to meet the needs of this special population. The stated priorities of the initiative are employment, education, and wellness. These priority areas have been described in the scientific literature as cornerstones of a healthy community. Nursing theorists such as Orem and Henderson describe the efficacy of approaches to support self-care management. These theoretical constructs provide the underpinning for the nursing profession to take an active role in the Joining Forces initiative.

Virginia Henderson theorized that as a patient receives treatment and is on the road to recovery, it is important that the patient is able to take care of themselves after being released from medical care. To that end, nurses should be caring for the patient while, at the same time, be helping the patient become more independent and reach goals and milestones on the road to health. Virginia Henderson's Need Theory (1966) addresses this issue and helps nurses to help patients so that they can care for themselves when they leave the health care facility.

The Nursing Need Theory was derived from Henderson's practice and education. Henderson's goal was not to develop a theory of nursing, but rather to define the unique focus of nursing practice. This theory emphasizes the importance of increasing the patient's independence so that the progress after hospitalization would not be delayed. Her emphasis on basic human needs as the central focus of nursing practice has led to further theory development regarding the needs of the patient and how nursing can assist in meeting those needs.

Henderson (1966) identified three major assumptions in her model of nursing. The first is that "nurses care for a patient until a patient can care for him or herself," though it is not stated explicitly. The second assumption states that nurses are willing to serve and that "nurses will devote themselves to the patient day and night." Finally, the third assumption is that nurses should be educated at the college level in both sciences and arts.

The four major concepts addressed in Henderson's theory (1966) are the individual, the environment, health, and nursing. The introduction and background sections provided in this chapter identify the relationship between individual, environment, and health for military service members, their families, and veterans. Thus, Henderson's theory supports the role of nursing in addressing the needs of this unique population. Advanced practice registered nurses (APRNs) have and will continue to play a pivotal role in health care approaches supported by Henderson's theory.

According to Henderson (1966), individuals have basic needs that are components of health. She emphasizes the point that individuals may require assistance to achieve health and independence, or assistance to achieve a peaceful death. For the individual, mind and body are inseparable and interrelated, and the individual considers the biological, psychological, sociological, and spiritual components—a clear correlation to today's descriptions of health care needs of military service members, their families, and veterans. This theory presents the patient as a sum of parts with biophysical needs rather than as a type of client or consumer.

Henderson (1966) postulated that the environment (such as encountered through military experience) is made up of settings in which an individual learns unique patterns for living—all external conditions and influences that affect life and development. The environment also includes individuals in relation to families. This theory minimally discusses the impact of the community on the individual and family. Basic nursing care involves providing conditions in which the patient can perform independently.

"The unique function of the nurse is to assist the individual, sick or well, in the performance of those activities contributing to health or its recovery (or to peaceful death) that would perform unaided if he had the necessary strength, will, or knowledge—and to do this in such a way as to help him gain independence as rapidly as possible" (Henderson, 1966). Additional foundational concepts are provided by the work published in the Institute of Medicine (IOM) Report on *The Future of Nursing: Leading Change and Advancing Health* (2010). This report outlines the following four key messages that are relevant to this discussion on the role of APRNs in meeting the needs of military service members, their families, and veterans:

1. Nurses should practice to the full extent of their education and training.
2. Nurses should achieve higher levels of education and training through an improved education system that promotes seamless academic progression.
3. Nurses should be full partners, with physicians and other health professionals, in redesigning health care in the United States.
4. Effective workforce planning and policy making require better data collection and improved information infrastructure.

(IOM, 2010, p. 4)

APPLICATION TO APRNs

APRNs have advanced clinical knowledge and skills to provide direct care to patients in a defined component of practice. All APRNs have a significant component of education and practice focusing on direct care of individuals. The APRN Consensus Model (2008) defines APRNs as licensed independent practitioners who are expected to practice within the standards established or recognized by a licensing body. Each APRN is accountable to patients, the nursing profession, and the licensing board and must comply with the requirements of the state nurse practice act and the quality of advanced nursing care rendered; for recognizing limits of knowledge and experience, planning for the management of situations beyond the APRN's expertise; and for consulting with or referring patients to other health care providers as appropriate.

The work and commitment of APRNs are essential to advance the intentions of the Joining Forces initiative. APRNs have expertise across the continuum of care and their demonstrated leadership capabilities are vital characteristics that the nursing profession relies upon to enhance the health of America's citizens. With focused attention on military service members, their families, and veterans, APRNs can lead the way in meeting the needs of this deserving population. It is suggested that APRNs seek a sound understanding of the unique aspects of health and well-being in the context of education, employment, and wellness for this population. The importance of interprofessional interdependence must be recognized as APRNs advance health and lead change for our nation's heroes. Collective efforts across nursing communities and multidisciplinary teams will bring a coordinated effort to the forefront. Advanced practice nurses should engage nursing administration, nursing management, clinical nurse leaders (CNLs) who shape practice at the microsystem level working with teams at every point of care, and all staff nurses. In addition, APRN-led partnerships across thought leaders in practice, academic, research, and community settings would be effective approaches to mobilize all sectors of society to give service members, their families, and veterans the opportunities and support they have earned. This has already proven to be effective by the earlier efforts of key officials in nursing organizations such as the American Nurses Association (ANA), the American Academy of Nurse Practitioners, the American Psychiatric Nurses Association, the American Association of Colleges of Nursing, and the National Association of Clinical Nurse

Specialists. These organizations have developed specific strategies to raise awareness of their members and provide resources to members in areas of mental health, TBI, and PTSD. APRN members of these organizations can play an active role in advancing the health of this special population. Many APRNs fill faculty positions at academic institutions. It is important for these practicing APRN faculty members to bring their specialized knowledge and expertise regarding military service and veteran specific needs to the next generation of nurses through their academic studies and clinical experiences. Launching health system workgroups, community groups, or on-campus programs (grade school, high school, and higher education settings) to address the needs of military service members, their families, and veterans will have significant impact on elevating awareness and ability to support this deserving population.

EVALUATION CONCEPTS

Metrics aligned with successful outcomes of APRN involvement in advancing the objectives of the Joining Forces initiative are essential aspects to consider. Individual and groups of APRNs can and should consider actions that will realize a positive impact on the understanding of the special needs of military service members, their families, and veterans, and more importantly, move citizens of the nation and their communities to provide the deserved support to these heroes. APRN engagement in their practice settings, networks of colleagues, friends, and families along with their professional organizations will result in the enhanced engagement in support of these heroes in communities across the nation.

Success will be defined by having citizens of all ages well informed about the laudable characteristics and risks and challenges faced by military service members, their families, and veterans. Teachers in all settings will include didactic and experiential offerings to students in elementary, secondary, graduate, and postgraduate coursework. Professional nursing organizations will focus strategic initiatives on objectives of the Joining Forces initiative with consideration to relevant references and evidence-based practice scenarios on their websites as well as include appropriate information in general communication and conference planning activities. Faith communities will come to understand the unique needs and skills that military service members and veterans bring to their work. Employers will seek opportunities to support this special population by recognizing their skills and competencies developed through their military life experiences. Community engagement will include development of special interest groups for military service members, their families, and veterans allowing for self-awareness and mutual support with the assistance of references or resources based on best practices. Bottom line—the success of the Joining Forces initiative will be evident when these deserving citizens are recognized, understood, and supported during peace time as well as during war and international conflicts.

THOUGHTS FOR DISCUSSION

Behavioral health disorders are common among troops that have returned from war zones. This observation is not new. A report based on health records of Civil War Veterans showed life-long health consequences of combat even among those who escaped traumatic injury. Surveys of U.S. combat units returning from the war in Iraq (Hoge et al., 2004) found that as many as one in four soldiers met criteria for a behavioral health disorder. Among this group, less than one in three soldiers had received help from a behavioral health or primary care professional. The gap between the need for treatment and receiving it deserves urgent attention by APRNs.

According to experts from the Uniformed Services University stated, there is a need to put into practice a systematic primary care approach to the management of depression. The advanced practitioner leads change and advances health by example and through active involvement in systems redesign and continuous improvement. This places the APRN community in a unique position of being a catalyst for policy setting at a care delivery level by leading programs and projects targeted to support military service members, their families, and veterans. The unique contributions of APRNs should focus on local policy setting in practice sites as well as community services and governance. APRNs can lead policy efforts to include military experiences in admission assessments and plans of care to include strategies for spouses and children of service members and veterans. The cumulative impact of multiple deployments is associated with more emotional difficulties among military children and more mental health diagnoses among spouses (Lester et al., 2010).

Reducing these negative effects requires a robust psychological health plan, such as better data collection, reducing stigma-related barriers, and stronger involvement from the chain of command (Mansfield et al., 2010). APRNs should consider targeted efforts to address these needs. Special attention should also be paid to advanced practice nursing competencies related to prevention of suicide because research has shown that veterans who have attempted suicide not only have an elevated risk of further suicide attempts, but also face mortality risks from all causes at a rate three times greater than the general population (Richmond, 2012). Richmond (2012) further urged rigorous efforts to identify and support at-risk veterans, especially those who have previously attempted suicide. APRNs are well positioned to influence academic preparation of future health professionals by providing mentorship and preceptorship for students and trainees. In addition, APRNs have appropriate avenues to be involved in curriculum development with academic affiliates through adjunct faculty roles and practice/academic partnerships that are not necessarily available to other segments of the nursing workforce.

APRNs providing care to school-age children need to recognize that according to Blue Star Families (2010), "there are 1.9 million children with a parent serving in the military. 220,000 of these children had a parent deployed in 2011. At that time, there were 153,669 single parents serving in the military. The demands of the extended conflict added to the challenges faced by military families. Research suggests that children of deployed parents experience more stress than peers. While they are often described as a resilient group, the cumulative effects of multiple moves and significant parental absences can erode this resilience. Too many of our military children in public schools feel like their classmates and teachers do not understand what they are going through. Between frequent moves and service member time away from home, many parents worry about their children getting a good education and staying healthy. A recent survey found 34% are 'less or not confident' that their children's school is responsive for the unique aspects of military family life."

The ANA, in partnership with the Office of Nursing Service (ONS), Department of VA hosted a Leadership Summit for the Joining Forces initiative (April, 2011). Key participants and contributors at that summit included national organizations representing APRNs across the nation. The American Academy of Nurse Practitioners and the American Psychiatric Nurses Association played a prominent role at the summit providing useful resources and commitment to several activities to enhance and sustain the efforts to support our national heroes. ANA pledged to host a public website (www.ANAJoiningForces.org) for coordination of efforts between nursing organizations and academic institutions. Representatives from the American Association of Nurse Anesthetists, American College of Nurse Midwives, and International Nurses

Society on Addictions were among the many voices that came together to represent the work of APRNs that could be dedicated to the Joining Forces initiative. A summary of guided tabletop discussions around what is being done, what can be done, and how best to partner was developed and is available on the ANA portal to Joining Forces (www.nursingworld.org). Dissemination of ongoing efforts continues to be supported by a list serve of interested organizations, academic institutions, and practice settings. In addition, Joining Forces partnered with Medscape, the leading provider of online continuing medical education, as well as the National Association of Community Health Centers, which represent the health centers that provide health care for more than 20 million individuals in over 8,000 locations across the country. Several hundred professional and educational associations have enthusiastically partnered with Joining Forces by pledging (Figure 12.2) to make commitments

---

Nursing Pledge

Support our Military Service Members, Veterans, and their Families

Joining Forces is First Lady Michelle Obama's comprehensive national initiative to mobilize all sectors of the community to give our service members, veterans, and their families the support they deserve, particularly when it comes to employment, education, and wellness (http://www.whitehouse.gov/joiningforces).

Our military service members, veterans, and their families have made a significant contribution to our nation's safety and security. This contribution has been at great cost to each veteran and her or his family. The profession of nursing has a long and established history of meeting and supporting the physical and mental health needs of our nation's military service members, veterans, and their families. So, the profession of nursing has pledged to inspire and prepare each nurse to recognize the unique health and wellness concerns of this population.

And with this pledge, the profession of nursing is committed to:

- Educating America's future nurses to care for our nation's veterans, service members, and their families facing post-traumatic stress disorder, traumatic brain injury, depression, and other clinical issues;

- Enriching nursing education to ensure that current and future nurses are educated and trained in the unique clinical challenges and best practices associated with caring for military service members, veterans, and their families;

- Disseminating the most up-to-date information as it relates to traumatic brain injury (TBI) and psychological health conditions, such as post traumatic stress disorder (PTSD);

- Growing the body of knowledge leading to improvements in health care and wellness for our military service members, veterans, and their families; and

- Leading and advancing the supportive community of nurses, institutions, and health care providers dedicated to improving the health of military service members, veterans, and their families.

By Joining Forces, the profession of nursing will inspire and prepare each nurse to recognize the unique health and wellness concerns of the population, and thereby improve the lives of those who have sacrificed in the service of our country.

FIGURE 12.2 Nursing Pledge.

and launch efforts to help to educate their members about military and veterans' health issues. Collectively, these organizations represent more than 4 million future or currently practicing health professionals. Specifically, nursing schools and groups pledged to educate their students and members on the most common health issues facing veterans, such as PTSD and TBI; to disseminate effective models of care and share the most up-to-date information across academic and practice settings; and to partner with others to expand the body of clinical knowledge in these areas. APRNs across the nation are engaged and are a vital force within the initiative.

ETHICAL CONSIDERATIONS

Ethical considerations are those moral principles that govern our behavior with honesty and integrity. APRNs are reminded of the rules of conduct that guide their practice as described by the ANA (2010) Code of Ethics, which are a written set of guidelines issued to help practitioners conduct their actions in accordance with the primary values and standard of the profession. The nurses' primary commitment is to the patient, whether an individual, family, group, or community. The Joining Forces initiative has sharpened our focus on a commitment to the individuals, families, and populations of military service members, and veterans. It is not acceptable to overlook or neglect the unique needs of these deserving individuals. So, there is a clear ethical imperative for APRNs to engage in further learning regarding this important segment of society and to develop appropriate strategies to embed appropriate practice standards to meet their needs. The ANA (2010) Code of Ethics further delineates ethical requirements for collaboration. The ANA (2010) Code of Ethics identified that:

> ...collaboration is not just cooperation, but it is the concerted effort of individuals and groups to attain a shared goal. In health care, that goal is to address the health needs of the patient and the public ... Nurses should work to assure the relevant parties are involved and have a voice in decision making about patient care issues. Nurses should see that the questions that need to be addressed are asked and that the information needed for informed decision making is available and provided. Nurses should actively promote the collaborative multidisciplinary planning required to ensure the availability and accessibility of quality health services to all persons who have needs for health care.
>
> *(ANA, 2010, p. 5)*

APRNs have played a pivotal role in shaping ethical approaches for collaboration among community partners as a key aspect of their engagement in the Joining Forces initiative.

DISCUSSION QUESTIONS

1. What are current policies in your practice setting that focus on military service members, families, and veterans?
2. Are you aware of typical needs of children of military service members or veterans? Do you know how to access reliable resources to gain a better understanding of veterans' typical health care needs?
3. Are standards and criteria established for APRN practice related to veterans? Who develops these standards? How and by whom are APRNs evaluated against these standards?

4. Should APRN certification and/or licensing examinations include aspects of caring for military service members, their families, and veterans?
5. What does Veterans Day mean to you, your family, your faith community, your children's school, and your spouse's workplace?
6. Have you pledged to support the Joining Forces initiative?

SYNTHESIS EXERCISES

1. Conduct a focus group of military service members to gain an understanding of the impact of this service.
2. Conduct a focus group of veterans of different eras/age groups to gain understanding of the impact of their service.
3. Interview an elected official of an APRN professional organization to discuss veteran-specific strategies.
4. Develop a sample model for educating and empowering veterans and their families through a proactive outreach by leveraging partnerships.
5. Discuss strategies to improve the perception and understanding of VA care in the private sector.
6. Develop and disseminate best practices to professional colleagues in your practice setting to support veterans and their families.
7. Speak to a leader of a faith community to provide advice on potential strategies to strengthen support for service members, their families, and veterans.
8. Develop a self-care tool for service members, families, or veterans.
9. Develop a list of research questions to advance care delivery options for veterans.

REFERENCES

American Nurses Association (ANA). (2010). *Code of ethics for nurses* (p. 5). Retrieved from http://www .nursingworld.org

APRN Joint Dialogue Group Report. (2008, July). *Consensus model for APRN regulation: Licensure, accreditation, certification & education* (p. 5).

Blue Star Families. (2010, May). *Military family lifestyle survey*. Retrieved from http://www.bluestarfam .org

Henderson, V. (1966). *The nature of nursing*. London: Collier MacMillan Ltd.

Hoge, C. W., Castro, C. A., Messer, S. C., McGurk, D., Cotting, D. I., & Koffman, R. L. (2004). Combat duty in Iraq and Afghanistan, mental health problems, and barriers to care. *New England Journal of Medicine, 351*, 13–22.

Institute of Medicine (IOM). (2010). Retrieved on October 27, 2013 from http://www.iom.edu /Reports/2010/The-Future-of-Nursing-Leading-Change-Advancing-Health.aspx

Lester, P., Peterson, K., Reeves, J., Knauss, L., Glover, D., Mogil, C., ... Beardslee, W. (2010). The long war and parental combat deployment. *Journal of the American Academy of Child and Adolescent Psychiatry, 49*(4), 310–320.

Mansfield, A. J., Kaufman, J. S., Marshall, S. W., Gaynes, B. N., Morrissey, J. P., & Engel, C. C. (2010). Deployment and the use of mental health services among U.S. Army wives. *New England Journal of Medicine, 362*, 101–109.

Richmond, T. S. (2012). A war inside: Saving veterans from suicide. *Penn Medicine News*, 19. Retrieved from http://www.nursing.upenn.edu

Spelman, J., Hunt, S., Seal, K., & Burgo-Black, A. L. (2012, September). Post deployment care for returning combat veterans. *Journal of General Internal Medicine, 27*(9), 1200–1209.

ADDITIONAL RESOURCES

Clark, M. E., Scholten, J. D., Walker, R. L., & Gironda, R. J. (2009). Assessment and treatment of pain associated with combat-related polytrauma. *Pain Medicine, 10,* 456–469.

Frayne, S. M., Chiu, V. Y., Iqbal, S., Berg, E. A., Laungani, K. J., Cronkite, R. C., ... Kimerling, R. (2011). Medical care needs of returning Veterans with PTSD: Their other burden. *Journal of General Internal Medicine, 26,* 33–39.

Hoge, C. W., Castro, C. A., Messner, S. C., McGurk, D., Cotting, D. I., & Koffman, R. L. (2004). Combat duty in Iraq and Afghanistan, mental health problems, and barriers to care. *New England Journal of Medicine, 351,* 13–22.

Hoge, C. W., McGurk, D., Thomas, J. L., Cox, A. L., Engel, C. C., & Castro, C. A. (2008). Mild traumatic brain injury in U.S. soldiers returning from Iraq. *New England Journal of Medicine, 358,* 453–463.

Institute of Medicine of the National Academies. (2010). *Returning home from Iraq and Afghanistan: Preliminary assessment of readjustment needs of veterans, service members, and their families.* Washington, DC: National Academies Press.

Killgore, W. D., Cotting, D. I., Thomas, J. L., Cox, A. L., McGurk, D., Vo, A. H., ... Hoge, C. W. (2008). Post-combat invincibility: Violent combat experiences are associated with increased risk-taking propensity following deployment. *Journal of Psychiatric Research, 42*(13), 1112–1121.

Mansfield, A. J., Kaufman, J. S., Marshall, S. W., Gaynes, B. N., Morrissey, J. P., & Engel, C. C. (2010). Deployment and the use of mental health services among US army wives. *New England Journal of Medicine, 362,* 101–109.

Milliken, C. S., Auchterlonie, J. L., & Hoge, C. W. (2007). Longitudinal assessment of mental health problems among active and reserve component soldiers returning from the Iraq war. *Journal of the American Medical Association, 298,* 2141–2148.

Sayer, N. A., Norbaloochi, S., Frazier, P., Carlson, K., Gravely, A., & Murdoch, M. (2010). Reintegration problems and treatment interests among Iraq and Afghanistan combat veterans receiving VA medical care. *Psychiatry Service, 61*(6), 589–597.

Sayers, S. L., Farrow, V. A., Ross, H., & Oslin, D. W. (2009). Family problems among recently returned military veterans referred for mental health evaluation. *Journal of Clinical Psychiatry, 70*(2), 163–170.

Schniederman, A. I., Braver, E. R., & Kang, H. K. (2008). Understanding sequelae of injury mechanisms and mild traumatic brain injury incurred during the conflicts in Iraq and Afghanistan: Persistent postconcussive symptoms and posttraumatic stress disorder. *American Journal of Epidemiology, 167,* 1446–1452.

Seal, K. H., Metzler, T. J., Gima, K. S., Bertenthal, D., Maguen, S., & Marmar, C. R. (2009). Trends and risk factors for mental health diagnoses among Iraq and Afghanistan veterans using Department of Veterans Affairs health care, 2002–2008. *American Journal of Public Health, 99,* 1651–1658.

Sellig, A. D., Jacobson, I. G., Smith, B., Hooper, T. I., Boyko, E. J., Gackstetter, G. D., ... Millennium Cohort Study Team. (2010). Sleep patterns before, during, and after deployment to Iraq and Afghanistan. *Sleep, 33,* 1615–1622.

Smith, T. C., Zamorski, M., Smith, B., Riddle, J. R., LeardMann, C. A., Wells, T. S., ... Blaze, D. (2007). The physical and mental health of a large military cohort: Baseline functional health status of the Millennium Cohort. *BMC Public Health, 7,* 340.

Tanielian, T., & Jaycox, L. H. (Eds.). (2008). *Invisible wounds of war: Psychological and cognitive injuries, their consequences, and services to assist recovery.* Santa Monica, CA: RAND Center for Military Health Policy Research.

The White House Report. (2011, January). *Strengthening our military families: Meeting America's commitment.* Washington, DC: Author.

AANP's Joining Forces. www.joiningforces.aanp.org
www.afterdeployment.org
www.allabouttbi.com
www.centerforthestudyoftraumaticstress.org
www.citizensoldiersupport.org/initiatives/health.php
www.dcoe.health.mil/ForHealthPros.aspx

www.mentalhealthamerica.net
www.ptsd.va.gov/professional/index.asp
www.warwithin.org
www.whitehouse.gov/joiningforces/resources

National Center for PTSD Professional Section. This comprehensive resource offered by the VA offers access to training material, information, and tools to assist health care providers with assessment and treatment of PTSD. Select resources from this site include: www.ptsd.va.gov/professional/index.asp

- **PTSD Overview.** Reviews statistics and history of PTSD, diagnostic criteria, treatment factors, and much more. www.ptsd.va.gov/professional/pages/fslist_ptsd_overview.asp
- **Printable Materials.** Includes handouts and posters that can be used to increase awareness and educate about PTSD for families, military personnel, and others. www.ptsd.va.gov/about /print-materials/Materials_for_Printing.asp
- **Women Who Served in Our Military: Insights for Interventions.** A 70-minute video presenting perspectives regarding women who have served in the military, how they are impacted by stress, and treatment options. www.ptsd.va.gov/professional/videos/emv-womenvet-mhcp .asp
- **Online Iraq War Clinician Guide.** A Department of Defense manual published to address the needs of Iraq and Afghanistan war veterans. www.ptsd.va.gov/professional/manuals/iraq -war-clinician-guide.asp
- **Working with Families.** Resources for spouses, children, and other family members of patients with PTSD and how to incorporate the family in treatment plans. www.ptsd.va.gov/profes sional/pages/fslist-tx-family.asp
- **Citizen Soldier Support.** Home to an initiative providing resources related to "citizen soldiers," who serve in our Reserve and National Guard, including many designed to increase access to improved health care. www.citizensoldiersupport.org/initiatives/health.php
- **War Within.** Provides a database through which users can identify health care providers who accept service members in need of assessment or treatment. The site also provides means through which health care providers may register in the database. www.warwithin.org
- **Mental Health America.** Provides resources to help all people live mentally healthier lives, including those addressing issues among soldiers and their families. www.mentalhealthamer ica.net
- **Defense Centers of Excellence for Psychological Health and Traumatic Brain Injury.** Provides extensive resources for service members, families, and clinicians on psychological health and TBI. www.dcoe.health.mil/TraumaticBrainInjury/TBI_Information.aspx
- **After Deployment.** Provides a range of resources on topics ranging from PTSD, TBI, stress, health and wellness, work adjustment, and much more. www.afterdeployment.org

GENERAL RESOURCES FOR PROVIDERS

VA/DoD Clinical Practice guidelines: provides access to specific clinical practice guidelines on various topics including concussion/mTBI, PTSD, and medically unexplained symptoms. www.healthquality.va.gov

Provides assistance with diagnosis and management of PTSD, depression, and integrated treatment. Recommendations are consistent with and support applications of VA/DoD Clinical Practice Guidelines for PTSD and for depression. www.pdhealth.mil/respect-mil/index.asp

Search engine for services and resources at the national, state, and local levels that support recovery, rehabilitation, and reintegration. www.nationalresourcedirectory.gov

Deployment Health Clinical Center (DoD) with comprehensive information and a good section on military sexual trauma. www.pdhealth.mil/hcc/sapr.asp

RESOURCES FOR PATIENTS

Comprehensive link to multiple resources for returning service members. www.oefoif.va.gov

A site to help service members maximize their support systems. www.Militaryonesource.mil

Evidence-based self-help resource for veterans and families in addition to a provider resource portal and handouts. www.afterdeployment.org

MENTAL HEALTH RESOURCES

Vet Centers: individual, group, and family counseling to all veterans who served in any combat zone. www.va.gov/rcs

PTSD care with information for veterans and providers including training on military culture. www.ptsd.va.gov; www.centerforthestudyoftraumaticstress.org

Veteran Suicide Hotline 800-273-TALK. www.veteranscrisisline.net

Depression resources. www.nimh.nih.gov/health/publications/depression/complete-index .shtml

National Institute on Drug Abuse. www.drugabuse.gov

TBI/EXPOSURE/PAIN MANAGEMENT RESOURCES

Defense Centers of Excellence for Psychological Health and Traumatic Brain Injury (DCoE) www.dcoe.health.mil; also find comprehensive TBI information www.dvbic.org

Information on deployment exposure concerns. www.publichealth.va.gov/exposures/index.asp

Information from Institute of Medicine report on burn pit exposures. www.iom.edu/reports/2011 /long-term-health-consequences-of-exposure-to-burn-pits-in-iraq-and -afghanistan.aspx

VHA national pain management. www.va.gov/painmanagement

SMART PHONE AND I-PAD APPLICATIONS

PTSD Coach, provides reliable information on PTSD, tools for screening and tracking symptoms, and self-management skills.

Breath2Relax teaches the relaxation response, Co-Occurring Conditions Toolkit (CCT) and mTBI pocket guide providing screening VA/DoD guideline tool.

CHAPTER 13

Effective State-Level Advanced Practice Registered Nursing Leadership in Health Policy

Christine Filipovich

Becoming an effective advocate requires experiences in the real world where policy is made. This chapter provides information and suggestions to prepare the reader for effective interaction with policy and decision makers. The content is intended to help the advanced practice nurse to be a knowledgeable and effective advocate in their own state, where much policy affecting health care, nursing, and advanced practice nursing originates.

Legislation, regulation, and court rulings related to health care service delivery and reimbursement are types of government "policy" that directly impact nurses and nursing practice. The focus of this chapter is to overview how an advanced practice registered nurse (APRN) can identify issues of health policy and then work with the legislature and agencies under the jurisdiction of the governor to advance the practice of nursing at the state level.

HEALTH POLICY AND PUBLIC POLICY DEFINED

Broadly speaking, health policy is a course of action that influences health care decisions (www.aacn.org). Public policy refers to policy that is generated by governmental agencies and enacted through legislation. Public policy is made on behalf of the citizens and is influenced by factors such as economics, social issues, research, and technology. Health policy influences decisions about the health of a society. Similar to public policy, health policy is also influenced by factors such as health status of the citizens, research, and economics. Health policy can be developed and implemented as follows:

1. on an institutional level to address workplace issues, such as in hospitals to establish limitations on the number of patients a registered nurse can care for;

2. to shape nursing practice through professional organization policies by established standards of care or a code of ethics; or
3. to promote healthy communities through community, regional, or national policies (e.g., improving air quality or implementing health-screening processes).

New Jersey Collaborating Center for Nursing
Workforce Development (2003)

APRN IS AN EXPERT

Registered nurses prepared at the advanced practice level, by definition, possess knowledge and skill for expert practice in a specialized field of nursing. As most professionals, APRNs are lifelong learners because advances in science, technology, and theoretical foundations of nursing practice require continuous learning in order to remain professionally competent.

Most undergraduate and graduate nursing education programs include learning experiences that expose students to some aspects of legal and regulatory matters affecting nursing, such as the state's licensing law and regulations. However, neither formal education programs nor years of clinical practice are likely to equip the APRN for effective policy advocacy. This expertise comes from experience and real-time exposure to the policy-making process.

The APRN has expert knowledge of the health care delivery system and advanced clinical nursing skills. In addition, the APRN has well-developed critical thinking skills and both knowledge and experience in applying change theory and principles to effectively lead system transformation. Historically, education of clinical nurse specialists (CNSs) has emphasized preparation to be a change agent. More recently, the doctor of nursing practice (DNP) has incorporated aspects of both change management and systems-level analysis into preparation for all four of the APRN roles.

Through leadership and influence, APRNs impact policy making and policy decisions within an agency or health system. Thus, the APRN has an excellent foundation for effectively impacting and influencing health policy and policy decisions in a broader scope. Health policy within the scope of state government and the implications of the APRN to influence that policy will be discussed.

APRN POLICY/ADVOCACY COMPETENCIES

Practice competencies published by national organizations representing APRNs outline the role expectations and activities of APRNs in policy advocacy. Each of the four roles of CNS, certified nurse practitioner (CNP), certified nurse midwife (CNM), and certified registered nurse anesthetist (CRNA) have defined competencies within their core documents for educational preparation for the role.

CNSs are expected to evaluate the impact of legislative and regulatory policies as they apply to nursing practice and patient or population outcomes. CNSs also are expected to advocate for the CNS/APRN role and for positive legislative response to issues affecting nursing practice (National Association of Clinical Nurse Specialists [NACNS], 2010). Nurse practitioners are expected to participate in the health policy activities at the local, state, national, and international level (American Academy of Nurse Practitioners [AANP], 2010). CNMs are expected to know issues and trends in health care policy and systems, and to evaluate women's health policy issues within a variety of jurisdictions (local to federal), and demonstrate the ability to develop remedies to promote health improvement for women and newborns (American College of Nurse Midwives, 2011).

Until recently, public health nurses were considered to be a part of the CNS role but their professional organization made the decision to exclude components of the evolving definition of APRN. For that reason, they are no longer considered to be APRNs but do provide advanced nursing care. Although not currently considered APRNs, public health nurses are also expected to demonstrate expertise in understanding and interpreting health policy, as defined by the Quad Council's 2011 competencies intended to guide public health nursing education and practice at all levels. The Quad Council of Public Health Nursing Organizations is composed of the Association of Community Health Nurse Educators (ACHNE), the Association of State and Territorial Directors of Nursing (ASTDN), the American Public Health Association Public Health Nursing Section (APHA), and the American Nurses Association's Congress on Nursing Practice and Economics (ANA). They made the decision to not include core educational elements from the APRN Consensus Model (2008) and so determined that the public health and community health nurses would no longer be considered as APRNs.

According to the American Association of Colleges of Nursing (AACN), APRNs who earn a DNP degree are educationally prepared to assume a leadership role in the development of health policy and DNP graduates have the capacity to engage proactively in the development and implementation of health policy at all levels, such as institutional, local, state, regional, federal, and international levels (AACN, 2006).

The APRN leadership role in health policy may take many forms and may be carried out by the individual APRN or by groups of individuals who work together to accomplish a common goal. Leadership in any form requires current knowledge of the issues that affect nursing and health care as well as how policy decisions pertaining to those issues are made. Federal legislation, such as the Affordable Care Act, is enacted in large measure at the state level and often the effects are directly evident in clinical care at the bedside. For example, the increased focus on quality measures and value-based payment models creates the perfect environment for APRN leaders to demonstrate the value of APRN care. In fact, it demands that APRNs lay claim to their essential role in promoting wellness and improving chronic disease management. When APRNs can demonstrate the value of their work in terms of cost savings and improved patient outcomes, policy makers listen. Finding an open door to the arenas where policy is made and, once inside, proving to be an effective advocate will lead to influence.

INTERACTING WITH POLICY MAKERS AND POLICY-MAKING BODIES

Nursing's concerns are related to all three branches of government: the administration, the legislature, and the courts. The infrastructure of policy making in each state revolves around government bodies—the legislature, agencies, and regulatory boards—that are unique to each state. For example, a governor's decision to expand Medicaid is a legislative matter with potential for significant impact at the agency level where Medicaid programs are administered, and perhaps also impacting scope of practice decisions by the APRN-licensing board. Through state-level advocacy, APRNs can raise the awareness of both government officials and the public about the role that APRNs play in expanding access to care for Medicaid recipients.

Two foundational steps toward effective advocacy are identifying the key policy leaders at the state level and gaining a clear understanding of the detailed processes through which state legislation and regulations are made. This includes knowing who sets the policy agenda, who determines policy goals and alternatives, who formulates policy, and who implements and evaluates policy.

In the governor's office, the governor, lieutenant governor, attorney general, and secretary of state all have roles that influence nursing. In the legislature, the licensing committees take the lead in matters affecting professional licensure, but other committees such as health and consumer safety blaze the trail for nurses and nursing issues. For example, public discussion of a proposal to authorize unlicensed, minimally trained health aids to provide services to elderly residents in their homes may be initiated in a legislative committee responsible for consumer safety.

Each state in the United States passes its own laws regulating APRNs based on the health care environment within that state. Hence the reason that rules and regulations governing the practice of the APRN vary in each state.

Legislatures differ from state to state. Two key differences among states are (a) some legislatures are full time and others are part time and (b) the frequency with which the state legislature meets to conduct business varies. Some state legislatures are similar to Congress in that an elected seat in the legislature is considered as a full-time job and the legislatures meet in year-round session. California, New York, Michigan, and Pennsylvania top the list of states considered to have a "full-time" legislature, whereas the smaller, more rural states—Montana, New Hampshire, North Dakota, South Dakota, Utah, and Wyoming—have "citizen legislatures" made up of elected representatives who have full-time occupations in addition to being legislators (National Conference of State Legislatures, 2012).

Perhaps, the policy-making government agency most familiar to nurses is the state nurse-licensing board. The term "state board of nursing" will be used to refer to the state entity responsible for nurse licensing. The name of the nurse-licensing board varies among states, however, as does the composition of the state board and the position of the board within the regulatory structure of the state. For example, the Pennsylvania State Board of Nursing is one of the many licensing boards within the Pennsylvania Department of State's Bureau of Professional and Occupational Affairs. The North Carolina Board of Nursing is independent and self-supporting, but not part of another state government agency. In some states, the nurse practice act dictates the composition of the board by specifying a certain number of board seats to be filled by individuals with certain qualifications. For example, the Illinois nursing law establishes four board seats for advanced practice nurses representing CNS, CNP, CNM, and CRNA practice.

To effectively impact state governance of the nursing profession, all APRNs must understand the role of the state board and know both the state nursing law (known as the Nurse Practice Act or similar name) and rules and regulations promulgated by the board to carry out the Act. It is also important to clearly understand the composition of the board and the process through which individuals gain seats on the board. Appointment to a licensing board is usually made by the governor. Often, endorsement by professional associations and other influential bodies is necessary for success in being selected by the governor for such an appointment.

In addition to knowing the composition of the board, it is very helpful to know the individual board members' alliances with special interest groups. In some states, these relationships are permitted, whereas in other states, a clear connection to an affected group of licensees or other interest group precludes eligibility to sit on the board. If these alliances are known, it may impact the decisions made by that individual and subsequently the board. This can have a significant impact on the rules and regulations that then affect all members of the nursing profession in that state.

State "Sunshine laws" provide for open meetings that allow members of the public to be present at board meetings. Attending and observing state board meetings is an excellent and easily available way to learn the functions, scope, and limits of regulatory agencies. Remember that there are a lot of "behind the scenes" discussions that you are not privy to that will influence the decisions made at the board meetings. See if you can sit with someone who is a long-term attendee who may be able and/or willing to mentor you or a lobbyist who has a vested interest in the outcomes of a particular decision. Their insights will be invaluable to you as you learn the processes.

Licensing boards typically make regulations and amend them in collaboration with stakeholder groups; however, boards vary with respect to how they interact with and communicate with their licensees and leaders who represent the licensees. Some state boards actively and routinely seek input from licensees when matters come before the board that affect or have the potential to impact on their practice. The interaction may be informal, with representatives of the licensees serving as subject matter experts with whom the board consults. The board may hold public hearings to more formally gather information and perspectives from an array of interested parties. In addition, an interested stakeholder or group may request to be placed on the board's meeting agenda to address the board in public session.

WHO SPEAKS FOR APRNs?

Every APRN should know the representatives of the nursing profession speaking as advanced practice nursing experts to the state board, to legislators, and to state agencies. In addition to knowing who those representatives are, it is important to know the topics they are discussing and the positions they are advancing. Those who have the ear of the decision makers may be promoting policy decisions that are not in the best interest of APRNs or advanced nursing practice. Never assume that a nurse or nursing organization will understand and advocate for the best interests of APRNs unless APRNs have contributed to the development of the underlying position.

An effective working relationship with legislators and state regulatory boards is critical for organizations that represent nurses. Often, the state nurses' association is the representative of nursing interests most recognized and consulted by state legislators and regulators. Although there may be many voices speaking for APRNs presenting varied positions on a given issue; in general, the state nurses' association is usually viewed as a key leader for carrying nursing's positions forward.

Agencies such as state health departments may have a designated office of policy or policy director responsible for developing major policy positions for the department, consistent with the governor's goals and objectives. The policy office or director ensures that policies and initiatives supported by the governor are implemented within the agency and, conversely, that the agency's positions and views are communicated to the governor's office for consideration in policy decision making.

Communications with stakeholders is an important function of the agency's policy office or director and that interaction typically takes place through contact with lobbyists representing the stakeholder groups. Bringing stakeholders into discussion of proposed legislation that the agency is negotiating with the legislature is a common strategy for garnering support for positions and proposals that satisfy the stakeholders' interests as well as the intent of legislators and agency leaders.

ADVOCACY STRATEGY TOOLS AND RESOURCES

Governments exist to protect the welfare of the public. Advocacy efforts with government officials and agencies should be built on this premise. It is strategically important to know the governor's priorities and priority initiatives and, if possible, to demonstrate how these priorities can be achieved or positively affected by the proposal or position being presented or recommended.

Many APRNs are very good at applying their advanced analytical skills to understanding a policy issue and then using their clinical reasoning to formulate a solution. However, the influence of state-wide politics and political positioning must be taken into consideration in order to be strategically effective. Detailed personal knowledge of a policy problem or issue and a logical solution are a good start, but will not necessarily lead to effective policy change. The knowledge and expertise of APRNs as individuals, combined with the knowledge and expertise of others who know the political landscape and how to navigate it, will likely be more effective.

In many cases, strategic alliances with other stakeholders are necessary for positioning a proposal or issue so that it will get attention and action. This requires building and maintaining collegial relationships with groups both within and outside of nursing. This does not necessarily include just those groups that share priorities and perspectives supportive of nursing or advanced practice nurses. In the course of daily practice, APRNs are likely to interact with leaders of organizations such as the state medical society, the hospital association, the long-term care association, and other groups that have interest and influence in state health care matters. Cultivating those individual relationships is beneficial for both the information exchange and sharing of perspectives on policy issues that can result. APRNs and practitioners of disciplines outside nursing who interact positively as colleagues in clinical settings are likely to engage comfortably in conversation about policy issues, even if they espouse differing views. Even though APRNs and other practitioners, such as physicians, often have conflicting positions with regard to policy matters pertaining to scope of practice, they can also easily coalesce around other current policy issues that have direct, high impact on health care delivery, for example, gun violence. It is equally important to know the reasons driving antagonists to oppose your position. Knowing the basis of adversarial positions is a key factor in successful negotiation of more compatible working relationships.

By working with state leaders in disciplines other than nursing to learn about their priorities and activities, nurses and nursing groups can identify potential allies and adversaries who may pursue policy initiatives that impact APRNs and APRN practice. It is important to recognize opportunities to informally or formally support them. Participating in other organizations' activities provides the opportunity to develop acquaintances that promote collegial relationships and greater familiarity with how and why others take the positions that they do.

Both active involvement in the groups that represent APRNs' interests at the state level and development of one's own skills are important for effective advocacy. APRNs who belong to these organizations support effective policy leadership by their individual contributions and leadership within these organizations. Individuals' skills develop over time and are built on exposure to and experience in a variety of policy arenas.

The ability to write and speak clearly and concisely in a style that can be understood by the public and legislators is critical for effective advocacy. Understanding the frame of reference of the intended audience and presenting information in terms that have meaning within that frame of reference will increase the effectiveness of communications. APRNs can develop skill in preparing issue briefing papers that outline a problem or concern in a manner that reaches beyond the clinical patient care world and makes the matter meaningful to the public, the legislator, or the regulator.

APRNs clearly understand the critical value of data. Facts and figures presented in an easily understood manner can make it easier to garner support for a policy position. Telling an audience what "should" happen and why from the perspective of the health care provider or patient is often more effective when accompanied by undeniable, unemotional statements of fact about how supporting an issue or position will result in better outcomes—that is, lives saved, public spending reduced or eliminated, costs to the citizens or to the government minimized. Citations from the law or literature are important components of an effective advocacy presentation. A position supported by precedent set in law or a citation from the law will have impact with policy decision makers and will contribute to evidence-based decision making. As an APRN faced with trying to influence policy makers, be prepared with your clear, rational, and well-thought out discussion of the facts in the situation that would sway the decision in the direction you feel it needs to go.

In addition to effective communications, relationships are also a valuable tool. Creating and maintaining relationships with those who make policy and influence decision making is an important strategy for nurses as individuals and for nursing groups collectively. By introducing themselves to elected representatives who serve in the state legislature and becoming acquainted, APRNs can establish an identity as an expert resource among the representative's constituents. Ongoing communication with elected representatives and/or their staff, based on issues of mutual concern or about matters that fall within the APRN's scope of expertise, will help that relationship develop. The APRN who has specialized expertise in chronic illness, for example, or violence prevention can be a valuable source of information as an unpaid consultant for their legislator when proposed legislation or policy decisions relating to those topics are developing or are presented.

Nursing knowledge is intellectual capital that APRNs should feel comfortable sharing. For example, a perinatal CNS can talk to a legislator about the importance of funding preterm birth prevention programs based on the authority of their own experience and knowledge. While speaking to an audience of policy makers who are not health professionals, the nurse is likely to be the person in the room most qualified to address topics pertaining to the delivery of health care.

Negotiating skills and understanding how negotiation works in the political and policy environment are also important. Understanding who has the power to set policy and to make policy decisions is critical. Understanding who is in the decision-making role and their scope of authority and appealing to the right agency or the right office or person within the agency will also prevent time wasting that undermines efforts to influence change. Knowing and working with other stakeholders to gain strength from shared positioning is an important part of negotiation.

Along with negotiation, patience is more than just a virtue—it is essential for effective advocacy. The APRN who has a mindset based in clinical reasoning and is accustomed to making rapid, decisive actions in response to a need for change may find a high level of frustration with the plodding nature of negotiation and the perceived expectation to "give away" some pieces of a policy proposal in order to gain support for other remaining pieces of it. The essence is acquiring one small gain each time the issue is brought forward to the legislative process and not taking an "all or nothing" stance.

Policy initiatives that require legislation are often subject to extensive and complex negotiation. These are most effectively managed by professional lobbyists whose daily work enables them to have depth and breadth of knowledge of the players and the power structure. The opportunity to do advocacy work in collaboration with a lobbyist contributes to the APRNs knowledge of the bigger picture, the views held by policy leaders in the world outside of health care who are making decisions that affect nursing and patient care.

Timing is crucial. Those who work in policy day-in and day-out have the best knowledge about when the state political climate and broader policy direction are amenable to a policy proposal and when a proposal, no matter how well conceived and planned, will not succeed and why. APRNs and other nursing leaders must collaborate with individuals and groups who are connected, are sensitive, and can speak the language and negotiate the complexities of the state government on their behalf. Even though a policy proposal may be perfectly sound, thoroughly supported with logic and good for the public, there may be some political reasons that will make it impossible to move forward. Policy is based on both politics and rational, evidence-based logic.

In addition to working with personnel who have expertise in government relations to lead and advise APRN policy initiatives, individuals who want to develop expertise can access other resources. Most states' statutes are accessible for free online, offering the actual text of existing laws. Licensing boards' laws, such as the state nurse practice act, and the administrative rules/regulations promulgated by the board may be accessed by the board's web pages. Likewise, a state agency web pages may offer access to the specific statutes and regulations that establish the agency's duties, responsibilities, and programs. When legislators develop a statute, committee conference notes are documented. These conference notes reflect discussion about the wording, text, staff thoughts, and decisions made as the law was drafted. They are available to the public and offer valuable insight and understanding about the intended meaning of the statutory language.

Information about current policy initiatives of interest to APRNs is likely to be available through the state professional organizations that are sponsoring them. Access to some information may be offered only to the organization's members. When activity is occurring in the legislature on bills that the professional organization has sponsored or supported, the organization may provide regular updates for members and/or for the public via the website.

Professional organizations also provide specific materials for individuals' advocacy efforts. Examples include the NACNS "Starter Kit for Impacting Change at the Government Level: How to Work with Your State Legislators and Regulators," materials developed by the Oregon Nurses Association that address reimbursement for Nurse Practitioners, the Pennsylvania State Nurses Association's advocacy training entitled "Advocacy 101: Advocating for your future," and a study of the economic impact of greater utilization of APRNs publicized in May, 2012, by the Texas Coalition of Nurses in Advanced Practice (CNAP). By taking advantage of these resources, you become a better advocate for your discipline and the health care provided in your state.

TEACH/MENTOR/MODEL

Leadership in policy issues is a critical role for advanced nursing leaders globally. Noting that nursing and therefore nursing leadership is shaped dramatically by the impact of politics and policy, a Royal College of Nursing study concluded that effective nursing leadership currently is a vehicle through which *both* nursing practice and health policy can be influenced and shaped (Antrobus & Kitson, 1999). The APRN is in a position to serve as a teacher, mentor, and role model for colleagues, students, staff, and other health care workers. Just as nursing practice expertise evolves over time through continuous search for new knowledge and opportunities, expertise in policy leadership can develop for the APRN who seeks these opportunities either as an individual or as a member of a professional organization. Modeling this role for other APRNs new to practice and supporting their development of skills in this area are critical for nursing's advancement in the health care marketplace.

CONCLUSION

This chapter has presented information to stimulate more thinking about how APRNs can assume a position to lead health care policy efforts. The current significant focus on transparency in government, legislative, and regulatory affairs offers a wealth of opportunity for those who want to learn more. State government is highly visible through the internet, with proposed rulemaking, regulations, and other policies available on the government's website. A motivated APRN constituency can become a powerful force in exerting control of APRN practice at the state level. Competent professional practice includes knowledge and competence in policy and advocacy to benefit nursing practice and health care. APRNs should be leaders who seek and accept every opportunity for visibility, for advocacy, and for taking ownership of their own professional practice.

DISCUSSION QUESTIONS

1. What do newspaper and/or university public opinion polls indicate about the public's perceptions of nursing? On what basis does the public form these opinions?
2. Who are the nurses in your state legislature and what are their educational and clinical backgrounds?
3. What are the sources of rules in your state regarding APRN reimbursement? (State law or regulations? Agency policies or policy interpretation?)
4. What organizations outside nursing share a stake in policy matters that concern APRNs? How do they stand to benefit from being involved in and/or influencing policy decisions that affect nursing practice or nursing education?

SYNTHESIS EXERCISES

1. Identify the current state governor's priorities and learn about the initiatives the governor is supporting.
2. Meet with the lobbyist for the state nurses association. Discuss the lobbyist's view of the most influential leaders driving the health care agenda in the state and their priorities.
3. Identify at least one board or advisory panel convened by state government (a state agency other than the state licensing board) that makes decisions affecting your practice. Investigate how appointments to that board/advisory panel are made and whether or not nurses serve on it.
4. Identify the agency in your state that administers the state's Medicaid program. Learn how decisions are made regarding provider reimbursement for APRNs.

REFERENCES

American Academy of Nurse Practitioners. (2013). *Standards of practice for nurse practitioners*. Retrieved from http:www.aanp.org

American Association of Colleges of Nursing. (2006). *The essentials of doctoral education for advanced nursing practice*. Retrieved from http:www.aacn.nche.edu

American College of Nurse Midwives. (2011). *The practice doctorate in midwifery*. Retrieved from http:www .midwife.org

Antrobus, S., & Kitson, A. (1999). Nursing leadership: Influencing and shaping health policy and nursing practice. *Journal of Advanced Nursing, 29*, 746–753. doi:10.1046/j.1365-2648.1999.00945.x

APRN Consensus Work Group & the National Council of State Boards of Nursing APRN Advisory Committee. (2008). *Consensus model for APRN regulation: Licensure, accreditation, certification & education*. Retrieved from http:www.ncsbn.org

National CNS Core Competency Task Force. (2010). *Clinical nurse specialist core competencies*. Retrieved from http:www.nacns.org

National Conference of State Legislatures. (2008). *Full and part time legislatures*. Retrieved December 21, 2012 from http://www.ncsl.org/legislatures-elections/legislatures/full-and-part-time-legislatures.aspx

New Jersey Collaborating Center for Nursing Workforce Development. (2003). *Nursing in public and health policy*. Retrieved October 12, 2012 from www.njccn.org

CHAPTER 14

Funding of Advanced Practice Registered Nurse Education and Residency Programs

Suzanne Miyamoto

AN HISTORICAL PERSPECTIVE

The political roots for nursing education funding can be traced back to the Administration of President John Adams when the Public Health Service (PHS) was created in 1798 (Kalisch & Kalisch, 1982). To date, nurses are a vital part of the PHS and the use of health care professionals to provide public services spans the centuries as well as the investment by the federal government. In 1902, the U.S. PHS was created and eventually the division of nursing (Kalisch & Kalisch, 1982), currently housed within the U.S. Department of Health and Human Services (HHS), Health Resources and Services Administration (HRSA).

However, the nation's attention to the importance of nurses became increasingly evident during World War I. Nurses who were a part of the PHS were deployed to military camps and asked to care for the civilian populations around the camps by teaching proper sanitation, treating children, and investigating communicable diseases (Kalisch & Kalisch, 1982). The care these nurses provided during wartime demonstrated the critical importance of public health nursing.

> In general, the public health expenditures of the 1920s proved that public health nursing could be a purchasable commodity: The public health nursing programs, which had grown up in the first quarter of the 20th century, had helped to lower the mortality rate, to increase life expectancy and reduce significantly the morbidity rate from tuberculosis, typhoid fever, smallpox, malaria, and most infant diseases.
>
> *Kalisch and Kalisch (1982, p. 170)*

The Great Depression, the next chapter in U.S. history, caused federal funding for PHSs to be slashed. In 1933, the New Deal allowed the federal government to invest in programs that were cut during the Great Depression, which included nursing.

Congress established the Federal Emergency Relief Administration and the Civil Works Administration, which significantly invested in nursing (Kalisch & Kalisch, 1982). It was during this era that the federal government provided postgraduate training for public health nurses. Yet, one of the most notable federal investments for nursing education policy came in the 1940s. The United States had entered World War II and again, the call for nursing care had intensified.

During this time, the PHS funded a national nursing survey and allocated dollars to support nursing programs for the imminent increase in students. This work was conducted by the Nursing Council for National Defense that was created by the nation's nursing leaders (Kalisch & Kalisch, 1982). A total of $1.2 million was allocated for basic training and administered by the Public Health Nursing section of the Division of States Relations of the PHS. This marked the first federal investment in nursing education. But it was the creation of the U.S. Cadet Nurse Corps in 1943 that established more comprehensive funding for nursing education (Kalisch & Kalisch, 1982).

Nurses were being drafted to serve in the military and this in turn led to a shortage of nurses in civilian hospitals, marking the first American nursing shortage. Given this demand for nurses in both the military and civilian sectors, proposals were offered to shorten nursing education programs. However, these were strongly opposed by nursing leaders as they feared a "…massive collapse of the already meager educational standards" (Kalisch & Kalisch, 1982, p. 173). The initial objections were quickly overshadowed by the great need for nurses. In 1943, the U.S. Cadet Nurse Corps was introduced by Congresswoman Frances Payne Bolton (R-OH) and signed into law by President Roosevelt on June 15 of that year. Nursing students entering this 24- or 30-month program received free tuition, a monthly stipend, and uniforms. To oversee the corps, the PHS Surgeon General created the Division of Nursing Education (DNE). The U.S. Cadet Nurse Corps was the "largest experiment in federally subsidized education in the history of the United States up to that time" (Kalisch & Kalisch, 1982, p. 174).

The U.S. Cadet Nurse Corps was a major success, but the importance of this program as well as the DNE ended after the war. Congress viewed this particular federal investment as part of the war effort and phased out both programs. This result made a drastic impact on nursing school enrollments and the nation's hospitals experienced severe nursing shortages (Kalisch & Kalisch, 1982). Moreover, the effects created a shortage of nursing faculty and many nursing leaders were concerned over the academic standards.

Ninety-seven percent of nursing education was hospital-based programs (Kalisch & Kalisch, 1982). The profession needed to investigate its trajectory. In 1948, the Carnegie Corporation and the Russell Sage Foundation sponsored the report *Nursing for the Future* (Kalisch & Kalisch, 1982). The recommendations included one that has survived decades, nursing programs should be housed in colleges and universities and sub-par programs should be closed. In 1948, the American Medical Association concurred with this recommendation through its *Committee on Nursing Problems* that investigated patient care standards and stressed the importance of nursing education at the baccalaureate level (Kalisch & Kalisch, 1982).

Although no major funding streams from Congress were appropriated for nursing education during this time, support on Capitol Hill was gaining momentum. As Kalisch and Kalisch (1982) noted, "…their [nursing legislation] recurring appearance before each session of Congress indicated that they had acquired a permanent base of support" (p. 180). The only federal support for nursing from 1948 to 1956 was through the National Mental Health Act of 1946 that provided funding for psychiatric nursing education (Kalisch & Kalisch, 1982). The next major Congressional action to support nursing education (beyond mental health nursing) was through the Health Amendments Act of 1956. In its first year, this legislation authorized $2 million in traineeships for approximately 3,800 nurses pursuing a career in education or administration (Kalisch & Kalisch, 1982). However, nursing leaders knew the piecemeal approach to funding nursing education would not be sufficient. The demand had surfaced for consistent federal funding for nursing education.

CONGRESSIONAL ACTION TO ESTABLISH CONSISTENT FUNDING FOR NURSING EDUCATION

The U.S. faced its second significant nursing shortage in the late 1950s and early 1960s as the nation's hospitals reported high registered nursing (RN) vacancy rates (Buerhaus, Staiger, & Auerbach, 2009). In 1961, the reported vacancy rate soared to 23.2% (Yett, 1975). The shortage was driven by expanding positions for nurses in the hospital setting. As Kalisch and Kalisch (1982) noted:

> In the 1940s, hospitals had about one professional nurse for every fifteen beds and one practical nurse, or other auxiliary, for every ten beds. By the 1960s, one professional nurse was required for every five beds and one auxiliary for every three beds. Health care was given to a greater variety of people, and the primary focus of care had shifted from the home to the institution. (p. 186)

The nursing shortage impacted quality nursing care. Without the supervision of licensed RNs, non-professional personnel were providing direct patient care resulting in dangerous errors (Yett, 1966). The impact of the nursing shortage on patient care was quickly rising to the national agenda. Its effects were highlighted in medical, nursing, and public health journals, in magazines, and in public newspapers (Yett, 1966). As cited by Yett (1966), "Gradually, and inevitably, an awareness of this situation has become a part of what John Kenneth Galbraith so aptly has described as our 'conventional wisdom'" (p. 190). The RN vacancy rate was on the rise from 5% in the 1940s to 10–15% in the 1950s and eventually 20% in the 1960s (Yett, 1966). It was at this time in history that hospitals lobbied Congress to enact legislation that would fund nursing education and help address the demand for nurses (Buerhaus et al., 2009).

In 1963, the Surgeon General released the report *Toward Quality in Nursing, Needs and Goals* (Congressional Research Service [CRS], 2005). This report signified the need for comprehensive legislation for nursing workforce development. It recommended that the supply of practicing RNs should be increased to 850,000 by 1970, which would have resulted in a growth of 55%. It also recommended that nursing school graduates increase by 75% to meet this goal and more specifically noted that nurses with graduate degrees should increase by 194%, baccalaureate prepared nurses by 100%, and licensed practical nurses by 50% (Kalisch & Kalisch, 1982).

The Nurse Training Act (NTA) of 1964 (Pub. L. No. 88-581) established Title VIII of the Public Health Service Act (PHSA), which is known today as the Nursing Workforce Development programs. While the legislation authorized a total of $238 million for five programs over five years, when it was signed into law by President Johnson on September 4, 1964, it received $9.92 million in its first year (Kalisch & Kalisch, 1982). "On signing the act, President Johnson observed that the NTA of 1964

TABLE 14.1 Title VIII Programs and Authorization Levels

PROGRAMS	AUTHORIZATION	PURPOSE
Nursing student loans	$85 million	Those who received the awards agreed to work for 5 years after graduation and would be forgiven half of their loan
Professional nurse traineeship	$50 million	Continuation of existing professional nurse traineeship programs
Construction grants	$90 million	Construction and improvement of nursing facilities $55 million for diploma and associate degree programs $35 million for baccalaureate programs
Project grants	$17 million	Improvements to teaching methodologies and other special projects
Formula grants to diploma schools	$41 million	Improvements to hospital-based nursing programs such as the quality of instruction

Source: Kalisch and Kalisch (1982); Scott (1967).

was the most significant nursing legislation in the history of the country" (Kalisch & Kalisch, 1982, p. 188). Furthermore, "…he believed that it would enable the nation to attract more qualified young people to this 'great and noble calling'" (Kalisch & Kalisch, 1977, p. 855).

The five programs included nursing student loans, professional nurse traineeships, construction grants, project grants, and formula grants to diploma schools (Scott, 1967) (see Table 14.1).

To administer the new authorities, the Division of Nursing created the Nursing Education and Training Branch (Kalisch & Kalisch, 1982). The programs made a significant impact. Between the years of 1964 and 1967, the Nursing Student Loan Program supported over 32,000 nursing students (Scott, 1967). The Professional Nurse Traineeship Program was expanded to include long-term and short-term traineeships for graduate nurses seeking a clinical specialty track and from 1964 to 1967, a total of 17,000 RNs were supported (Scott, 1967).

The other Title VIII programs were focused more on the didactical as well as the "brick and mortar" of nursing education. Scott (1967) noted that the construction grants were established to help to address the overcrowding of the nation's nursing schools and the obsolete buildings. Sixty-two schools were funded to renovate their buildings between 1964 and 1967, which resulted in 2,600 more students to be enrolled (Scott, 1967). In addition, nine new nursing schools were developed because of the construction grants. The project grants, which were created by the NTA, awarded 116 schools federal dollars and benefited 33,000 students (Scott, 1967). The grant money was used for projects such as investing in multimedia to enhance education and teaching students in the community, away from the hospital setting. The final program created through the NTA went to support a total of 414 diploma programs given the high costs incurred by the hospitals in administering them (Scott, 1967).

Nursing experts of the 1960s noted that the NTA would significantly help alleviate the nursing shortage. However, others felt that the original projections made in 1963 to increase the profession to 850,000 practicing nurses were not achievable. Yett's (1966) analysis of the NTA and the Surgeon General's report revealed a discrepancy of 170,000 nurses. According to the Surgeon General's Consultant Group on Nursing, who wrote the 1963 report,

...a feasible goal for 1970 is to increase the supply of professional nurses in practice to about 680,000 and that to meet this goal schools of nursing must produce 53,000 graduates a year by 1969 (including 13,000 baccalaureate, and an additional 3,000 at the master's level)

U.S. PHS, 1963 as cited in Yett (1966)

Adding to the shortfall, Kalisch and Kalisch (1977) described in their unpublished study for the Division of Nursing that "It soon became obvious that unless the shortage of classroom and other training space in hospital schools of nursing and junior college nursing programs was corrected, it would stand in the way of the nation's goal of having 680,000 nurses in active practice by 1970" (p. 834).

When the NTA was up for reauthorization in 1969, a committee was established to evaluate the five authorities. They found them to be effective in addressing the national nursing shortage through investments in nursing education, but noted that the NTA should be expanded to address planning, recruitment, and research (Kalisch & Kalisch, 1982). Congressional hearings were held on the NTA and other legislation supporting health professionals to determine how to act on the recommendations of the various committees. The Health Manpower Act of 1968 reauthorized the NTA. The reauthorization weakened the accreditation standards (the original bill required accreditation by the National League for Nursing, which at the time only accredited baccalaureate programs, weakening federal support for diploma programs) due in large part to the associate degree lobby, but it did increase the number of scholarship provisions (Kalisch & Kalisch, 1982).

In the 1970s and 1980s, the Title VIII programs saw a number of amendments and reauthorizations. The NTA of 1971 (Pub. L. 92-158) and 1975 (Pub. L. 94-63), for the first time, provided grants for all types of nursing education programs (Kalisch & Kalisch, 1977). Known as capitation grants, they were "... based on the well-established need to maintain the quality of education in schools of nursing by establishing a firm core of financial support" (Kalisch & Kalisch, 1977, p. 1135). Capitation grants provided formula grants based on enrollment rates in schools of nursing (American Association of Colleges of Nursing [AACN], 2008a). Schools were awarded the grants if they could demonstrate enrollment growth over the previous year and could use the funds to hire faculty, recruit students, enhance clinical laboratories, expand school of nursing buildings, or for other learning equipment (AACN, 2008a). For collegiate schools of nursing, Congress provided "...$400 for each full-time baccalaureate student enrolled in the last 2 years of a nursing program, and approximately $275 for each student enrolled in an associate degree or diploma program" (AACN, 2008a, p. 3). Capitation grants received significant funding support from Congress and in fiscal year (FY) 1977 and FY 1978 the program was appropriated $55 million (AACN, 2008b).

The capitation grant program proved to be a powerful source of funding for the nation's nursing schools. However, politics played a significant role in their eventual elimination. The program was endorsed by the liberal Congress, but not the conservative Nixon Administration. While President Nixon signed the Nursing Training Act into law in 1971, continual debates between the Administration and Congress over the appropriate funding levels for nursing education led President Nixon to veto a number of bills that would have created higher levels of support (Kalisch & Kalisch, 1982). In 1972 and 1973, Congress passed continual resolutions (appropriations bills funded at the previous year's level) but President Nixon impounded $73 million nursing appropriations that were later recovered through a federal court case (Kalisch & Kalisch, 1982). Funding for nursing education continued to be a target. In

1974, President Nixon's budget request slashed the $160 million appropriated to Title VIII in 1973 to $49 million (Kalisch & Kalisch, 1982). Although Congress was able to secure funding for Title VIII above the President's request and $139 million was finally appropriated for the NTA programs in FY 1974 (Division of Nursing, 2008), nursing would continue to fight for necessary federal support.

The Ford Administration also made cuts to nursing education funding. President Ford vetoed the NTA of 1974 claiming that it was too expensive (Kalisch & Kalisch, 1982). In addition, the Administration felt that the nurse scholarship and loan programs were unnecessary as nursing students were eligible for other federal loans (Kalisch & Kalisch, 1982). The NTA of 1975 attempted to find a middle ground with the Administration. It decreased federal funding for the Title VIII programs, but extended their authorization through FY 1978. However, the most notable difference of the NTA of 1975 was the creation of the Advanced Nurse Training Program. This legislation provided funding for the expansion of master's and doctoral nursing education programs, most notably those for advanced practice registered nurses (APRNs). President Ford vetoed this bill, but Congress was able to override his veto (Kalisch & Kalisch, 1982).

The nursing community fought with their Congressional champions to keep the legislation intact and funded. When President Carter took office, he viewed the programs similarly to his predecessors Presidents Nixon and Ford. He believed that nursing students could obtain funding from other federal programs, the NTA had helped to address the nursing shortage, and the funding levels were too excessive (Kalisch & Kalisch, 1982). In President Carter's FY 1978 budget, he provided no funding for nurse training "…and foreboded the probable end of the Division of Nursing had his administration continued" (Kalisch & Kalisch, 1977, p. 1225). Congress did pass an extension to the NTA in 1978, but it was pocket-vetoed on November 11, 1978, by President Carter (Kalisch & Kalisch, 1982). This move ignited outrage from the nursing community.

The following year, a new version of the legislation was drafted. It required a national study to be conducted by the Institute of Medicine (IOM) to determine if the federal government should continue to provide institutional support, if there was an actual nursing shortage, if the government should subsidize all of a nursing student's loan, and how should Congress address the unequal distribution of nurses and the increase in nursing specialization (Congressional Research Service [CRS], 2005). The NTA of 1979 was signed into law by President Carter on September 29 of that year given the provision of the study (Kalisch & Kalisch, 1982). The IOM report, *Nursing and Nursing Education: Policies and Private Actions*, found that the federal support for the "overall supply of nurses was not needed, but that generalist education programs should continue to help to sustain the nursing supply" (CRS, 2005, p. CRS-2). The results of this report caused further cuts to the Title VIII programs and eliminated the construction grants, capitation grants, and scholarships at schools of nursing. Laws passed in 1981 and 1982 repealed most of the programs that were created in the 1960s and 1970s (CRS, 2005).

CURRENT FEDERAL FUNDING FOR APRNs

Despite the political battles the Title VIII Nursing Workforce Development programs faced over the years, they still represent the largest dedicated source of federal funding for nursing education (Nursing Community, 2012). They also continue to support APRNs through consistent funding. To date, the Title VIII programs have seven authorities as follows: (a) Advanced Nursing Education (ANE) grants (Section 811), (b) Nursing Workforce Diversity (Sec. 821), (c) Nursing Education, Practice, Quality, and Retention (Sec. 831), (d) Nursing Student Loan Program (Sec. 835), (e) Nurse Loan Repayment and Scholarship program (Sec. 846), (f) Nurse Faculty Loan Program (Sec. 846A), and (g) Comprehensive Geriatric Education Grants (Sec. 855). Each of these programs has the potential to support APRNs. However, one major program within Title VIII focuses on APRN training, the ANE Grants.

ANE Grants (Sec. 811 of the PHSA) are modeled after the traineeship programs that were originally created in the 1960s and 1970s. There are three distinct programs authorized under this section. First, they provide schools of nursing, academic health centers, and other nonprofit entities funding to improve the education and practice of nurse practitioners (NPs), certified nurse midwives (CNMs), certified registered nurse anesthetists (CRNAs), clinical nurse specialists (CNSs), nurse educators, nurse administrators, public health nurses, and other nurses pursuing ANE (Pub. L. 107-205).

Second, they provide full or partial traineeship support for graduate nursing students to help with the expense of tuition, books, program fees, and other reasonable living expenses (Pub. L. 107-205). This program is known as the Advanced Education Nursing Traineeships (AENT). Finally, the ANE section of Title VIII also funds the Nurse Anesthetist Traineeship (NAT), which provides the same type of support as the AENT to students in nurse anesthetist programs. Funding for the ANE programs is a substantial portion of Title VIII funding. As seen in Table 14.2, the average percent of funding allocated for the program over the last decade is 38.5%. The decrease in funding seen after 2002 could be attributed to the enactment of the Nurse Reinvestment Act of 2002 in which a number of new programs were added to Title VIII, which impacted future allocations.

Two additional sources of federal support for APRN education and training are funded through the National Health Service Corps (NHSC) and the U.S. PHS. The NHSC was created through the Emergency Health Personnel Act (Pub. L. 91-623) in 1970 (Politzer et al., 2000). The intent of the legislation was to create a program that would direct commissioned officers and civil service personnel to the nation's health professional shortage areas (HPSAs). The health care professionals were to provide primary care to those in rural and underserved areas. The goal was to ensure that

TABLE 14.2 Percent of ANE Funding Compared With Total Title VIII Dollars

FISCAL YEAR	TOTAL TITLE VIII FUNDING (IN MILLIONS)	FUNDING FOR ANE (IN MILLIONS)	ANE % OF TITLE VIII FUNDING
2002	92.74	60.04	64.7
2003	112.76	50.17	44.5
2004	141.92	58.65	41.3
2005	150.67	58.17	38.6
2006	149.68	57.06	38.1
2007	149.68	57.06	38.1
2008	156.05	61.88	39.7
2009	171.03	64.44	37.7
2010	243.87	64.44	26.4
2011	242.39	64.05	26.4
2012	231.10	63.93	27.7

Source: AACN (2012a).

after the health care professional finished their tour, they would find the work to be rewarding and would choose to stay and practice in the communities (Redman, 1973, as cited in Politzer et al., 2000). The first cohort of 20 commissioned officers began in 1972 and included two nurses. As the importance of this effort grew, the federal government established a scholarship and loan repayment program within the NHSC.

Based on each school year, the scholarship program provides financial support if health professional students agree to serve in a NHSC-approved site that is located in an HPSA. For each full or partial school year that is reimbursed, the program requires a minimum of a two-year commitment (U.S. Department of Health and Human Services, HRSA, 2012a). The NHSC scholarship program supports NPs and CNMs.

The loan repayment program offers three options for primary care providers. The NHSC loan repayment program is offered to primary care providers who seek to work in an approved NHSC site. The students to service loan repayment program provides loan repayment to medical students in their fourth year. Finally, this program is a "federally funded grant program to states and territories that provides cost-sharing grants to assist them in operating their own state educational loan repayment programs for primary care providers working in HPSAs within their state" (U.S. Department of Health and Human Services, HRSA, 2012b, p. 1). Currently, the NHSC loan repayment program funds primary care NPs, CNMs, and psychiatric CNSs.

As noted, the U.S. PHS began in 1798 under the Adams Administration and was designated as one of the nation's seven uniformed services. Nearly a century later, in 1889, the Commissioned Corps was officially established. But it was in 1944 that the PHS Act authorized nurses and other health professionals into the commissioned corps (Debisette, Martinelli, Couig, & Braun, 2010). In 1949, when the PHS was restructured, the Chief Nurse Officer position was created with the rank of Assistant Surgeon General (Rear Admiral) (Debisette et al., 2010). As a nurse in the U.S. PHS, such as the Army, Navy, and Air Force, loan repayment options are available.

THE PATIENT PROTECTION AND AFFORDABLE CARE ACT: INVESTING IN APRN EDUCATION

Beginning in 2008, the health care community was deeply engaged and excited by the potential for health care reform. Discussion regarding massive and overarching changes to increase health care access, reduce expenditures, and improve quality resonated inside and outside the capital beltway. The nursing community was no exception. It would be through this legislative vehicle that they could achieve substantial and even monumental provisions that would invest in nursing education and practice with the ultimate goal of helping to meet the nation's changing patient care needs.

One of the first coordinated efforts by the nursing community was the reauthorization of the Title VIII Nursing Workforce Development programs. On January 24, 2008, Senator Barbara Mikulski (D-MD), a long-time nursing champion, contacted nursing leaders and requested that they develop a single document that detailed the priorities for a standalone Title VIII reauthorization bill (Nursing Community, 2008). Headed by AACN, a Title VIII Reauthorization task force was created to develop the consensus document that Senator Mikulski's office had requested. The nursing organizations around the table had a short deadline of three weeks to agree on a set of priorities and set them to paper. By the end of the first week, nursing organizations participating had to submit priorities and recommendations for the reauthorization. During the second week, the task force voted on which of the presented recommendations would be appropriate for a Title VIII reauthorization. The final week was spent drafting the recommendations and their accompanying rationale.

The document included one overarching principle, increase funding for Title VIII—all other principles were contingent upon increased funding levels, and four guiding principles were given as follows: (a) increase support for nurse faculty education, (b) strengthen specific resources for the education of advanced practice nurses and advanced education nursing, (c) increase efforts to develop and retain a diverse and professional nursing workforce for the transforming health care delivery system, and (d) increase efforts of HRSA and the Division of Nursing to release timely and more comprehensive data on the nursing workforce (Nursing Community, 2008).

This document was signed by 37 national nursing organizations such as the American Association of Colleges of Nursing, the American Nurses Association, and major APRN organizations such as the American Academy of Nurse Practitioners (AANP) (Now the American Association of Nurse Practitioners), the American College of Nurse Practitioners (ACNP), the National Organization of Nurse Practitioner Faculties (NONPF), the American Association of Nurse Anesthetists (AANA), the American College of Nurse-Midwives (ACNM), and the National Association of Clinical Nurse Specialists (NACNS). It was presented to Senator Mikulski's office and while a standalone bill to reauthorize Title VIII was not introduced, the document was used as a tool by the Senator and the nursing community in preparing the Title VIII provisions that were included in the Patient Protection and Affordable Care Act or ACA (Pub. L. 111-148).

Near the end of May 2009, a total of 29 national nursing organizations, led by AACN, came together and agreed on a set of statutory language changes to Title VIII. Two significant changes were important to future APRN education funding. First, the ANE grant program included a clause under Section 296j(f)(2) that stated, "The Secretary may not obligate more than 10% of the traineeships under subsection (a) of this section for individuals in doctorate degree programs." Education for APRNs and those seeking advanced education in nursing was changing. The Doctorate of Nursing Practice (DNP) was gaining momentum across the country and the data clearly indicated a need for more nurse faculty with doctoral degrees (Title VIII Reauthorization, 2009). This clause severely limited the nation's nursing schools from supporting those who were enrolled in DNP or PhD programs. Second, under the ANE grant program, the definition of authorized midwifery programs was included to remain current with the changes in midwifery education. These provision changes were eventually included in the ACA.

In relation to the Title VIII ANE program, the ACA also led to the development of the Prevention and Public Health Fund (Sec. 4002). The fund, administered by HHS, provided support for programs authorized by the PHSA that focused on public health, wellness, and prevention (Pub. L. 111-148). It was through this fund that HRSA had the authority to create the ANE Expansion (ANEE) grant program in 2010. According to HRSA's 2010 funding opportunity announcement,

> The program's two purposes are (a) to increase the number of students enrolled full time in accredited primary care nurse practitioner and nurse midwifery programs, and (b) to accelerate the graduation of part time students in such programs by encouraging full time enrollment.
>
> *(U.S. Department of Health and Human Services, HRSA, 2010)*

In the rationale, HRSA noted,

> The need for primary care continues to grow because of expanded health care coverage for the un-insured and under-insured provided by the Affordable Care Act. The ANEE program will help meet this need by increasing the supply of primary care nurse practitioners and nurse-midwives.
>
> *(U.S. Department of Health and Human Services, HRSA, 2010)*

TABLE 14.3 APRN Enrollment[1] and Graduations[2] 2002–2012

Year		MASTER'S				PBDNP				PMDNP				DNP TOTAL			
		CNS	NP	NURSE MIDWIFERY	NURSE ANESTHESIA	CNS	NP	NURSE MIDWIFERY	NURSE ANESTHESIA	CNS	NP	NURSE MIDWIFERY	NURSE ANESTHESIA	CNS	NP	NURSE MIDWIFERY	NURSE ANESTHESIA
2002	Enrollment	3,730	16,675	677	2,198	-	-	-	-	-	-	-	-	-	-	-	-
	Graduation	1,072	5,785	334	510	-	-	-	-	-	-	-	-	-	-	-	-
2003	Enrollment	3,506	18,163	657	2,424	-	-	-	-	-	-	-	-	-	-	-	-
	Graduation	901	5,717	281	641	-	-	-	-	-	-	-	-	-	-	-	-
2004	Enrollment	3,597	19,488	562	2,498	-	-	-	-	-	-	-	-	-	-	-	-
	Graduation	978	5,589	239	680	-	-	-	-	-	-	-	-	-	-	-	-
2005	Enrollment	3,992	20,965	544	2,725	-	-	-	-	-	-	-	-	-	-	-	-
	Graduation	1,035	5,920	206	840	-	-	-	-	-	-	-	-	-	-	-	-
2006	Enrollment	3,932	23,980	771	2,793	6	80	5	1	-	-	-	-	-	-	-	-
	Graduation	1,031	6,475	234	844	0	0	0	0	-	-	-	-	-	-	-	-
2007	Enrollment	3,747	26,802	797	2,908	3	152	11	0	33	391	10	19	36	543	21	19
	Graduation	1,073	6,859	229	981	0	0	0	0	1	22	0	0	1	22	0	0
2008	Enrollment	3,768	29,323	951	3,247	12	324	21	9	112	1,158	23	64	124	1,482	44	73
	Graduation	965	7,613	251	989	1	17	2	0	4	110	2	1	5	127	4	1
2009	Enrollment	3,879	33,182	759	3,308	35	813	33	30	144	1,578	23	51	179	2,391	56	81
	Graduation	930	8,354	232	1,087	5	28	4	0	14	188	3	10	19	216	7	10
2010	Enrollment	3,424	38,858	1,168	3,690	33	1,570	41	82	117	1,812	24	33	150	3,382	65	115
	Graduation	903	9,633	327	1,256	1	28	5	0	13	409	11	13	14	437	16	13
2011	Enrollment	3,139	43,475	1,272	3,614	59	2,569	61	158	137	2,021	20	63	196	4,590	81	221
	Graduation	871	10,866	345	1,289	1	95	2	0	28	535	5	20	29	630	7	20
2012	Enrollment	2,557	48,685	1,370	3,653	83	3,793	61	252	136	1,867	18	57	219	5,660	79	309
	Graduation	821	12,785	398	1,347	1	222	9	19	13	514	17	11	14	736	26	30

[1]As of fall of the current year.

[2]August 1 of the previous year to July 31 of the current year.

CNS, clinical nurse specialists; DNP, Doctor of Nursing Practice; NP, nurse practitioner; PBDNP, Post-Baccalaureate Doctor of Nursing Practice; PMDNP, Post-Masters Doctor of Nursing Practice.

Source: AACN (2003–2013).

The total amount of funding was $30 million over a 5-year period and 26 grants were made to schools of nursing across the country (U.S. Department of Health and Human Services, HRSA, 2010). Although the program was not funded again through the Prevention and Public Health Fund, the noteworthy investment and recognition by the federal government to the important role NPs and CNMs play in providing primary care was substantial.

However, one of the most significant investments made to APRN education through the passage of the ACA was the Graduate Nurse Education (GNE) Demonstration (Sec. 5509). This program amended Title XVIII of the Social Security Act (SSA) to provide up to five hospitals with reimbursement for the clinical training of APRNs (Pub. L. 111-148). The road to achieve this important provision for APRN education was long, and demanded the attention of critical nursing champions and a strong coalition of health care expertise.

THE ROAD TO THE GNE DEMONSTRATION

To understand the development of the GNE demonstration, a historical base must be laid for mandatory APRN education funding. Mandatory funding for nursing education and attempts to secure mandatory funding for APRN education are long embedded in nursing's history. In fact, mandatory funding for nursing education dates back to the creation of Medicare through Title XVIII of the SSA (Thies & Harper, 2004). Graduate Medical Education, or GME, essentially reimburses hospitals for the care provided to Medicare patients by physician residents. Within GME, there also lies what is known as GME pass through dollars. These dollars fund nursing and other allied health prelicensure education programs (Thies & Harper, 2004). Section 413.85 of the SSA stipulates, however, that these education programs can only be supported if they "...are operated by providers as specified [hospitals], enhance the quality of inpatient care at the provider"; and meet the requirements of paragraph of this section for State licensure or accreditation. It is the first clause that clarifies GME pass through dollars. The nursing programs have to be owned and operated by the hospital. Therefore, this funding has traditionally been allocated to diploma programs and some CRNA programs operated by hospitals because of how nursing programs were administered in the 1960s (Aiken, Cheung, & Olds, 2009).

Nursing's advocacy to change the structure of this aspect was most notable during the 1990s when the Clinton Administration was debating health care reform. Many dialogues ensued on how the American health care systems should be restructured and nursing leaders were engaged in serious discussions concerning funding for nursing education. In the late 1990s, nursing and other health care leaders believed that it was the opportune time to discuss changes to GME reimbursement. Specifically, that Medicare funding should be directed to APRN education. At that point in history, diploma programs had been significantly phased out and most registered nurses obtained their nursing degree from an associate or baccalaureate program. Aiken, Cheung, and Olds (2009) noted that the "...rationale for Medicare support for graduate nursing education is the same as the rationale for GME: namely, that nurses in graduate programs are providing significant clinical care to Medicare beneficiaries in hospitals and other settings" (w653). The IOM (1997) released its report *On Implementing a National Graduate Medical Education Trust Fund* that made the recommendation that,

> Nursing DME (direct medical education) should be structured like physician DME and be paid to sponsoring institutions for the support of advanced practice, graduate clinical trainees. This provision should be neutral with respect to the proportion of

DME that has supported nursing; diploma, undergraduate nurse education support should be phased out in 4 years or less to allow present students to complete their training. (p. 16)

Inspired by national support for APRN education, AACN, ACNP, and NONPF released the *Statement on the Redirection of Nursing Education Medicare Funds to Graduate Nurse Education* on January 29, 1998. This document, intended for the *National Bipartisan Commission on the Future of Medicare Graduate Medical Education Study Group*, urged that Medicare dollars given to entry-level nursing education be directed to graduate nursing education and specifically APRN programs (AACN, 1998). The comprehensive document outlined the role of APRNs in health care delivery, educational trends of APRN students, nursing research demonstrating the effectiveness and high quality of APRN care, as well as citing outside support for the recommendation (AACN, 1998). The report noted that the Physician Payment Review Commission in 1995 and 1997 "recommended that advanced degree nursing programs operated by 4-year colleges and universities be eligible to receive Medicare funds that otherwise would be available only to hospital-operated programs" (p. 8). The Association of Academic Health Centers also supported the allocation of Medicare dollars to APRN education as well as the GNE Coalition that represented 11 national nursing organizations (AACN, 1998).

The battle to redirect the Medicare funding from entry-level nursing to APRN education continued in the early 2000s, as AACN's department of government affairs urged Congress to make this change through a legislative fix. However, no action was taken and the health care reform discussions under the Obama Administration opened the door for a unified approach. In 2009, health care reform discussions were heating up and nursing wanted to ensure the best possible legislative results for the profession and America's patients. One entity to join the campaign to demonstrate nursing's vital role in improving the nation's health care system was a collaboration between the Robert Wood Johnson Foundation and AARP. Together, these powerful health care voices formed a new entity called the Center to Champion Nursing in America (CCNA). Their goal was to work with the nursing community to help promote the exceptional contributions of RNs to improve health care access and quality, while reducing costs. In May 2009, AARP representatives met with nursing lobbyists to discuss the potential to secure mandatory funding for APRN education.

Initial dialogues between AARP began with AANP, AACN, AANA, ACNP, ACNM, NACNS, and NONPF. Throughout the spring and summer of 2009, they negotiated a proposal for the Medicare reimbursement for APRN education. This proposal was not to redirect the existing funding for nursing education, but a separate and distinct pot. While the nursing leaders clearly understood it would be ideal to direct the funding for APRN education to the schools of nursing, Medicare law was not structured for this type of funding allocation. Medicare reimbursed hospitals, not the school of health professions. Therefore, when legislation was introduced in the Senate and House by Senator Deborah Stabenow (D-MI) and Representative Lois Capps, RN (D-CA), respectively, the bill directed the reimbursement of hospitals and affiliated schools of nursing for APRN education (S. 1569, H.R. 3185, 110th Cong.). The legislation, titled *Medicare Graduate Nursing Education Act*, also clearly stated that the hospital must have an agreement with an accredited school of nursing offering APRN programs. Educational costs associated in the bill included faculty salaries, student stipends (if any), clinical instruction costs, and other direct and indirect costs (S. 1569).

The coalition that worked to develop the legislation also grew to a total of 14 organizations including a number of specialty NP organizations. The next steps to secure this program included meeting with key committee staff of the Senate Finance Committee and the House Ways and Means Committee (these committees have jurisdiction over changes to Medicare) to include the *Medicare Graduate Nursing Education Act* in the final health care reform legislation. Eight months of intense negotiations with key House and Senate Committee staff, particularly Senate Finance Committee staff, proved successful. When the ACA was signed into law on March 23, 2010, by President Barack Obama, the GNE demonstration was included.

Because of necessary negotiations, the final GNE demonstration was not the original proposal that AARP and the nursing community agreed upon in the summer of 2009. Given the uncertainty of total funding, complexity of its structure, and the new model for the Centers for Medicare and Medicaid (CMS), a demonstration or test was created. Up to five hospitals would be selected and a total funding level of $200 million over a 4-year period would be allocated. The funding could only be used for the reimbursement of APRN training. The law clearly stipulated that

> Qualified training means training that provides an advanced practice registered nurse with the clinical skills necessary to provide primary care, preventive care, transitional care, chronic care management, and other services appropriate for individuals entitled to, or enrolled for, benefits under part A of Title XVIII of the Social Security Act, or enrolled under part B of such title.
>
> *(Pub. L. 111-148, Sec. 5509)*

According to the GNE solicitation, "Costs associated with the didactic training component as well as the costs for certification and/or licensure are not eligible for reimbursement under this Demonstration" (U.S. Department of Health and Human Services, CMS, 2010, p. 3). As stipulated in the law, hospitals had to establish an agreement with at least one school of nursing and also had to include two or more non-hospital community-based care settings (Pub. L. 111-148, Sec. 5509). Because of the fact that CRNA education is almost exclusively administered in acute care settings, a waiver was included in rural and medically underserved communities where 50% of the education did not occur in a community-based care site.

On March 21, 2012, CMS announced the solicitation for proposals for the GNE demonstration program with a deadline of May 21, 2012. The GNE demonstration would be run through the Center for Medicare and Medicaid Innovation, which was created through the ACA.

In its personal communication to AACN members on March 21, 2012, the association stated, "AACN, along with our colleagues in the APRN community and AARP, have been advocating for this program since its inception and are excited to see the long-awaited solicitation for proposals released."

Upon the release of the solicitation, the coalition noticed a few problems with the program that would need to be corrected and, led by AACN, quickly advocated for their change. For example, DNP programs were excluded and there was confusion concerning APRN specialties. The solicitation was changed to allow only DNP programs where the students were not already licensed as an APRN. Essentially, postmaster's DNP programs were not applicable (U.S. Department of Health and Human Services, CMS, 2010). Both the GNE coalition and CMS held webinars to help to inform the hospital and nursing community about the demonstration.

After the proposals were collected (a short extension was granted), the final models were chosen and announced on July 30, 2012. They included the Hospital of the University of Pennsylvania (Philadelphia, PA), Duke University Hospital

(Durham, NC), Scottsdale Healthcare Medical Center (Scottsdale, AZ), Rush University Medical Center (Chicago, IL), and Memorial Hermann-Texas Medical Center Hospital (Houston, TX). Whereas Duke and Rush University hospitals only included their affiliated school of nursing, the proposals from Arizona and Texas included four schools of nursing and Pennsylvania included nine schools (AACN, 2012b). It remains to be seen if the demonstration will continue after its four-year period. This demonstration was a major success for nursing in achieving a program that, if successful, could help to make the case for mandatory APRN education funding in the future. By all accounts, it was a remarkable achievement for the profession as it came together under true collaboration and a unified voice.

APRN RESIDENCIES

In 2010, the Robert Wood Johnson Foundation and the IOM released the landmark report, *The Future of Nursing: Leading Change, Advancing Health.* The report was regarded by the nursing community as monumental and quickly became the rationale and support for initiatives the profession had strived to achieve for decades. The key messages focused on nurses practicing to the full extent of their education and training, nurses achieving higher levels of education, nurses being full partners with their colleagues in health delivery reform, and improving workforce planning and data collection (IOM, 2010). In considering the education of nurses and APRNs, the report was clear that residencies should be a vital part of their training.

The Future of Nursing report noted that in 2002, the Joint Commission "recommended the development of nurse residency programs—planned, comprehensive periods of time during which nursing graduates can acquire the knowledge and skills to deliver safe, quality care that meets defined (organization or professional society) standards of practice" (IOM, 2010, p. 5). Historically, residency programs have been focused on the acute care setting, but as the report urged, residencies must be developed and evaluated outside the acute care setting (IOM, 2010). Increasing demand for nurses who practice primary care and serve those in the rural and underserved communities required more focus on developing highly skilled practitioners. Therefore, the following recommendation was included in *The Future of Nursing* report:

> Recommendation 3: Implement nurse residency programs. State boards of nursing, accrediting bodies, the federal government, and health care organizations should take actions to support nurses' completion of a transition-to-practice program (nurse residency) after they have completed a prelicensure or advanced practice degree program or when they are transitioning into new clinical practice areas.
>
> *(IOM, 2010, p. 11)*

The report recommended that all levels of nurses should receive a residency program after graduation and offered a number of tactics to achieve this goal.

1. State boards of nursing, in collaboration with accrediting bodies such as the Joint Commission and the Community Health Accreditation Program, should support nurses' completion of a residency program after they have completed a prelicensure or advanced practice degree program or when they are transitioning into new clinical practice areas.

2. The Secretary of HHS should redirect all GME funding from diploma nursing programs to support the implementation of nurse residency programs in rural and critical access areas.
3. Health care organizations, the HRSA and Centers for Medicare and Medicaid Services, and philanthropic organizations should fund the development and implementation of nurse residency programs across all practice settings.
4. Health care organizations that offer nurse residency programs and foundations should evaluate the effectiveness of the residency programs in improving the retention of nurses, expanding competencies, and improving patient outcomes.

(IOM 2010, p. 12)

The actions to achieve residency programs require a significant commitment by both public and private investors.

In November 2010, the CCNA launched the Campaign for Action. Their mission is "to promote implementation of recommendations in the in the IOM report, *The future of nursing: Leading change, advancing health"* (Center to Champion Nursing in America [CCNA], 2013, p. 2). The Campaign for Action established State Action Coalitions in which nursing, health care, and industry leaders have committed to implementing various portions of the report in their state. A number of state coalitions are working to implement the need for nurse residencies at all educational levels.

At the federal level, one initiative to fund APRN residencies was signed into law through the ACA. Section 5316, Demonstration Grants for Family Nurse Practitioner Training Programs, was an attempt to provide NPs with a one-year residency after graduation from their program. These practitioners would provide primary care to those in federally qualified health centers (FQHCs) and nurse-managed health clinics (NMHCs). Grants would be awarded to eligible FQHCs and NMHCs to cover the cost of full-time paid employment and benefits of family NPs. The law authorized $600,000 for each grant and designated such sums as necessary for FY 2011 and 2014 (Pub. L. 111-148, Sec. 5316). However, like many programs and demonstrations created through the ACA, authorized does not equate to appropriated. It remains to be seen if this demonstration will be funded in the future.

CONCLUSION

Funding for RN and APRN education has ebbed and flowed throughout history. New programs are developed given the nursing demand and phased out as they relate to the national agenda. Political factors have and will continue to play a large role in federal support for nursing education. However, nursing leaders have adapted to and advocated based on the ever changing dynamics. They have become savvier by seeking partners outside the profession and have truly invested in the importance of coalitions. For example, the work to achieve the GNE demonstration could not have been accomplished by one entity. Legislators need to know that the proposal or nursing policy is the will of the entire community.

The health care system will continue to evolve and change. APRNs will be substantial players in ensuring access to the high-quality, cost-effective care that America's patients deserve. However, it is clear that the nation will not meet its goals of an improved system if federal investments in health professions education, including nursing, are not a priority.

REFERENCES

Aiken, L., Cheung, R., & Olds, D. (2009). Education policy initiatives to address the nurse shortage in the United States. *Health Affairs 28*(4), w646–w656.

American Association of Colleges of Nursing (AACN). (1998). *Statement on the redirection of nursing education Medicare funds to graduate nurse education to the National Bipartisan Commission on the Future of Medicare Graduate Medical Education Study Group.* Retrieved from http://www.aacn.nche .edu/government-affairs/resources/Statement_on_the_Redirection_of_Nursing_Education _Medicare_Funds_to_GNE.pdf

AACN. (2003–2013). *Enrollment and graduations in baccalaureate and graduate programs in nursing.* Washington, DC: AACN.

AACN. (2008a). *Capitation grants: A solution for improving nursing school capacity.* Retrieved from http:// www.aacn.nche.edu/Government/pdf/CapGrants.pdf

AACN. (2008b, October). *Government affairs report: October 2008.* Report presented at the meeting of the American Association of Colleges of Nursing, Washington, DC.

AACN. (2012a). *Historical funding for Title VIII by program.* Archives from the American Association of Colleges of Nursing. Retrieved from http://www.aacn.nche.edu/government-affairs/Historic-FY -Funding.pdf

AACN. (2012b). *Graduate nurse education (GNE) demonstration.* Retrieved from http://www.aacn.nche .edu/government-affairs/gne

Buerhaus, P. I., Staiger, D. O., & Auerbach, D. I. (2009). *The future of the nursing workforce in the United States: Data, trends, and implications.* Boston, MA: Jones & Bartlett.

Center to Champion Nursing in America. (2013). *About us.* Retrieved from http://www.campaignfor action.org/about-us

Congressional Research Service (CRS). (2005). *Nursing Workforce Programs in Title VIII of the Public Health Service Act* (Order Code RL32805). Washington, DC: Library of Congress.

Debisette, A. T., Martinelli, A. M., Couig, M. P., & Braun, M. (2010). US Public Health Service Commissioned Corps Nurses: Responding in times of national need. *Nursing Clinics of North America, 45*(2), 125–135.

Division of Nursing. (2008, May). *Historical appropriations.* Provided via electronic mail.

Institute of Medicine (IOM). (1997). *On implementing a national graduate medical education trust fund.* Washington, DC: National Academies Press.

IOM. (2010). *The future of nursing: Leading change, advancing health.* Washington, DC: National Academies Press.

Kalisch, B. J., & Kalisch, P. A. (1977). *Nurturer of nurses: A history of the U.S. Public Health Service and its antecedents: 1798–1977.* Unpublished study prepared for the Division of Nursing.

Kalisch, B. J., & Kalisch, P. A. (1982). *Politics of nursing.* Philadelphia, PA: J. B. Lippincott & Company.

Medicare Graduate Nursing Education Act of 2009, S.1569, 110th Cong. (2009).

Medicare Graduate Nursing Education Act of 2009, H.R. 3185, 110th Cong. (2009).

Nurse Training Act of 1964. Pub. L. No. 88-581.

Nursing Community. (2008). *Nursing Community Consensus Document: Reauthorization Priorities for Title VIII, Public Health Service Act* (42 U.S.C. 296 et seq.). Archives of the American Association of Colleges of Nursing.

Nursing Community. (2012, March). *Nursing Workforce Development Programs: Title VIII of the Public Health Service Act.* Retrieved from http://www.aacn.nche.edu/government-affairs/TitleVIII.pdf

Patient Protection and Affordable Care Act of 2010. Pub. L No. 111-148 (Sec. 5509).

Patient Protection and Affordable Care Act of 2010. Pub. L No. 111-148 (Sec. 5316).

Politzer, R. M., Trible, L. Q., Robinson, T. D., Heard, D., Weaver, D. L., Reig, S. M., & Gaston, M. (2000). The National Health Service Corps for the 21st century. *Journal of Ambulatory Care Management, 23*(3), 70–85.

Public Health Service Act. (2002). Pub. L. No. 107-205.

Scott, J. M. (1967). Three years with the Nurse Training Act. *American Journal of Nursing, 67*(10), 2107–2109.

Thies, K., & Harper, D. (2004). Medicare funding for nursing education: Proposal for a coherent policy agenda. *Nursing Outlook, 52*(6), 297–303.

Title VIII Reauthorization: Statutory Language Changes. (2009). Archives of the American Association of Colleges of Nursing. Washington, DC.

U.S. Department of Health and Human Services, Centers for Medicare and Medicaid, Center for Medicare and Medicaid Innovation. (2012). *Graduate nurse education demonstration solicitation*. Retrieved from http://www.innovation.cms.gov/Files/x/GNE_solicitation.pdf

U.S. Department of Health and Human Services, Health Resources and Services Administration. (2010, June 17). Affordable Care Act, Advanced Nursing Education Expansion (ANEE), New Competition. Announcement Number HRSA-10-281, Catalog of Federal Domestic Assistance No. 93.513.

U.S. Department of Health and Human Services, HRSA. (2012a). *NHSC scholarship*. Retrieved from http://www.nhsc.hrsa.gov/scholarships/index.html

U.S. Department of Health and Human Services, HRSA. (2012b). *NHSC loan repayment*. Retrieved from http://www.nhsc.hrsa.gov/loanrepayment/index.html

Yett, D. E. (1966). The nursing shortage and the Nursing Training Act of 1964. *Industrial and Labor Relations Review, 19*(2), 190–200.

Yett, D. E. (1975). An economic analysis of the nursing shortage. In P. I. Buerhaus, D. O. Staiger, & D. I. Auerback (Eds.), *The future of the nursing workforce in the United States: Data, trends, and implications*. Boston, MA: Jones & Bartlett.

CHAPTER 15

Interface of Policy and Practice in Psychiatric Mental Health Nursing: Anticipating Challenges and Opportunities of Health Care Reform

Kathleen R. Delaney and Andrea N. Kwasky

The Patient Protection and Affordable Care Act (PPACA) initiated the most significant upheaval in the health care system in 50 years. This chapter focuses on the PPACA provisions that impact the care of individuals with mental health issues and the mental health care system. We trace how these ideas grew from the realities of health care economics and the perceived problems in health care delivery, and eventually threaded through the PPACA via service innovation. Reform advocates have pushed for an organizing principle for health care reform, the triple aim which is: improving the experience of care, improving the health of populations, and reducing per capita costs of health care (Berwick, Nolan, & Whittington, 2008). Key implications of the PPACA and their ramifications for psychiatric mental health (PMH) nursing practice are highlighted along with suggestions for how PMH advanced practice registered nurses (APRNs) might thrive within service innovations and achieve this triple aim. The intent of the reform provision is emphasized, including how PMH APRNs might collect outcomes that are in line with that intent and, in turn, use that data to influence the development of policy aimed at helping individuals achieve mental health. Finally, we suggest how the specialty might respond to provisions of the PPACA which frame policy issues critical to both workforce development and mental health service delivery. We begin with a summary of the context for health care reform because U.S. citizens' overall health, poor coordination of service delivery, and cost are the driving forces of reform.

CONTEXT FOR HEALTH CARE REFORM

Each January for the past two decades, health care economists have anticipated the year-end reports on health care expenditures; data which indicated what sectors of health care costs (e.g., hospital, labor, pharmaceutical) were rising and what was being held in check (e.g., Hartman, Martin, Benson, Catlin & the National Health Expenditure Accounts Team, 2013). Although specific sector spending varies from year to year, the clearest trend has been the steady rise in health care spending, now at 17.9% of gross national product (Hartman et al., 2013). The need for health care system reform has been a concern for years, and current problems such as rising health care insurance premiums (Gabel et al., 2004), the uninsured (Hadley & Holahan, 2003), or the cost of chronic illness (Druss et al., 2001) have been in the making for the last decade. Most citizens will mark the beginning of the era of health care reform with the signing of the PPACA. While not minimizing the innovation brought with the PPACA, the APRN should understand that the payment/service system reform has been a process slowly evolving for over 20 years.

BRIEF HISTORICAL BACKGROUND

The PPACA institutes broad reform in how the business of health care is conducted and incentivized. With the help of public media, the PPACA has become synonymous with issues of expanding federal health insurance to those in particular income brackets and with state expansion of insurance coverage. Actually, the PPACA is a bill with 90 provisions that will be phased in over 5 years (see www.kff.org/interactive /implementation-timeline/). Taking this broader viewpoint, it becomes apparent that the bill was constructed to strengthen and innovate particular health care sectors such as primary care, long-term care, and mental health services; create new models of care—such as the medical home; incorporate quality as an element of reimbursement; and fundamentally change the fee-for-service payment structure (Chaikind, Copeland, Redhead, & Staman, 2011).

These fundamental reform elements are intertwined. For instance, strengthening primary care through payment reform is viewed as a way to address the needs of the chronically ill, reduce unnecessary hospitalization, and curtail emergency room treatment (Davis, Abrams, & Stremikis, 2011). Service models such as the patient-centered medical home are meant to encourage care coordination which is seen as a way to reduce the costs of persons with chronic illness and multiple comorbidities (Rittenhouse & Shortell, 2009). Within each of these practice models innovations are provisions that change the provider incentives from a strict fee-for-service system to one where quality becomes a factor in the payment structure (Berenson, 2010). The PPACA also contains provisions aimed at building the workforce, which will work within and engineer the reform of services. For example, PPACA provisions provide monies to increase the primary care workforce, which will be needed to address the increasing number of citizens eligible for health care due to the expansion of health insurance (Carrier, Yee, & Stark, 2011; Centers for Medicare and Medicaid Services [CMS], 2013a).

In line with this triple aim the PPACA is threaded with innovative philosophies of care, such as patient-centered care, which demands that consumer/family goals and treatment preferences are integrated into health care decision making (Epstein, Fiscella, Lesser, & Stange, 2010). Particular PPACA provisions shift the health care system to a focus on the health of the population, emphasizing prevention and wellness (Goodson, 2010). In integrated care/payment networks, such as Accountable Care Organizations, incentives make it profitable to keep people healthy. Thus, the PPACA is a complex compilation of payment restructuring, workforce initiatives, insurance reforms, penalties, and incentives designed to fundamentally change the business of health care.

PPACA AND MENTAL HEALTH CARE

The aims, innovations, and incentives of PPACA are moving into mental health care via integrated care models, parity in mental health insurance coverage, and initiatives to move Medicare and Medicaid into a capitated system (American Psychiatric Association [APA], 2012; Ebert et al., 2013). To reduce costs while maintaining quality, the PPACA strengthens and expands the primary care system, bringing more individuals into the system while addressing mental health and physical needs in a coordinated manner (Ebert et al., 2013). Individuals with mental illness represent a significant portion of the U.S. population and their service needs are largely unmet (see Box 15.1). As individuals dealing with mental illness are more likely to be uninsured, the PPACA provisions to expand health insurance coverage to individuals at 133% of poverty level should also expand coverage for mental health issues (Garfield, Zuvekas, Lave, & Donohue, 2011). The psychiatry community generally endorsed the PPACA, emphasizing the benefits of extending health coverage to 32 million more Americans, prohibitions on denying coverage based on preexisting conditions, and particularly that mental health and substance abuse disorder treatment were to be part of the basic package of benefits in the health insurance plans that would be part of state exchanges (APA, 2012; Mental Health America [MHA], 2011). However concerns exist regarding coverage for mental health treatment within these new state exchanges plans: particularly that rates may be structured to discourage enrollment of individuals with high mental health needs, and that insurance packages may not contain necessary benefits for those with serious mental illness (SMI) (Barry, Weiner, Lemke, & Busch, 2012).

The PPACA initiatives, particularly in mental health, are impacted by the broader federal strategic agendas of the Substance Abuse and Mental Health Services Administration (SAMHSA, 2011a) and Centers for Disease Control and Prevention (CDC, 2011b) and powerful agencies that set the language and principle for change, such as the Institute of Medicine (IOM) (2006). Dominant themes include

---

PREVALENCE OF MENTAL ILLNESS IN THE UNITED STATES AND TREATMENT RATES	BOX 15.1

- In 2010, an estimated 45.9 million adults aged 18 or older in the United States had any mental illness in the past year (SAMHSA, 2012).
- The reported rate of lifetime depression in one multistate survey was 16.1% in 2008 and the lifetime prevalence of anxiety was 12.3% in 2008 (CDC, 2011a).
- The lifetime diagnosis of bipolar disorder and schizophrenia results indicated 1.7% of participants had received a diagnosis of bipolar disorder, and 0.6% had received a diagnosis of schizophrenia (CDC, 2011a).
- Current data estimates 2.8 million U.S. citizens are dealing with substance use issues and that is expected to double in 2020, particularly with adults over 50 (Han, Gfroerer, Colliver, & Penne, 2009).
- In 2010, among the 20.3 million adults with a past year substance use disorder, 45.1% (9.2 million adults) had a co-occurring mental illness (SAMHSA, 2012).
- In 2010, of the 45.9 million adults with mental illness, more than 60% had not received mental health services (SAMHSA, 2012).
- In 2010, approximately 40% of the 11.4 million adults with SMI in the past year did not receive treatment (SAMHSA, 2012)

an emphasis on patient-centered care and recovery, the need to reduce disparities and promote resiliency, and a focus on building healthy communities that provide support for those in recovery. Similarly, a coalition of mental health organizations endorsed that reform in mental health care should be organized around increasing access, quality, and choice; building a system that recognizes recovery from mental illness and addictions is integral to health; and focusing on investment in prevention, early intervention, and research on mental health disorders and addictions (Manderscheid, 2010a).

It is within these economic, policy, and social contexts that key issues of the PPACA and its impact on mental health care are examined. We suggest that five areas of reform will have significant impact on service delivery and, in turn, psychiatric nursing and their future roles. These five areas are: the growth of integrated care, wellness emphasis, emergence of collaborative care models (including the behavioral health care home), health information technology (IT) systems, and patient-centered care. The main impacts on PMH practice of these five trends will be: *Integrated care* will diffuse the traditional practice role; *wellness emphasis* will demand new strategies to promote behavior change; *collaborative care models* will bring new roles for both PMH RNs and APRNs; *National health IT systems* will mine, organize, and make accessible PMH workforce and quality data; and *patient-centered care* is a natural fit with nursing ideology and should augment the PMH perspective of relationship-centered care. These areas of impact highlight how the PPACA addressed significant problems in health care by reorganizing incentive structures, particularly around payment reform and building new models of care.

CONCEPTUAL SUPPORT FOR IMPACTS

Integrated Health Care

Problem

The mental health care delivery system is generally depicted as fragmented, with significant gaps in coverage and care and the tendency to deliver care in highly specialized subsystems (President's New Freedom Commission on Mental Health, 2003). As the PPACA was being formulated, the publication of data on the medical comorbidities and decreased life expectancy of individuals with serious mental illness hastened calls for developing a system that integrated behavioral and primary care services (Horvitz-Lennon, Kilbourne, & Pincus, 2006). Related issues also emerged, including the costs of these comorbidities along with the increased risk of disability and poor health outcomes, particularly for those dealing with substance abuse issues (Melek & Norris, 2008; Najt, Fusar-Poli, & Brambilla, 2011; Scott et al., 2009).

Innovation

Integrated care is a strategy that makes sense given that an individual is more likely to see a primary care provider than engage in specialty care, and the consumer's preference for treatment in a less stigmatizing primary care setting (Manderscheid, 2010b). Even before the PPACA CMS money and SAMHSA grants funded innovations in integrated care delivery (SAMHSA, 2009). Initially, models of integrated care were forwarded with various collocations of services; the emphasis of treatments depended on the needs of the population (Butler et al., 2008). Integrated care models have evolved various ways to integrate services, from telepsychiatry to co-located models in a behavioral health care home (Collins, Hewson, Munger, & Wade, 2010; SAMHSA-HRSA Center for Integrated Health Care Solutions, n.d.).

Incentives

The PPACA has built-in incentives to strengthen integrated primary care, such as increased payment to primary care physicians to work with families and coordinate care (U.S. Department of Health and Human Services [HHS], 2011). The PPACA also hastened the transition to integrated care via provisions which called for expansion of insurance coverage and a reimbursement structure that favors primary care, particularly care coordination services (HHS, 2011), by awarding grants to explore models of integrated care (CMS, 2011) and the development of the Community-based Collaborative Care Network Program. While the latter was not funded, it did result in other innovation awards to create state-wide integrated care networks for vulnerable populations (Witgert & Hess, 2012).

Wellness

Problem

Beginning with changes at the beginning of the 20th century, the U.S. health care system became increasingly geared toward treating illness and not promoting health (Fani Marvasti, & Stafford, 2012). The result is a costly system which yielded poor health outcomes for our citizens, as indicated by the greater rates of morbidity and mortality of U.S. citizens compared to other industrialized countries (Commonwealth Fund, 2008). Additionally, the cost of health care was increasingly tied to health conditions brought on by modifiable risk factors such as obesity and stress (Thorpe, 2005).

Innovations

The PPACA focused on wellness, health promotion, and prevention. It initially established a prevention fund, and recently HHS launched its National Strategy for Quality Improvement in Health Care (2012), which included the key provisions they believed would make care safer, as well as more cost-effective and patient-centered. Within this document is the notion that health care organizations must focus on prevention and promoting the wellness of their members. Workplace wellness centers were also seen as a way to bend the cost curve on direct medical costs and boost productivity (Cohen, Boukus, & Tu, 2010). In the mental health arena, SAMHSA (2011b) published the eight dimensions of wellness and criteria that outline the physical health outcomes expected of all behavioral health care centers (SAMHSA-HRSA, 2012a).

Incentives

The PPACA incentivized wellness through grants to small businesses to start Wellness Programs (Cohen et al., 2010); CDC assistance in evaluating wellness programs (Tu & Mayrell, 2010); and a pay-for-performance system where a health care system will produce key outcomes, and based on their success in select areas of prevention/guideline adherence/wellness outcomes, they will be financially rewarded or penalized (Berenson, 2010). Funding for prevention activities includes state-based demonstration projects, funding for community health departments' prevention activities, and regulations stating that Medicare and Medicaid cannot impose costs on patients for services deemed beneficial by the Preventive Services Task Force (Hardcastle, Record, Jacobson, & Gostin, 2011).

Care Coordination

Problem

The portion of persons with two or more chronic conditions increased from 24% in 2001 to 28% in 2006 (Anderson, 2010). By 2009, Anderson estimated that 145 million Americans were living with a chronic condition — almost half of our population. The care of these individuals had become increasingly fragmented, ineffective, and costly (Anderson, 2010). The approach to these individuals was siloed, with practitioners focused on the individual chronic diseases specific to their practice (Parekh, Goodman, Gordon, & Koh, 2011).

Innovation

Several care coordination models were strengthened by the PPACA, such as the patient-centered medical home (PCMH): a primary care based model in which a team of professionals work to coordinate care for individuals with complex health needs (Rittenhouse & Shortell, 2009). A variation of the PCMH specific to mental health has also been devised: the behavioral health care home (SAMHSA-HRSA Center, 2012b). Disease management models, such as the Wagner chronic disease model, are proving to be effective (Woltmann et al., 2012), as well as innovations specific to behavioral health care which ensure that professionals communicate with each other regarding behavioral care as well as co-morbid medical issues (Sabo, Leviton, & McKaughan, 2012).

Incentives

Care coordination efforts are rewarded in the health care reform payment system by enhanced reimbursement to PCMH. The PPACA also established the CMS Innovation Center to pilot service delivery models, including care coordination efforts (Chaikind et al., 2011). There are notable disincentives for poor care coordination, particularly the penalties for 30-day preventable readmissions (Milstein & Shortell, 2012).

Health IT

Problem

One factor in poor care coordination between service sectors was the inability of clinicians to easily communicate across service sites, but even by 2009 only a percentage of providers were utilizing the full capabilities of their EHR systems (Robinson et al., 2009). Also, prior to the PPACA there was no national health IT platform to examine the relationship of EHR use and quality care. Health IT was seen as a means to facilitate patients receiving recommended care, as well as reducing medical errors. However, HIT dissemination was slow, partially due to cost, a factor with even greater impact in rural areas (Blumenthal et al., 2006).

Innovations

In 2003 electronic reporting and billing regulations were put in place, which have evolved into the development of the Electronic Data Interchange system, which collects, organizes, and reports on a broad range of encounter data (CMS, 2013b). The Federal Health IT Strategic Plan (2012) includes provisions for building systems that will allow service sectors to hold common information and use it to augment care coordination. In their vision, SAMHSA (2011a) plans to boost the information exchange between specialty behavioral health care and primary care. Within this initiative are plans for developing the infrastructure of an interoperable EHR, as well as addressing the accompanying privacy, confidentiality, and data standards issues.

Incentive

Stimulus money incentivized providers to develop an electronic health record. The PPACA added to these incentives by offering meaningful use payments to providers who met particular objectives, many of which demonstrated how they used their EHR to improve care (CMS, 2013c). Along similar lines, the Federal IT strategic plan called for the development of clinical IT which can serve as a platform for information exchange, quality improvement initiatives, and dissemination of health care reform innovation projects (DHHS Office of the National Coordinator for Health Information Technology, 2012).

Patient-Centered Care

Problem

In 2001, the Institute of Medicine set down six principles for improving the quality of care in America's health care system (IOM, 2001). Recognizing that treatment had become focused more on the needs of the system than the individual receiving care, they established the need for a new direction: patient-centered care. While there have been great strides in defining patient-centered care and its components, research demonstrates instances where clinicians are not listening to patient concerns (Tai-Seale, Foo, & Stults, 2013). Issues of patient-centered care magnify in behavioral health where stigma often creates a status differential that silences the patient's voice (Lawrence & Kisely, 2011).

Innovation

Patient-centered care is woven throughout many of the critical policy documents of the PPACA, such as the HHS National Quality Strategy and the Patient Centered Health Care (National Council for Community Behavioral Healthcare, 2009). Consumers have also been vocal in outlining how to effectively achieve collaboration, effective communication, and use of peer navigators in systems of care (CalMend, 2011). Finally the science and methods of shared decision making have been formalized, and its potential outcomes have become increasingly evident (SAMHSA, 2010).

Incentives

One provision of the PPACA is that patients' experience-of-care scores will be used (in part) to determine a hospital's bonus (Wolosin, Ayala, & Fulton, 2012). The PPACA also established the Patient-Centered Outcomes Research Institute which awards research monies for investigations into the mechanics and measurement of patient-centered care. An outgrowth of patient-centered care that is being incentivized in meaningful use stage 2 is patient engagement, which leads to a patient who participates in his or her treatment and thus achieves better outcomes (Pelletier & Stichler, 2013).

PMH NURSING PRACTICE: IMPACT AND ADJUSTMENT

Integrated Care

PMH APRNs have a skill set that fits well with integrated care: they have been educated in the sciences—e.g., medical, prevention, psychiatry/behavioral health, and neuroscience—(Hanrahan, Delaney, & Merwin, 2010), and thus have the education and training to monitor co-existing physical conditions and screen for emerging physical problems (Delaney, Robinson, & Chafetz, in press). While their role within traditional psychiatric models is clear, the exact function PMH APRNs have in providing assessments of medical needs and preventive care has not been well defined (Weinstein, Henwood, Cody, Jordan, & Lelar, 2011). Many agencies and payers are unaware of what PMH APNs actually do.

PMH APRNs must clearly articulate the skills they bring to new health care settings and identify the scope of their practice to providers who are engaged in primary care as well as patients who may not have had previous experience with mental health care providers (Delaney, 2013). Scope of practice parameters for assessment of physical issues, and integration of these issues in a plan of care is contained in the PMH Scope and Standards of Practice (ANA, in press). Specific competencies are contained in the National Organization of Nurse Practitioner Faculties (NONPF) Core Competencies (NONPF, 2011) and the PMH Nurse Practitioner Competencies (NONPF, 2013).

The latter document was written while the *Diagnostic and Statistical Manual of Mental Disorders, 4th edition, text revision* (*DSM-IV-TR*; APA, 2000) and ICD-9 taxonomies were in use. With the May 2013 publication of the *DSM-5*, PMH APRNs are in a position to educate our primary care practice partners about the modifications in diagnosis and assessment strategies. The ability of PMH APRNs to understand and communicate issues related to scope of practice, billing, coding, and reimbursement are paramount for their transition to integrated care.

Decisions regarding what is appropriately treated in primary care and what issues should be addressed in specialty care are an important element of integrated care. By working together with APRN groups, PMH APRNs can define the appropriate hand-offs in primary care so that when the patient's behavioral/medical treatment plan is devised there is an underlying logic matching the intensity of need with the intensity of services. There are existing systems for screening clients on both medical and mental health issues and, based on the professionals' assessment scores, assigning patients to a level of treatment that matches their service needs (Intermountain Healthcare, 2009). For the health of our clients, developing such systems of clinical decision-making in integrated care should be a PMH APRN priority. PMH APRNs must also be mindful of the inherent barriers to consumers and work to help them navigate these complex systems.

Wellness

In tandem with an emphasis on physical health, the PPACA focuses on wellness. NPs have been recognized for their provision of preventive care, health education, health promotion, and wellness care as well as their holistic approach (Hardcastle et al., 2011). PMH APRNs must bring their expertise with wellness into the mental health arena (Delaney et al., 2013). PMH nurses understand that the keys to healthy behaviors are increasing an individual's sense of self-efficacy and empowering them to move toward a self-constructed vision of health (Anthony, 2006). Helping individuals make healthier choices depends on an individual's willingness to engage with a clinician and adopt particular behaviors. Thus PMH APRNs should cultivate methods to increase patient engagement (Pelletier & Stichler, 2013).

For patients with SMI, a holistic approach also demands an understanding of their illness and the social determinants of health. Poverty and the related issues of nutrition, housing, and occupational status impact health and wellness (Onie, Farmer, & Behforouz, 2012). PMH APRNs should employ a holistic approach to put wellness in the context of an individual's lifestyle and beliefs (Delaney et al., 2013). This emphasis on wellness naturally involves prevention and early intervention by mental health practitioners, particularly with children. We are increasingly aware of the impact adverse childhood events can have on an individual's mental and physical health long into adulthood (Felitti et al., 1998), and that common mental disorders are likely to first emerge in childhood and adolescence (Kessler et al., 2007). Evidence-based programs exist that address early signs of major mental health issues such as anxiety, depression, and conduct disorders (Delaney & Staten, 2010). Psychiatric APRNs should focus on informing and implementing these EBPs with an eye on the emerging neuroscience research that supports building resiliency (Brown & Barila, 2012).

Care Coordination

Given the recognized need for improved care coordination for vulnerable populations, older adults and the chronically ill, new models of care are emerging which utilize NPs in both care coordination and direct service (Stanley, Werner, & Apple, 2009). As with other nursing specialties, PMH APRNs' competencies and scope of practice may be unclear to service organizations and payers (Lowe, Plummer, O'Brien, & Boyd, 2011). Historically, the caring practices rendered by nurses have not been deemed reimbursable, contributing to the "economic invisibility" of our profession (Safriet, 2011). Thus PMH nurses must clearly articulate their skill set and where it fits in effective care coordination.

To provide effective, quality care to patients dealing with complex conditions, PMH APRNs must invest in achieving seamless transitions between types of care and developing innovative models (including nurse-managed health centers) to meet the patients' holistic needs (Naylor & Kurtzman, 2010). As PMH APRNs collaborate with the care team, they must also demonstrate the added value they bring. PMH APRNs should not only participate in these models of care but initiate new strategies for care coordination that ensure each patient receives safe, quality, cost-effective care in the least restrictive setting.

PMH APRNs are able to provide the full scope of mental health services to consumers (ANA, 2007). Their ability to understand the multiple levels of need and interacting behavioral/medical systems puts PMH nurses in a distinctive position to bridge between hospital, home-specialty, and primary care. In this effort, affiliations will be key; with other professionals but more so with consumers and peer specialists, who have unique capabilities to partner with others in the recovery process (Faces and Voices of Recovery, 2013).

Health IT

The Federal Health IT Strategy illuminates the potential of IT systems to mine, organize, and report workforce, encounter, and quality data. Billing encounter forms may become a source of information on who provides care, where it is provided, and select outcomes of that care (Poghosyan et al., 2012). Currently there are financial incentives for billing a category of APRN encounters under the physician's name. Billing records also contain an APRN's National Provider Identifier (NPI) which will also become a source of workforce data, perhaps eventually tracking APRN concentrations and access to care (Kaplan, Skillman, Fordyce, McMenamin, & Doescher, 2012). PMH APRNs must be aware of how national encounter data will be an important source of reports on both outcomes and access, and thus assert the prerogative of billing under their own provider numbers.

Health IT clinical information systems hold similar promise given their potential to organize and communicate quality initiatives, best practices, and outcomes of service innovations. At this juncture, PMH APRNs should be documenting their use of practice guidelines and EBPs in treatment planning, particularly in the EHR. Efforts to increase quality could be enhanced by increasing the capacity of the system's EHR to provide data that would inform the APRN of the success of or problems with clinical processes or the achievement of health outcomes (Dennehy et al., 2011).

Patient-Centered Care

Health Care Reform initiatives around patient-centered care provide PMH APRNs with the opportunity to revitalize PMH traditions of relationship-based care and bring their skill with interpersonal connections to their work with individuals and their efforts to achieve wellness (Delaney et al., 2013). PMH nurses understand that achieving wellness benchmarks for individuals with SMI may require additional strategies, given the lifestyle habits the patients may have developed to cope with their illness and its treatment (Delaney et al., 2013). For instance obesity and metabolic syndrome are increasingly understood in relation to particular atypical antipsychotics (Pramyothin & Khaodhiar, 2010). Lifestyle also comes into play with regards to smoking, which may to some extent be "self medication" and thus cannot be adequately addressed without concurrent attention to psychiatric symptom management (Delaney et al., 2013). The new emphasis on Doctor of Nursing (DNP) degrees provides PMH nurses with opportunities to shape wellness initiatives in line with what patients need and to collect data on their efforts (Tierney & Kane, 2011).

As PMH nurses move into new roles in integrated care they must be guided by the needs of the consumer and the consumer's expression of what will help them lead a more meaningful life in the community. Recovery adds an additional dimension to patient-centered care; working through mental health issues requires the APRN to convey hope, encouragement, and therapeutic optimism (Stickley & Wright, 2010). These interpersonal elements; positive emotions as well as sensitivity to and capacity for tolerating and understanding distress (Gilbert, 2009), are all components of the person-centered care APRNs must cultivate.

EVALUATION OF APRN PRACTICE INITIATIVES

Cost, quality, and access are three of the underlying principles for evaluation of APRN practice. Cost outcomes of APRN practice are increasingly emerging in the literature (AANP, 2013a). Cost benefits can operate at the level of savings-related factors such as decreased length of stay (Newhouse et al., 2011) or the cost benefits of an individual model (Allen, Himmelfarb, Szanton, & Frick, 2013). Similar cost outcomes of PMH APRN practice could be assessed, such as the cost savings related to care coordination and decreased use of emergency services or hospitalization.

Quality outcomes are also available in the literature, particularly for NP practice (AANP, 2013b). Outcomes for integrated care are limited; mainly isolated to outcomes for specific conditions, such as somatoform and depression, and for specific models, such as IMPACT (van der Feltz-Cornelis, Van Os, Van Marwijk, & Leentjens, 2010). What remains unknown are the effects of specific strategies, and how outcomes correlate with levels of integration or care coordination processes (Miller, Kessler, Peek, & Kallenberg, 2011). By defining the scope of their practice and roles,

PMH APRNs can begin to measure quality metrics, such as how care coordination relates to patient satisfaction, and how a particular health coaching technique relates to patient engagement in care (Pelletier & Stichler, 2013) (see Table 15.1).

APRNs are critical to improving access to primary care for U.S. citizens (Naylor & Kurtzman, 2010). The PPACA, along with the Mental Health Parity Laws, expands coverage for mental health services to the majority of Americans. The payment changes anticipated by the PPACA, particularly Medicaid expansion, will potentially bring more individuals into the MH system. However, funded individuals may be impacted by the scarcity of MH providers. One outcome of APRN practice should be the ability to increase access to care and provide services; particularly in rural areas where there is often a low density of mental health providers (Hanrahan & Hartley, 2008).

PMH AND POLICY: UNIFYING EFFORTS

Alignment of APRN practice with the principles of health care reform will depend on our specialty's resilience, but equally on the alliances we develop with consumers, advocacy groups, APRN professional organizations, and other behavioral health care professionals. It will require that the PMH APRNs see themselves as a single workforce with their PMH RN colleagues and other APRN groups. This perspective is essential if APRNs are to engineer systems where persons are treated holistically, and mental health, wellness, and medical needs are acknowledged with equal vigor. By bringing this focus on connectivity to the nursing community, health care reform helps to achieve a public health model of mental health care, wherein individuals would receive mental health interventions at multiple points in the health care delivery system (Delaney, 2011). This will require unifying nurses from a wide range of disciplines to bring care to the individual's home environment and for constructing patient-centered outcome measures.

Within this broad vision two policy issues demand particular attention. To create a coordinated, integrated system of care will require APRNs practicing at their full scope of practice (Newhouse et al., 2011; Stanley et al., 2009). In the APRN community it is broadly acknowledged that recognizing the capacity of APRNs to improve access to and quality of care will also necessitate attention to barriers to practice arising from restrictive state regulations and payer recognition of APRNs (Poghosyan et al., 2012). PMH APRNs must join the state nursing groups that are focused on APRN issues. APRNs need to monitor government initiatives, the problems which motivate them, and how they connect to innovations and payment incentives. The specialty as a whole must focus on mining national IT banks to create sources of data to produce PMH outcomes that impact the direction of federal policy streams. They must gauge the national agenda in order to anticipate workforce needs and understand their leverage.

The second critical area is health insurance and payment reform. There are particular concerns regarding the impact of insurance reform on access to care and benefits for persons in need of mental health services—particularly adverse selection, wherein plans "cherry pick" healthy individuals to keep the cost of services low (Barry et al., 2012). There is also concern about the actual breadth of benefits being offered in state insurance exchange plans (Garfield et al., 2011). APRNs need to embrace their advocacy role by becoming educated on each state's insurance structure, and work to clarify mental health benefits within the state insurance pool.

TABLE 15.1 Practice Reform and APRN Outcomes and Core Competencies

PRACTICE REFORM	PATIENT OUTCOMES	SERVICE DELIVERY OUTCOMES	APRN-RELATED OUTCOMES	APRN CORE COMPETENCY
Integrated care	Functional status Patient experience Symptom relief	Increased access Cost effectiveness SAMHSA PBHCI measures	Care coordination Quality indicators Safety indicators	Analyzes organizational structure, functions, and resources to improve the delivery of care Assesses impact of acute and chronic medical problems on psychiatric treatment
Wellness and prevention	Progress on select wellness indicators, e.g., PROMIS measures Received EPB prevention/health promotion Patient engagement	Percent of patients screened for mental health issues Longitudinal health indicators of populations Cost utility	Use of EBP in wellness promotion Patient engagement	Applies principles of self-efficacy/empowerment and other self-management theories in promoting behavior change Modifies treatment approaches based on the ability and readiness to learn
Care coordination roles	Patient connected to services they want and need Use of services within a behavioral health care home	Reduction of unnecessary rehospitalization Reduced use of ED for episodic care needs Cost minimization	APRN planning and monitoring APRN role on care team and relation to outcomes APRN added value	Collaborates in planning for transitions across the continuum of care Considers motivation and readiness to improve self-care and healthy behavior when teaching
Health IT to improve care	Patient population served and health indicators measured Patient risk delineated	Evidence that health information drives quality initiative Evidence on use of EBP and practice guidelines	Data on patients receiving APRN interventions, APRN practice alignment with practice guidelines	Contributes to the design of clinical information systems that promote safe, quality, and cost effective care Uses technology systems that capture data on variables for the evaluation of nursing care
Patient-centered care	Patient experience Patient engagement	Improvement in core health indicators related to patient engagement/activation measures (e.g., PROMIS measure)	APRN documentation of shared decision making, APRN provision of recovery support	Provides leadership to foster collaboration with multiple stakeholders (e.g., patients, community, integrated health care teams, and policy makers) to improve health care

EPB, evidence-based practices; PBHCI, primary and behavioral health care integration; PROMIS, patient-reported outcomes measurement information system; SAMHSA, Substance Abuse and Mental Health Services Administration.

The economic pressures on mental health services have never been greater. Between 2009–2012, the fiscal crisis forced cuts in states' mental health budgets of approximately $4.35 billion and health care reform's innovations are only a partial response (NASMHPD, 2012). Since sites that provide acute care were particularly affected the entire mental health system was impacted since a reduction in hospital beds is tied to increases in homelessness, emergency room use, and use of prisons as de-facto psychiatric hospitals (Treatment Advocacy Center, 2008). PMH nurses must educate themselves and advocate for the policies that ensure access to the full range of services for individuals with mental health needs.

ETHICAL CONSIDERATIONS

The innovations introduced by health care reform promise to improve the health of individuals with SMI and expand access to mental health services to individuals who may not have had prior access to those services. The need for inpatient services for those in crisis is also recognized (NAMI, 2011). However, as state mental health care budgets shrink—particularly in the wake of the financial downturn of 2008—there may not be sufficient acute care beds or services for those in crisis. As PMH nurses engage in the development of integrated care, they should not lose sight of the ethical principle of professional stewardship of resources. PMH nurses should advocate for funding to maintain the mental health inpatient beds needed by those experiencing an acute exacerbation of their illness.

Mental health records have been traditionally subject to additional privacy safeguards. Depending on the orientation, PPACA brings some degree of threat to that confidentiality. Efforts to reduce preventable hospitalizations will invite inspection of an individual's pattern of accessing mental health services. The promise of integrated and coordinated care naturally leads to communication between clinicians and across service agencies. Integrated care networks for vulnerable populations open up the records of those enrolled in the program (Witgert & Hess, 2012). As PMH APRNs practice within these networks, they must be mindful of confidentiality, involving patients in decisions about sharing health information and taking time to explain the ramifications of signing releases of information versus the benefits of restricting communication between providers.

For the past decade, recovery has been a grounding principle of the mental health system. According to the National Consensus Statement on Mental Health Recovery (SAMHSA, 2011c), recovery is a journey of healing that enables a person with a mental health problem to live a meaningful life in his or her community. Inherent in this statement is the principle of autonomy: honoring the individual's movement along the healing trajectory. In the PPACA world of population outcomes and system benchmarks, the PMH nurse must be mindful of the principle of protecting that autonomy and the patient's right to map their journey toward health.

Stigma is an enduring ethical issue and it is the APRN's duty to be aware of how stigma operates within systems of care, both subtle and overt (Lawrence & Kisely, 2011), and how it affects individuals with mental health issues (Hinshaw, 2007). From a nursing perspective, stigma is a major roadblock—along with poverty and victimization—to completing the recovery journey and gaining access to services (Perese, 2007). Combating stigma is bound with the ethics of distributive justice, which requires that all citizens have access to the health care needed for living a full human life (Lamont & Favor 2013). For PMH APRNs to combat the ubiquitous effects of stigma, awareness and advocacy are critical (Delaney, 2012).

CONCLUSION

At this juncture, it is essential that those in the PMH specialty refine their vision, articulate it clearly, and disseminate it widely. The PMH workforce has a unique combination of education and training that makes them particularly suited for integrated care, collaborative team models, and wellness initiatives. The key to creating and sustaining these newer models of care may not lay in any particular structure, but in designing a model with an evaluation system that offers timely data on its effectiveness (Milstein & Shortell, 2012). As PMH nurses expand their vision of mental health within a community of support, their alliances within a network of providers, consumers, and the community will be crucial to building an environment of health, recovery, and resilience. The impact of PMH APRN practice will come from this collective vision of psychiatric nurses, working to integrate evidence-based interventions into their practice sites, and engaging with consumers and communities to build health.

DISCUSSION QUESTIONS

1. How might changes in health care policy encourage creation of the nurse-managed health care center?
2. What is the biggest impact of your state nursing regulations on your future APRN practice?
3. What are the biggest hurdles to achieving effective integrated care in your state? How could policy address those hurdles?
4. Name one way that stigma impacts mental health care service delivery.
5. What are the major advocates for mental health in your state? How can you join with them to improve mental health care?

ANALYSIS AND SYNTHESIS EXERCISES

1. How do lifestyle and psychotropic medications combine to create risk for medical complications in individuals with serious mental illness?
2. What are the factors that create difficulty when isolating APRN outcomes in the patient-centered medical home?
3. Why would psychiatric clients be excluded from data collection on the patient experience?
4. Should there be a separate set of physical health benchmarks for individuals with serious mental illness?

CLINICAL APPLICATION CONSIDERATIONS

1. Investigate and compare among students, in the populations served by clinical practicum sites, the most common medical/psychiatric/substance use co-morbidities.
2. What is the current policy(s) in the state legislature that will likely impact the APRN workforce?
3. Name one strategy used in your clinical site to promote healthy behaviors among individuals with serious mental illness.
4. Investigate data in your state on access to services for individuals with mental illness.
5. Compare and contrast the mental health benefits in three policies in your state insurance exchange.

REFERENCES

American Academy of Nurse Practitioners. (2013a). *Nurse practitioner cost-effectiveness*. Retrieved from http://www.aanp.org/images/documents/publications/costeffectiveness.pdf

American Academy of Nurse Practitioners. (2013b). *Quality of nurse practitioner practice*. Retrieved from http://www.aanp.org/images/documents/publications/qualityofpractice.pdf

American Nurses Association (ANA). (2007). *Psychiatric-mental health nursing: Scope and standards of practice*. Silver Spring, MD: Author.

American Psychiatric Association (APA). (2012). *Health care reform: A primer for psychiatrists*. Washington, DC: Author.

Allen, J. K., Himmelfarb, C. R. D., Szanton, S. L., & Frick, K. D. (2013). Cost-effectiveness of nurse practitioner/community health worker care to reduce cardiovascular health disparities. *Journal of Cardiovascular Nursing*. Epub ahead of print. doi: 10.1097/JCN.0b013e3182945243

Anderson, G. (2010). *Chronic conditions: Making the case for ongoing care*. Robert Wood Johnson Foundation. Retrieved from http://www.rwjf.org/content/dam/farm/reports/reports/2010/rwjf54583

Anthony, W. A. (2006). What my MS has taught me about severe mental illness. *Psychiatric Services, 57*, 1081–1082.

Barry, C. L., Weiner, J. P., Lemke, K., & Busch, S. H. (2012). Risk adjustment in health insurance exchanges for individuals with mental illness. *American Journal of Psychiatry, 169*, 704–709.

Berenson, R. A. (2010). *Moving payment from value to volume: What role for performance measurement—Timely analysis of immediate health policy issues*. Robert Wood Johnson, Urban Institute. Retrieved from http://www.rwjf.org/content/dam/farm/reports/issue_briefs/2010/rwjf69037

Berwick, D. M., Nolan, T. W., & Whittington, J. (2008). The triple aim: Care, health and cost. *Health Affairs, 27*, 759–769.

Blumenthal, D., DesRoches, C., Donelan, K., Ferris, T. G., Jha, A. K., Kaushal R., … Shield, A. (2006). *Health information technology in the United States: The information base for progress*. Princeton, NJ: Robert Wood Johnson Foundation. Retrieved from http://www.rwjf.org/files/publications/other/EHRReport0609.pdf

Brown, M., & Barila, T. (2012). *Children's resilience initiative: One community's response to adverse childhood experiences*. Retrieved from http://www.acmha.org/summit_reports_2012.shtml

Butler, M., Kane, R. L., McAlpine, D., Kathol, R. G., Fu, S. S., Hagedorn, H., & Wilt, T. J. (2008, October). *Integration of mental health/substance abuse and primary care no. 173* (Prepared by the Minnesota Evidence-based Practice Center under Contract No. 290-02-0009). AHRQ Publication No. 09-E003. Rockville, MD: Agency for Healthcare Research and Quality.

CalMend. (2011). *Integration of mental health, substance use and primary care services: Embracing our values from a client and family member perspective* (Vol. 1). Retrieved from http://www.calmed.org.

Carrier, E. R., Yee, T., & Stark, L. (2011). Matching supply to demand: Addressing the US primary care workforce shortage. *Looking Ahead, 5*, 4. NIHCR Policy Brief. Retrieved from http://www.nihcr.org/PCP_Workforce

Centers of Disease Control and Prevention (CDC). (2011a). Mental illness surveillance among adults in the United States. *Morbidity and Mortality Weekly Report, 60*(3), 1–32. Retrieved from http://www.cdc.gov/mmwr/preview/mmwrhtml/su6003a1.htm?s_cid=su6003a1_w

Centers for Disease Control and Prevention (CDC). (2011b). *Public health action plan to integrate mental health promotion and mental illness prevention with chronic disease prevention, 2011–2015*. Atlanta, GA: U.S. Department of Health and Human Services.

Centers for Medicare and Medicaid Services (CMS). (2011). *Active projects report. Research and demonstrations in health care financing. A comprehensive guide to CMS research activities*. Retrieved from http://www.cms.gov/Research-Statistics-Data-and-Systems/Statistics-Trends-andReports/ActiveProjectReports/Downloads/2011_Active_Projects_Report.pdf

CMS. (2013a). *Graduate nurse education demonstration*. Retrieved from http://innovation.cms.gov/initiatives/gne

CMS. (2013b). *Electronic billing & EDI transactions*. Retrieved from http://www.cms.gov/Medicare/Billing/ElectronicBillingEDITrans/index.html?redirect=/electronicbillingeditrans

CMS. (2013c). *CMS EHR incentive programs*. Retrieved from http://www.cms.gov/Regulations-and-Guidance/Legislation/EHRIncentivePrograms/index.html?redirect=/EHRIncentivePrograms/

Chaikind, H., Copeland, C. W., Redhead, C. S., & Staman, J. (2011). *PPACA: A brief overview of the law, implementation, and legal challenges.* Congressional Research Services, Report for Congress. Retrieved from http://www.nationalaglawcenter.org/assets/crs/R41664.pdf

Cohen, G. R., Boukus, E. R., & Tu, H. T. (2010). *Workplace clinics: A sign of growing employer interest in wellness.* HSC Research brief, No. 17. Retrieved from http://www.hschange.com/CONTENT/1166/

Collins, C., Hewson, D. L., Munger, R., & Wade, T. (2010). *Evolving models of behavioral health integration in primary care.* New York, NY: Milbank Memorial Fund.

Commonwealth Fund Commission on a High Performance Health System. (2008). *Why not the best? Results from the National Scorecard on U.S. Health System Performance, 2008.* Retrieved from http://www.commonwealthfund.org/Publications/Fund-Reports/2008/Jul/Why-Not-the-Best--Results-from-the-National-Scorecard-on-U-S--Health-System-Performance--2008.aspx

Davis, K., Abrams, M., & Stremikis, K. (2011). How the Affordable Care Act will strengthen the nation's primary care foundation. *Journal of General Internal Medicine, 26,* 1201–1203.

Delaney, K. R. (2011). Child mental health care workforce: What vision are we working towards? *Journal of Child and Adolescent Psychiatric Nursing, 24,* 1–2.

Delaney, K. R. (2012). Stigma that we fail to see. *Archives of Psychiatric Nursing, 26,* 333–335.

Delaney, K. R. (2013). Psychiatric mental health nurses: What should we be "called" in the broad health care arena? *Journal of the American Psychiatric Nurses Association, 19,* 176–178.

Delaney, K. R., Robinson, K. M., & Chafetz, L. (in press). Development of integrated mental health care: Critical workforce competencies. *Nursing Outlook.* Retrieved from http://www.sciencedirect.com.ezproxy.rush.edu/science/journal/aip/00296554. doi: http://dx.doi.org/10.1016/j.outlook.2013.03.005

Delaney, K. R., & Staten, R. T. (2010). Prevention approaches in child mental health disorders. *Nursing Clinics of North America, 45,* 521–539.

Department of Health and Human Services Office of the National Coordinator for Health Information Technology. (2012). *Federal Health Information Technology Strategic Plan 2011–2015.* Retrieved from http://www.healthit.gov/policy-researchers-implementers/health-it-strategic-planning

Dennehy, P., White, M. P., Hamilton, A., Pohl, J. M., Tanner, C., Onifade, T. J., & Zheng, K. (2011). A partnership model for implementing electronic health records in resource-limited primary care settings: Experiences from two nurse-managed health centers. *Journal of the American Medical Informatics Association, 18,* 820–826.

Druss, B. G., Marcus, S. C., Olfson, M., Tanielian, T., Elinson, L., & Pincus, H. A. (2001). Comparing the national economic burden of five chronic conditions. *Health Affairs, 20,* 233–241.

Ebert, M. H., Findling, R. L., Gelenberg, A. J., Kane, J. M., Nierenberg, A. A., & Tariot, P. N. (2013). The effects of the affordable care act on the practice of psychiatry. *Journal of Clinical Psychiatry, 74,* 357–367.

Epstein, R. M., Fiscella, K., Lesser, C. S., & Stange, K. C. (2010). Why the nation needs a policy push on patient-centered health care. *Health Affairs, 29,* 1489–1495.

Faces and Voices of Recovery. (2013). *Why peer integrity and recovery orientation matters.* Reform and Peer Recovery Support Service Faces and Voices of Recovery, Issues Brief #3. Retrieved from http://www.facesandvoicesofrecovery.org/pdf/Health_Reform/6.14.13_Issue_Brief_No_3.pdf

Fani Marvasti, F., & Stafford, R. S. (2012). From sick care to health care—Reengineering Prevention into the US System. *New England Journal of Medicine, 367,* 889–891.

Felitti, V. J., Anda, R. F., Nordenberg, D., Williamson, D. F., Spitz, M., Edwards, V., … Marks, J. S. (1998). Relationship of childhood abuse and household dysfunction to many of the leading causes of death in adults. *American Journal of Preventive Medicine, 14,* 245–258.

Gabel, J., Claxton, G., Gil, I., Pickreign, J., Whitmore, H., Holve, E., … Rowland, D. (2004). Health benefits in 2004: Four years of double-digit premium increases take their toll on coverage. *Health Affairs, 23,* 200–209.

Garfield, R. L., Zuvekas, S. H., Lave, J. R., & Donohue, J. M. (2011). The impact of national health care reform on adults with severe mental disorders. *American Journal of Psychiatry, 168,* 486–494.

Goodson, J. D. (2010). Patient Protection and Affordable Care Act: Promise and peril for primary care. *Annals of Internal Medicine, 152,* 742–744.

Gilbert, P. (2009). *The compassionate mind: A new approach to life's challenges.* Oakland, CA: New Harbinger Publications.

Hadley, J., & Holahan, J. (2003). How much medical care do the uninsured use, and who pays for it? *Health Affairs (Project Hope), W3*, w66–w81.

Han, B., Gfroerer, J. C., Colliver, J. D., & Penne, M. A. (2009). Substance use disorder among older adults in the United States in 2020. *Addictions, 104*, 88–96.

Hanrahan, N., Delaney, K. R., & Merwin, E. (2010). Health care reform and the federal transformation initiatives: Capitalizing on the potential of Advanced Practice Psychiatric Nurses. *Policy, Politics and Nursing Practice, 11*, 235–244.

Hanrahan, N. P., & Hartley, D. (2008). Employment of advanced-practice psychiatric nurses to stem rural mental health workforce shortages. *Psychiatric Services, 59*, 109–111.

Hardcastle, L. E., Record, K. L., Jacobson, P. D., & Gostin, L. O. (2011). Improving the population's health: The Affordable Care Act and the importance of integration. *Journal of Law, Medicine & Ethics, 39*, 317–327.

Hartman, M., Martin, A. B., Benson, J., Catlin, A., & the National Health Expenditure Accounts Team. (2013). National health spending in 2011: Overall growth remains low, but some payers and services show signs of acceleration. *Health Affairs, 32*, 87–99.

Hinshaw, S. P. (2007). *The mark of shame: Stigma of mental illness and an agenda for change.* New York, NY: Oxford Press.

Horvitz-Lennon, M., Kilbourne, A. M., & Pincus, H. A. (2006). From silos to bridges: Meeting the general health care needs of adults with severe mental illnesses. *Health Affairs, 25*, 659–669.

Institute of Medicine (IOM), Quality of Health Care in America. (2001). *Crossing the quality chasm: A new health system for the 21st century.* National Academy Press.

Institute of Medicine (IOM), (US) Committee on Crossing the Quality Chasm, Adaptation to Mental Health, & Addictive Disorders. (2006). *Improving the quality of health care for mental and substance-use conditions.* Washington, DC: National Academy Press.

Intermountain Healthcare. (2009). *Overview of scoring and evaluating child/adolescent MHI forms.* Retrieved from http://www.intermountainhealthcare.org/ext/Dcmnt?ncid=520702514&tfrm=default

Kaplan, L., Skillman, S. M., Fordyce, M. A., McMenamin, P. D., & Doescher, M. P. (2012). Understanding APRN distribution in the United States using NPI data. *Journal for Nurse Practitioners, 8*, 626–635.

Kessler, R. C., Amminger, G. P., Aguilar-Gaxiola, S., Alonso, J., Lee, S., & Ustun, T. B. (2007). Age of onset of mental disorders: A review of recent literature. *Current Opinion Psychiatry, 20*(4), 359–364.

Lamont, J., & Favor, C. (2013). Distributive justice. In E. N. Zalta (Ed.), *The Stanford encyclopedia of philosophy* (Spring 2013 edition). Retrieved from http://www.plato.stanford.edu/archives/spr2013/entries/justice-distributive

Lawrence, D., & Kisely, S. (2011). Inequalities in healthcare provision for people with severe mental illness. *Journal of Psychopharmacology, 24*, 61–68.

Lowe, G., Plummer, V., O'Brien, A. P., & Boyd, L. (2012). Time to clarify–The value of advanced practice nursing roles in health care. *Journal of Advanced Nursing, 68*, 677–685.

Manderscheid, R. (2010a). Moving our agenda forward. *Behavioral Healthcare, 30*(7), 9. Retrieved from http://www.behavioral.net/article/moving-our-agenda-forward

Manderscheid, R. W. (2010b). Evolution and integration of primary care services with specialty services. In B. Levin, K. Hennessy, & J. Petrila (Eds.), *Mental health services: A public health perspective* (3rd ed., pp. 389–400). New York, NY: Oxford University Press.

Melek, S., & Norris, D. (2008). *Chronic conditions and comorbid psychological disorders.* Seattle, WA: Milliman.

Mental Health America (MHA). (2011). *Position Statement 71: Health Care Reform.* Retrieved from http://www.mentalhealthamerica.net/go/position-statements/71

Miller, B. F., Kessler, R., Peek, C. J., & Kallenberg, G. A. (2011). *A national agenda for research collaborative care: Papers from the collaborative care research network.* Research Development Conference. AHRQ Publication No. 11-0067. Rockville, MD: Agency for Healthcare Research and Quality.

Milstein, A., & Shortell, S. (2012). Innovations in care delivery to slow growth of US health spending. *Journal of the American Medical Association, 308*, 1439–1440.

Najt, P., Fusar-Poli, P., & Brambilla, P. (2011) Co-occurring mental and substance abuse disorders: A review of the potential predictors and clinical outcomes. *Psychiatry Research, 186*, 159–164.

National Alliance on Mental Illness. (2011). *State mental health cuts: A national crisis.* Retrieved from http://www.nami.org/ContentManagement/ContentDisplay.cfm?ContentFileID=126233

National Association of State Mental Health Program Directors. (2012). *Proceedings on the State Budget Crisis and the Behavioral Health Treatment Gap: The Impact on Public Substance Abuse and Mental Health Treatment Systems*. Retrieved from http://www.nasmhpd.org/docs/Summary Congressional%20 Briefing_March%2022_Website.pdf

National Council for Community Behavioral Healthcare. (2009). *Behavioral health/Primary care integration and the person-centered healthcare home*. Retrieved from http://www.thenationalcouncil.org /galleries/resources-services%20files/Integration%20and%20Healthcare%20Home.pdf

National Organization of Nurse Practitioner Faculties. (2012). *Nurse practitioner core competencies*. Retrieved from http://www.nonpf.com/associations/10789/files/NPCoreCompetenciesFinal 2012.pdf

National Organization of Nurse Practitioner Faculties. (2013). *Population focused nurse practitioner competencies. Psychiatric-mental health nurse practitioner competencies*. Retrieved from http://www.nonpf .org/associations/10789/files/PopulationFocusNPComps2013.pdf

Naylor, M. D., & Kurtzman, E. T. (2010). The role of nurse practitioners in reinventing primary care. *Health Affairs, 29*, 893–899.

Newhouse, R. P., Stanik-Hutt, J., White, K. M., Johantgen, M., Bass, E. B., Zangaro, G., … Weiner, J. P. (2011). Advanced practice nurse outcomes 1990–2008: A systematic review. *Nursing Economics, 29*(5), CNE series, 1–21.

Newhouse, R. P., Weiner, J. P., Stanik-Hutt, J., White, K. M., Johantgen, M., Steinwachs, D., … Bass, E. B. (2012). Policy implications for optimizing advanced practice registered nurse use nationally. *Policy, Politics, & Nursing Practice, 13*, 81–89.

Onie, R., Farmer, P., & Behforouz, H. (2012). Realigning health with care. *Stanford Social Innovation Review, 10*, 28–35. Retrieved from http://www.ssireview.org/articles/entry/realigning_health _with_care

Parekh, A. K., Goodman, R. A., Gordon, C., & Koh, H. K. (2011). Managing multiple chronic conditions: A strategic framework for improving health outcomes and quality of life. *Public Health Reports, 126*, 468–471.

Pelletier, L. R., & Stichler, J. F. (2013). Action brief: Patient engagement and activation: A health reform imperative and improvement opportunity for nursing. *Nursing Outlook, 61*, 51–54.

Perese, E. F. (2007). Stigma, poverty, and victimization: Roadblocks to recovery for individuals with severe mental illness. *Journal of the American Psychiatric Nurses Association, 13*, 285–295.

Poghosyan, L., Lucero, R., Rauch, L., & Berkowitz, B. (2012). Nurse practitioner workforce: A substantial supply of primary care providers. *Nursing Economics, 30*, 268–274, 294.

Pramyothin, P., & Khaodhiar, L. (2010). Metabolic syndrome with the atypical antipsychotics. *Current Opinion Endocrinology, Diabetes, and Obesity, 17*, 460–466.

President's New Freedom Commission on Mental Health. (2003). *Achieving the promise: Transforming mental health care in America. Final Report*. DHHS Pub. No. SMA-03-3832. Rockville, MD.

Rittenhouse, D. R., & Shortell, S. M. (2009). The patient-centered medical home. *Journal of the American Medical Association, 301*, 2038–2040.

Robinson, J. C., Casalino, L. P., Gillies, R. R., Rittenhouse, D. R., Shortell, S. S., & Fernandes-Taylor, S. (2009). Financial incentives, quality improvement programs, and the adoption of clinical information technology. *Medical Care, 47*, 411–417.

Sabo, J., Leviton, L., & McKaughan, M. (2012). *Diffusion of a model for addressing behavioral health issues in primary care practices*. Robert Wood Johnson Foundation, Diffusion series. Retrieved from http://www.rwjf.org/content/dam/farm/reports/program_results_reports/2012/rwjf403130

Safriet, B. (2011). Federal options for maximizing the value of advanced practice nurses in providing quality, cost-effective health care. Committee on the Robert Wood Johnson Foundation Initiative on the Future of Nursing, at the Institute of Medicine. *The future of nursing: Leading change, advancing health* (443–476). Retrieved from http://www.healthforceminnesota.org/Partnership-Council /documents/SafrietArticle2010.pdf

SAMHSA-HRSA Center for Integrated Health Care Solutions. (n.d.). *List: Integrated care models*. Retrieved from http://www.integration.samhsa.gov/integrated-care-models/list

SAMHSA-HRSA Center for Integrated Health Care Solutions. (2012a). *PBHCI Candidate Measures*. Retrieved from http://www.integration.samhsa.gov/clinical-practice/PBHCI_Candidate_Measures _RAND.pdf

SAMHSA-HRSA Center for Integrated Health Care Solutions. (2012b). *Behavioral health homes for people with mental health & substance use conditions. The core clinical features.* Retrieved from http://www.integration.samhsa.gov/clinical-practice/CIHS_Health_Homes_Core_Clinical_Features.pdf

Schiff, M. (2012). *The role of nurse practitioners in meeting increasing demand for primary care.* National Governors Association for Best Practices. Retrieved from http://www.nga.org/cms/home/nga-center-for-best-practices/center-publications/page-health-publications/col2-content/main-content-list/the-role-of-nurse-practitioners.html

Scott, K. M., Von Korff, M., Alonso, J., Angermeyer, M. C., Bromet, E., Fayyad, J., ... Williams, D. (2009). Mental–physical co-morbidity and its relationship with disability: Results from the World Mental Health Surveys. *Psychological Medicine, 39,* 33–43.

Stanley, J. M., Werner, K. E., & Apple, K. (2009). Positioning advanced practice registered nurses for health care reform: Consensus on APRN regulation. *Journal of Professional Nursing, 25,* 340–348.

Stickley, T., & Wright, N. (2010). The British research evidence for recovery, papers published between 2006 and 2009 (inclusive). Part One: A review of the peer-reviewed literature using a systematic approach. *Journal of Psychiatric and Mental Health Nursing, 18,* 247–256.

Substance Abuse and Mental Health Services Administration (SAMHSA). (2009). *FY 2009 grant announcement—CMHS grants for primary and behavioral health care integration.* Retrieved from http://www.samhsa.gov/grants/2009/sm_09_011.aspx

Substance Abuse and Mental Health Services Administration (SAMHSA). (2010). *Shared decision-making in mental health care: Practice, research, and future directions.* HHS Publication No. SMA-09-4371. Rockville, MD: Center for Mental Health Services, Substance Abuse and Mental Health Services Administration.

Substance Abuse and Mental Health Services Administration (SAMHSA). (2011a). *Leading change: A plan for SAMHSA's roles and actions 2011–2014.* HHS Publication No. (SMA) 11-4629. Rockville, MD: Author.

Substance Abuse and Mental Health Services Administration (SAMHSA). (2011b). *SAMHSA's wellness initiative: Eight dimensions of wellness.* Retrieved from http://www.store.samhsa.gov/product/SAMHSA-s-Wellness-Initiative-Eight-Dimensions-of-Wellness/SMA12-4568

Substance Abuse and Mental Health Services Administration (SAMHSA). (2011c). *National consensus statement on mental health recovery.* Retrieved from http://www.apna.org/files/public/National_Consensus_Statement_trifold.pdf

Substance Abuse and Mental Health Services Administration (SAMHSA). (2012). *Results from the 2010 National Survey on Drug Use and Health: Mental Health Findings,* NSDUH Series H-42, HHS Publication No. (SMA) 11-4667. Rockville, MD: Author.

Tai-Seale, M., Foo, P. K., & Stults, C. D. (2013). Patients with mental health needs are engaged in asking questions, but physicians' responses vary. *Health Affairs, 32,* 259–267.

Tierney, K. R., & Kane, C. F. (2011). Promoting wellness and recovery for persons with serious mental illness: A program evaluation. *Archives of Psychiatric Nursing, 25,* 77–89.

Thorpe, K. E. (2005). The rise in health care spending and what to do about it. *Health Affairs, 24,* 1436–1445.

Treatment Advocacy Center. (2008). *Severe shortage of psychiatric beds sounds national alarm bell.* Retrieved from http://www.treatmentadvocacycenter.org/home-page/71/81

Tu, H. T., & Mayrell, R. C. (2010). *Employer wellness initiatives grow, but effectiveness varies widely.* National Institute for Health Care Reform Research Brief, (1). Retrieved from http://www.ihbaonline.org/documents/Employer-Wellness-Programs.pdf

United States Department of Health and Human Services (HHS). (2011). *HHS launches new initiative to strengthen primary care.* Retrieved from http://www.hhs.gov/news/press/2011pres/09/20110928a.html

United States Department of Health and Human Services (HHS). (2012). *2012 Annual Progress report to congress: National Strategy for Quality Improvement in Health Care.* Retrieved from http://www.ahrq.gov/workingforquality/nqs/nqs2012annlrpt.pdf

van der Feltz-Cornelis, C. M., Van Os, T. W., Van Marwijk, H. W., & Leentjens, A. F. (2010). Effect of psychiatric consultation models in primary care: A systematic review and meta-analysis of randomized clinical trials. *Journal of Psychosomatic Research, 68,* 521–533.

Weinstein, L. C., Henwood, B. F., Cody, J. W., Jordan, M., & Lelar, R. (2011). Transforming assertive community treatment into an integrated care system: The role of nursing and primary care partnerships. *Journal of the American Psychiatric Nurses Association, 17,* 64–71.

Witgert, K., & Hess, C. (2012). *Including safety-net providers in integrated delivery systems: Issues and options for policymakers.* Commonwealth Fund, Issues Brief, Retrieved from http://www.mhnchicago .org/sites/default/files/including_safety_net_providers_in_integrated_delivery_systems _commonwealth_aug_2012_.pdf

Wolosin, R., Ayala, L., & Fulton, B. R. (2012). Nursing care, inpatient satisfaction, and value-based purchasing: Vital connections. *Journal of Nursing Administration, 42,* 321–325.

Woltmann, E., Grogan-Kaylor, A., Perron, B., Georges, H., Kilbourne, A. M., & Bauer, M. S. (2012). Comparative effectiveness of collaborative chronic care models for mental health conditions across primary, specialty, and behavioral health care settings: Systematic review and meta-analysis. *American Journal of Psychiatry, 169,* 790–804.

HEALTH POLICY AND SPECIAL POPULATIONS

CHAPTER 16

The Aging Population

Pat Kappas-Larsen

An increase in aging of the population is one of the most dramatic demographic trends in the world today. By 2030, older adults are expected to comprise one-fifth of the world's population (Institute of Medicine [IOM], 2008). Over the next three decades, the number of persons over 65 will double. From 2000 to 2050, the number of older adults will increase from 12.5% to 20% in the United States alone (Center for Health Workforce Studies, 2006). The average age of the old is also increasing—the over-86 age group is the fastest growing segment of the U.S. population (Bennett & Flaherty-Robb, 2003). This trend is important as a significant number of these individuals are likely to be disabled, use multiple medications, or need at least some level of care management. As identified in the IOM (2008) report, these older adults consume a disproportionately large share of American health services when compared with younger population segments so demand for service will most likely grow.

Responding to this demand is expected to be compounded as legislators have worked to bring comprehensive change in U.S. health care by increasing access for the nation's more than 32 million under- and uninsured with the passage of the Patient Protection and Affordable Care Act (ACA). A significant number of those under- and uninsured include older adults such as those who are living with more health problems. The reforms driven by this act, combined with the surge of new health care consumers, are expected to tap a system already challenged by the expanding numbers of elderly with divergent needs needing care in a wide variety of settings.

One possible approach to responding to these issues is greater use of advanced practice registered nurses (APRNs). The ACA has several provisions that affect this group of professionals and will increase the demand for their services and thus create a need to broaden their scope of practice (O'Grady & Brassard, 2011). The clinical nurse specialists (CNSs) and nurse practitioners (NPs) included in this group of professionals have a demonstrated ability to provide affordable, accessible, quality care (Naylor & Kurtzman, 2010). They have proven ability to provide services in homes, community health centers, nurse-managed clinics, and other traditional and nontraditional settings, and can address the unmet need for primary care, disease management, and care coordination (Robert Wood Johnson Foundation [RWJF], 2011).

As the act unfolds over the coming years, key provisions undergird the need for these highly qualified APRNs.

There is a broad support for APRNs and an interest in increasing access to these vital providers. Consumer demand for APRN-provided care is growing thanks to a shortage of physicians, the soaring cost of health care, and a population that is aging and living longer with more acute and chronic conditions. Access, however, can only increase if there is modernization of the regulations and administrative mandates that limit their scope of practice and thus impact their availability or how they function in various settings of care.

SCOPE OF PRACTICE, REIMBURSEMENT, AND PRESCRIPTIVE AUTHORITY: PRACTICE CONSTRAINTS IMPACTING CARE OF THE OLDER ADULT

Currently, state and federal regulatory issues that most directly affect care for older adults are scope of practice, reimbursement, and prescriptive authority. These issues are interrelated and when combined are referred to as constraints to practice. APRNs have a graduate level of education and are trained in preventing, diagnosing and treating illness, prescribing medications, and care coordination inclusive of referral management to specialists. CNSs and NPs are trained to provide primary care. Although APRNs are already working in a wide variety of settings—from long-term care to acute care and from offices to the home—care they can provide in each of these venues is governed by conflicting and restrictive regulatory restrictions and by fragmented and limiting standards. These are not new issues. Nearly a decade ago, Safriet (2008) noted the underlying problem of state-by-state variations in regulatory restrictions that impacted scope of practice and prescriptive authority compounded by federal policy that limited reimbursement. These issues have been associated with the nation's elderly experiencing hardships related to lack of access to health care and delays in treatments (Horton & Johnson, 2010).

Eighteen states plus the District of Columbia have liberalized and standardized their scope-of-practice regulations and allow NPs to practice and prescribe independently (Fairman, Rowe, Hassmiller, & Shalala, 2011). In those states, APRNs can therefore treat and prescribe without a physician's supervision or collaboration. However, there are considerable differences among the states regarding CNSs and NPs (Newhouse, Weiner, Stanik-Hutt, White, et al., 2012) with some states significantly restricting the scope of practice of CNSs.

This is important as CNSs are expert clinicians that specialize in an area of nursing practice. The specialty may be identified in terms of a population (e.g., geriatrics); a setting (e.g., emergency room); or a disease (e.g., diabetes). They are instrumental in the integration of nursing practice, which focuses on assisting patients in prevention or resolution of illness, with medical diagnosis and treatment of disease, injury, and disability. They, along with the NPs, are a vital part of the health care workforce.

Seven states require physician's oversight of prescribing and 25 states require oversight of diagnosis, treatment plans, and prescribing (Phillips, 2013). There is a high degree of variation in the oversight requirement and again variation in how it can impact the NP versus the CNS. The requirement for physician oversight interferes with patient access to care, fosters delays in treatment, and may result in care duplication. The latter can also impact costs of care for the older adult when they are required to have face-to-face visits by both providers or require a specialist's involvement prior to ordering medications or diagnostic tests. State practice acts that restrict patients' access to APRNs impede the APRN's ability to achieve positive health outcomes.

Regardless of this impact, significant state-by-state variation exists and is driven by the fact that APRNs practice under the laws of the state in which they are licensed and each state has its own licensing and certification criteria. In some states, state boards of nursing and medicine may jointly oversee APRNs licensing. The issue of scope of practice becomes one of the reliance on availability of physicians to provide the required oversight and collaboration and the degree of oversight that the regulations demand. In those states requiring oversight, APRNs are more likely to have work delegated to them to satisfy the oversight and collaboration requirement. The result is often co-management of the patient panel rather than the APRN acting as the sole, designated care provider. This becomes an issue for older adults who may require immediate visits when a physician is not available or require visits in a setting of care or a geographic area where the physician does not desire to practice.

In addition to the issue of physician's oversight requirements, other state-to-state variations in practice include maximum "collaboration ratios" for APRNs working with physicians, an inability to certify home health care visits or stays in skilled nursing facilities or hospice, ordering of durable medical equipment, admitting of patients to hospitals, or prescribe medications (Fairman et al., 2011). These variations not only create barriers for patients but also the care they receive in one state does not mirror the care in another. This impacts the mobile older adult who spends time in more than one state.

For the older adult who is often dealing with multiple health issues and is fragile, timely access to care is an even greater issue. Any delays or limits on access to care may well result in the use of higher cost settings of care and negative health outcomes. It has been documented that quality of health care received by older adults varies from one condition and type of care to another. In part, this occurs because of the critical shortage of health care providers who are educated in the unique health needs of older adults (IOM, 2008). The challenge in caring for the older adult is not limited to managing the chronic conditions they present with but also understanding the existence and impact of geriatric-specific conditions.

Researchers have noted that adherence to quality indicators for geriatric conditions—such as dementia, urinary incontinence, and falls, which primarily affect the older population—is even lower than adherence for such general medical conditions as diabetes and hypertension (IOM, 2008; Rand Health, 2004). Given the existence of chronic and geriatric conditions, demand for care is high. Older adults account for more than 13 million visits per year to outpatient departments and use a disproportionate share of emergency services (Hing, Cherry, Woodwell, & Division of Health Care Statistics, 2006). Managing chronic illness and the conditions associated with aging requires a complex set of skills and continuous management, which is an integral part of APRN education.

In addition to the array of identified practice constraints that challenge APRNs in their role, they are underutilized as primary care providers in settings that are used with frequency by the older adult such as the hospital setting or long-term care facilities. These barriers occur at both the federal and state levels where laws and regulations exert authority over hospital-admitting privileges for APRNs as well as their designation as the primary care provider of record. Although nearly all states defer to individual hospitals to set their own policies they do influence them. State scope-of-practice constraints may inadvertently encourage hospitals to block hospitalized patients' access to their provider of choice, if that provider is an APRN (Brassard & Smolenski, 2011). The issue is not only can the APRN, who is the provider of choice, follow the individual in the hospital but also those hospitals who allow only physicians to admit create challenges for care continuity upon return to the community as the discharge information goes to the physician of record and NOT to the APRN provider in the community.

Regulations established by the Centers for Medicare and Medicaid Services (CMS) also preclude APRNs from being designated as the primary care provider in long-term care facilities. As a result, the practice model in those settings is a medical model of care which often precludes the APRN from providing patient-centered, health-focused, and holistic care. These role impediments restrict access to patients and may well inhibit a wellness, quality-of-life approach for a very vulnerable group of older adults that would benefit from that type of care model.

In addition to settings of care restraints and requirements regarding oversight, the regulations regarding prescriptive authority may have significant impact on the older adult. For the older adult in those states that do not allow NPs to prescribe independently or those that do not allow for CNS authority, timely response to their needs becomes an issue as care interventions may well be delayed because of lack of physician provider availability. In states such as Massachusetts and Arkansas where collaborative agreements with physicians are required to diagnose, treat, and prescribe, it is even more problematic and again limited availability of physicians adds to the issue. In those states with these restrictive requirements, the NP is "tethered to the physician" and cannot go out into rural communities or into settings of care that physicians are unwilling to go. At a minimum, this may well reduce the APRN's efficiency and ability to respond to immediate needs as well as limit settings of care. Immediate care needs are even more problematic in such states as Arkansas and Michigan, which prohibit or restrict how APRNs prescribe Schedule II controlled substances often used to treat pain. Given these restrictions, patients may encounter delays in securing much needed medication and it is often that the older adult is in need of such medications, individuals who can least afford delays in treatment.

In summary, limitations on prescriptive authority and the vastly different regulations from state to state suggest that the regulatory framework for APRN practice is not evidence based and the states are not promulgating regulations with the patient in mind (O'Grady & Brassard, 2011). Restrictive policies impede continuity of care and may therefore negatively impact health outcomes.

Payer policies and reimbursement may well have an even greater impact on practice than scope-of-practice issues even those inclusive of prescriptive authority limitations. Payers set reimbursement levels and they are based on their own determination of place of service. This is true of both public and private payers. Since mid-2000s, Hansen-Turton has been highlighting the issue of managed care companies' lack of recognition of APRNs as primary care providers. Even for those who have allowed for the designation or have allowed for incident-to-billing that requires physician supervision the reimbursement remains lower (Hansen-Turton, Ritter, & Torgan, 2008a, 2008b; Yee, Boukas, Cross, & Samuel, 2013). Private payers tend not to recognize the APRN as a primary care provider, and may also decline to credential or directly pay for their services. Private payers' regulations and Any Willing Provider laws vary from state to state but in general do little to facilitate the ability of APRNs to be reimbursed for their services or to be recognized as primary care providers (Chapman, Wildes, & Spetz, 2010). This can limit their ability to provide services in certain areas or settings and therefore limits access, fosters care duplication, and increases costs. Lack of adequate reimbursement from private payers is compounded by declining reimbursements by public payers such as Medicare and Medicaid, the key insurance programs utilized by the older adult. The discounting reimbursements provided to APRNs along with overall declining rates makes it difficult to sustain a practice thus once again impacting access.

Reimbursements, prescriptive authority, and scope-of-practice issues impact access to those who require home health, hospice, and even x-rays. State and federal regulations have prohibited APRNs to sign certification documents or orders that allow consumers to receive these needed services. Older adults are high users of hospice and home care services with at least 10% of Medicare beneficiaries using some level of home health services each year (Brassard & Smolenski, 2011) yet their ability to access services may be delayed or the services may not be able to be delivered. Until January of 2013, APRNs were unable to order x-rays again resulting in delays in the assessment of patients, delays in intervention, and increasing costs. An aging population requires timely access to all of these services to prevent disease progression and associated functional deterioration, and to decrease the use of high-cost care settings.

HEALTH CARE NEEDS OF THE OLDER ADULT

Delivery of high quality, cost-effective care requires comprehensive care across care settings and coordination among providers. APRNs are capable of providing safe, effective care to those with acute and chronic conditions. They are better at communicating with patients about self-managing their conditions offering advice, providing screenings, counseling, and ensuring follow-up care is provided (Naylor & Kurtzman, 2010). For about five decades, they have been utilized to deliver primary care, traditionally in underserved areas or to vulnerable populations (Poghosyan, Lucero, Rauch, & Berkowitz, 2012). They have delivered care to the older adult in assisted living settings, in their homes, in nursing facilities as well as in traditional care settings.

The health of older adults in the United States is a critical issue and as a country, we may need to rethink about how and who provides health care to older adults with chronic conditions and those who deserve a focus on preventive health. Simply treating disease will no longer be sufficient. The growing number of older adults, and the families who care for them, will need emotional, educational, and preventive services that are not currently available and not addressed in a medical model of care.

Today, considerable differences exist regarding scope of practice, prescriptive authority, and reimbursement across states and they are exacerbated by those imposed at the federal level or by private payers. APRNs, therefore, are not being utilized as fully as they could be. They can be a big part of the solution to the growing needs of the older adult population and respond to the opportunities now provided in the ACA. With an emphasis on prevention, chronic care management, and quality care, the ACA promotes many of the priorities of advanced practice nursing and those of the older adult.

The need to transform care of the older adult is demonstrated by discussing Ms. E, a 79-year-old adult who lives alone in an apartment. She has chronic obstructive pulmonary disease (COPD), which for many years has resulted in frequent hospital admissions with each admission resulting in a subsequent physical decline. She is taking multiple medications that are taken 3 to 4 times a day that she reports are difficult to manage. She has no regular schedule of care with her primary care physician and has not participated in any care transition program, disease management, or complex care management programs.

During her last hospitalization, she was seen by CNSs specializing in COPD management who enrolled her in a complex, case management program. As a result, she received regular phone calls from a case management nurse who provided education, support, and coordination of care. Ms. E's living situation has been transformed to a safe, comfortable environment where she receives care in the least restrictive setting. Every morning she receives a phone call and her responses are compared with those of the previous day. When she reports respiratory symptoms her medication dosage is adjusted and the information is sent to her NP. The constant monitoring has allowed her to avoid readmissions for COPD. Phone support and site visits have allowed her to achieve a higher quality of life and reduce her use of high-cost care settings. This is care transformation at its best and can only work for all with elimination of current practice constraints that exist today.

Older adults have reduced physiological reserve requiring that decisions about interventions take into account the physiologic disturbances that may be related to illness or aging and the more subtle response that the older adult has to illness. The care provider must also consider if the presenting problem is related to an adverse reaction or treatment, or is triggered by environmental or social factors. Many will lead active, productive lives whereas others will experience limitations in daily activities, hospitalizations, transitions to long-term care facilities, and poor quality of life. They all will require health care.

APRNs are prepared and educated to consider all factors impacting the health care needs of the older adult as well as focus on their preventive health needs. The APRN's holistic approach can yield increased, vital information that impacts intervention decisions that may well impact quality of life. Furthermore, APRNs are focused on the assessment of functionality, development of goals of care, and outlining strengths that can be maximized to ensure the achievement of a positive response to planned interventions. Beyond this approach that APRNs bring to the assessment and planning process, they are also prepared to engage patients in the decision-making process. Older adults who often are researching their treatment options prior to visits to care providers are increasingly involved in decisions about their health care. There is an expectation that they are provided the time to ask questions and share their thoughts. They need to have time spent on health promotion activities that focus on prevention, screening, and counseling. APRNs are educated and prepared to address these issues. Multiple studies in fact confirm that APRNs consistently achieve better results on measures of patient follow-up; consultation time; satisfaction; and the provision of screening, assessment, and counseling (Naylor & Kurtzman, 2010). Providing this type of care to older adults is however complicated by their increasing numbers, their increasing complexity, and the array of needs previously described.

The unprecedented growth in this segment of the population fuelled by the aging of the Baby Boomers is compounded by the fact that people are living longer. When the youngest of the nation's 77 million Baby Boomers turn 65 years of age in 2030, they can expect to live about 20 more years (Chin Hansen, 2013). They will also be living with more health problems, such as chronic disease and progressive diseases.

Although not every older adult requires the same level of intensity of care, they all require care. Consider a 75-year-old adult with a long history of high blood pressure that follows a healthy diet and exercises daily. He has a primary care physician that he sees at least every 6 months and he receives an annual wellness visit. Follow-up reminders are required to ensure that he receives his vaccinations and preventive tests. He is an ideal candidate for having an APRN function as a primary care provider. Consider another adult, also 75 years old who has high blood pressure, severe arthritis, and diabetes. He has not seen a primary care provider in over a year because of mobility limitations. He resides in assisted living. Home visits for him may well avoid the emergency room. He is an ideal candidate for having an APRN doing those visits in his home.

Despite reimbursement and scope-of-practice issues, APRNs have been and are delivering services in rural and underserved areas, where primary care physicians are the hardest to find (RWJF, 2011) and have developed care models that allow them to be cost-effective in a variety of settings. They have provided care to the types of older adults just described. Their focus on care versus cure, prevention, and coordination are methodologies that have driven their ability to impact costs of care while ensuring high satisfaction with the care delivered. Most importantly, APRNs have demonstrated positive health outcomes across care settings and documented their approach of blending counseling with clinical care, and coordinating of health services in diverse settings. They have contributed to the accessibility of health care. Older adults can and do benefit from their expertise and deserve access to their clinical expertise in all settings of care and regardless of what their health care needs are.

NEW OPPORTUNITIES: RESPONDING TO THE NEEDS OF THE OLDER ADULT

In spite of practice constraints, the APRN workforce is predicted to grow (Poghosyan et al., 2012) and new opportunities are emerging that will support the efforts to increase access to effective, quality, and cost-sensitive care by these practitioners. These new opportunities include initiatives focused on transitional care, complex care management, disease management, retail clinic services, hospital at home programs, telehealth, and medical homes.

Care transition programs support the older adult who has experienced a hospitalization until they are stable at home. Such programs may provide access to APRNs who do home visits, reconcile medications, coach patients about their condition, and ensure care is coordinated. Programs such as these respond to the needs of individuals such as Mr. N who is an 82-year-old adult who lives in an apartment with his wife. He has a history of hypertension, peripheral vascular disease with a left below-knee amputation, COPD, and diabetes. Despite having lower-leg prosthesis, he is nonambulatory and unable to shop, do housekeeping, drive, or use public transportation. He is taking eight medications and has been admitted to several hospitals and long-term care facilities over the past 2 years on multiple occasions for respiratory infections. He has no provider of record and uses the emergency room for acute issues. During his last visit to the emergency room, he was seen by an acute care NP who initiated treatment for an upper respiratory infection and referred him to a house call program available through the hospital system. He was seen at his home within 24 hours of discharge and on-going care was launched. He was seen thereafter in his home on a regular basis by the NP/MD team and after 6 months of continuing care had no admissions nor had he utilized the emergency room.

In contrast to the complex care needs of Mr. N, Mrs. S is a 70-year-old woman who retired from her job as a factory worker. She lives alone in a modest senior housing complex and is able to drive. She has hypertension that requires monitoring and takes two medications daily. She receives her annual influenza vaccinations at her local pharmacy. She has had neither preventive screening tests nor any other vaccinations. She admits to urinary incontinence issues and is concerned about her history of breast cancer some 10 years ago. Her primary care clinic is about six blocks from her home but the last time when she was called for an appointment she was told there were no available timeslots for at least 6 weeks. She has chosen not to call again. She did however take advantage of a retail clinic in her area. The APRN in the clinic provides her with the needed vaccinations and coordinates needed follow-up visits with a primary care provider that is accessible inclusive of arranging for scheduling of needed preventive care screening visits. She benefits from retail clinic care that is responding to consumers' desire for more ready access. Expansion of these clinics will be supported under ACA.

Disease management and chronic care are areas of need that APRNs can respond to and that again will be expanded under certain provisions in ACA. The APRNs can and have demonstrated the ability to optimize health by improving adherence to evidenced-based guidelines. For the older adult, this has resulted in decreased hospitalization and rehospitalization rates. Expansion will improve quality, reduce complications, and impact the use of higher costs services.

Medical homes and other types of coordination programs are intended to become major features of the U.S. health care delivery system. The inclusion of APRNs who are able to utilize all of their skills and competencies is a crucial component.

Tele-health, the use of technology, allows for virtual visiting and on-going monitoring for individuals who live remotely or have difficulty physically getting to a clinic setting. APRNs, with their expertise in communication and education, can monitor patients for changes in condition and responses to interventions. They can treat symptoms proactively prior to escalation to a degree that would require hospitalization.

Long wait times, high use of the emergency room, inattention to preventive care, substandard chronic disease management, and lack of attention to preventive health needs impact the older adult. All of these issues contribute to the use of hospitals and other institutional settings of care, drive costs of care, and decrease satisfaction. APRNs can be part of the solution. They have demonstrated results with innovations that have resulted in positive health outcomes. Given the results demonstrated by these programs a growing number of states have allowed APRNs to function as primary care providers and even lead primary care practices (Newhouse et al., 2012). The ACA includes NPs and CNSs as primary care practitioners and contains extensive provider neutral language that will serve to support the removal of restrictions on scope of practice. In addition to these language changes, there are projects underway that will further respond to the needs of the older adult and raise the issue of regulatory constraints on APRN practice.

FOUNDATIONAL WORK UNDERWAY

In an effort to validate the concepts of home visitation programs, the federal CMS in 2011 launched the Independence At Home Demonstration to test the effectiveness of delivering primary care to Medicare beneficiaries with multiple conditions (MediServe, 2001). The Patient Protection and ACA also contained measures that supported this type of demonstration and the delivery of care in the home (Peterson, Landers, & Bazemore, 2012). This demonstration is a part of an emerging trend of clinician visits in the home or incorporated into residential settings. The care models associated with these trends require integrated teams and interprofessional collaboration, such as APRNs, with each profession contributing at the highest level of its competencies (Bookbinder et al., 2011). These are the models that are needed to address the issues of the complex older adult and are intended to provide regular oversight that can lower hospital admissions, shorten length of stay, and lower readmissions.

The Patient Protection and ACA also provided $50 million in fiscal year 2010, with contingencies to extend funding through 2014, to expand nurse-managed clinics (Naylor & Kurtzman, 2010). These nurse-managed clinics utilize APRNs and have served the uninsured and vulnerable populations. Their continuing existence not only provides access for the older adults they serve in medically underserved inner city areas but also allows for the development of evidence-based practices through continuing research. It allows for continuing validation of the need, the outcomes achieved by use of APRNs, and for validation of the issues surrounding the impact of scope-of-practice variations.

The Joint Commission, the national organization certifying hospitals for adherence to quality standards, and the Patient Self-determination Act have identified requirements that address dignified, self-directed, quality patient care. These requirements include a focus on advance directives during the course of hospitalizations.

This provides an opportunity to utilize CNSs who are involved in direct clinical practice, function as consultants, provide coaching and guidance, and provide leadership. They are prepared to initiate organizational changes that are needed to meet mandates and requirements. The CNSs can use basic core competencies to facilitate the change and institute new processes and policies (Meehan, 2009). Older adults experiencing a hospitalization are often the very patients in need of respect for their choices and need advocates that can assist in the design, confirmation, and implementation of advance directives. CNSs have been utilized in the hospital settings to avert just such occurrences and to design programs and processes that educate all about advance directives, how to obtain them, how to validate them, and how to ensure they are followed. Structured initiatives such as this will promote research and therefore validation of the vital role the CNS plays in the management of key issues that impact the older adult.

In addition to the aforementioned opportunities that provide for *kairos* moments in advanced practice nursing—a time when current events align in such a way that significant and rapid change is possible—APRNs have the opportunities to provide care equal to that of their physician counterparts and perhaps demonstrate even more relevant care. To respond to the increasing needs and demands of the older adults, change must occur now or current regulations will thwart the innovations underway. APRNs must be recognized as primary care, independent practitioners. Current regulations that were developed 20 or 30 years ago are outdated and no longer useful. They will need to change to allow APRNs to practice to the fullest of their education and preparation and doing so may have significant impact on health care.

According to Safriet (2008), removing barriers to APRN practice and care can accomplish many outcomes that are important to the older adult. These outcomes include:

- Increased access to highly qualified health care provider
- Decreased costs (unnecessary duplication, additional visits, etc.)
- Increased patient satisfaction
- Improved continuity of care
- Improved health outcomes
- Enhanced flexibility in delivery of care

Older adults are among the fastest growing age group and are at high risk for developing chronic diseases and related disabilities. Many of them will experience hospitalizations, nursing home admissions, and low-quality care. On a global basis, overall spending for a person with one chronic condition is three times higher than someone without and 17 times higher for someone who has five or more conditions. The rising numbers combined with the rise in chronic disease in the Medicare population will severely strain the current health care system. The need to utilize all professionals and allow them to function at the highest level of their education and credentialing will be even more critical. To address the increasing demand and ensure that a larger group of professionals are prepared to care for the needs of the expanding population of older adults, the APRN Consensus Model was developed and will help to provide a possible solution. This emerging regulatory model for APRNs promotes uniformity on credentialing and licensure (Hamric, Spross, & Hanson, 2009) and will be foundational to ensuring APRNs can provide care in more than one state and drive changes in academic preparation that will increase the number of APRNs who are academically prepared to care for the older adult population. It is anticipated that this regulatory model will eliminate the state-by-state variations that currently limit APRNs' capacity to practice to the full extent of their education, training, and competence.

THE FUTURE: THE APRN CONSENSUS MODEL

The APRN Consensus Work Group and the National Council of State Boards of Nursing (NCSBN) APRN Advisory Committee published the *Consensus Model for APRN Regulation: Licensure, Accreditation, Certification, and Education* in July 2008. In this model, they acknowledged the increasing need for providers with expertise to care for older adults. The stagnant number of providers prepared as gerontological NPs contributed to the decision to eliminate both the GNP as well as the ANP (acute and primary care) as preparation for licensure. The same situation was occurring with the gerontological CNS. Instead the new population focus was described as a "marriage" of the two and the population was defined as adult gerontology. New competencies were developed for both the A-GNP acute care and primary care NP that reflected the specialty content. An adult gerontology CNS population focus was also developed with corresponding competencies. These competencies, along with recommended adult gerontology competencies for family and women's health NPs can be found on the American Association of Colleges of Nursing (AACN) website at www.aacn.nche.edu/education-resources/competencies-older-adults. The Consensus Model also includes the opportunity for postlicensure recognition as a gerontological specialist that could be even more narrowly defined as care of frail elders, long-term care specialist, etc., because this designation is not for licensure and is administered by the professional organization. In addition to this new population, the consensus model directs programs that prepare the other population majors, family, women's health, and psychiatric, also to include more gerontological content to meet the need of the growing number of older adults.

CONCLUSION

This new model is in the process of implementation. Schools have changed their curricula and the certification bodies have revamped their exams to reflect the changes. In theory, it is a good model and hopefully will increase the number of providers with geriatric expertise. Its impact is yet to be seen. Efforts to broaden the legal authority of APRNs to provide a level of health care that matches their education, training, and competencies is vital as the U.S. health care delivery system transforms and attempts to achieve the goal of providing accessible, high-quality, cost-effective care.

Perhaps, the most notable support for this model and the drive for reform of scope-of-practice regulations are found in the publication of the IOM of the National Academies report. Recommendation 1 in this report calls for removal of scope-of-practice constraints and advocates APRNs to "be able to practice to the full extent of their education and training" (Kugler, Burhans, & George, 2010).

In caring for the older adult population, all potential providers will need to be engaged and utilized. A retooling of the health care system, over the next several

years, is required if the country is going to respond to the needs of the fastest growing segment of the population.

DISCUSSION QUESTIONS

1. Over the last several years, as the number of older adults in the United
   States with complex and multiple health problems has begun growing
   markedly, so have concerns that the number of professionals who
   understand the field of geriatrics might fall considerably short of the need.
   In response, what strategies are required to generate interest in the field and
   increase numbers? What can we do to provide the care these patients need?
   What are universal gerontology competencies that can be used for training
   in all health care disciplines?
2. As the IOM recommended in the landmark report, Crossing the Quality
   Chasm (2001), care for those with complex and multiple health problems
   should be delivered by integrated teams. What are the issues and challenges
   that must be confronted to develop integrated teams and what role can
   APRNs play in the elimination of unnecessary barriers?
3. A promising initiative focused on caring for the older adults who require
   care in their home setting is the Independence at Home Demonstration.
   APRNs can play a vital role in the delivery of primary care at home and
   in such demonstrations. What role do you see them playing, what level of
   autonomy is required to deliver timely care, and what education is required
   to deliver care in such settings?
4. The application of evidence that drives practice has long been challenging.
   The Rand report on quality found that the care of the older adult frequently
   does not match evidence-based guidelines. What role can APRNs play in
   the development, implementation, and adherence to evidence and ensure
   evidence-based practice in all care settings?
5. The health of the older adults in the United States is a critical national issue.
   As a country, we need to rethink fundamental values about the meaning
   of providing health care to older adults with chronic conditions. How can
   APRNs lead the way in embracing the importance of quality of life as an
   integral component of health care of older adults?
6. Transforming chronic care for older adults will require the development of
   new care models and the launching of innovative programs. Complex care
   management and tele-monitoring may be opportunities for those models
   and programs. What skills and competencies will be required of APRNs to
   be at the forefront of innovation, to develop the business models associated
   with new programming, and to validate the program outcomes?

REFERENCES

Bookbinder, M., Glaichen, M., McHugh, M., Higgins, P., Budis, J., Solomon, N., ... Portenoy, R. K. (2011).
    Nurse practitioner-based models of specialist palliative care at home: Sustainability and evalua-
    tion of feasibility. *Journal of Pain and Symptom Management, 41*(1), 24–34.
Brassard, A., & Smolenski, M. (2011, September). Removing barriers to advanced practice registered
    nurse care: Hospital privileges. *AARP Public Policy Institute. Insight on the Issues,* (55), 1–12.
Bennett, J. A., & Flaherty-Robb, M. K. (2003). Issues affecting the health of older citizens: Meeting
    the challenge. *Online Journal of Issues in Nursing, 8*(2). Retrieved from www.nursingworld.
    org/MainMenuCategories/ANAMarketplace/ANAPeriodicals/OJIN/TableofContents/
    Volume82003/No2May2003/OlderCitizensHealthIssues.aspx

Center for Health Workforce Studies. (2006). *The impact of the aging population on the health workforce in the United States: Summary of key findings*. Rensselaer, NY: Author.

Chapman, S. A., Wildes, C. D., & Spetz, J. (2010). Payment regulations for advanced practice nurses: Implications for primary care. *Policy, Politics & Nursing Practice, 11*(2), 89–98.

Chin Hansen, J. (2013). *Senior report–Working together to care for an aging nation* (pp. 98–101). America's Health Rankings Senior Report. Retrieved from http://www.americashealthrankings.org /Commentaries/Hansen-AGS-WorkingTogether

Fairman, J. A., Rowe, J. W., Hassmiller, S., & Shalala, D. (2011). Broadening the scope of nursing practice. *New England Journal of Medicine, 364*, 193–196.

Hamric, A. B., Spross, J. A., & Hamson, C. M. (2009). *Advanced practice nursing: An integrative approach* (4th ed., pp. 606–607). St. Louis, MO: Elsevier

Hansen-Turton, T., Ritter, A., Rothman, N., & Valdez, B. (2008a). Insurer policies create barriers to health care access and consumer choice. *Nursing Economics, 24*(4), 204–211.

Hansen-Turton, T., Ritter, A., & Torgan, R. (2008b). Insurers' contracting policies on nurse practitioners as primary care providers. *Policy, Politics, & Nursing Practice, 9*(4), 241–248.

Hing, E., Cherry, D. K., Woodwell, D. A., & Division of Health Care Statistics. (2006). *National ambulatory medical care survey: 2004 summary*. Advanced data from Vital and Health statistics, No. 374. Hyattsville, MD: National Center for Health Statistics.

Horton, S., & Johnson, R. (2010). Improving access to health care for uninsured elderly. *Public Health Nursing, 27*(4), 362–370.

MediServe. (2011). *Independence at home demonstration–Where health care is headed*. Retrieved from http://www.mediserve.com/blog/outpatient-rehab/independence-at-home-demonstration -where-health-care-is-headed

Institute of Medicine (IOM). (2008). *Retooling for an aging America: Building the health care workforce*. Washington, DC: National Academies Press.

Kugler, E. C., Burhans, L. D., & George, J. L. (2010). Removal of legal barriers to the practice of advanced practice registered nurses. *NC Medical Journal, 72*(4), 285–288.

Meehan, K. A. (2009). Advance directives: The clinical nurse specialist as a change agent. *Clinical Nurse Specialist CNS, 23*(5), 258–264.

Naylor, M. D., & Kurtzman, E. T. (2010). The role of nurse practitioners in reinventing primary care. *Health Affairs, 29*(5), 893–899.

Newhouse, R. P., Weiner, J. P., Stanick-Hutt, J., White, K. M., Johantgen, M., Steinwachs, D., & Bass, E. B. (2012). Policy implications for optimizing advanced practice registered nurse use nationally. *Policy, Politics & Nursing Practice, 13*(2), 81–89.

O'Grady, E. T., & Brassard, A. (2011). Health care reform; Opportunities for APRNs and urgency for modernizing nurse practice acts. *Journal of Nursing Regulation, 2*(1), 4–9.

Peterson, L. E., Landers, S. H., & Bazemore, A. (2012). Trends in physician house calls to Medicare beneficiaries. *Journal of the American Board of Family Medicine: JABFM, 25*(6), 862–868.

Phillips, S. (2013). 25th annual legislative update: Evidence-based practice reforms improve access to APRN care. *Nurse Practitioner, 38*(1), 18–42.

Plager, K. A., & Conger, M. M. (2007). Advanced practice nursing: Constraints to role fulfillment. *Internet Journal of Advanced Nursing Practice, 9*(1), 1–7. Retrieved from http://www.ispub/journal /the-internet-journal-of-advanced-practice

Poghosyan, L., Lucero, R., Rauch, L., & Berkowitz, B. (2012). Nurse practitioner workforce: A sustainable supply of primary care providers. *Nursing Economics, 30*(5), 269–284.

Rand Health. (2004). The quality of health care received by older adults. *Research Highlights*. Retrieved from http://www.rand.com

Reuben, D. B. (2007). Saving primary care. *American Journal of Medicine, 120*(1), 99–102.

Robert Wood Johnson Foundation (RWJF). (2011). *APRNs a "Big Part of the Solution" to the primary care provider shortage*. Retrieved from http://www.rwjf.org/newsroom

Safriet, B. J. (2008). *Federal options for maximizing the value of advanced practice nurses in providing quality, cost-effective health care*. Retrieved from http://www.nap.edu/openbook.php?record_id=12956& page=443

Yee, T., Boukas, E. R., Cross, D., & Samuel, D. R. (2013). *Primary care workforce shortages: Nurse practitioner scope-of-practice laws and payment policies* (pp. 1–10). National Institute for Health Care Reform Brief No. 13. Retrieved from http://www.nihcr.org/PCP-Workforce-NPs

CHAPTER 17

The Certified Nurse Midwife in Advanced Nursing Practice

Janelle Komorowski

Midwives have a long history of advocating for women and their infants. In America's early years, lay midwives often served as the only health care provider in the community. As physicians increasingly assumed dominance over the field of obstetrics in the early 20th century, demand for lay midwives dwindled. The majority of midwives who remained active were forced out of practice by legislation that made it nearly impossible to meet the qualifications for licensure. Some states went so far as to criminalize the practice of midwifery.

Although the birth place had predominately moved from the home to the hospital setting by the early 1900s, there remained populations of women unable to access prenatal care or hospital delivery due to socioeconomic, religious, cultural, or racial disparities. In 1925, Mary Breckinridge determined to improve the condition of underserved women and children and founded what would later become the Frontier Nursing Service. Mary had served as a public health nurse during World War I and was touched by the masses of underserved women and children she encountered. She returned to England for additional training in midwifery and came back to the United States with a plan. Nurses would travel on horseback in order to reach even the most remote families, providing midwifery and public health nursing care for those who would otherwise find such services inaccessible. Mary organized a system of nurses and recruited a physician to provide consultation at a central hospital location. Within a few years, over 1,000 families were being cared for by the nurses (Breckinridge, 1981). In 1929, Mary brought British nurse-midwives to America to work alongside her public health nurses. Around the same time in New York City, the Maternity Center Association and Lobenstein Clinic founded the first nurse midwifery educational program in the United States, followed in 1939 by the Frontier Graduate School of Midwifery (Rooks, 1997). The profession of nurse midwifery grew rapidly, with seven schools established by the 1950s. Nurse midwives excelled at providing care for disadvantaged women, but their popularity also grew among the affluent as women began to recognize the benefits of the midwifery model of care.

Nurse-midwives in the United States today provide care for a disproportionately large number of women who are considered higher risk during pregnancy: adolescents, single mothers, economically disadvantaged women, the uninsured, women of color, women of low education, immigrants, and women who for various reasons seek prenatal care late in their pregnancies or not at all. Given a higher-risk population and access to fewer resources, one would expect high rates of undesirable outcomes among the women and infants for whom nurse-midwives provide care, when compared with women of means who have access to physician care. The opposite is actually the case. Nurse-midwives in the Frontier Nursing Service significantly reduced some of the highest maternal and neonatal mortality rates in the country at the time, while providing care in very remote and impoverished settings (Frontier Nursing Service, 1958).

In 1960, nurse midwives were introduced to a hospital in Madera County, California, a medically underserved area with a high proportion of migrant workers. Half of the workers typically received either late prenatal care or none at all. Because midwifery was illegal in California at that time, a special law was passed to permit the midwives to practice in one hospital. Prematurity and neonatal death rates dropped significantly during the 3 years that the midwives cared for the indigent women. Funding for the project ended in 1963. When physicians took over the practice, prematurity and neonatal death rates returned to preproject levels (Rooks, 1997). Although many reasons for the drop and subsequent rise in prematurity and neonatal death rates were proposed, none were adequate to explain the change. Levy et al. (1971) asserted that the reason for the changes was the introduction and subsequent removal of nurse-midwives from the area. Prematurity and neonatal death rates had remained unchanged at other hospitals in the area during the time that the nurse-midwives worked, lending credence to the theory that midwifery care made the difference.

Today, certified nurse midwives (CNMs) caring for the underserved continue to achieve excellent outcomes. The Family Health and Birth Center in Washington, DC, has a 9% preterm birth rate, compared with 14.2% in the area, and a low birth weight rate that is half of that of the region's (Family Health and Birth Center, 2007). The contribution of nurse-midwives to improved primary health care services for underserved women has been affirmed by the Institute of Medicine (IOM) (2011), which recommends expanding the responsibilities of nurse-midwives as primary care providers for women.

CONCEPTUAL AND THEORETICAL SUPPORT FOR NURSE MIDWIFERY PRACTICE

The conceptual basis for nurse midwifery practice is reflected in the Philosophy of Care outlined by the American College of Nurse Midwives (ACNM, 2010). The Philosophy of Care emphasizes the partnership of the nurse midwife with women, recognizes the woman as the expert in her own life and needs, and encourages the advocacy and support of the CNM for the woman's choices for her health care. Kennedy, Rousseau, and Low (2003) identified four common themes of midwifery care as follows:

- the midwife as an instrument of care
- the woman as a partner in care
- the alliance between the woman and her midwife
- the environment of care

These themes are also identified in the ACNM's Philosophy of Care. Emphasis on the normalcy of birth resonates throughout midwifery literature. Carolan and Hodnett (2007) voiced concern that this emphasis of nurse midwifery on the normal could lead to an exclusionary model, leaving out women with higher needs. Midwives do serve a disproportionate number of at-risk women, a number that is expected to increase as physicians leave the practice of obstetrics or limit their practices to privately insured patients. Although emphasis on the normal is a hallmark of midwifery care, CNMs have proven their ability to achieve superior outcomes even when caring for higher risk women. As midwifery caseloads shift to include larger numbers of medically indigent women, the emphasis on normalcy must be extended to include those who fall into higher risk categories.

Rooks (1997) contrasted the midwifery and medical models of care, asserting that the two often overlap and are not mutually exclusive, and that the optimal intertwining of the two models of care is a collaborative relationship between the nurse midwife and the physician. However, she emphasizes the unique contributions of the nurse midwifery model in preservation of normalcy in birth, avoidance of unnecessary interventions, and the acknowledgement of needs often unaddressed by the medical model. Perhaps, the most significant validation of Rooks' assertions comes from Stapleton, Osborne, and Illuzzi (2013). The researchers examined records of 15,574 births that occurred in midwife-led birth centers. Outcomes show significant cost savings, a cesarean section rate of only 6% as compared with a national average of U.S. cesarean section rate for 2011 was 32.8% (Centers for Disease Control, 2011), fewer routine interventions, and perinatal outcomes comparable with physician-attended, hospital-based birth.

Although there is ample evidence to support the benefits of midwifery care, the development of a theoretical basis for midwifery knowledge is relatively recent. Credit for the beginnings of midwifery theory is given to Ernestine Wiedenbach, a nurse midwife and nurse theorist whose work was the basis for the first written philosophy of the ACNM. Wiedenbach is credited with focusing nursing research on a patient-centered versus medical model. She theorized that nurse midwifery should focus on meeting the patient's "need-for-help," which she defined as interventions either wanted or needed by the patient that can improve her coping abilities (Nickel, Gesse, & MacLaren, 1992).

Three middle-range theories of midwifery practice each incorporate the nurse midwifery philosophy of care in development of their theories. Lehrman (1981) developed the first nurse midwifery theory to be tested. Her work focused on six constructs depicting midwifery practice and drawn from ACNM philosophy. Congruent with ACNM philosophy, Lehrman's center of focus is the patient, either the parturient or the neonate. A descriptive study by Morten et al. (1991) validated Lehrman's prenatal care theory and suggested a correlation between the positive attitude of the nurse midwife and desirable patient outcomes. Because she links the nurse midwifery care processes with outcomes, Lehrman's work is a strong basis for future nurse midwifery practice theory and research.

Thompson et al. (1989) sought to develop a middle-range theory that could explain the difference nurse midwifery care makes in patient outcomes. Thompson identified six core principles of nurse midwifery practice based on the ACNM philosophy. Thompson's broad theory includes specific behaviors for each concept, which will benefit future researchers in identifying correlations between nurse midwifery care practices and patient outcomes, and may guide development of future practice guidelines.

Kennedy's theory (2000) also links superior patient outcomes to nurse midwifery practices, but identifies a lack of knowledge as to why such practices produce exemplary outcomes. Two assumptions underlying Kennedy's model are that exemplary practice is associated with positive outcomes for women and infants, and that core philosophies and standards for the practice of nurse midwifery are the foundation of exemplary midwifery practice. Echoing Lehrman and Thompson, a central focus of Kennedy's theory is the woman as an active participant in her care, with the nurse midwife cast in a supporting role. Kennedy has proposed that her model be tested to confirm whether specific nurse midwifery behaviors affect patient outcomes. She has continued to develop her theory, which is recognized by many nurse midwives and nurse midwifery educators as the best description of the essence of nurse midwifery practice.

Berg (2005) proposed a theory of "Genuine Caring in Caring for the Genuine" and stressed the importance of balancing care for the high-risk woman in a way that meets her medical needs while still acknowledging her right to give birth in a way that honors the natural process of becoming a mother. Emphasis in Berg's model is placed on a synthesis of medical science and traditional midwifery care, which she asserts is best achieved in collaborative practice between physicians and midwives.

Fahy and Parratt (2006) proposed the concept of "Birth Territory," which encompasses the birth environment, the locus of control over the birth, and the woman's physical and psychological experience of the birth. They juxtapose the concept of "midwifery guardianship" with "midwifery domination." Midwifery guardianship assumes a supportive role on the part of the midwife, whose goal is to facilitate the woman's desires and her ability to give birth normally in a physiologic manner. Midwifery domination is any action on the part of the midwife that requires the woman to submit to the midwife's directives rather than rely on her own inner knowledge. The woman may react by abandoning her intuitive ability to give birth, or by responding aggressively toward the midwife in an effort to protect her intuitive abilities to give birth.

Doherty (2009) introduced the concept of the midwife–patient relationship as a "therapeutic alliance" in which the midwife and the client work together to achieve mutually agreed-upon goals for client care. A therapeutic alliance is subtly differentiated from a collaborative relationship in that collaboration may be more midwife-directed; in other words, the midwife may propose to the client options from which she may choose, versus working together with the client to identify options the client would like to choose from. In the collaborative relationship, the midwife still retains the role of leader, whereas the therapeutic alliance is more a partnership of equals with differing skills.

The common thread among midwifery theories and care models is the theme of preserving the normalcy of pregnancy and birth insofar as possible, the midwife in partnership with the woman versus an authoritarian relationship, and keeping the woman as the central focus of care. As these models are tested and refined, future research will further contribute to the development of nurse midwifery practice and philosophy.

CORE COMPETENCIES

The practice of nurse midwifery in the United States is guided by the Core Competencies of the ACNM. Although many of the competencies describe essential clinical skills for nurse midwifery practice, significant attention is also given to recognition of parturition as a normal process, and avoidance of technological interventions in the absence of clear medical need. Advocacy for the woman's right to informed choice and self-determination, health promotion, and family-centered care are also included in the Core Competencies. Although these ideals are widely espoused by nurse-midwives, Lange and Kennedy (2010) found significant discrepancies between ideal and actual practice, as identified by 245 new CNMs. In describing their final clinical practice settings prior to graduation, study participants reported a disconnect between the espoused core philosophy of preserving normal birth and actual clinical practices. Differences between theory and practice in the demonstration of caring behaviors were insignificant, but wide variations between theory and practice were apparent in the frequency of routine interventions and infrequent choice of nontechnological approaches when appropriate. In addition, continuous support in labor was not observed in actual practice to the degree it is emphasized in the midwifery model of care.

Vedam et al. (2007) states that "there are unique competencies in perinatal management that characterize, promote, and preserve the midwifery model of care." Certainly, the ACNM Core Competencies reflect the College's belief in the uniqueness of the midwifery model; why then is there such a gap between theory and practice? The answer may lie in the barriers to practice facing today's midwives. Many of these barriers relate to health policy and can be categorized as regulatory, collegial, and financial barriers.

REGULATORY BARRIERS

As of 2012, 32 states required nurse practitioners (NPs) to have some degree of physician involvement in their practices. In some states, physician involvement is limited to a formal "collaborative agreement," in which the physician agrees to be available for consultation and collaboration for patients whose care falls outside the midwife's scope of practice. Other states require a supervisory relationship, with the physician signing admission and discharge orders, and cosigning all inpatient care and medication orders. Only 18 states and the District of Columbia grant primary care and prescriptive privileges to NPs without requiring any level of physician involvement. Thus, whereas certification attests that the midwife is qualified to practice independently as a primary care provider, state regulations may significantly restrict the midwife's ability to practice to the full extent of her or his training and certification.

Sonenberg (2010) attempted to assess the impact of differing state regulations on CNMs. The project was challenging due to the practice of putting the supervisory physician's name on medical records, obscuring data pertaining to midwife-attended births and outcomes. Inability to determine from records when a midwife was the care provider creates a barrier to ascertaining the effect of state regulations on midwifery practice. It also obscures data about who is providing care for disadvantaged women and the impact of CNM care on perinatal outcomes.

In addition to dealing with restrictive state regulations, the midwife who works near state borders faces additional problems. Lugo et al. (2007) stated, "Disease doesn't respect geographic boundaries, but even though patient condition, diagnosis, and management don't change, the regulations for NPs do change [between states]. When you read all 51 Nurse Practice Acts, you can't help but have an emotional reaction. There are some very strange stipulations and arbitrary limitations put on NPs, which speaks to how NP regulation is not evidence-based and needs to be cleaned up."

Safriet (2011) gives the example of an advanced practice registered nurse (APRN) licensed in two states, with differences in authority to practice between the two states. The APRN's competency does not change when they cross the state line, but reimbursement and scope of practice may be significantly different. Much of the difference can be attributed to politics, rather than sound policy. Safriet identified further problems with inconsistent state regulations as follows:

- Decision makers, even in progressive states, will often adopt the policies of the most restrictive jurisdictions. Safriet termed this as a "race to the bottom" (2011, p. 450).
- Patients living in rural or underserved areas, or those without insurance, may find themselves without adequate care due to lack of physicians who are willing and/or able to enter into a collaborative or supervisory agreement.
- Competent, well-trained APRNs may become discouraged when they are unable to practice to the full scope of their training and may relocate to more favorable practice areas leaving underserved areas even more destitute.
- Costs of care increase and creative ideas for health care delivery are stifled.
- APRNs may fear disciplinary action when even mundane activities, such as a phone consult or a birth control prescription refill, cross state lines.
- Technological advancements are restricted. For example, APRNs are increasingly utilizing telemedicine innovations, but working across state lines presents a barrier to practice and reimbursement.

Forty-one states regulate APRNs through a board of nursing, one state (Nebraska) has an advanced practice board to oversee APRN practice, and eight states have combined board of nursing and board of medicine oversight. Working to establish the board of nursing as the regulatory body for NPs in every state is a step toward increasing autonomy for APRNs. With the annual number of primary care visits expected to increase by 15.07 million to 24.26 million visits by 2019, an anticipated 4,307 and 6,940 new primary care providers will be needed to meet the demand (Hofer, Abraham, & Moscovice, 2011). Projections do not take into account changes in demand because of population growth and changes in demographics. Hauer et al. (2008) suggests projected needs for primary care providers may be grossly underreported as a result of declining numbers of medical students choosing primary care specialties. With these anticipated shortfalls, the APRN is likely to be ever more in demand, as their lower salary, shorter educational time, and the willingness of more APRNs to serve in primary care capacities can help meet the anticipated needs. It is even more critical that state regulation of advanced practice nurses become uniform, as primary care advanced practice nurses in rural areas may rely heavily on telemedicine, raising questions of licensing and scope of practice across state borders. Although physicians must also be licensed separately from state to state, they are given authority to diagnose, treat, and prescribe equally in all 50 states and the District of Columbia. In order for APRNs to step in and fill the need for primary care providers, it is imperative that they achieve uniform authority to diagnose, treat, and prescribe in all jurisdictions.

COLLEGIAL BARRIERS

As we evaluate the need for uniform scope-of-practice authority for NPs, collegial barriers must be considered. With 32 states currently requiring varying degrees of collaboration with a physician in order for the APRN to practice, physicians have significant influence on accessibility of advanced practice nurses to the general public. Perhaps, in no specialty has this been more apparent than in that of obstetrics. Throughout the history of midwifery, physicians have been content to allow midwives to care for the patients they did not wish to manage, often because it was not financially lucrative. As the midwifery model of care became better known and the excellent outcomes achieved with midwifery care were studied and published, significant numbers of privately insured women began to seek out midwives for their primary care provider for obstetrics and gynecology. Numerous accounts exist of profitable nurse-midwifery practices abruptly shut down because of physician pressure (Garloch, 2012; Pleticha, 2004; Shaver, 2007), yet the IOM, citing the cost savings and excellent outcomes of nurse midwifery care, urged the expanded use of nurse-midwives and utilization of nurse practitioners as patient-centered medical home (PCMH) leaders (IOM, 2011). Despite studies suggesting equal to better outcomes with advanced practice nurse care (Newhouse et al., 2011) and nurse midwifery care (Cragin & Kennedy, 2006; Newhouse et al., 2011), some physician groups have vehemently opposed expansion of APRNs into independent primary care and leadership of PCMHs. Citing the shorter duration of APRN education, the American Medical Association (AMA) insisted that only a physician is qualified to lead a PCMH and that the NPs should only work under the supervision or collaboration of a physician (AMA, 2010). The American Academy of Family Physicians (AAFP) (2010) agreed. Both organizations cite patient safety as their overarching concern, despite ample evidence establishing the quality outcomes of NPs in primary care roles (Newhouse et al., 2011).

The fact that many states still require some level of physician involvement in a nurse midwife's practice poses a significant practice barrier for many midwives. Even in states that grant midwives independent practice status, individual hospitals still retain the option to restrict nurse midwifery credentialing to those midwives who have a "sponsoring" physician agreement or are employees of a physician. Hospitals are not at liberty to grant midwives *more* privileges than state regulations allow, but are permitted to be as restrictive as they wish in *limiting* midwifery privileges and scope of practice. Even in hospitals that only require a collaborative agreement, midwives may often feel compelled to practice in a way that violates the tenets of the ACNM philosophy. If minor complications of labor arise, which by hospital protocols mandate consultation with an obstetrician, the obstetrician may make recommendations based on the medical model of care. The nurse midwife may be compelled to comply with the obstetrician's recommendations, even when they are not evidence based, and to disregard the ACNM philosophy of care.

A further constraint to collaborative relationships is the perception of many physicians that collaboration means the APRN functions in a dependent role under a delegating physician (similar to the physician relationship with a registered nurse, but with expanded scope of practice for the APRN). In contrast, APRNs view collaboration as the consultation of one health care professional with another (Cairo, 1996), just as a family physician might consult with an obstetrician for a laboring patient in need of cesarean delivery. Shaw et al. (2005) identified the persistence of a dominant medical hierarchy, despite efforts to create team collaboration between physicians and NPs. Nurse midwives, especially, may perceive this as a lack of respect for the differences between the midwifery and medical models of care, which can lead to job dissatisfaction and further widen the theory–practice gap.

In a literature review examining collaboration between physicians and NPs, Clarin (2007) identified several barriers to collaborative practice as follows:

- Lack of knowledge about NP scope of practice
- Lack of knowledge about NP role
- Poor physician attitude
- Lack of respect
- Poor communication
- Patient and family reluctance to receive NP care

Clarin asserts that a strategy for improving collaboration between physicians and APRNs is increased communication and education regarding the role of the APRN. Other authors disagree suggesting that rather than focusing on increased communication and education about APRN roles, the focus should be on removing legislative barriers to completely independent APRN practice (Van Soeren et al., 2009). When the ability of CNMs to practice independently is restricted, it limits the full potential of their benefit to vulnerable populations and underserved women. One successful APRN practice rose out of a shortage of providers for over 30,000 patients in Ontario. Eight unemployed APRNs proposed creating an APRN-led clinic. By going public with their idea, they garnered the support of the community, the media, and professional nursing organizations. The pilot project has been successful in Ontario (Heale, 2012) and could be a model for similar projects in the United States. The AARP-sponsored webinar (2012) finding seem to support Heale's findings, suggesting that a power shift involving consumers and stakeholders is the means to achieving regulatory changes.

The IOM (2011) has recommended state and federal changes that will allow NPs to exercise their full scope of practice. It is recommended that state legislatures bring their scope-of-practice regulations in line with the National Council of State Boards of Nursing Model Nursing Practice Act and Model Nursing Administrative Rules, which provide a template for the scope of advanced practice nursing. In addition, the IOM recommends that states require fee-for-service plans to cover NP services and that the Federal Trade Commission pinpoint state regulations that present barriers to practice without increasing public health and safety, and pressure states to change these regulations based on their anticompetitive effect. The IOM recommends that the Centers for Medicare and Medicaid Services (CMS) require hospitals which participate in Medicare/Medicaid programs to give NPs full medical staff eligibility and clinical/admitting privileges. Such changes would largely eliminate the collegial barriers APRNs face today.

FINANCIAL BARRIERS

NPs typically earn less than half of their closest physician counterparts, family practice physicians. Midwives have been at the forefront of fighting for equal Medicaid and Medicare reimbursement for NPs. Although the battle is not fully over, the ACNM has made great strides toward equal compensation. Nurse midwives are now compensated equally with their physician counterparts for the same services. Even with equity in compensation, nurse midwives still provide less costly care, because of less frequent use of expensive diagnostic tests and technological interventions during childbirth, as well as a significantly lower cesarean section rate.

Private insurers are mixed in their payment for nurse midwife services, varying from not covering midwifery care, to excluding birth centers and home birth, to fully covering all birth options. Medicaid now covers 41% of all prenatal patients (March of Dimes, 2013), and although it grants compensation for all birth settings (where legal) and providers, the rate of compensation is so low that many practitioners cannot break even unless they have enough private-pay patients to balance out the Medicaid loss (New York Times, 2010). This can lead to rationing of Medicaid services, where clinics limit the proportion of Medicaid patients to private-pay patients in order to survive financially; in many cases, physician practices have stopped accepting Medicaid patients entirely (Hogberg, 2012; Jackson Healthcare, 2013).

Hospital budgets can present a barrier to ideal midwifery practice. Need for quick turnover of labor and delivery rooms can lead to pressure on the midwife to schedule inductions, to encourage repeat cesarean section rather than a trial of labor after cesarean (TOLAC), and to encourage patients to agree to interventions intended to hurry the normal process of labor, effecting faster delivery and consequently making more labor rooms available. Collaborating physicians, schooled in the medical model of obstetric care, may struggle to understand why the midwife objects to financially based interventions, while nursing staff may empathize with the midwife's perspective but struggle with the demands of staying within a budget while still maintaining adequate staffing for patient needs.

Additional financial barriers to midwifery practice come in the guise of safe medical care. Although midwives order fewer diagnostic tests and perform fewer technological interventions, they can still fall prey to fear of litigation, and the "I did everything I could" mentality that prompts many providers to order tests and procedures that are likely unnecessary, in an effort to protect themselves from lawsuits. Midwives especially, because of their unique practice philosophy, are likely to feel the theory–practice gap as they find themselves utilizing tests and procedures in order to protect themselves rather than to serve in the best interests of the patient.

For some midwives, even obtaining malpractice insurance is difficult at best. Washington state is one of a few that have enacted legislation mandating that insurers take turns offering affordable coverage to NPs. In other states, insurance is mandated yet prohibitively expensive, presenting a significant economic barrier to practice. Although insurance is generally available (albeit costly) to NPs, midwives as a specialty group are often entirely excluded from coverage if they offer any intrapartum care, and even the coverage offered by the ACNM, which supports home birth as a viable choice for women, has periodically excluded home birth midwives from qualifying for professional liability insurance. This becomes an insurmountable barrier to practice if the midwife is unable to contract with insurers as a preferred provider because they mandate liability coverage for their contracted providers. To further complicate matters, some insurers have refused coverage for physicians who collaborate with midwives, citing the myth of vicarious liability (Booth, 2007). This concept suggests that the physician who collaborates with a midwife will be responsible for any actions they take prior to transferring care of a patient to the obstetrician, even when there is not a formal, signed collaborative agreement between the midwife and the physician. In an already-litigious atmosphere, obstetricians are understandably hesitant about any collaboration they fear could increase their risk of liability.

Finally, no discussion of financial barriers would be complete without mention of the marginalized women in our society: women who have neither the financial resources to purchase health insurance, or if they qualify for Medicaid have other financial disparities that limit their access to appropriate care. These women often experience a lack of resources such as transportation, lack of funds to purchase nonprescription items that Medicaid will not cover, lack of money to pay for services Medicaid either does not cover or for which they cannot find a provider who accepts Medicaid (dental care in pregnancy is a prime example), and lack of funds to provide even the most basic necessities of life for themselves: food, heat, telephone, clothing, and shelter. These are the women to whom midwives are uniquely qualified to reach out and make a difference. The PPACA purposes to make care accessible for these women, but during the time it takes to establish the system, there will continue to be women who fall through the cracks. Even after the system is in place, it is likely that new financial barriers to care will be identified; midwives need to be prepared to address these barriers. The focus of midwives on woman-centered care and serving the underserved positions them to be at the forefront of health care changes over the next decade.

OUTCOME MEASURES FOR CNM PRACTICE

The ACNM initiated a Benchmarking Project (Collins-Fulea, Moore, & Tillett, 2005) with the intended goal of practice improvement and risk reduction. In 2011, the ACNM reported on 15 outcome measures (ACNM, 2011) as follows:

- Total rate of vaginal births
- Rate of spontaneous vaginal births
- Primary C-section rate
- Total C-section rate
- VBAC success rate
- Intact perineum rate
- Episiotomy rate
- Neonatal intensive care unit admission rate
- Preterm birth rate
- Low birth weight infant rate
- Breastfeeding initiation rate
- Breastfeeding continuation rate
- Total induction rate
- Less than 41 weeks induction rate
- Epidural use rate

Any actions that CNMs take to remove barriers to practice must always be with the goal in mind of improving quality of care. Interestingly, the benchmarking project has found that the highest proportion of practices reporting benchmark data were midwife-led and managed practices, as opposed to those practices that are collaborative practices or physician-owned. A possible reason for this could be reflected in the numerous studies indicating better outcomes with midwifery care, considering many of the above outcome measures (Cragin & Kennedy, 2006; Johantgen et al., 2012; Newhouse et al., 2011). Certified nurse midwives have a clear vision of ACNM core competencies and philosophy of care. The challenge today is to remove the barriers standing in the way of successfully implementing the midwifery model of care.

Every CNM has an ethical imperative to become involved in removing barriers that prevent midwives from practicing in accordance to the midwifery model of care. Practice constraints from collaborative agreements, financial constraints, or legislative barriers can no longer be used as a reason for providing patient care that is not in sync with one's philosophy of practice. Each CNM can become a grassroots advocate for midwifery, women, and children (ACNM, 2012a).

LOOKING AHEAD: THE IMPACT OF THE PATIENT PROTECTION AFFORDABLE CARE ACT (PPACA) ON THE FUTURE OF MIDWIFERY

Although health policy experts have offered differing opinions regarding the impact of the PPACA on health care, the state of Massachusetts serves as an example of likely outcomes of PPACA implementation. Structured similarly to the PPACA, the Massachusetts law initially resulted in an increase in emergency department visits as patients struggled to find primary care providers. To help meet the shortfall of PCPs, Massachusetts enacted legislation facilitating the recognition and reimbursement of APRNs as primary care providers. With an anticipated increased need for primary care providers as the PPACA is implemented, now is the time to press for legislative and regulatory changes recognizing APRNs as independent, primary care providers nationwide. The recent CMS decision to reimburse CNMs at 100% of the physician fee scale for Medicare patients opened the door for expanded nurse midwifery services to disabled women of childbearing age, and to senior women who also benefit from midwifery's "with women for a lifetime" approach to care. Several other facets of the PPACA will also impact midwifery as follows (PPACA, 2010):

- Educational funding: Anticipating increased demand for registered nurses and advanced practice nurses, the PPACA provided for an increase in funding, not only in loans available to nursing students, but also in reimbursements for graduates who are employed as nursing faculty. The increased funding helps meet the need for more nurse-midwives to provide primary care to low-risk pregnant women and Medicare/Medicaid insured women.
- Grants for nurse-managed health clinics: The CMS is offering a number of grants and support through its Center for Medicare and Medicaid Innovation (CMS) (n.d.). In accordance with the recommendations of the IOM for an increase in the number of nurse-led clinics and PCMHs, CMS Innovation Models provide incentives for multiples types of practices, as well as proposals for innovative practice.
- Changes in how primary care is delivered: Nursing as a whole and midwives as a specialty have always emphasized preventive care and wellness. Now practices which promote wellness will be at the cutting edge of changes in the way care is delivered. Increased emphasis will be placed on cultural competency in delivery of care, with a shift to community care. Home visits for women and infants are supported by CMS, with other insurers likely to follow suit (CMS, n.d.). Midwives are the ideal leaders for care models serving vulnerable populations of women and infants. Their unique focus on pregnancy and childbirth as a normal part of a woman's life, rather than a disease, and their emphasis on keeping childbirth free of unnecessary medical interventions position midwives to make significant contributions to a holistic model of primary health care for women.
- Increased recognition of CNMs as primary care providers. Advanced practice nurses are often excluded from preferred provider lists, making them less visible to the public. With the emphasis of increased utilization of advanced practice nurses as primary care providers, more options will be offered to patients as APRNs are included on preferred provider lists.

One area where the PPACA currently poses a problem for nurse-midwives is initiation of wellness exams for Medicare and Medicaid patients. Although termed an "exam," the wellness exam is not a physical examination. Rather, it is a visit that includes collection of medical and family history, medication history, list of medical providers, routine measurements such as blood pressure, weight, and body mass index (BMI), a cognitive assessment, development of a screening schedule for the next 5 to 10 years, health education, and referrals for education and preventive care as indicated. Under the current language of the PPACA, nurse-midwives are not authorized to perform the initial wellness exam. CNMs may still perform the annual well-woman physical exam, which also includes collection of much of the same information comprising the wellness exam. At the time of this writing, the ACNM is in discussion with the Secretary of CMS in an effort to revise the current language to be inclusive of CNMs as approved providers of the initial wellness exam (ACNM, 2012c).

In order for midwives to realize the full benefit of the PPACA to independent APRN practice, they must succeed not only in changing language that excludes midwives from recognition as providers of the initial wellness exam, they must work within their home states to achieve legislative and regulatory changes allowing them to practice to the full extent for which the PPACA provides. An example can be found in the recent success of the ACNM's Maryland chapter in passage of the Maryland Birth Options Preservation Act. The Act removed supervisory language and replaced it with the ACNM guideline that calls for midwives to have a written plan for collaboration, consultation, and referral (ACNM, 2008). Other state chapters have achieved similar successes (ACNM, 2012b). For midwifery to remain a viable and growing profession in the coming years, every midwife must give serious consideration to becoming personally involved in working to remove barriers to practice.

REMOVING BARRIERS TO PRACTICE

Clarin (2007) proposed six strategies for removing barriers to APRN practice as follows:

- Educate physicians to understand the APRN role and scope of practice
- Train medical students with graduate nursing students
- Work toward uniformity of education and certification requirements for APRNs
- Apply integrated collaboration models when developing new APRN positions
- Require all team members to be responsible for improvement of communication
- Practice interdisciplinary rounds with APRNs and physicians to demonstrate the APRN's ability and involvement in medical management

Quinn (in AARP, 2012) asserts that change will require an advocacy approach. In order to remove practice barriers, CNMs will need to make a power shift. This can be performed by creating a coalition of multiple stakeholders: nurses, advanced practice nurses, consumers, payers, and businesses affected by the practice barriers. In most states that have outdated practice laws, the power lies with those who have the most money. Policy makers will vote according to who is supporting them financially and who is voting for them. Although nurses do not have as strong an economic base as physicians, they have the numbers to significantly influence a vote for or against a politician. Consumers can also significantly impact a vote by sheer numbers. As demonstrated in the Ontario NP clinic project (Van Soeren et al., 2009), concerned consumers were able to effect a change in outdated practice laws simply by their vote.

Restrepo (2012) suggested ways that the individual APRN can become involved in removing barriers to practice as follows:

- Discontinue use of the term "mid-level practitioner" as it implies a lesser quality care provider
- Emphasize our professional standing and our unique contributions to health care, especially in the areas of health promotion, coordination of care, disease prevention, and palliative care
- Become actively involved in your specialty professional organization, whether by contributing financially, politically, or both
- Contribute to research contributions submitted not only to nursing journals but also to other nonnursing publications in order to reach a larger professional audience

Whether by educating physician colleagues, becoming active in grassroots advocacy campaigns, contributing financially to professional organizations, providing information to legislators, or sharing information on the professional capabilities of APRNs on a one-to-one basis with consumers, each CNM has the ability—and the obligation—to fight for the future of midwifery and advanced practice nursing.

DISCUSSION QUESTIONS

1. What are the specific barriers to CNM practice in your state? What needs to be changed?
2. What are the typical requirements for credentialing of CNMs at hospitals in your area? Are they equivalent to state requirements, or more restrictive?
3. Discuss the ways that you can become involved in helping remove barriers to advanced practice nursing in your community.
4. How might you use social media to help remove barriers to CNM practice?
5. Review the information at the Grassroots Advocacy page of the American College of Nurse Midwives website at www.midwife.org/Grassroots-Advocacy. How many of the suggested actions could you carry out?
6. Discuss collaborative practice with CNMs in your area.
   - Is their collaborative relationship formal (as in a written agreement) or informal?
   - Have the CNMs you talk with ever felt compelled, due to the hierarchical nature of their collaborative relationship, to practice in a way that conflicted with the ACNM philosophy of care?
   - What do they feel would improve collaboration in their practice setting?

7. Imagine your ideal practice setting a decade from now. How will it be different than your practice today? What steps can you take now to achieve that ideal practice?

CLINICAL APPLICATION QUESTIONS

1. Ellen is a nurse midwife caring for a 22-year-old G1P0 in early labor. Two hours ago, the patient's exam was 4 cm/70%/-3/posterior with 30-second contractions every 7 minutes. The patient was smiling and talking through contractions. Ellen's exam now shows the patient to be 4 cm/100% effaced/0 station/anterior, with 45-second contractions every 3 minutes. The patient is breathing hard with each contraction and expressing doubt that she can handle natural labor. The charge nurse of the labor and delivery unit informs Ellen that they need the bed for this patient, and urges her to either augment labor to expedite delivery or discharge the patient to home because "she is not progressing." The patient does not want to go home, does not want augmentation, and is relying on Ellen's support to help her have a natural birth. Ellen knows that augmentation will make it more difficult for her patient to have a natural birth.
   - Which aspects of the ACNM philosophy of care are important to consider in Ellen's situation?
   - Which core competencies apply in this situation?
   - How can Ellen advocate for her patient in this situation?
   - Can Ellen be an advocate for her patient while still being supportive of the charge nurse's concerns? Why or why not?

2. Judith has just started a new job as a certified nurse midwife on a busy labor unit. The hospital bylaws require her to consult with an obstetrician in the event a patient has a baby suspected to be larger than 4000 g. Her patient's baby is estimated at 4200 g by a 39-week ultrasound performed today. The patient has otherwise been healthy, negative for gestational diabetes, and had a 22-pound weight gain with a starting BMI of 24. This is the woman's first baby and her Bishop's score is 2. The consulting obstetrician instructs Judith to admit her patient and begin an induction for suspected macrosomia. Judith knows that the evidence does not support the benefit of induction of labor for suspected macrosomia in the absence of gestational diabetes, and that an induction may increase her patient's risk of needing a cesarean birth.
   - Which aspects of the ACNM philosophy of care are important to consider?
   - Which core competencies apply in this situation?
   - How should Judith respond to the obstetrician's instructions?
   - If the obstetrician insists that Judith needs to induce the patient, regardless of evidence presented, what ethical principles apply to the situation?

3. Mary Beth has been one of four midwives in an all-midwifery practice at a busy city hospital for the last 8 years. The midwives in her group deliver about 35% of the babies born in the hospital each year and collaborate with two private groups of obstetricians. The midwives' practice is the only one in the city that accepts Medicaid. The obstetricians will take Medicaid referrals that are too high-risk for midwifery care, but otherwise will not see Medicaid patients due to low reimbursement. Mary Beth's friend in the hospital credentialing department tells her the physicians are discussing rescinding their collaborative agreement for "sponsorship" of hospital privileges for midwives. They want the midwives to perform all the prenatal and postpartum care for the Medicaid patients, while the obstetricians will manage intrapartum care, allowing them to collect the majority of the Medicaid fee. The midwives do not want to stop attending births, but need their collaborative agreement with the obstetricians in order to continue to practice in their state.
   - Which aspects of the ACNM philosophy of care are important to consider?
   - Which core competencies apply in this situation?
   - What strategies can Mary Beth and her group use in approaching the obstetricians?
   - Imagine Mary Beth practices in a state that authorizes independent practice of nurse midwives. Would the obstetricians' proposal present a regulatory barrier or a collegial barrier, or both? Why?
   - What strategies might Mary Beth and her group use to approach hospital administrators about a bylaw revision that would allow the midwives to practice independently, without a physician "sponsor"?

REFERENCES

American Academy of Family Physicians (AAFP). (2010). *AAFP takes issue with IOM report calling for greater nursing role*. Retrieved from http://www.aafp.org/online/en/home/publications/news/news-now/professional-issues/20101006iomnursingreport.html

American Association of Retired Persons (AARP). (2012, October 17). *Removing barriers to APRN practice and care: The consumer perspective*. Future of Nursing: Campaign for Action, at the Center to Champion Nursing in America. Retrieved from http://www.campaignforaction.org/webinar/removing-barriers-aprn-practice-and-care-consumer-perspective

American College of Nurse Midwives (ACNM). (2008). *Supplement to ACNM annual report 2008*. Retrieved from http://www.midwife.org/ACNM/files/ccLibraryFiles/Filename/000000000522/annualreport2008_supplement.pdf

ACNM. (2010). *Our philosophy of care*. Retrieved from http://www.midwife.org/Child-Page-3

ACNM. (2011). *2011 ACNM benchmarking project: Summary data—Preliminary report*. Retrieved from http://www.midwife.org/ACNM/files/ccLibraryFiles/Filename/000000002152/2011%20ACNM%20Benchmarking%20Preliminary%20Summary.pdf

ACNM. (2012a). *Grassroots advocacy*. Retrieved from http://www.midwife.org/Grassroots-Advocacy

ACNM. (2012b). *Legislative developments archives*. Retrieved from http://www.midwife.org/2012-Legislative-Developments-Archives

ACNM. (2012c). *Midwives and Medicare after health care reform*. Retrieved from http://www.midwife.org/Midwives-and-Medicare-after-Health-Care-Reform

American Medical Association (AMA). (2010). *AMA responds to IOM report on future of nursing*. Retrieved from http://www.ama-assn.org/ama/pub/news/news/nursing-future-workforce.page

Berg, M. (2005). A midwifery model of care for childbearing women at high risk: Genuine caring in caring for the genuine. *Journal of Perinatal Education, 14*(1), 9–21.

Booth, J. W. (2007). An update on vicarious liability for certified nurse midwives/certified midwives. *Journal of Midwifery and Women's Health, 52*(2), 153–157.

Breckinridge, M. (1981). *Wide neighborhoods* (2nd ed.). Lexington, KY: University Press of Kentucky.

Carolan, M., & Hodnett, E. (2007). 'With woman' philosophy: Examining the evidence, answering the questions. *Nursing Inquiry, 14*(2), 140–152.

Cairo, M. J. (1996). Emergency physicians' attitudes toward the emerging NP role: Validation versus rejection. *Journal of the American Academy of Nurse Practitioners, 8*(9), 411–417.

Centers for Disease Control. (2011). *Births: Method of delivery*. Retrieved from http://www.cdc.gov/nchs/fastats/delivery.htm

Centers for Medicare and Medicaid Services (CMS). (n.d.). *Innovation models*. Retrieved from http://www.innovation.cms.gov/initiatives/index.html#_Expand

Clarin, O. A. (2007). Strategies to overcome barriers to effective nurse practitioner and physician collaboration. *Journal for Nurse Practitioners, 3*(8), 538–548.

Collins-Fulea, C., Moore, J. J., & Tillett, J. (2005). Improving midwifery practice: The American College of Nurse-Midwives' benchmarking project. *Journal of Midwifery and Women's Health, 50*(6), 461–471. Retrieved from http://www.midwife.org/ACNM/files/ccLibraryFiles/Filename/000000000189/PIIS1526952305003302.pdf

Cragin, L., & Kennedy, H. P. (2006). Linking obstetric and midwifery practice with optimal outcomes. *Journal of Obstetric, Gynecologic, and Neonatal Nursing, 35*(6), 779–785.

Doherty, M. E. (2009). Therapeutic alliance: A concept for the childbearing season. *Journal of Perinatal Education, 18*(3), 39–47.

Fahy, K. M., & Parratt, J. A. (2006). Birth territory: A theory for midwifery practice. *Women Birth, 19*(2), 45–50.

Family Health and Birth Center. (2007). *Briefing Statement to the Committee on Health of the Council of the District of Columbia, 2/22/07*. As cited in ACNM (2007). Issue brief: *Reducing health disparities*. Retrieved from http://www.midwife.org/siteFiles/education/Health_Care_Disparities_Issue_Brief_10_07.pdf

Frontier Nursing Service. (1958). Summary of the first 10,000 confinement records of the Frontier Nursing Service. *QBull Frontier Nursing Service, 33*, 45–55.

Garloch, K. (2012). Seven nurse midwives lose physician supervision; expecting moms left looking for birthing care. *News and Observer*. Retrieved from http://www.newsobserver.com/2012/06/03/2108042/seven-nurse-midwives-lose-physician.html

Hauer, K. E., Durning, S. J., Kernan, W. N., Fagan, M. J., Mintz, M., O'Sullivan, P. S., & Schwartz, M. D. (2008). Factors associated with medical students' career choices regarding internal medicine. *Journal of the American Medical Association, 300*(10), 1154–1164.

Heale, R. (2012). Overcoming barriers to practice: A nurse practitioner-led model. *Journal of the American Academy of Nurse Practitioners, 24*(6), 358–363.

Hofer, A. N., Abraham, J. M., & Moscovice, I. (2011). Expansion of coverage under the Patient Protection and Affordable Care Act and primary care utilization. *Milbank Quarterly, 89*(1), 69–89.

Hogberg, D. (2012, August). *The next exodus: Primary-care physicians and Medicare*. National Policy Analysis. Retrieved from http://www.nationalcenter.org/NPA640.html

Institute of Medicine (IOM). (2011). *The future of nursing: Leading change, advancing health*. Retrieved from http://www.iom.edu/Reports/2010/The-Future-of-Nursing-Leading-Change-Advancing-Health.aspx

Jackson Healthcare. (2013). *Physician practice trends survey 2012*. Retrieved from http://www.jacksonhealthcare.com/media-room/surveys/physician-practice-trends-survey-2012.aspx

Johantgen, M., Fountain, L., Zangaro, G., Newhouse, R., Stanik-Hutt, J., & White, K. (2012). Comparison of labor and delivery care provided by certified nurse-midwives and physicians: A systematic review, 1990 to 2008. *Women's Health Issues, 22*(1), 73–81.

Kennedy, H. P. (2000). A model of exemplary midwifery practice: Results of a Delphi study. *Journal of Midwifery & Women's Health, 45*(1), 4–19.

Kennedy, H. P., Rousseau, A. L., & Low, L. K. (2003, September). An exploratory metasynthesis of midwifery practice in the United States. *Midwifery, 19*(3), 203–214.

Lange, G., & Kennedy, H. P. (2010). Student perceptions of ideal and actual midwifery practice. *Journal of Midwifery & Women's Health, 51*(2), 71–77.

Lehrman, E. J. (1981). Nurse-midwifery practice: A descriptive study of prenatal care. *Journal of Nurse Midwifery, 26*, 27–41.

Levy, B. S., Wilkinson, F. S., & Marine, W. M. (1971). Reducing neonatal mortality rates with nurse-midwives. *American Journal of Obstetrics and Gynecology, 109*, 50–58.

Lugo, N. R., O'Grady, E. T., Hodnicki, D. R., & Hanson, C. M. (2007). Ranking NP state regulation: Practice environment and consumer healthcare choice. *American Journal for Nurse Practitioners, 11*(4), 8–24.

March of Dimes. (2013). *Medicaid coverage of births: U.S. 2001–2003*. PeriStats. Retrieved from http://www.marchofdimes.com/peristats/level1.aspx?reg=99&top=11&stop=154&lev=1&slev=1&obj=1&dv=cr

Morten, A., Kohl, M., O'Mahoney, P., & Pelosi, K. (1991). Certified nurse-midwifery care of the postpartum client: A descriptive study. *Journal of Nurse-Midwifery, 36*(5), 276–288.

Newhouse, R. P., Stanik-Hutt, J., White, K. M., Johantgen, M., Bass, E. B., Zangaro, G., & Weiner, J. P. (2011). Advanced practice nurse outcomes 1990–2008: A systematic review. *Nursing Economics, 29*(5), 1–22.

New York Times. (2010, December 11). Following the money, doctors ration care. *New York Times*. Retrieved from http://www.nytimes.com/2010/12/12/business/12view.html?_r=0

Nickel, S., Gesse, T., & MacLaren, A. (1992). Ernestine Wiedenbach: Her professional legacy. *Journal of Nurse-Midwifery, 37*(3), 161–167.

Patient Protection and Affordable Care Act (PPACA). (2010). *One Hundred Eleventh Congress of the United States of America at the Second Session*. Retrieved from http://www.gpo.gov/fdsys/pkg/BILLS-111hr3590enr/pdf/BILLS-111hr3590enr.pdf

Pleticha, K. (2004). The birth battle: Doctors, midwives, and the politics of pregnancy. *Parent: Wise, 1*(1). Retrieved from: http://www.parentwiseaustin.com/Archive/2004-04/Birth-Battle-Doctors-Midwives-and-Politics-Pregnancy

Restrepo, G. (2012, October 25). *Advanced practice nursing: The future is now*. The Clinical Advisor. Retrieved from http://www.clinicaladvisor.com/advanced-practice-nursing-the-future-is-now/article/265419/#

Rooks, J. (1997). *Midwifery and childbirth in America*. Philadelphia, PA: Temple University Press.

Safriet, B. (2011). Appendix H: Federal options for maximizing the value of advanced practice nurses in providing quality, cost-effective health care. *The future of nursing: Leading change, advancing health*. Washington, DC: National Academies Press.

Shaver, K. (2007, May 18). Birth centers' closures limit delivery options. *The Washington Post*, pp. B1–B5.

Shaw, A., deLusignan, S., & Rowlands, G. (2005). Do primary care professionals work as a team: A qualitative study. *Journal of Interprofessional Care, 19*(4), 396–405.

Sonenberg, A. (2010). Medicaid and state regulation of nurse-midwives: The challenge of data retrieval. *Policy, Politics, and Nursing Practice, 11*(4), 253–259.

Stapleton, S. R., Osborne, C., & Illuzzi, J. (2013). Outcomes of care in birth centers: Demonstration of a durable model. *Journal of Midwifery and Women's Health, 58*(1), 3–14.

Thompson, J. E., Oakley, D., Burke, M., Jay, S., & Conklin, M. (1989). Theory building in nurse-midwifery. *Journal of Midwifery & Women's Health, 4*(3), 120–130.

Van Soeren, M., Hurlock-Chorostecki, C., Goodwin, S., & Baker, E. (2009). A primary healthcare nurse practitioner in Ontario: A workforce study. *Nursing Leadership, 22*(2), 59–72.

Vedam, S., Goff, M., & Marnin, V. N. (2007). Closing the theory–practice gap: Intrapartum midwifery management of planned home births. *Journal of Midwifery & Women's Health, 52*(3), 291–300.

CHAPTER 18

Health Policy Implications for Advanced Practice Registered Nurses Related to End-of-Life Care

Judy Lentz

The process of dying and the ultimate death experience over the past 100 years has changed dramatically (Table 18.1). In the early 20th century, generally deaths followed short-term illnesses such as pneumonia, end-stage cancers, strokes, and so on. In the 21st century, those diseases are either cured or controlled for prolonged periods of time.

In 1900, the average life span was 48.23 years as compared with 78.3 in 2010, more than a century later (Bakitas et al., 2010; Centers for Disease Control and Prevention [CDC], 2012a; Infoplease, 2012). Only 4% of Americans in the early 1900s were over 65 years of age (Hoefler, 2010). Today, more than 12.8% of Americans are 65 years and over, and this percentage is projected to increase to 19.3% by 2030, more than quadrupling in the past 100 years (Jackson et al., 2012). Again, in the early 20th century, the dying trajectory was short term following an acute illness. However, in mid-century, a short 50 years later, circumstances changed. With the advent of anti-neoplastics, antimicrobial agents, and technological advances, acute illnesses were treatable and life-threatening illnesses could be ameliorated. Many life-threatening acute illnesses became chronic in nature and Americans began to believe most diseases could be cured or at least controlled for long periods. The extended life span in the 21st century has confirmed this belief.

As a result of these advances, illnesses progressed more slowly, treatment options caused more suffering, pain was frequently unrelieved, and the dying process became protracted. Physicians who had taken the Hippocratic Oath sought to prolong life and family members became death-denying by urging the medical staff to try "one more'" approach. Dying with dignity became an unfulfilled wish. In its place was isolation, pain, and suffering.

Today, more than 2.5 million people die in the United States annually (CDC, 2012b). Most of these deaths are caused by heart disease, cancer, cerebrovascular diseases, pulmonary diseases, and renal syndromes. Providing quality end-of-life care is a huge challenge given the many variations of disease processes, ages, settings, and health care professionals, for those who face these challenges daily. Assuring

TABLE 18.1 Changes in Death Processes in the Last 100 Years

CRITERIA	1900	2010
Average life expectancy	48.23 years	78.3 years
Place of death	Majority at home	Majority at hospital
Family acceptance	Openly discussed	Death-denying society
Expenses paid by	Family	Medicare
Disease trajectory prior to death	Acute—short term	Chronic—long term

palliative care services begin at the time of diagnosis and include hospice care over the final 6 months for every one of the 2.5 million people is the goal of the palliative care health care professionals.

DRIVING FORCES

Changes in the way Americans view end-of-life care have been influenced over the past 35 years by a death-denying society, family value changes, financial cost escalations, geography, and political influences. Let us begin with why Americans are a death-denying society. Technology has driven this sociological change. Americans have witnessed an explosion of technology and advanced treatment modalities. With the development of automatic implantable cardiac defibrillators (AICDs), the perfection of transplantation of organs and bone marrow, the advancements in surgical procedures through robotics, as well as the advancement of genomics, Americans believe any disease can be cured and life can be prolonged hopefully indefinitely. Just look at the statistics describing the number of people living well beyond 100 years of age. If we continue to perfect and advance medical management of diseases, we strengthen this myth of infinite living.

Family value changes are evidenced by egocentricity, belief of the rights of individuals, an educated society, and family advocacy. Again, technological advances through social media, the internet, global communication, and natural inquisitiveness drive the individual to demand a certain level of expectation of medical treatment regardless of cost.

The financial impact of this level of care is driving our country into an extreme debt. In 2012, health care in the United States was 17.3% of the gross national product. This level of cost is unsustainable. If unchecked, the rates are projected to increase another 17% in the next 70 years (Hixon, 2012). Yet, in a recent Economist Intelligence Unit (EIU) report, the United States ranked ninth in the end-of-life care only slightly ahead of Hungary and Poland. In terms of funding palliative/end-of-life care, the United States ranked 31st of 40 (Hoefler, 2010). One analyst in the EIU report commented about the United States saying it is "the epicenter for the technologies that allow us to keep people alive for 60 additional days with no improvement in outcome but with substantial increase in costs" (Hoefler, 2010). The Hospice Medicare Benefits (HMBs) spending in 2007 for an average of 67 days per patient was more than $10 billion. Only 1.2 million Americans received hospice care in 2008, less than half of those who die annually. This cost is expected to be double for the same number of people over the next 10 years (Buck, 2011). Extrapolating from this, if all dying Americans received end-of-life care, the costs would quadruple. Ironically, studies have demonstrated that cost savings of nearly $1,700 per admission for live discharges and $5,000 per admission for patients who died can be realized through hospital-based palliative care teams who through advance care planning (ACP) allow the patient to shift the chosen course of care (Morrison et al., 2008). For an average 400 bed hospital, these savings translate to nearly $1.3 million net savings per year.

Where one lives can also influence end-of-life care (Buck, 2011; Giovanni, 2012; Meier & Beresford, 2008a; Sherman & Cheon, 2012). The number of hospital beds and physicians there are per patient population can directly influence whether patients are admitted to hospitals to die or are cared for at home (Meier & Beresford, 2008a). For example, statistics of those dying in hospitals in rural areas of the Western and Northwestern states were lower as compared with Southern and Eastern states where large urban medical centers were easily accessible (Giovanni, 2012; Sherman & Cheon, 2012).

The political environment has also negatively influenced end-of-life care in the United States. Understandably, as legislators and their aides are representatives of the death-denying society in which they live, they are naturally influenced by their constituencies. When the 2010 Patient Protection and Affordable Care Act (PPACA) recommended reimbursement for advance care planning, adversaries interpreted this recommendation as rationing care and the language was removed from the final document (Giovanni, 2012; Zeytinoglu, 2011). The positive impact on quality of end-of-life care is directly dependent on having the conversations with the patient, their family, and the legislators who create laws that determine the right to have life-saving or ending treatment. Removing the incentives to do so, negatively impacts the outcomes of care—physically, psychosocially, and economically.

NEED FOR POLICY CHANGES IN END-OF-LIFE CARE

Although there has been extensive political debate about end-of-life care, the number of policy changes has been negligible. According to the *Approaching Death: Improving Care at the End-of-Life* report written by a panel from the Institutes of Medicine in 2007, "…people have come both to fear a technologically over-treated and protracted death and to dread the prospect of abandonment and untreated physical and emotional distress" (Zeytinoglu, 2011).

Several studies have suggested that patients and families believe end-of-life care is inadequate (Giovanni, 2012; Hoefler, 2010; Jackson et al., 2012; Morrison et al., 2011; Pace & Lunsford, 2011; Sherman & Cheon, 2012). Access alone is a major problem. Millions of Americans are denied palliative care services because none are available where they live even though we have experienced tremendous growth in the number of programs over the past decade. According to the 2008 Center to Advance Palliative Care (CAPC) Report card and consistent in 2011, 85% of large hospitals with 300 or more beds have a palliative care team (Morrison et al., 2011). Palliative care is most prevalent in the Northeast and lowest in the South (Morrison et al., 2011). The overall grade for palliative care across the nation improved from a C in 2008 to a B in 2011 (Morrison et al., 2011). Only two states received failing grades—Mississippi and Delaware. More than 50% of the states received As or Bs (Morrison et al., 2011).

Just as in the 1980s when legislators saw the opportunity to improve quality and to reduce the cost of care in end-of-life by establishing the Medicare Hospice Benefit, in 2012, we once again saw the opportunity to advance palliative care nationally through policy change. What those changes should be is a national debate currently underway.

Studies continue to show that treatments fail to align with patient wishes (Giovanni, 2012; Morrison et al., 2008). Curtis et al. (Jackson et al., 2012) defines quality of dying and death as "the degree to which a person's preferences for dying and the moment of death are consistent with observations of how the person actually died as reported by others" (p. 304). Having conversations with patients and family members when serious illnesses have been detected provides the insight to what the patient/family preferences are, allows the burden of decision making for the family to be decreased, and assures the treatments to match the patient's wishes. Although these conversations are difficult for the generalist, experienced palliative care professionals are experts and can make all the difference in achieving quality of dying and death in end-of-life care (Boucher et al., 2010).

HISTORY

In the early 1960s, as Dr. Elisabeth Kubler-Ross was beginning her teaching career at the University of Colorado Medical School, she was distressed to find nothing in the medical school curricula regarding how to care for the dying. In an effort to introduce medical students to the needs and concerns of the dying patient, she invited a young 16-year-old girl with leukemia to come to her lecture. Dr. Kubler-Ross encouraged the students to ask the young girl anything they would like. Their questions were directed only to her medical condition. The young girl became angry and began talking about what mattered most to her—like what it would be like to never get married or have children or even attend her senior prom. This encounter led Kubler-Ross to extensively study and publish research regarding the responses of those who were experiencing the dying process (Biography.com, 2012).

At the same time, Dame Cicely Saunders, who started the hospice movement in England, was invited to Yale University to lecture about her new philosophy of care for the dying. Dean of the School of Nursing at Yale University at that time was Dr. Florence Wald. Dr. Wald was so impressed after hearing Dame Saunders's lecture, she resigned her position at Yale and returned to her beloved public health nursing where she focused on the care of young dying breast cancer patients. In her effort to improve their quality of life, she, along with other health care professionals, initiated the Connecticut Hospice in 1972 (Buck, 2011; Pace & Lunsford, 2011). This occurrence determined the inauguration of the hospice philosophy in the United States.

Soon after, legislators began to look for ways to reimburse this new model of care. In 1986, the Medicare Hospice Benefit was made a permanent entitlement under Medicare (Buck, 2011). Those hospices receiving reimbursement for medical care have to be certified through the Centers for Medicare and Medicaid Services (CMS) and are required to strictly adhere to the Conditions of Participation (CoPs) to prevent sanctions (Federal Register, 2012). The CoPs are frequently revised through the Federal Registry and continue to serve as the regulatory standards of hospice care. Nonadherence leads to financial penalties and certification removal.

This was the same period of time that the Hospice Nurses Association was incorporated. Thirty-eight hospice nurses established the specialty nursing organization to "lead the way" in hospice nursing through education. The organization quickly grew and soon thereafter spawned the National Board for Certification of Hospice Nurses in 1992. In 1998, both of these organizations added the word "palliative" to their name, becoming the Hospice and Palliative Nurses Association (HPNA) and the National Board for Certification of Hospice and Palliative Nursing (NBCHPN®) recognizing the significance of palliative care that was simply providing the hospice philosophy earlier in the disease trajectory.

As legislators worked to improve end-of-life care in America, a new policy was written called the Patient Self-Determination Act of 1991 (Hayes, 2004). The intent of the act was to give Americans a voice in end-of-life decisions through the completion of advance directives (Giovanni, 2012). The law required every Medicare-participating organization to ask patients upon admission if they had an advance directive and if not, would they like assistance in completing one. The advance directive was then supposed to become a part of the permanent medical record. As well intentioned as it was, the law failed miserably. Despite more than 20 years of promoting advance directives, only 20% to 30% of Americans currently have written one (Derby, O'Mahony, & Tickoo, 2010).

In 1995, a study underwritten by Robert Wood Johnson Foundation became the first of three sentinel studies to serve as springboards to the introduction of palliative care in America. The study was called *The SUPPORT Study: A Controlled Trial to Improve Care for Seriously Ill Hospitalized Patients—The Study to Understand Prognoses and Preferences for Outcomes and Risks of Treatment* (Pace & Lunsford, 2011). The objectives of this study were to seek ways to improve the end-of-life decision making and improve the quality of life of the dying. Several outcomes highlighted the abysmal circumstances that existed for the dying. Communications were lacking regarding patient preferences and choices, do-not-resuscitate orders were being written within 2 days of death, patients wanted to die at home yet were dying in intensive care units, and patients/family members were reporting excessive levels of pain being experienced by their dying loved one.

Soon thereafter, the Institute of Medicine published the second sentinel study called *Approaching Death: Improving Care at the End-of-Life*. One outcome of this study confirmed the findings of the SUPPORT Study—pain was undertreated in the dying. Other outcomes focused on the need to gather more data, remedy the impediments to quality care, and research the many gaps in scientific knowledge (Chiarella & Duffield, 2007; Pace & Lunsford, 2011).

The third sentinel study was the Last Acts Report called *Means to a Better End: A Report on Dying in America Today* again underwritten by the Robert Wood Johnson Foundation. This study graded each state in the nation on eight criteria that described the availability and quality of end-of-life care in America (Bakitas, Bishop, & Caron, 2010; Pace & Lunsford, 2011). The results of this study were very discouraging. Our nation was failing miserably.

The previous studies launched a national campaign for moving hospice care upstream. In 2001, Dr. Diane Meier convened a group of national leaders in palliative care and challenged them to create a set of palliative care guidelines. With representation from the four leading organizations—American Academy of Hospice and Palliative Medicine (AAHPM), CAPC, HPNA, and the National Hospice and Palliative Care Organization—the National Consensus Project (NCP) work began. The first edition of the *Clinical Practice Guidelines for Quality Palliative Care* was published in 2004 and revised in 2009. A third edition is currently underway. These guidelines are intended to be initiated at the time of diagnosis and continue throughout the disease trajectory, the death, and the bereavement period thereafter, therefore, inclusive of hospice care representing the end of the palliative care continuum (Figure 18.1). The guidelines espouse eight domains of care—structure and process, physical aspects, psychosocial and psychiatric aspects, social aspects, spiritual/religious/existential aspects, cultural aspects, care of the imminently dying, and ethical/legal aspects of care (National Consensus Project for Quality Palliative Care, 2009). For more details, visit www.nationalconsensusproject.org. These core elements serve as the conceptual framework of quality palliative care in America.

In 2006, the National Quality Forum (NQF), the nonprofit agency charged with building consensus on performance improvement through measurement, reporting, education, and outreach programs, developed a more formal definition by naming 38 preferred practices published in a document known as *A National Framework and*

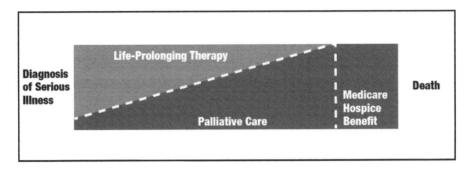

FIGURE 18.1 Palliative Care's Place in the Course of Illness.

Source: National Consensus Project for Quality Palliative Care (2009, p. 6).

Preferred Practices for Palliative and Hospice Care Quality and can be found at www. qualityforum.org (Meier & Beresford, 2008b; National Consensus Project for Quality Palliative Care, 2009; NQF, 2012b). The preferred practices were synergistic to the NCP Clinical Practice Guidelines and can be easily cross-walked with the eight domains. This document becomes the first step toward the development of quality indicators as required by CMS.

PALLIATIVE CARE IN THE 21ST CENTURY

Over the past decade, palliative care has achieved significant momentum spurred by the negative outcomes of the SUPPORT Study (Chiarella & Duffield, 2007; Forero et al., 2012). The development of the clinical practice guidelines by the National Consensus Project and the preferred practices published by the NQF generated a great deal of attention among health care professionals. A broad dissemination of the guidelines with requests for endorsement yielded positive responses. The work of the CAPC to establish palliative care delivery models in hospitals across the nation created the incentives to establish these highly successful programs. The momentum gave great hope to the leaders in the field. But were the programs reflective of the tenets of the hospice philosophy as described in the clinical practice guidelines?

The tenets of palliative care are many: holistic care inclusive of mind, body, and spirit aspects; 24/7 coverage; interprofessional team specifically including the physician, nurse, social worker, chaplain, and any other health care professionals indicated; ACP as a continuous and dynamic process; patient/family as the unit of care; and assurances that treatments match the patient-stated wishes. To assure program development matched the guidelines, The Joint Commission established a palliative care certification initiated in August, 2011. The written standards for this certification match the 2009 clinical practice guidelines. Thus far, several hospital programs have achieved palliative care certification recognition as an add-on option. The rights of the dying supersede all others issues and palliative care professionals are the team to assure these rights are acknowledged and honored. *The American Journal of Nursing* published a "Dying patient bill of rights" widely used by practitioners in the field of hospice/palliative care (Table 18.2).

Several successful programs have come out of demonstration projects, research studies, and exemplar practice settings. These programs have served as pioneers,

TABLE 18.2 Dying Bill of Rights

I have the right to be treated as a living human being until I die.
I have the right to maintain a sense of hopefulness, however changing its focus may be.
I have the right to be cared for by those who can maintain a sense of hopefulness, however changing this might be.
I have the right to express my feelings and emotions about my approaching death in my own way.
I have the right to participate in decisions concerning my care.
I have the right to expect continuing medical and nursing attention even though "cure" goals must be changed to "comfort" goals.
I have the right not to die alone. I have the right to be free from pain.
I have the right to have my questions answered honestly.
I have the right to not be deceived.
I have the right to have help from and for my family in accepting my death.
I have the right to die in peace and dignity.
I have the right to retain my individuality and not be judged for my decisions that may be contrary to beliefs of others.
I have the right to discuss and enlarge my religious and/or spiritual experiences, whatever these may mean to others.
I have the right to expect that the sanctity of the human body will be respected after death.
I have the right to be cared for by caring, sensitive, knowledgeable people who will attempt to understand my needs and will be able to gain some satisfaction in helping me face death.

Source: Launer (n.d.).

role models, and benchmarks for new developing programs. Take for instance, the Safe Conduct Study performed in 2000–2002. Awarded a demonstration project from Robert Wood Johnson Foundation, the Ireland Cancer Center in Cleveland, Ohio, and the Hospice of the Western Reserve teamed together to offer a unique palliative care service for newly diagnosed Stage 4 lung cancer patients. Patients were randomized into the study group or the control group. This study group received care by a palliative care nurse practitioner, social worker, and chaplain every visit they made to the facility from the time of diagnoses throughout the disease trajectory, death, and bereavement thereafter. The control group received standard care. The outcomes of this study were most surprising. Not only did patients and families rate the quality of their care as highly satisfactory, but also they rated their quality of life highly satisfactory while the control group rated the quality of their care much lower. An interesting review of the data, not intentionally studied, was that the amount and kind of care received by the study group was only half of that of the control group yet rated much higher (Pitorak & Armour, 2003).

A similar study was conducted in 2009 by Dr. Jennifer Temel at the Massachusetts General Hospital Palliative Care service. Although the outcomes of the Temel study replicated those of the Safe Conduct Study, one additional benefit was noted in the Temel study. For unexplainable reasons, the patients in the study group lived 2.7 months longer than the control group (Kelly & Meier, 2010). Although unexplainable, it is believed that the reasons may be because the patient's symptoms were better controlled, the patient's depression was treated, and there was a reduction in patient hospitalizations (Kelly & Meier, 2010). This was a landmark study because it refuted the general public suspicions that those receiving palliative care may have life short-ened by withdrawal or withholding of care by the medical team.

Other studies conducted by Dr. Joan Teno, Bon Secours, Mt. Sinai/Franklin Health, and the Institute of Healthcare Improvement's Triple Aim have established credible outcomes to prove the value of palliative care in improving quality of end-of-life care (Gelfman et al., 2008; Giovanni, 2012; Meier et al., 2004; Meier & Beresford, 2010; Nelson et al., 2011). These success stories stress values in terms of patient and family satisfaction, quality practice emphasizing quality of life for the patient and family, cost effectiveness, and performance improvement.

CONCEPTUAL AND THEORETICAL FRAMEWORK

Historically, palliative care has been based on the hospice philosophy. The core elements for hospice are replicated in palliative care. The management of serious illness is very different than the management of acute care. The theoretical frame-work recommends introduction of palliative care at the time of diagnosis, increasing the concentration of the palliative care team based on the disease progression and the patient wishes, ultimately assuming 100% of the care management through the dying phase, death, and bereavement thereafter (National Consensus Project for Quality Palliative Care, 2009).

Two distinct elements make palliative care unique—the interprofessional team and ACP. Care is delivered by an interprofessional team composed of the physi-cian, nurse, social worker, and chaplain at a minimum of health care professionals as required by the Medicare Hospice Benefit CoPs and replicated by palliative care as written in the clinical practice guidelines. The nurse becomes pivotal to this team serving as the care coordinator, assures the care plan reflects the patient and family wishes and goals, assures the team knows and honors the patient's stated care goals, coordinates the plan-of-care meetings, and continually evaluates the effectiveness of treatments prescribed to relieve the physical, psychosocial, and spiritual distresses experienced by the patient.

The success of the interprofessional team is assured by hiring the right people, demonstrating mutual respect and humility, building a quality team, and assuring healthy group dynamics occur during debriefing sessions. The conceptual frame-work for the interprofessional team is based on interprofessional collaboration that is defined by Bronstein as "an interpersonal communication process leading to the attainment of specific goals not achievable by any single team member alone" (Baldwin, Wittenberg-Lyles, Oliver, & Demiris, 2011, p. 173). Team training, conflict resolution, and team building are critical processes to define for a successful team. Seeking ways to support one another, balancing workloads, and providing self-care options are some examples of team building (Egan City & Labyak, 2010; Krammer, Martinez, Ring-Hurn, & Williams, 2010; Meier & Beresford, 2008b).

ACP is a process of conversations based on what the needs of the patient and family might be. In palliative care, this mantra is frequently heard: "it's all about the conversation." Make no mistake, it sounds simple but is far from it. Acquiring skill in these kinds of conversations is what makes palliative care professionals unique.

The American Academy of Nursing published a policy brief (2010) titled *Advance Care Planning as an Urgent Public Health Concern.* Collaborating with HPNA leaders, the task force made several recommendations: (a) to pay for the conversa-tions, (b) to utilize the electronic medical record to record the patient's preference, (c) to update the advance directives and expand the requirements of the Patient Self Determination Act of 1991, and finally (d) to provide health professionals with education and training for caring of the dying (American Academy of Nursing Policy Brief, 2010).

Even though death is inevitable for all of us, discussing the possibility is difficult for all of us. And yet, when diagnosed with a serious illness, patients and families will emphatically say, decision making is simplified by ACP discussions. These discussions occur frequently based on the individual and the situation beginning with the first conversation to establish the patient/family goals of care. In palliative care, the patient is the driver of the treatment directions. There are several steps to each conversation beginning with knowing what the patient/family understands about the situation. Next, the palliative care professional must establish how much the patient wants to know and who will make decisions if he or she is unable. The conversations from then on should be frequent, transparent, based on what the patient/family wants and cover the benefits and burdens of each treatment being considered. Shared decision making from patients/families that have been fully informed is the hallmark of quality palliative care. It is a dying patient's right (American College of Healthcare Executives, 2009; Giovanni, 2012; HPNA, 2012d; Jackson et al., 2012; Launer, n.d.; Schaffer et al., 2012; Zeytinoglu, 2011).

And yet, with all the uniqueness of palliative care, Carlson sums up the current thinking with the following quote: "Improving end-of-life care should be a national priority, not just from a cost-perspective, but from a quality perspective, because we can do much better" (Carlson, 2010). Studies have shown little evidence that treatments match patient wishes. Why? Access, fear, educational curricula failing to address end-of-life care, and workforce issues are some of the reasons (Giovanni, 2012). Providing the right care to the right patient at the right time defines quality according to Giovanni.

HEALTH POLICY

Since the inception of hospice in America, health policy has served as an impetus for change in the care of the dying. Health policy is often guided by the research. Although the availability of quantitative and qualitative research has the potential to drive decisions in health policy, in a field as new as palliative care, there is as yet a paucity of research (Lunney, 2011; Scanlon, 2010). But this trend is changing as evidence-based research is growing rapidly. However, the research continues to have a minimum impact indicated by a low level of attention (Forero et al., 2012).

Several noted nursing researchers have contributed heartily to the field of hospice/palliative care—Jeanne Quint Beneliel, Florence Wald, Ida Martinson, Marylin Dodd, Elizabeth Clipp, Virginia Tilden, Betty Ferrell, Joy Buck, Mary Ersek, and June Lunney are several notable historic end-of-life nursing research leaders. A 2010 review of the published research literature revealed that 14% had been contributed by nursing in that year (Lunney, 2011). The lack of funding seems to be the most prominent barrier to nursing research (Ferrell, Grant, & Sun, 2010).

The majority of funds received for early research came from private funders—Robert Wood Johnson Foundation and George Soros contributed millions of research dollars (Martinez, 2011). Although funding from governmental sources was limited in the early years, the National Institutes of Health has substantially increased their support to the study of hospice and palliative research over the recent years. Funded projects increased from less than 50 in 1990 to over 350 in 2010 (Lunney, 2011). The National Institute of Nursing Research (NINR) is the agency that provides the focus of all palliative care research currently—medical and nursing. The NINR recently funded two initiatives in 2011, one called the *End-of-Life and Palliative Care Needs*

Assessment and the other a *Summit on the Science of Compassion: Future Directions in End-of-Life and Palliative Care*. These initiatives will help to shape the future research needs in palliative care (Lunney, 2011).

The HPNA Scope and Standards of Practice document has always defined research as an expected area of participation for hospice and palliative nurses. Hospice nurses in earlier years hesitated to allow their patients to participate in research because of the severity of their illness. It was later discovered that patients wanted the opportunity to participate in an effort to advance the field for their loved ones. Defining areas of research need has long been attributed to the clinician as well as assisting with data collection (Lunney, 2011). Every hospice and palliative nurse can contribute to research in meaningful ways.

Until 2009, the HPNA had no research agenda even though the organization's leaders valued the need (HPNA, 2012b). Through the efforts of a core group of palliative nursing researchers, the first HPNA research agenda was published in 2011. The focus was to encourage research on dyspnea, fatigue, constipation, and heart failure (Lunney, 2011). Then in 2012, the HPNA Board of Directors published the second research agenda that is available at www.hpna.org. New areas of focus include Domains I (Structure and Processes), II (Physical Aspects of Care), and III (Psychological and Psychiatric Aspects of Care) of the Clinical Practice Guidelines in Quality Palliative Care. The physical symptoms specifically are fatigue, dyspnea, and constipation (HPNA, 2012b).

Nurses led the policy changes with hospice care. As noted earlier, it was Dr. Florence Wald who spearheaded the hospice movement in America. Through stories told by nurses, many policies have been generated in an effort to improve the care of the dying (Buck, 2011). The HMB reimbursement was probably the most significant change so far. Although offering financial security for hospices in America at the time the HMBs were initiated, these benefits have been attributed as the cause for many reimbursement issues that exist today (Buck, 2011; CMS, 2012).

In 2004, the HPNA Board of Directors recognizing the critical need for nursing advocacy established a Public Policy Committee. One of the very first efforts of this committee was to recommend "Public Policy Guiding Principles." Originally written in 2006 and revised in 2010 (Figure 18.2), the concept of guiding principles continues today (HPNA, 2010).

The public policy issues that continue to hinder the field of hospice/palliative care are many. Access is the most significant one (NQF, 2012a). Not only do individuals not have access to palliative care in many areas of the nation, but also 45 million individuals do not have health care insurance and another 25 million are underinsured for such care. Awareness is another issue. As many health care professionals do not understand what palliative care is, how can we expect the lay public to comprehend its complexity? A third area of concern is the death-denying society that precludes having the conversations. When the PPACA was approved in 2010, the legislators removed the language recommending advanced care planning conversations (Giovanni, 2012). However, the PPACA did expand coverage to over 30 million Americans previously uninsured (Sherman & Cheon, 2012).

Other public policy issues focus on pain management, workforce issues, educational needs, physician and advanced practice nurse fellowships, ACP, comparative effectiveness research, health information technology, payment reform, health delivery reform, and chronic care coordination (Meier & Beresford, 2009). The list is long and much work is needed.

Several statewide initiatives are demonstrating success—New Hampshire's *Reclaiming the End-of-Life Citizens Forum* (Meier & Beresford, 2009) and Maryland's

HPNA acts independently and with collaborating organizations to address hospice and palliative care issues at the national, state, local and regional levels. HPNA bases its public policy positions and actions on the following guiding principles.

1. HPNA asserts that it is the responsibility and obligation of clinicians to address hospice/palliative care public policy and regulatory issues that impact the health related quality of life of patients and caregivers living with progressive chronic and/or life limiting illnesses and conditions.

2. HPNA takes a leadership and advocacy role to ensure equitable access to comprehensive palliative care as defined by the National Consensus Project Clinical Practice Guidelines for Quality Palliative Care, across the life span and illness continuums.

3. HPNA works independently and collaboratively to promote ethical and competent provision of hospice/palliative care based upon the expressed goals of the patient and family/caregivers as the unit of care.

4. HPNA takes a leadership and advocacy role in regulatory issues and public education regarding the legitimate use and the misuse of prescription medication.

5. HPNA advocates for nursing workforce and professional education issues as they impact hospice and palliative care.

6. HPNA advocates for equitable funding for hospice/palliative care research.

7. HPNA supports improved access to comprehensive health care for appropriate management of physical and emotional symptoms that allows patients to achieve the highest quality of life through the relief of suffering in all of its manifestations.

FIGURE 18.2 HPNA 2010 Public Policy Guiding Principles.

Action Plan for Palliative and Hospice Care (Sherman & Cheon, 2012) are just two that are currently generating positive outcomes. New York recently passed the Palliative Care Information Act (2012) that requires physicians and nurse practitioners to offer counseling regarding end-of-life options such as risks and benefits, prognosis, and the patient's legal rights to pain and symptom management. This must be offered to every New York patient (or health care proxy for those without capacity) with an illness or condition that is expected to end in death within the next 6 months (Palliative Care Information Act, 2012).

ROLE OF THE PALLIATIVE CARE ADVANCED PRACTICE REGISTERED NURSE

The role of the advanced practice palliative care nurse is growing rapidly as indicated by the increased demand. Historically, the American Academy of Nurse Practitioners argued that APRNs demonstrated their ability to be cost-effective and provide high-quality care (Reifsnyder, & Yeo, 2011). In palliative care, APRNs spearhead the palliative care delivery service through development, implementation, and evaluation of services, and are considered as highly valued members of the interprofessional team (Rapp, 2003; Sherman & Cheon, 2012). Dr. Ira Byock, a highly acclaimed palliative care physician, has often stated, "If you want a good palliative care service, you need to find a good palliative care nurse" (personal communication, August 12, 2011).

The significance to the value of palliative care increased in January 2009 when the CMS finally recognized the new specialty. With this approval came a new code for physicians and nonphysician practitioners to bill for their services (Meier & Beresford, 2008b; Pace & Lunsford, 2011). Advanced practice palliative care nurses are poised for success with the recognition of the palliative care specialty in the medical community, regulatory recognition by CMS for palliative care billing purposes, and legal recognition by CMS in terms of the approval of the palliative care nursing certification body (NBCHPN®) that finally occurred in 2007 (Horton & Indelicato, 2010).

In addition to their clinical practice role, APRNs serve as administrators, educators, health policy makers, and researchers Figure 18.3 (Sherman & Cheon, 2012). As administrators, they assure the implementation and evaluation of the programs and assure that they remain viable and eventually eligible for The Joint Commission certification. As educators, they are called upon to assist staff with the dying process and to educate the patient and family to be fully informed and able to understand the disease process and the subsequent prognosis and treatment options in terms of benefits and burdens. They also educate the lay public about the value of palliative care and educate other health care professionals to improve communication and quality of life for all patients (Jackson et al., 2012).

As health policy advocates, the adage "all politics are local" becomes a mantra of nursing advocacy (Meier & Beresford, 2009). Reaching out locally, influencing state lawmakers as well as federal senators and representatives can be very effective. The more committed nurses are to public policy, the louder our voice of advocacy will be heard. It is through stories told by nurses that regulatory and legislative changes occur. In 2009, the Federal Drug Administration (FDA) mandated that morphine can be pulled from the manufacturing process to comply with current

Clinical consultant

- Leads the team as coordinator, leads family conferences, updates plan of care, monitors and revises treatments to achieve stated patient goals

Administrator

- Designs, implements and evaluates program delivery
- Advocates business model to administration

Educator

- Educates staff, patients, family members, other health care professionals and lay public

Health care policy maker

- Advocates for policy changes internally and externally on the local, state and national levels

Researcher

- Recommends clinical issues to study
- Advocates for research participation and assists in data collection
- Designs research studies, seeks funding and implements research

FIGURE 18.3 Palliative Care Advanced Practice Roles.

Source: Sherman and Cheon (2012).

approval requirements of new drugs. Morphine, a long-established drug, had no previous approval requirements. The FDA had no idea of the unintended consequences of their mandate. Pain management for the terminally ill became a nightmare. Opioid shortages occurred as a ripple effect. Opioid rotations became more difficult. Practitioners scrambled to achieve pain control. In an effort to effectively communicate the subsequent havoc, letters with attached surveys were sent to nurses and physicians. The survey data achieved were significant but it was the impact of the dramatic stories told by the nurses in the field that reversed the new FDA mandate and morphine became immediately available once again. According to Dr. Douglas Throckmorton of the FDA, it was the stories from the nurses that convinced the FDA of the need to make a sudden process change. Finally, in terms of research, the role of the APRN is not only to define areas of needed research but also to participate in research through data collection, prevention of "gatekeeper" mentality of coworkers, and education of the patient/family in terms of participation to increase the base of evidence for practice.

In July 2012, HPNA held a Congressional Briefing with legislative aids discussing the importance of being able to make informed choices in palliative care. A panel of patients and family members participated expressing their concerns. An issue brief titled *Assuring Choice for Seriously and Progressively Ill Patients* was distributed that recommended the following: "Include in future legislative language a requirement that advanced practice nurses and physicians offer seriously, progressively ill patients information and counseling concerning palliative and end-of-life options for care and treatment" (HPNA, 2012a).

The education of advanced practice palliative care nurses began with Ursuline College in 1997. Soon after, New York University established an advanced degree program. Although 10 additional programs followed, many have since converted to postgraduate certificate programs or have become tracks in the Adult-Geriatric programs that currently exist (HPNA, 2012c). Although APRNs work in all arenas of palliative care, it is difficult to identify the total number because of expansiveness of care settings. As a result of the Advanced Practice Registered Nursing Consensus Work Group with what is referred to as the Licensure, Accreditation, Certification, and Education (LACE) project, subspecialty emphasis lies outside the mandated educational components. The four groups represented by the LACE acronym have been working collaboratively since 2006 to design an advanced practice model that will satisfy all four advanced practice nursing roles (Pace & Lunsford, 2011). In this model, palliative care is defined as a specialty. Beginning in 2015, APRN education will focus on one of the four roles and one of six primary population foci. Certification for licensure purposes will be focused on the two components of role and population (e.g., Adult-Gerontology Nurse Practitioner) and then the individual will be permitted to become certified in a specialty (e.g., palliative care). As a result, the educational curricula has been modified accordingly and any emphasis on specialties becomes self-education, postgraduate, or at the discretion of the faculty.

Certification for the APRN is critical to practice. The National Board for Certification of Hospice and Palliative Nurses (NBCHPN®) offers an advanced practice certification with the credential ACHPN, the acronym for Advanced Certified Hospice and Palliative Nurse (Lentz & Sherman, 2010; NBCHPN®, 2012). As of 2012, 765 advanced practice palliative care nurses hold this credential. The ACHPN exam is accredited by the Accreditation Board of Specialty Nursing Certification (ABSNC) (NBCHPN®, 2012). Accreditation is an important distinction not only acknowledging the adherence to 18 stringent standards (Martinez, 2011; American Board of Nursing

Specialties [ABNS], 2012) but also is required by the state to achieve recognition for advanced practice licensure as well as being approved for billing by CMS.

Although certification is the focus of its mission, NBCHPN® (2010) undertook a major initiative seeking a singular broadly endorsed definition for continuing competence for nurses at all levels of practice recognizing the need to apply this definition to certification. In the field of nursing education, competence usually represents the knowledge, skills, and ability to practice in one's specialty. Competency refers to the skillful art of actual practice. Both competence and competency are especially important to the APRN as well as the safety of the public. As noted in the Institute of Medicine report (2010) entitled *Future of Nursing: Leading Change, Advancing Health,* lifelong learning is one of the recommendations. The American Nurses Association (ANA), the National Council of State Boards of Nursing (NCSBN), the ABNS, and the Citizen Advocacy Coalition (CAC) have long sought ways to prove continuing competence through portfolios, self-assessments, examinations, simulated judgment exams, and personal improvement plans (Martinez, 2011).

As NBCHPN® (2010) sought to implement a plan to establish continuing competence, they recognized the variations of definitions in the literature and decided to undertake this initiative. With a team of experts from both inside and outside of hospice and palliative care, the work began. Nearly a year later, the agreed upon definition titled "Statement on Continuing Competence for Nursing: A Call to Action" was presented to the Accreditation Board for Specialty Nursing Certification (ABSNC) and ABNS for endorsement. ABNS further committed themselves to seek an even broader endorsement through their 32 member organization and, to date, 10 organizations have endorsed this document (ABNS website). The American Association of Colleges of Nursing (AACN) has also voted to endorse this definition that will drive the implementation throughout the graduate programs for advanced practice nurses nationally.

With this milestone complete, NBCHPN® launched a yearlong study of how the newly endorsed definition (Figure 18.4) could be implemented in palliative care. The study includes a variety of methodologies, a feedback loop for the certificant, and a certification renewal process that clearly defines the individual's unique continuing education and competence.

Simultaneously, a new initiative is underway with AACN in terms of future continuing education. Spawned from the Institute of Medicine report conducted in 2009 indicating the need to revamp the entire educational process for health care professionals, AACN has joined five other major organizations to provide recommendations to establish a new approach—interprofessional education (AACN, 2012). Ironically, palliative care has long participated in interprofessional education being a hallmark for the field and thus for advanced practice nursing. For example, for the past 9 years, physicians, nurses, social workers, chaplains, pharmacists, and others co-present and attend the annual cosponsored educational conference. This mirrors the education occurring daily in the field.

> "Continuing competence is the ongoing commitment of a registered nurse to integrate and apply the knowledge, skills, and judgment with the attitudes, values, and beliefs required to practice safely, effectively, and ethically in a designated role and setting."   (NBCHPN.org website)

FIGURE 18.4 Definition of Continuing Competence.

OUTCOME MEASURES

Under the current Affordable Care Act, starting in 2014, hospices will be required to publicly report quality data to the federal government (NationalQualityForum.org website). The NQF has developed the "Triple Aim" that will help to define directions for this new requirement and will extend the public reporting to the hospice community similar to the requirements for other practice settings. The Triple Aim represents (a) healthier people, (b) better care, and (c) more affordable care. In 2011, NQF convened a group of 60 organizations called the Measure Applications Partnership (MAP) to function as an advisory role to the Department of Health and Human Services. MAP has offered 28 measures, nearly half of which are ready for immediate use (NQF, 2012a). Two of the nonclinical measures are person- and family-centered care and care coordination—easily prioritized to hospice care. Of the other measures, seven of the recommended measures apply to both hospice and palliative care, three apply only to hospice, and three apply only to palliative care (Table 18.3).

A group of experts convened by the CAPC agree with many of these measures and suggested specific ways to assess the needs of patients at admission with a potentially life-limiting or life-threatening condition. They recommend beginning with a checklist that contains primary criteria (Weissman & Meier, 2011). The primary criteria are the minimum indicators that hospitals should use in screening patients on admission and they include palliative care's most effective question called the "surprise question"—"would you be surprised if the patient died within 12 months or before adulthood" (Weissman & Meier, 2011, p. 19). Other criteria include frequent admissions, admissions due to uncontrolled symptoms, complex care requirements, and a significant decline in function, weight, or feeding.

IMPLICATIONS FOR APRN PRACTICE

End-of-life care is long overdue for social change. In 2010, in a letter to the editor of *Journal of Pain and Symptom Management*, Dr. James M. Hoefler, Policy Studies Program at Dickinson College wrote: "The United States lags behind other countries

TABLE 18.3 Measure Application Partnership (MAP) Measures

MEASURE	HOSPICE CARE	PALLIATIVE CARE	BOTH
Experience of care			X
Comprehensive assessment (holistic)			X
Physical aspects—pain, dyspnea, constipation, etc.			X
Care planning			X
Implement patient/family goals			X
Prevent avoidable admissions to ED and hospital			X
Manage anxiety, depression, delirium, other psychological			X
Timeliness/responsiveness of care	X		
Access to health care team on 24-hour basis	X		
Avoiding unwanted treatments	X		
Sharing medical records and advance directives		X	
Patient education and support		X	
Access to palliative care		X	

Adapted from NQF MAP data 2012.

of the world when it comes to providing palliative care to patients at the end-of-life" (Hoefler, 2010). He cited specific areas such as pain and suffering, the short median length of stay in hospices (less than 3 weeks), and the expected dramatic rise in the "chronic, disabling, and often painful conditions" in the coming years. Lastly, he cited underfunding of palliative care in the United States (Hoefler, 2010).

Society values health care and finds ways to seek improvements through public policy changes. Reporting quality measures is one way to track and evaluate quality measures to allow society to initiate ways to improve policies in support of palliative care. Nurses, especially APRNs, are in the perfect position to advocate for policy changes and to conduct research that will provide the evidence base for practice changes.

According to Coleen Scanlon, "nurses are unequally positioned to influence the development of public policy that benefits patients, families and communities" because APRNs are uniquely positioned in the work they do—especially in palliative care (Scanlon, 2010, p. 1180). Dr. Karin Dufault states, "Advocacy goes hand in hand with the privilege of being called a nurse—a palliative care nurse—and new doors are now opening to be heard" (Ferrell & Coyle, 2010, p. 1173).

HPNA's branded motto is "leading the way." Palliative care nurses must be at the forefront leading the way to change through public policy. Nurses have the ability, knowledge, and power to make a difference in shaping the future of end-of-life care and the time is now. With more than 2,000 researchers and APRN palliative care nursing members of HPNA, the collective influence for policy changes created by their voices would be powerful.

ETHICS

Due to the complexity of the patient's condition as well as the vulnerability of these patients, ethical dilemmas can be expected. How we handle these situations is an area needing a great deal of attention in hospice and palliative care directly led by palliative APRNs.

Ethical dilemmas such as double effect, competency versus capacity, benevolent deception with informed consents, futility, withholding/withdrawing, goals of care, and substituted judgment are just a few of the myriad of ethical concerns facing hospice and palliative nurses daily as they assist the terminally ill patient and their family through critical decisions (Hayes, 2004). Moral distress occurs in nurses who have neither the power of autonomy nor the power of futility (Hayes, 2004). Dr. Ira Byock stated it best: "Clinicians can serve the dying person by being present. We may not have the answers for the existential questions of life and death any more than the dying person does. We may not be able to assuage all feelings of regret or fears of the unknown. But it is not our solutions that matter. The role of the clinical team is to stand by the patient, steadfastly providing meticulous physical care and psychological support, while people strive to discover their own answers" (Hayes, 2004, p. 43).

The advanced practice palliative care nurse is the coordinator of the interprofessional team and therefore uniquely positioned to assure the meticulous care of which Byock refers and thereby allowing the patient and family to discover their own answers. As an APRN in palliative care, offering nonjudgmental support, genuine compassion, education about the benefits and burdens of options, and most importantly, having the expertise to relieve physical, emotional, and spiritual suffering provides the experience and knowledge to advocate for health policy changes that improve the quality of life for these most vulnerable patients.

CONCLUSION

With a $2.4 trillion health care industry that fails to meet the needs of those experiencing end-of-life, the need for health care reform and availability of palliative care is obvious. Unacceptable outcomes continue to exist—unrelieved suffering, failure to acknowledge and honor wishes, benevolent deception, and death without dignity. The need for change is now.

What should that change look like? The call to action white paper called *Call to Action: Health Care Reform 2009* offered one model emphasizing three legs of reform. The design advocates weeding out waste and overpayment, focusing on quality, value, and less costly care, and finally ensuring meaningful coverage and care to all Americans (Meier & Beresford, 2009).

Others recommend changing the educational preparation of all health care professionals creating a new culture. A cultural change is needed in the lay public as well. It is the belief of many in the field of palliative care that the baby boomers will be instrumental in creating this cultural change. As a sandwich generation, they struggle to meet the needs of aging parents as they raise their young children. The 55-year-old daughter who is working full time is frustrated with the complexity of the health care system and the compassion needed to meet the demands of dying parents. In fear of losing her job, she searches Google for answers. Once she is guided to palliative care and recognizes the value palliative care has offered her loved ones as well as herself, she becomes an ambassador for having palliative care available for all. It is just a matter of time until the tipping point is reached and the consumer becomes the driver of change.

Again the sage advice of Byock guides us in our thinking with this statement of his:

> Our field knows a great deal that would be of value in the health care reform process. We know where the excesses are, and the deficiencies that should be addressed—if only we were asked. The public clearly wants what we have to offer. But if there's no voice speaking for the public on these matters, who is going to advance these goals? Unless and until our field is able to translate what we know is possible to improve care into terms that can be used by a consumer-driven movement, we will not realize what is possible in health care reform. We must make key expectations about care for frail elders and the seriously ill part of the citizen and consumer rights agenda, that patients' wishes are known and honored, that continuity of care is assured, that pain is managed, and that families are supported in their caregiving and in their grief.
>
> *Meier & Beresford (2009, p. 595)*

APRNs possess the skills, knowledge, and ability to teach the public so the public can give "sound" to the silent consumer voice. In the meantime, palliative care advanced practice nurses will continue to start the conversations and continue to talk as needed, learn about patient/family wishes, preferences, and goals, and advocate to assure these wishes are honored and treatments matched. They will continue to keep the patient/family fully informed, be fully transparent, and coordinate the interprofessional team to achieve the patient stated goals. Palliative care advanced practice nurses are experts and as such serve as the beacon to lead social change through policy change so that palliative care is accessible to all.

DISCUSSION QUESTIONS

1. What are the critical issues requiring legislative changes?
2. Discuss the regulatory impact on managing pain in palliative care.
3. What are examples of barriers to practice for the palliative care APRN?
4. What is the impact of the PPACA on palliative care?
5. Name three major workforce issues in palliative care.
6. How can a palliative care APRN get involved in policy on a local level?
7. Aside from survey success with the FDA/Morphine mandate, are there other research examples that led to changes in palliative care?
8. What do you do to facilitate research in your work setting?
9. Discuss your concerns for the need for caregiver support in palliative care.
10. How can changes in legislation improve quality of end-of-life care?
11. Talk to an ACHPN to get ideas on how you can get involved in advocacy.

REFERENCES

American Academy of Nursing Policy Brief. (2010). *Advance care planning as an urgent public health concern.* Retrieved from http://www.aan.org

American Association of Colleges of Nursing (AACN). (2012). *Core competencies for interprofessional collaborative practice: Report of an expert panel.* Retrieved from http://www.aacn.nche.edu /education-resources/IPECReport.pdf

American Board of Nursing Specialties (ABNS). (2012). *Promoting excellence in nursing certification.* Retrieved from http://www.nursingcertification.org

American College of Healthcare Executives [Policy Statement]. (2009). Decisions near end of life. *Frontiers of Health Services Management, 27*(3), 49–50.

Bakitas, M., Bishop, M. F., & Caron, P. A. (2010). Hospital-based palliative care. In B. R. Ferrell & N. Coyle (Eds.), *Oxford textbook of palliative nursing* (pp. 53–86). New York, NY: Oxford University Press.

Baldwin, P. K., Wittenberg-Lyles, E., Oliver, D. P., & Demiris, G. (2011, May/June). An evaluation of interdisciplinary team training in hospice care. *Journal of Hospice and Palliative Nursing, 13*(3), 172–182.

Biography.com. (2012). *Elisabeth Kubler-Ross—Biography: Facts, birthday, life story.* Retrieved from http://www.biography.com/people/elisabeth-kubler-ross-262762

Boucher, J., Bova, C., Sullivan-Bolyai, S., Theroux, R., Klar, R., Terrien, J., & Kaufman, D. (2010, January/February). Next-of-kin's perspectives of end-of-life care. *Journal of Hospice and Palliative Nursing, 12*(1), 41–50.

Buck, J. (2011, November/December). Policy and the reformation of hospice. *Journal of Hospice and Palliative Nursing, 13*(6S), S35–S43.

Carlson, J. (2010). Not finished yet: Coalition wants end of life care to be a priority. *Modern Healthcare, 40*(43), 17–18.

Centers for Disease Control and Prevention (CDC). (2012). *Average life span.* Retrieved from http://www .cdc.gov/nchs/data/nvsr/nvsr60/nvsr60_09.pdf

CDC. (2012). *FastStats—Death and mortality.* Retrieved from http://www.cdc.gov/nchs/fastats/deaths .htm

Centers for Medicare and Medicaid Services (CMS). (2012). *Medicare benefit policy manual: Chapter 9—Coverage of hospice services under hospital insurance.* Retrieved from http://www.medicare.gov /Pubs/pdf/02154.pdf

Chiarella, M., & Duffield, C. (2007, November/December). Workforce in palliative and end-of-life care. *Journal of Hospice and Palliative Nursing, 9*(6), 334–341.

Curtis, J., Patrick, D., Engelberg, R., Norris, K., Asp, C., & Byock, I. (2002). A measure of the quality of dying and deaths: Initial validation using after-death interviews with family members. *Journal of Pain and Symptom Management, 24*(1), 17–31.

Derby, S., O'Mahony, S., & Tickoo, R. (2010). Elderly patients. In B. R. Ferrell & N. Coyle (Eds.), *Oxford textbook of palliative nursing* (pp. 713–743). New York, NY: Oxford University Press.

Egan City, K. A., & Labyak, M. J. (2010). Hospice palliative care for the 21st century: A model for quality end-of-life care. In B. R. Ferrell & N. Coyle (Eds.), *Oxford textbook of palliative nursing* (pp. 13–52). New York, NY: Oxford University Press.

Federal Register. (2012). *Hospice conditions of participation*. Retrieved from http://www.federalregister .gov/.../medicare-and-medicaid-programs

Ferrell, B. R., Grant, M., & Sun, V. (2010). Nursing research. In B. R. Ferrell & N. Coyle (Eds.), *Oxford textbook of palliative nursing* (pp. 1211–1223). New York, NY: Oxford University Press.

Forero, R., McDonnell, G., Gallego, B., McCarthy, S., Mohsin, M., Shanley, C., … Hillman, K. (2012). A literature review on care at end-of-life in the emergency department. *Emergency Medicine International, 2012,* 1–11.

Gelfman, L., Meier, D. E., & Morrison, R. S. (2008, July). Does palliative care improve quality? A survey of bereaved family members. *Journal of Pain and Symptom Management, 36*(1), 22–28.

Giovanni, L. A. (2012). End-of-life care in the United States: Current reality and future promise—A policy review. *Nursing Economics, 30*(3), 127–134.

Hayes, C. (2004, January–March). Ethics in end-of-life care. *Journal of Hospice and Palliative Nursing, 6*(1), 36–43.

Hixon, T. (2012). The U.S. does not have a debt problem... It has a health care cost problem. Retrieved from http://www.forbes.com/sites/toddhixon/2012/02/09/the-u-s-does-not-have-a-debt-problem -it-has-a-health-care-cost-problem

Hoefler, J. M. (2010). United States lags on palliative care at the end of life. *Journal of Pain and Symptom Management, 40*(6), e1–e2.

Horton, J. R., & Indelicato, R. A. (2010). The advanced practice nurse. In B. R. Ferrell & N. Coyle (Eds.), *Oxford textbook of palliative nursing* (pp. 1121–1129). New York, NY: Oxford University Press.

Hospice and Palliative Nurses Association (HPNA). (2010). *HPNA public policy guiding principles*. Retrieved from http://www.hpna.org/DisplayPage.aspx?Title=Guiding Principles

HPNA. (2012a). *Congressional issues brief: Assuring choice for seriously and progressively ill patients*. Retrieved from http://www.hpna.org/DisplayPage.aspx?Title=Congressional Issue Briefs

HPNA. (2012b). *HPNA research agenda*. Retrieved from http://www.hpna.org/DisplayPage.aspx ?Title=Research

HPNA. (2012c). *Palliative care graduate programs*. Retrieved from http://www.hpna.org /DisplayPage.aspx?Title=Graduate Program Listing

HPNA. (2012d). *Role of hospice and palliative nurses in research* [Position Statement]. Retrieved from http:// www.hpna.org/DisplayPage.aspx?Title=Position Statements

HPNA. (2012e). *The nurse's role in advance care planning* [Position Statement]. Retrieved from http://www .hpna.org/DisplayPage.aspx?Title=Position Statements

Infoplease. (2012). *Life expectancy by age, 1850–2004*. Retrieved from http://www.infoplease .com/ipa/A0005140.html

Institute of Medicine. (2010). *The future of nursing leading change, advancing health report recommendations*. Retrieved from http://www.iom.edu/nursing

Jackson, J., Derderian, L., White, P., Ayotte, J., Fiorini, J., Hall, R. O., & Shay, J. T. (2012). Family perspectives on end-of-life care. *Journal of Hospice & Palliative Nursing, 14*(4), 303–311.

Kelly, A., & Meier, D. E. (2010). Palliative care—A shifting paradigm [Editorial]. *New England Journal of Medicine, 363*(8), 781–782.

Krammer, L. M., Martinez, J., Ring-Hurn, E. A., & Williams, M. B. (2010). Nurse's role in interdisciplinary palliative care. In M. Matzo & D. W. Sherman (Eds.), *Palliative care nursing: Quality care to the end of life* (pp. 97–106). New York, NY: Springer Publishing Company.

Launer, L. (n.d.). The dying patient bill of rights. *American Journal of Nursing*. Philadelphia, PA: Lippincott Williams & Wilkins. Retrieved from http://www.lynnlauner.com/articles

Lunney, J. (2011, November/December). Hospice and palliative nursing research. *Journal of Hospice and Palliative Nursing, 13*(6S), S3–S7.

Lentz, J., & Sherman, D. W. (2010). Development of the specialty of hospice and palliative care nursing. In M. Matzo & D. W. Sherman (Eds.), *Palliative care nursing: Quality care to the end of life* (pp. 107–117, 3rd ed.). New York, NY: Springer Publishing Company.

Martinez, J. (2011, November/December). Hospice and palliative nursing certification: The journey to defining a new nursing specialty. *Journal of Hospice and Palliative Nursing, 13*(6S), S29–S34.

Morrison, R. S., Augustin, R., Souvanna, P., & Meier, D. E. (2011). America's care of serious illness: A state-by-state report card on access to palliative care in our nation's hospitals. *Journal of Palliative Medicine, 14*(10), 1094–1096.

Morrison, R. S., Penrod, J. D., Cassel, J. B., Caust-Ellenbogen, M. S., Litke, A., Spragens, L., … for the Palliative Care Leadership Centers' Outcome Group. (2008, September 8). Cost savings associated with US hospital palliative care consultation programs. *Archives of Internal Medicne, 168*(16), 1783–1790.

Meier, D. E., & Beresford, L. (2008a). Dartmouth Atlas data can support palliative care development [Notes from the field]. *Journal of Palliative Medicine, 11*(7), 960–962.

Meier, D. E., & Beresford, L. (2008b). The palliative care team. *Journal of Palliative Medicine, 11*(5), 677–681.

Meier, D. E., & Beresford, L. (2009). Palliative care seeks its home in national health care reform. *Journal of Palliative Medicine, 12*(7), 593–597.

Meier, D. E., & Beresford, L. (2010). Health systems find opportunities and challenges in palliative care development [Notes from the field]. *Journal of Palliative Medicine, 13*(4), 367–370.

Meier, D. E., Thar, W., Jordan, A., Gordhirsch, S. L., Siu, A., & Morrison R. S. (2004). Integrating case management and palliative care. *Journal of Palliative Medicine, 7*(1), 119–134.

National Board for Certification of Hospice and Palliative Nurses (NBCHPN®). (2012). *ACHPN examination information.* Retrieved from http://www.nbchpn.org/DisplayPage.aspx?Title=APRN Overview

NBCHPN®. (2010). *Definition of continuing competence.* Retrieved from http://www.nbchpn.org

National Consensus Project for Quality Palliative Care. (2009). *Clinical practice guidelines for quality palliative care* (2nd ed.). Pittsburgh, PA: Author.

Nelson, J. E., Cortez, T., Curtis, J. R., Lustader, D., Mosenthal, A., Mulkerin, C., & Puntillo, K. (2011, March/April). Integrating palliative care in the ICU. *Journal of Hospice and Palliative Nursing, 13*(2), 89–94.

National Quality Forum (NQF). (2012a, June). *Measure application partnership: Performance measures coordination strategy for hospice and palliative care* [Final Report] (pp. 2–25). Washington, DC.

NQF. (2012b). *Mission and vision.* Retrieved from http://www.qualityforum.org/About_NQF/Mission_and_Vision.aspx

Pace, J. C., & Lunsford, B. (2011, November/December). The evolution of palliative care nursing education. *Journal of Hospice and Palliative Nursing, 13*(6S), S8–S19.

Palliative Care Information Act. (2012). Retrieved from http://www.health.ny.gov/professionals/patients/patient_rights/palliative_care/information

Pitorak, E., & Armour, M. B. (2003). Project safe conduct integrates palliative goals into comprehensive cancer care. *Journal of Palliative Medicine, 6*(4), 645–655.

Rapp, M. (2003, November/December). Opportunities for advanced practice nurses in the nursing facility. *Journal of the American Medical Directors Association, 4,* 337–343.

Reifsnyder, J., & Yeo, T. P. (2011). Continuity of care. In D. B. Nash, J. Reifsnyder, R. J. Fabius, & V. P. Pracilio (Eds.), *Population health: Creating a culture of wellness* (pp. 63–88). Sudbury, MA: Jones and Bartlett.

Scanlon, C. (2010). Public policy and end-of-life care: The nurse's role. In B. R. Ferrell & N. Coyle (Eds.), *Oxford textbook of palliative nursing* (pp. 1173–1183). New York, NY: Oxford University Press.

Schaffer, M. A., Keenan, K., Zwirchitz, F., & Tierschel, L. (2012, January/February). End-of-life discussion in assisted living facilities. *Journal of Hospice and Palliative Nursing, 14*(1), 13–24.

Sherman, D., & Cheon, J. (2012, May–June). Palliative care: A paradigm of care responsive to the demands for health care reform in America. *Nursing Economics, 30*(3), 153–166.

Weissman, D. E., & Meier, D. E. (2011). Identifying patients in need of a palliative care assessment in the hospital setting. *Journal of Palliative Medicine, 14*(1), 17–22.

Zeytinoglu, M. (2011). Talking it out: Helping our patients live better while dying. *Annals of Internal Medice, 154*(12), 830–832. Retrieved from http://www.lynnlauner.com/yahoo_site_admin/assets/docs/The_Dying_Persons_Bill_of_Rights.114130706.pdf

Health Policy Implications for Advanced Practice Registered Nurses Related to Oncology Care

Cynthia Abarado, Kelly Brassil, Garry Brydges, and Joyce E. Dains

ONCOLOGY AS A SPECIALTY NURSING PRACTICE

Oncology advanced practice registered nurses (APRNs) are a uniquely specialized branch of health care providers. Specialized through education, certification, the population with whom they work, or a combination of these factors, the oncology APRN has a distinct place in a health care specialty that provides for 13.7 million individuals living with cancer in the United States (American Cancer Society [ACS], 2012). Although cancer incidence continues to grow, with an estimated 1.6 million new cases expected to be diagnosed each year (ACS, 2012), the availability of specialized advanced practice providers is challenged by policy-related changes in how these professionals are educated, certified, and licensed from state-to-state. As a result, an understanding of how the role of the APRN in oncology care will be impacted by current and future policy shifts is pivotal to understanding how and by whom individuals living with cancer in the United States will be treated and managed across the cancer continuum.

Oncology Advanced Practice Registered Nurse Competencies

The Oncology Nursing Society (ONS), a professional organization of more than 35,000 nursing and health care professionals, establishes the competencies for oncology nurse practitioners and clinical nurse specialists (Table 19.1, ONS, 2013a). The focus on health promotion, disease prevention, and managing illness, as well as the emphasis on negotiating health care systems, may be significantly influenced by evolving health and institutional policies. These include, but are not limited to, the APRN Consensus Model, the Patient Protection and Affordable Care Act (ACA),

TABLE 19.1 ONS APRN Competencies

NURSE PRACTITIONER (ONS, 2007)	OUTCOMES	CLINICAL NURSE SPECIALIST (ONS, 2008)	OUTCOMES
Health promotion, health protection, disease prevention and treatment	Increased access to care; decreased health care costs	The patient/client sphere of influence Assessment and diagnosis of health status Development of plan of care and interventions Evaluation of outcomes	Improved delivery of care through individualized care planning that leads to increased patient satisfaction and improved health outcomes
Nurse practitioner–patient relationship	Improved patient satisfaction achieved through fostering collaborative relationships with patients and their caregivers as partners in care	The nursing practice sphere of influence Assessment, diagnosis, outcomes identification and planning related to oncology nursing practice Intervention and evaluation of evidence-based oncology nursing practice Professional role development in oncology nursing	Generation of evidence for and implementation of evidence-based practice; development of self and colleagues toward competence and excellence in oncology nursing
Teaching–coaching function	Patient compliance; improved patient satisfaction	The organization/system sphere of influence Assessment, diagnosis, outcomes identification and planning related to organization practice settings Intervention and evaluation of oncology care delivery systems	Improvement in work environmental outcomes that impact the ability of the oncology APRN and interprofessional colleagues to deliver high-quality oncology care
Professional role	Generation of evidence for and implementation of evidence-based practice		
Negotiating health care delivery systems	Delivery of clinical services within an integrated system of health care that improves health outcomes for patients		
Monitoring and ensuring the quality of health care practice	Decreased length of stay, admission rates, emergency care visits, and health care costs		
Caring for diverse populations	Provision of culturally competent care that incorporates evidence-based practice to best meet population needs and reduce health disparities		

and the Health Information Technology for Economic and Clinical Health (HITECH) Act. Such legislation affects the manner in which the APRN is prepared for practice and how the APRN may deliver, manage, and support the care of oncology patients through engagement in Affordable Care Organizations (ACOs) and the use of electronic health records (EHRs) and ultimately meet the needs of a growing population of cancer patients and survivors across the cancer trajectory.

The APRN Consensus Model and Its Impact on Licensure, Accreditation, Credentialing, and Education

The APRN Consensus Work Group and the National Council of State Boards of Nursing Advanced Practice Nurse Advisory Committee (2008) developed the APRN Consensus Model to guide the licensure, accreditation, certification, and education of APRNs. The document served to delineate a generalist approach to APRN education, licensure, and credentialing that significantly impacts how oncology APRNs are prepared for and recognized in practice. The Consensus Model clearly defines four generalist APRN roles as nurse anesthetists, nurse-midwives, clinical nurse specialists (CNS), and nurse practitioners with licensure occurring at the levels of the role and population focus (APRN Consensus Work Group and the National Council of State Boards of Nursing Advanced Practice Nurse Advisory Committee, 2008). Because oncology is defined as a specialty area, preparation as an oncology specialist is optional and must build upon the APRN role and population focus. Competency for oncology specialization will be assessed and regulated by professional organizations instead of the state board of nursing (APRN Consensus Work Group and the National Council of State Boards of Nursing Advanced Practice Nurse Advisory Committee, 2008). As a result, oncology specialization in the form of education, certification, and licensure is significantly affected by changes associated with this regulatory model.

Education

As of 2012, 28 graduate programs throughout the United States offered primary degrees, concentration studies, or postmaster's certification in oncology. As a result of the APRN Consensus Model, educational institutions are moving away from specialized degree programs, although optional concentrations or postmaster's certification may still be offered. APRN education programs will be increasingly standardized and will require accreditation and approval by the U.S. Department of Education and/ or the Council for Higher Education Accreditation to ensure that the curriculum prepares graduates for certification and licensure (APRN Consensus Work Group and the National Council of State Boards of Nursing Advanced Practice Nurse Advisory Committee, 2008). Such changes will require individuals to pursue additional credits in order to obtain specialized oncology education and may prove to be both time- and cost-prohibitive, thereby limiting the number of oncology APRNs specialized by virtue of educational preparation.

A second consideration is the movement toward standardization of the Doctor of Nursing Practice as the entry-level degree for APRNs. Although the curriculum format for such degrees may limit opportunities for specialized course content, the emphasis on clinical immersion may enable individuals to obtain a focused clinical perspective on specific populations such as oncology. The transition away from specialty-focused educational preparation of the APRN raises the question of whether fellowship training can provide a viable avenue for specialized oncology APRNs, similar to the training of medical fellows. Oncology APRN fellowships such as those offered at the University of Texas MD Anderson Cancer Center, the Huntsman Cancer

Institute at the University of Utah, and Memorial-Sloan Kettering Cancer Center provide avenues for APRNs interested in specializing after receiving their degree to develop clinical expertise and to prepare for oncology certification through focused clinical rotations within this patient population.

Certification

Specialty certification will not be regulated by or recognized for practice by licensing boards; instead, it will be granted through specialty organizations, such as the Oncology Nurse Certification Corporation (ONCC). Currently, three oncology advanced-practice certifications are supported by the ONCC—Advanced Oncology Certified Nurse Practitioner (AOCNP®), Advanced Oncology Certified Clinical Nurse Specialist (AOCNS®), and Advanced Oncology Certified Nurse (AOCN®). Although pediatric oncology certification is available for registered nurses, no advanced practice pediatric oncology certification exists at this time. In addition, certified registered nurse anesthetists (CRNAs), who function in a specialized capacity distinct from other APRNs, may obtain oncology certification as an AOCNP®. However, no distinct certification specific to anesthetists practicing in oncology exists at this time.

One of the challenges of obtaining specialty certification within an increasingly generalist educational focus is that specialty education obtained concurrently with the generalist curriculum may not provide the number of clinical hours necessary for certification. Currently, oncology certification for both nurse practitioners (NPs) and clinical nurse specialists (CNSs) requires 500 to 1,000 hours of adult oncology nursing practice within the 5 years preceding the test registration date (ONCC, 2013).

The Role of Oncology APRNs in the Evolving Health Care Practice Setting

The Role of the Oncology APRN in Accountable Care Organizations

Accountable Care Organizations (ACOs), a derivative of the Patient Protection and Affordable Care Act of 2010, are defined as groups of doctors, hospitals, and other health care providers who come together voluntarily to give coordinated, high-quality care to Medicare patients. The goals of ACAs are to ensure that these individuals receive care at the right time, without duplication of services, and are aimed at preventing medical errors (Centers for Medicare and Medicaid Services [CMS], 2013). The ACA recognizes NPs and CNSs as ACO professionals who may participate in group practice arrangements to provide such care (American Nurses Association [ANA], 2013). As specialists, coordinating care for oncology patients is a significant priority for oncology APRNs as they collaborate with community-based primary care and other specialty providers to ensure continuity of care for this patient population. A key requirement of ACOs is that they serve at least 5,000 Medicare patients (ANA, 2013). With individuals aged 65 and older anticipated to account for more than 60% of the cancer cases in the United States (Repetto & Balducci, 2002), providing fluid transitions from screening through active treatment and into survivorship, chronic, or palliative care will be essential in ensuring quality care for this vulnerable population. As essential clinicians in both acute and primary care settings, APRNs will play a significant role in ensuring this continuity of care through interprofessional collaboration within and between care settings.

The Use of EHRs to Facilitate Collaborative Oncology Care

Like other APRNs, those specializing in oncology will be impacted by the HITECH Act, which requires use of a portable EHR. Oncology APRNs and their patient population stand to gain a significant advantage in restructuring care as a result of such technology. Identified benefits of EHRs for oncology clinicians include streamlining patient care within and across oncology, specialist, and primary care practice settings; facilitating data collection and monitoring protocols related to clinical trials; and improving fiscal efficacy through simplification of scheduling and claims (Ambinder, 2005). Perhaps, most significant is the ability to facilitate more consistent information sharing among the many specialists managing an oncology patient. This would include, but not be limited to, the patient's primary care provider, surgical oncologist, radiologist, radiation oncologist, cardiologist, pulmonologist, medical oncologist, and a host of other individuals who co-manage patient care. This communication and facilitation of shared patient care information may help to reduce errors and duplication of procedures and could increase collaborative decision making to support the oncology clinician at the point of care (Ambinder, 2005).

INTERPROFESSIONAL COLLABORATIVE PRACTICE AND THE CANCER CARE CONTINUUM

Introduction

Cancer, once associated with high mortality rates, is increasingly becoming a chronic condition that requires management across the cancer trajectory. APRNs are integral participants in the delivery of safe, high-quality care, including risk assessment, primary prevention, screening, detection, diagnosis, treatment, recurrence, surveillance, and end-of-life care (Zapka et al., 2003). As participants in interprofessional collaborative practice APRNs work with patients, families, caregivers, and communities to deliver the highest quality of care (World Health Organization [WHO], 2010). Oncology APRNs are charged with "provid[ing] leadership to improve outcomes for patients with cancer and their families by increasing health care access, promoting clinical excellence, improving patients' quality of life, documenting patient outcomes, and increasing the cost effectiveness of care" (ONS, 2013b). The oncology APRN has a responsibility, therefore, to assist patients in the transitions and interfaces in the delivery of health care across the cancer continuum, consistent with advanced practice competencies put forth by ONS (ONS, 2007; Taplin & Rodgers, 2010).

The health policy environment has a significant impact on the cancer care, most significantly in preventive care and surveillance, diagnosis and genetic testing, disease management, and reimbursement for care (National Cancer Institute [NCI], 2011). Understanding the influence of U.S. health policies, international and national practice guidelines, standards, laws, rules, and regulations on the oncology APRN is essential to delivering quality cancer care.

The Impact of Cancer as a Chronic Condition

Cancer diagnosis, treatment, and management as a chronic disease involve significant financial and productivity challenges (Box 19.1). The change in the cancer care trajectory from what was once a largely terminal illness, to what is now often a chronically managed condition is expected to strain Medicare expenditures and significantly impact the health care delivery system. Added to this burden are the health care needs of an aging population often affected by multiple chronic conditions.

The chronic care model (CCM) is one of the strategies expected to transform health care delivery in the United States. The CCM provides a framework within which aspects of effective health systems and community supports are identified to

CANCER BURDEN IN THE UNITED STATES	BOX 19.1

- Each year more than 1.6 million individuals are diagnosed with cancer.
- Annual cancer-related deaths total 577,000.
- Cancer accounts for $263.8 billion in medical costs and lost productivity annually.
- Nearly 13 million individuals are living with a cancer history.
- Approximately 41% of individuals born today will develop cancer.
- Overall cancer survival rate is 65.4%.

NCI (2012)

promote productive interactions that strengthen the provider–patient relationship, with the goal of improving health outcomes (Coleman et al., 2009). The CCM may be applied to care across the cancer trajectory with particular attention to the importance of care coordination, health information systems management, and health profession education. The oncology APRN role in the CCM includes care coordination and assumes competence in health information management. Mitigating and even reducing the severity of chronic disease occurs in the context of primary care and preventive medicine, a focus of the ACA. The oncology APRN may work directly with cancer patients to help them to control or change behaviors associated with health risks (e.g., smoking, physical inactivity, poor diet, and excessive drinking), and to encourage the use of preventive health-care services (i.e., cancer screening and prevention).

Cancer Prevention

The Patient Protection and Affordable Care Act of 2010 established the National Prevention, Health Promotion and Public Health Council, which will coordinate federal departments and agencies regarding prevention, wellness, and health promotion; the public health system; and integrative health care. The Council's aim is to develop a national strategy to be enacted no later than 1 year after the ACA is implemented. The ACA provides coverage for annual wellness visits, which will include the creation of a personalized prevention plan; an individualized health risk assessment, including medical and family history; evaluation of current providers and medications; physical and cognitive assessment; and review of a screening schedule. The ACA provides mandatory coverage of evidence-based practices in prevention services, specifically smoking cessation, weight control, stress management, and the promotion of healthy lifestyles. In the context of cancer care, this approach focuses on identifying and remediating behavioral, environmental, and genetic risk factors—areas in which oncology APRNs can use their expertise and skills to influence patient behavior.

The emphasis on smoking cessation is an example of this type of initiative. Effective October 1, 2010, all state Medicaid programs must provide tobacco cessation services for pregnant women as part of the Patient Protection and Affordable Care Act of 2010 (Sec. 4107), but in some states coverage is still limited for other nonpregnant populations. Coverage of pharmacotherapy for all Medicaid enrollees will be enhanced by January 2014, when smoking cessation drugs will no longer be excluded from covered benefits (NCI, 2012). The goal of enhanced access to treatment for tobacco dependence among Medicaid recipients is to help users to quit with the expectation of a reduction in cancer deaths and cancer-related health disparities in this population (NCI, 2012). The Family Smoking Prevention and Tobacco Control Act, commonly referred to as the Tobacco Control Act, gives the Food and Drug Administration (FDA) authority to regulate the manufacturing, distribution, and marketing of tobacco products as a means of protecting public health (FDA, 2013). The WHO Framework Convention on Tobacco Control (FCTC) produced the first treaty negotiated under the auspices of the WHO. The FCTC was developed in response to the globalization of the tobacco epidemic and is an evidence-based treaty that reaffirms the right of all people to have access to the highest standard of health (Division of Cancer Control and Population Sciences [DCCPS], 2011).

Initiatives such as these involve practices that have evolved from policies that aim to reduce risk factors and therefore occurrence and mortality related to preventable cancers. APRNs practicing in oncology are integral in capitalizing on these initiatives as a means of improving care and reducing cancer incidence.

Screening

The DCCPS of the NCI plans, implements, and maintains a comprehensive research program to promote the appropriate use of cancer screening tests, as well as strategies for informed decision making regarding cancer screening technologies, in both community and clinical practice. The U.S. Preventive Services Task Force uses the evidence from the Cancer Intervention and Surveillance Modeling Network (CISNET), funded by DCCPS, as they revise screening recommendations for breast and colorectal cancers (NCI, 2012). A component of the ACA supports increased awareness and early detection of breast cancer, as well as a national evidence-based educational media campaign to expand young women's knowledge of breast health and breast cancer awareness and occurrence. An advisory committee will be established to provide health information to young women diagnosed with breast cancer and preneoplastic breast diseases (Allbright et al., 2011).

Cancer Risk Assessment and Counseling

A significant component of cancer prevention is risk assessment. The NCI (2012) defines a risk factor as a behavioral, environmental, biological, or hereditary factor that increases an individual's predisposition toward developing a disease. Comprehensive cancer risk assessment includes clinical assessment, genetic/genomic testing when appropriate, and risk management (NCI, 2012). A defining component of cancer risk assessment in the future is the use of personalized medicine. Personalized medicine is an emerging practice that utilizes an individual's genetic profile to guide decisions related to the prevention, diagnosis, and treatment of disease (National Institutes of Health [NIH], 2013). An APRN competency, as defined by ONS, includes performance of a relevant cancer risk assessment for general populations, at-risk populations, newly diagnosed patients with cancer, cancer survivors, and patients with a past, current, or potential diagnosis of cancer. APRNs are also charged with educating patients, caregivers, and the community about cancer risk, screening, and early detection (ONS, 2007, 2008).

Cancer Genetic and Genomic Testing

The ANA (2009) has specified practice and education essentials in its *Essentials of Genetic and Genomic Nursing: Competencies, Curricula Guidelines, and Outcome Indicators.* ONS has endorsed these essentials for oncology care and further specifies in their position statement (ONS, 2012) that oncology APRNs also provide patient and community education and nursing practice that is consistent with the ANA Essentials and with the International Society of Nurses in *Essential Genetic and Genomic Competencies for Nurses with Graduate Degrees* (Greco, Tinley, & Seibert, 2012). Oncology APRN practice may include comprehensive cancer genetic risk assessment, education, facilitation and interpretation of genetic testing, pre- and post-test counseling and follow-up, and provision of personally tailored cancer risk recommendations and management, along with psychosocial counseling and supportive services. These guidelines constitute a powerful policy imperative for APRNs involved in oncology care to demonstrate educational preparation in the principles of human genetics and genomics, to integrate evidence-based genetic and genomic information into their practice, and to be cognizant of the ethical, legal, social, emotional, and advocacy issues in the application of personalized health care in oncology.

Testing in oncology may include both genetic testing (single gene testing, such as that performed for BRCA1 and BRCA2) to identify predisposition to inherited cancers, and genomic testing to identify multiple genes, DNA sequences, and gene expression of proteins and their interactions with one another. Results of these tests help to determine an individual's risk of cancer, cancer recurrence, and treatment response. The issue of whom and when to test is paramount in oncology care and involves legal, ethical, and clinical considerations. Both the American Society of Clinical Oncology (ASCO) (2003) and ONS (2012) provide guidelines that assist the oncology APRN in the decision process.

Direct-to-consumer (DTC) genetic testing is a method of marketing genetic tests to consumers via the Internet, television, and other media without involving an independent health care provider. Potential benefits of DTC testing include increased consumer awareness of and access to testing. Critics of DTC genetic testing have expressed concern that consumers may choose testing without adequate context or counseling, obtain tests from laboratories that are not of high quality, and could be misled by tests that lack adequate analytic validity or clinical utility (American College of Medical Genetics, 2008; Hudson, Javitt, Burke, & Byers, 2007; Robson, Storm, Weitzel, Wollins, & Offit, 2010). APRNs and other health care providers may be challenged when individuals who have obtained DTC tests come to them for help in interpreting the test results. ASCO states that it is appropriate to explain the lack of proven usefulness of the test and to base medical follow-up recommendations solely on established cancer risk factors, such as family history, possible exposures to cancer-causing substances, and behavioral factors, as well as scientifically validated tests for cancer risks (Robson et al., 2010).

An evidence-based resource that APRNs can use in evaluating a particular test is the Evaluation of Genomic Applications in Practice and Prevention (EGAPP). The EGAPP was launched in 2004 by the Centers for Disease Control and Prevention (CDC) to establish and test a systematic, evidence-based process for evaluating genetic tests, and other applications of genomic technology that are in transition from research to clinical and public health practice (CDC, 2013). This information enables health care providers and payers, consumers, policy makers, and others to distinguish genetic tests that are safe and useful (EGAPP, 2013).

Genetics-based discrimination by employers and health insurance companies has been a significant barrier to the use of genetic and genomic testing services. This has been particularly true in testing for susceptibility to inherited cancers. In 2008, the Genetic Information Nondiscrimination Act (GINA) established significant protections from genetics-based discrimination by health insurers and employers. The law prohibits health insurance carriers from denying coverage based on genetic information or because an individual took or refused to take a genetic test. This law also prohibits employers from using genetic information as the basis for employment decisions. Currently, no special protections guard against the use of genetic information for life insurance, disability insurance, or long-term care insurance. Oncology APRNs have a role in educating patients about the protections of the law and the law's limitations.

Cancer Treatment

Provisions of the ACA will significantly impact treatment options for cancer patients. These include, but are not limited to, legislation regarding biologic drugs, translational research, clinical trials coverage, comparative effectiveness research, and the removal of insurance caps for cancer treatment. Cancer treatment and the development of new therapies are largely dependent on successfully conducting of clinical trials. Several components of the ACA impact research and clinical trials. For example, as of 2012, the ACA prevents insurance companies from denying cancer patients participation in clinical trials and covers all clinical trial stages for cancer. This allows more individuals to participate in clinical trials that may benefit the patient or further the development of future treatments (American Association for Cancer Research [AACR], 2012). APRNs have an important role in educating patients about clinical trials and in facilitating their participation in a trial. The ACA also provided funding for the establishment of the Patient-Centered Outcomes Research Institute. This institute conducts and oversees research comparing the effectiveness of medical treatments, with the goal of improving patient outcomes by delivering the best treatment to the appropriate patient populations (AACR, 2012). This coincides with the ONS competency for APRNs to participate in clinical and nursing research to promote positive outcomes for cancer patients and their caregivers (ONS, 2007).

Funding also has been appropriated to support the translation of basic scientific discoveries into cancer treatment through grants to academic and industry researchers (AACR, 2012). Attention is directed toward health disparities research, with an emphasis on discovering the underlying causes of these disparities in order to reduce the burden of cancer in these populations across the United States (AACR, 2012). In addition, the NIH has been charged with conducting research to develop and validate new screening tests for breast cancer as a means of improving prevention and early detection, particularly among young women (AACR, 2012). APRNs must develop their roles as clinicians, educators, and researchers in order to engage in research that will generate evidence for practice, implement evidence-based care for best outcomes, and educate patients and their caregivers about treatment and clinical research options that may now be available to them as a result of health care reform.

Palliative Care and Survivorship

Survivorship and palliative care are integral components of cancer care, both during and after active cancer treatment. Emphasis on interprofessional collaboration, communication, increased adoption of quality improvement programs, expanded research, and health care provider and patient education in both survivorship and palliative care is consistent with the policies addressed throughout this chapter. The IOM report "From Cancer Patient to Cancer Survivor: Lost in Transition" identified the need for care planning and led to ASCO's development of recommendations for improving survivor care (Box 19.2) (Hewitt, Greenfield, & Stovall, 2005). The reauthorization of the DHHS's patient navigator program through the Patient Protection

AMERICAN SOCIETY FOR CLINICAL ONCOLOGY RECOMMENDATIONS FOR IMPROVING SURVIVOR CARE	BOX 19.2

- Promote patient-centered coordinated care through the use of shared-care models, which allow for collaboration among practitioners of different disciplines or with different skills and knowledge.
- Increase adoption of quality improvement programs, such as ASCO's Quality Oncology Practice Initiative (QOPI®), which help physicians to monitor and improve care for all survivors.
- Expand research on long-term and late effects to expand the evidence base required to define optimal survivor care.
- Strengthen education of health care providers on survivorship care to keep pace with growing evidence on the long-term follow-up care needs of different types of cancer.
- Educate and empower cancer survivors and their families to advocate for their unique needs and to ensure optimal long-term health.

and Affordable Care Act of 2010 (Sec. 3510) assists patients and survivors in maneuvering the health care system and addresses needs that may affect compliance with screening, surveillance, and treatment.

Similarly, the National Consensus Project (NCP) for Quality Palliative Care guidelines is based on the underlying tenets of palliative care as outlined in Box 19.3 (NCP for Quality Palliative Care, 2013). An ONS competency for oncology APRNs includes coordination of palliative and end-of-life care in collaboration with patients, families, caregivers, and other members of the multidisciplinary health care team (ONS, 2008). The IOM report, "Improving Palliative Care for Cancer," notes that in the United States half of dying cancer patients suffer from physical and psychosocial symptoms, such as pain, shortness of breath, and distress, which can reduce quality of life (Foley & Gellband, 2003). ACA provisions requiring enhanced coordination of NIH pain research and grants to improve clinicians' understanding of pain and their ability to assess and appropriately treat pain (Patient Protection and Affordable Care Act of 2010, Sec. 4305) are critical to improving quality of life for cancer survivors and individuals receiving palliative care. This area is particularly suitable for APRN involvement as research initiators and/or collaborators.

NATIONAL CONSENSUS FOR QUALITY PALLIATIVE CARE GUIDELINES	BOX 19.3

- Patient- and family-centered palliative care
- Comprehensive palliative care with continuity across health settings
- Early introduction of palliative care at diagnosis of a serious disease or life-threatening condition
- Interprofessional collaborative palliative care
- Clinical and communication expertise among palliative care team members
- Relief of the physical, psychological, emotional, and spiritual suffering and distress of patients and families
- A focus on quality and equitable access to palliative care services

As essential providers of cancer care, APRNs must understand how health policy affects their practice as well as their patients' access to care. Recognizing how critical interprofessional collaboration is in the ever-changing health care climate, APRNs must remain at the forefront as advocates and educators for patients undergoing cancer care and for their families. APRNs can benefit from career development awards with funding appropriated through the ACA, as well as from engaging in interprofessional collaboration to provide care to cancer patients throughout the treatment and into survivorship. Consistent with the ONS competencies, the oncology APRN is accountable and responsible for contributing to a comprehensive plan of care as patients transition from active treatment to survivorship, palliative care, or end-of-life care (ONS, 2008).

PRESCRIPTIVE AUTHORITY

Overview

Prescriptive authority is a component of oncology APRN practice that involves both clinical and licensure considerations. Limitations to prescriptive authority are one of the major barriers to APRN practice (Kaplan & Brown, 2007).

In many states, APRNs are not permitted to prescribe schedule II-controlled substances, which are a mainstay of practice for oncology APRNs who manage acute and chronic pain and hospice care. Prescribing authority in states that permit APRNs to prescribe schedule II-controlled substances can still be complicated by federal, local, and institutional requirements. Drug Enforcement Agency (DEA) registration is mandatory for prescribing APRNs, with some states requiring further state-regulated registrations prior to applying for a DEA number (Plank, 2011). Given the extent to which cancer patients may experience pain throughout the treatment and into survivorship and palliative care, policy restrictions that limit an APRN's caring for an oncology patient pose significant challenges to effective care. Other limitations include restrictions on prescribing for investigational drugs, chemotherapeutic agents, radiation therapy, and radiopharmaceuticals, and for patients receiving in-home hospice care (Kelvin et al., 1999; Lynch, Cope, & Murphy-Ende, 2001).

Barriers to Practice

APRN scope of practice, state nursing practice acts, limited prescriptive authority through state laws and regulations, and limited financial reimbursement are legislative barriers limiting APRN prescriptive authority (Plank, 2011).

Health care facility policy and procedures for APRN privileges must comply with federal laws, state laws, state board of nursing regulations, and APRN organizational scopes of practice. Ultimately, health care facility policy and procedures govern what an APRN is able to prescribe in that facility and can limit APRNs' full prescriptive authority through restrictive institutional policies. Some health care entities maintain policies stricter than those established by the state law.

Physician opposition to full prescriptive authority, which may reflect lack of knowledge, reluctance to collaborate, and lack of professional respect for the APRN roles in health care, also serves as a barrier (Brown & Kaplan, 2012; Plank, 2011). APRNs may contribute to barriers of their own with respect to prescriptive authority by resisting independent practice, increased accountability, and responsibility for health care delivery (Kaplan & Brown, 2007).

One example of the critical nature of prescriptive authority to oncology APRNs is in the area of radiation therapy. APRNs are critical in radiation therapy delivery and symptom management during radiation treatment (Kelvin et al., 1999). For example, anxiolytics and pain management are mainstays in the management of patients undergoing radiation therapy (Carper & Haas, 2006). Although radiation oncologists perform the core prescription of radiation therapy, APRNs are integral in the education and management of this patient population.

Medical Marijuana

The prescribing of medical marijuana in the context of cancer care is a source of significant debate. Although cannabinoids have shown antiemetic, appetite-stimulating properties, and efficacy in alleviating moderate neuropathic pain in cancer patients, concern remains about associated upper respiratory tract cancers resulting from their use (Hall, Christie, & Currow, 2005). In 2013, Washington and Colorado became the first states to legalize marijuana. Medical marijuana is considered a schedule I-controlled substance or an illegal drug. It is important to recognize that marijuana is not legal under federal law for any reason (Brown & Kaplan, 2012). Therefore, state laws that provide immunity from prosecution for practitioners who appropriately recommend the use of medical marijuana to oncology patients do not extend the same immunity to practitioners under federal law. Currently, 13 states and the District of Columbia maintain medical marijuana laws (Brown & Kaplan, 2012). Washington and New Mexico are the only two states that allow APRNs to be involved in the process of prescribing medical marijuana. Medical marijuana is an expanding adjunctive therapy for cancer and pain management (Brown & Kaplan, 2012). Such pharmacological adjuncts are limited to physicians in all states except Washington and New Mexico.

CONCLUSIONS

Oncology APRNs, like other generalist and specialist advanced practice clinicians, are affected by health policy regulated at federal, state, and institutional levels. However, oncology APRNs are uniquely affected by policies governing their education and licensure, provision of clinical services across the cancer care continuum, and ability to prescribe pharmacologic agents unique to this patient population. The impact of the APRN consensus model in moving educational preparation of the oncology APRN to an optional specialization, and subsequent inability of specialized clinicians to be licensed with oncology as the primary certification may impact the number of individuals who are educationally trained and certified to treat this unique population. APRN fellowships may provide the opportunity to achieve more focused clinical training in oncology. The impetus for interprofessional collaboration will encourage the oncology APRN to participate in or network with ACOs to ensure continuity of care for cancer patients in primary care settings. Understanding the ACA's impact on oncology research, cancer prevention, and insurance coverage for both providers and patients is essential to the APRN's ability and obligation to communicate these changes with colleagues and patients. Advocating for policies and legislation that support APRNs' ability to function to the fullest extent of their education and training is consistent with the Institute of Medicine's (2011) *Future of Nursing* recommendation, which emphasizes consistent licensure, title protection, and prescriptive authority. By engaging in and serving as advocates for APRN practice, the oncology APRN will benefit clinicians as well as improve patient care.

SYNTHESIS EXERCISES

Case Study 1: Gero-Oncology

Mr. Smith is a 71-year-old African American male who is being followed with "watchful waiting" for prostate cancer initially diagnosed 3 years ago. During his recent clinic visit, he reported bone pain and requested that a prostate-specific antigen (PSA) test be performed. The last PSA testing was a year earlier.

- Would your care of this patient, as an APRN, be reimbursed by Medicare?

From his medical history you know that Mr. Smith's father died of prostate cancer. He has two sons, one aged 50 and the other aged 30.

- Would genetic testing be appropriate for the sons and, if so, as an APRN are you qualified to provide genetic counseling?

PSA results showed a marked increase from 4 to 50. Your collaborating physician requested a staging work-up. Radiologic studies reveal bone metastasis and the patient verbalizes the presence of uncontrolled pain. The oncologist recommends that the patient participate in a clinical trial.

- As an APRN, what is your prescriptive authority to prescribe and/or manage pain medications?
- How does the ACA affect your cancer care delivery, specifically during treatment in a clinical trial?

The patient wished to continue treatment with a local oncologist for the second and third cycle of treatment.

- What other provisions of the ACA would promote safe, effective, and efficient care in transitioning this patient to community-based care?

Two weeks after the third cycle of treatment, the patient returns to the clinic with poor performance status and poor nutritional intake and decides against further treatment. He would like to go home with hospice care.

- What authority and responsibility by virtue of privileging and licensure do you have to manage this patient's hospice care?
- What are the provisions of the ACA affecting palliative and end-of-life care?

Case Study 2: Care of the Young Adult Across the Cancer Care Continuum

Kathleen is a 24-year-old Caucasian female who is referred to a cancer center by her gynecologist after a lump is discovered in her left breast on routine examination during her annual well-woman visit. Radiologic testing and biopsy confirm a Stage III-invasive ductal carcinoma. As part of her work-up, her oncologist, with whom you work as an oncology-certified APRN, feels that because of her age, genetic screening is appropriate to determine what mutations, if any, are present and might influence her treatment. The results of this testing reveal a BRCA2 mutation and she will require surgery, radiation, and chemotherapy. Kathleen is worried about insurance coverage for her treatment because she is no longer a student and works part time and is therefore not eligible for benefits.

- How might health information about this patient be communicated between the gynecologist and the oncologist?
- As an oncology APRN, what role might you play in the management of Kathleen's care, beginning at the time of her referral, based on the competencies for certified oncology APRNs?
- What authority would you have to provide genetic testing and counseling based on your licensure and institutional policies?
- What impact does the ACA have on Kathleen's insurability?

Once Kathleen's insurance coverage is cleared, she begins the treatment with neo-adjuvant chemotherapy. During her treatment, you are responsible for assessing Kathleen during her clinic visit, ordering labs and medications, such as antiemetics, and educating her and her parents about what to expect in the course of treatment. After six cycles of treatment, she is restaged and it is discovered that the disease has not responded. Her oncologist suggests a clinical trial.

- To what degree of autonomy would you be able to manage Kathleen's care and medication management based on licensure and prescriptive authority regulations in your state/institution?
- What parameters of the ACA would impact Kathleen's ability to participate in a clinical trial?

After discussions with her parents and oncologist, Kathleen consents to participation in the study. She is started on a different chemotherapy and a study drug and will be followed to evaluate tumor response. Because of increasing pain, Kathleen is concurrently managed by the Palliative Care Service for pain and symptom control. You collaborate with a CRNA who is a member of the Palliative Service to manage her pain and symptom needs.

- What prescriptive authority does the CRNA have for managing your patient's pain outside the OR setting?
- How might you collaborate across services to ensure continuity of care?

At her 3-month checkup, Kathleen has some regression of her tumor, but unfortunately it is also discovered that her cancer has metastasized to her liver, thereby disqualifying her for continued participation in the protocol. Recognizing that no additional treatment options are feasible, the APRN must discuss transition of care with Kathleen. An additional concern is that Kathleen will turn 26 in 1 month, at which time she will no longer qualify for her parents' insurance coverage. Because of her now preexisting condition, Kathleen is worried about whether or not she will be able to purchase insurance and at what cost.

- What authority do you have within your institution to share prognostic information with Kathleen?
- Can you refer Kathleen for home hospice services by virtue of licensure and insurance reimbursement parameters?
- What impact does Kathleen's age (now 26 years) have on her insurability given her employment and educational status?
- How might future legislation impact reimbursement for and coverage of palliative and hospice services?

REFERENCES

Advanced Practice Registered Nurse Consensus Work Group & the National Council of State Boards of Nursing Advanced Practice Nurse Advisory Committee. (2008). *Consensus model for APRN regulation: Licensure, accreditation, certification & education*. Retrieved from http://www.ncsbn.org/Consensus _Model_for_APRN_Regulation_July_2008.pdf

Allbright, H. W., Moreno, M., Feeley, T. W., Walters, R., Samuels, M., Pereira, A., & Burke, T. W. (2011). The implications of the 2010 Patient Protection and Affordable Care Act and the Health Care and Education Reconciliation Act on cancer care. *Cancer, 1117*(8), 1564–1574. doi: 10.1002 /cncr.25725

Ambinder, E. P. (2005). Electronic health records. *Journal of Oncology Practice, 1*(2), 57–63.

American Association for Cancer Research (AACR). (2012). *Health care reform & cancer research*. Retrieved from http://www.aacr.org/home/public--media/science-policy--government-affairs /health-care-reform--cancer-research.aspx

American Cancer Society. (2012). *Cancer facts and figures 2012*. Atlanta, GA: Author. Retrieved from http:// www.cancer.org/acs/groups/content/@epidemiologysurveilance/documents/document /acspc-031941.pdf

American College of Medical Genetics. (2008). *ACMG statement on direct-to-consumer genetic testing*. Author. Retrieved from http://www.acmg.net/AM/Template.cfm?Section=Policy_Statements &Template=/CM/ContentDisplay.cfm&ContentID=2975

American Nurses Association (ANA). (2009). *Consensus panel on genetic/genomic nursing competencies— Essentials of genetic and genomic nursing: Competencies, curricula guidelines, and outcome indicators* (2nd ed.). Silver Spring, MD: Author.

ANA. (2013). *Accountable care organizations (ACOs)—101*. Retrieved from http://www.nursingworld .org/MainMenuCategories/Policy-Advocacy/Positions-and-Resolutions/Issue-Briefs/ACOs /ACOs-101.pdf

American Society of Clinical Oncology (ASCO). (2003). American Society of Clinical Oncology policy statement update: Genetic testing for cancer susceptibility. *Journal of Clinical Oncology, 21*(12), 2397–2406.

Brown, M. A., & Kaplan, L. (2012). *The advanced practice registered nurse as a prescriber*. Chichester, West Sussex, UK: Wiley-Blackwell.

Carper, E., & Haas, M. (2006). Advanced practice nursing in radiation oncology. *Seminars in Oncology Nursing, 22*(4), 203–211.

Centers for Disease Control and Prevention (CDC). (2013). *Public health genomics 2013 at a glance: Realizing opportunities for genomics to improve health*. Retrieved from http://www.cdc.gov/genomics/about /AAG/index.htm

Centers for Medicare and Medicaid Services (CMS). (2013). *Accountable care organizations*. Retrieved from http://www.cms.gov/Medicare/Medicare-Fee-for-Service-Payment/ACO/index.html ?redirect=/aco

Coleman, K., Austin, B. T., Brach, C., & Wagner, E. H. (2009). Evidence on the chronic care model in the new millennium. *Health Affairs, 28*(1), 75–85. doi: 10.1377/hlthaff.28.1.75

Division of Cancer Control and Population Sciences (DCCPS). (2011). *Informing policy & programs 2011 update*. Bethesda, MD: National Cancer Institute.

Evaluation of Genomic Applications in Practice and Prevention (EGAPP). (2013). *About EGAPP*. Retrieved from http://www.egappreviews.org/about.htm

Foley, K. M., & Gelband, H. (Eds.). (2003). *Improving palliative care for cancer: National Council Policy Board & National Research Council*. Washington, DC: National Academies Press.

Food and Drug Administration (FDA). (2013). *Overview of the Family Smoking Prevention and Tobacco Control Act: Consumer fact sheet*. Retrieved from http://www.fda.gov/tobaccoproducts/guidance complianceregulatoryinformation/ucm246129.htm

Greco, K., Tinley, S., & Seibert, D. (2012). *Essential genetic and genomic competencies for nurses with graduate degrees*. Silver Spring, MD: American Nurses Association and International Society of Nurses in Genetics. Retrieved from http://www.nursingworld.org/MainMenuCategories /EthicsStandards/Genetics-1

Hall, W., Christie, M., & Currow, D. (2005). Cannabinoids and cancer: Causation, remediation, and palliation. *Lancet Oncology, 6*(1), 35–42.

Hewitt, M., Greenfield, S., & Stovall, E. (Eds.). (2005). *From cancer patient to cancer survivor: Lost in translation.* Committee on Cancer Survivorship: Improving Care and Quality of Life, Institute of Medicine, & National Research Council. Washington, DC: National Academies Press.

Hudson, K., Javitt, G., Burke, W., & Byers, P. (2007). ASHG statement on direct-to-consumer genetic testing in the United States. *American Journal of Human Genetics, 81*(3), 635–637. doi: 10.1086/521634

Institute of Medicine. (2011). *The future of nursing: Leading change, advancing health.* Washington, DC: The National Academies Press.

Kaplan, L., & Brown, M. A. (2007). The transition of nurse practitioners to changes in prescriptive authority. *Journal of Nursing Scholarship, 39*(2), 184–190. doi: 10.1111/j.1547-5069.2007.00165.x

Kelvin, J. F., Moore-Higgs, G. J., Maher, K. E., Dubey, A. K., Austin-Seymour, M. M., Daly, N. R., & Kuehn, E. F. (1999). Non-physician practitioners in radiation oncology: Advanced practice nurses and physician assistants. *International Journal of Radiation Oncology Biology Physics, 45*(2), 255–263.

Lynch, M. P., Cope, D. G., & Murphy-Ende, K. (2001). Advanced practice issues: Results of the ONS advanced practice nursing survey. *Oncology Nursing Forum, 28*(10), 1521–1530.

National Consensus Project (NCP) for Quality Palliative Care. (2013). *Clinical practice guidelines for quality palliative care* (3rd ed.). Pittsburgh, PA: Author.

National Cancer Institute (NCI). (2011). *Cancer control continuum.* Retrieved from http://www.cancer control.cancer.gov/od/continuum.html

NCI. (2012). *Cancer trends progess report—2011/2012 update.* Retrieved from http://www.progressreport .cancer.gov

National Institutes of Health (NIH). (2013). *Genetics home reference.* Retrieved from http://www.ghr.nlm .nih.gov/glossary=personalizedmedicine

Oncology Nursing Certification Corporation (ONCC). (2013). *Oncology nursing certification testing bulletin.* Pittsburgh, PA: Author. Retrieved from http://www.ons.org/media/oncc/docs /testbulletin_2013.pdf

Oncology Nursing Society (ONS). (2007). *Oncology nurse practitioner competencies.* Pittsburgh, PA: Author.

ONS. (2008). *Oncology clinical nurse specialist competencies.* Pittsburgh, PA: Author.

ONS. (2012). *Oncology nursing: The application of cancer genetics and genomics throughout the oncology care continuum. ONS positions—Health care policy and consumer advocacy.* Retrieved from http://www .ons.org/Publications/Positions/HealthCarePolicy

ONS. (2013a). *About ONS.* Retrieved from http://www.ons.org/about

ONS. (2013b). *Position on the role of the advanced practice nurse in oncology care.* Retrieved from http://www. ons.org/Publications/Positions/APNrole

Patient Protection and Affordable Care Act of 2010, Pub. L No. 111-148 (Sec. 2702), 124 Stat. 119, 318–319.

Plank, L. S. (2011). Governmental oversight of prescribing medications: History of the U.S. Food and Drug Administration and prescriptive authority. *Journal of Midwifery and Women's Health, 56*(3), 198–204. doi: 10.1111/j.1542-2011.2011.00062.x

Repetto, L., & Balducci, L. (2002). A case for geriatric oncology. *Lancet Oncology, 3*(5), 289–297.

Robson, M. E., Storm, C. D., Weitzel, J., Wollins, D. S., & Offit, K. (2010). American Society of Clinical Oncology policy statement update: Genetic and genomic testing for cancer susceptibility. *Journal of Clinical Oncology, 28*(5), 893–901. doi: 10.1200/JCO.2009.27.0660

Taplin, S. H., & Rodgers, A. B. (2010). Toward improving the quality of cancer care: Addressing the interfaces of primary and oncology-related subspecialty care. *Journal of the National Cancer Institute Monographs, 40*, 3–10. doi: 10.1093/jncimonographs/lgq00

World Health Organization (WHO). (2010). *Framework for action on interprofessional education & collaborative practice.* Geneva, Switzerland: Author. Retrieved from http://www.whqlibdoc.who.int /hq/2010/WHO_HRH_HPN_10.3_eng.pdf

Zapka, J. G., Taplin, S. H., Solberg, L., & Manos, M. M. (2003). A framework for improving the quality of cancer care: The case of breast and cervical cancer screening. *Cancer Epidemiology, Biomarkers & Prevention, 12*(1), 4–13.

HEALTH POLICY AND ITS IMPACT ON ADVANCED PRACTICE REGISTERED NURSE-DRIVEN QUALITY

Policy Implications for Advanced Practice Registered Nurses: Quality and Safety

Mary Jean Schuman

The last decade has seen substantial national policy devoted to the improvement of health care quality and safety. Driven by *To Err Is Human* (Institute of Medicine [IOM], 1999) and *Crossing the Quality Chasm* (IOM, 2001), continuous quality improvement is every health provider's business, regardless of educational preparation or role. For advanced practice registered nurses (APRNs), this emphasis on quality and safety requires a dual responsibility. First, APRNs are responsible for the safety and quality of care for their patients in a manner similar to their physician counterparts. That means APRNs need to be alert to quality outcome measures, evaluating the management outcomes of conditions such as congestive heart failure, pneumonia, diabetes, and asthma. For APRNs who work in acute care settings managing patients who are Medicare or Medicaid beneficiaries with these conditions, their institutions are being rewarded for following the best clinical practices for these conditions and enhancing patients' experiences of care. Physician and APRN care is being monitored and institutions reimbursed according to Centers for Medicare and Medicaid Services (CMS) values-based purchasing parameters that are based upon quality outcome measures. For APRNs who work in primary care settings providing preventive and primary care services, the quality of their care is measured through the Healthcare Effectiveness Data and Information Set (HEDIS) measures developed by the National Committee for Quality Assurance (NCQA). Those results are available to plan purchasers and employers through a *quality compass* (NCQA, 2013). However, every APRN does not manage the same patient population. Although adult/gerontology-focused nurse practitioners and clinical nurse specialists may be accountable for appropriate management of heart failure and diabetes, nurse midwives practice with different measures in mind. They are held accountable to the new standard of eliminating elective deliveries before 39 weeks gestation, for instance. Nurse anesthetists are evaluated on metrics that include OR checklists alongside their OR team.

APRNs are also accountable as nurses, and the expectations for all nurses, as for other health professionals, regardless of the level of education and practice, is to be proficient in knowledge, skills, and strategies that improve the quality and safety of care to all consumers of health and health care. This includes being accountable for driving health care-acquired infection (HAI) rates to zero, for eliminating medication errors, and for employing knowledge of health literacy, patient engagement and activation, motivational interviewing, shared decision making and decision aids, along with public reporting of comparative performance information. These are not skills that can be assumed left to others. APRNs, along with physicians and other health professionals, must be proficient in practicing these skills effectively, in setting the example for others, and in driving the health care system to respond positively and appropriately to patients and families.

APRNs must recognize that quality and safety exist in a very fluid landscape. What is not measured today in terms of patient outcomes of care could be the new electronic measure (e-measure) next year. Conversely, quality indicators may be retired from use if the quality outcome they are meant to measure is achieved successfully 100% of the time or if another indicator for the same outcome is tested and found more effective. This chapter is not about providing lists and recipes for how to score well on measures. It is about understanding the context in which APRNs possess accountability in the quality arena. It discusses acquiring new knowledge and skills that improve quality of care for patients; employing strategies for staying abreast of the changing trends in quality, performance measurement, and safety issues; and utilizing the payment reform provisions that incorporate measures of performance.

ARTICULATING THE CONNECTIONS BETWEEN POLICY AND QUALITY

Every discussion of policy needs to start with an assumption that policy is not only or even mostly about legislation. State and federal legislative agendas do drive payment reform strategies, reimbursement strategies, and often state practice acts. Yet, it is more often in the regulatory and standard setting processes that policy will be generated, dictating parameters of reimbursement eligibility and rates. In today's environment, the equation for reimbursement includes the quality of the care delivered, primarily based on outcome measures. As a result, a provider may make a conscious choice to focus on certain patient populations based upon reimbursement. Policies on quality-related priorities for performance-based reimbursement may influence which patients get more time with a provider or follow-up care by a registered nurse (RN). Decisions may give priority patients more listening time, more education about options in care, and even increased RN staff to support those patients in following through with mutually agreed upon plans of care. In a period of scarce resources and decreasing reimbursement based upon fees for service, the unintended consequence of policy can be that health disparities are exacerbated, or decreases in patient care quality occur in new populations or for diseases that are deemed less expensive to the bottom line.

So, in today's health systems, quality and policy are inextricably tied. High-quality health care is critically important. Although it has made the lives of APRNs more complicated, it is not the bad guy in the room. Without high quality and safe care, patients suffer preventable harm and even death. Quality driven by appropriate policy is intended to be beneficial to patients. In this context, it is very important for APRNs to understand the systems for generating policy that affect their practices and to stay linked into the development of new policy or proposed changes in existing policy before policy adoption. It is critical that APRNs examine those proposed policies to ascertain if they really can improve the quality and safety of the patients served. APRNs would benefit from devoting even a limited amount of time to reading, dissecting, and speaking out about how proposed policy will impact their patients, their practice, and the health of their community.

GROWTH OF THE IMPORTANCE OF QUALITY TO HEALTH CARE DELIVERY

Historically, even though the Japanese manufacturing world was introduced to the notion of quality by Edwards Deming in the 1950s, it took several decades to find its way to the United States and ultimately to the health care industry (Deming, 1986). The manufacturing world recognized that individual employees did not set out at the beginning of the work day to make auto parts that fit together improperly or cars that malfunctioned once assembled. Yet, mishaps would occur on the factory line, causing waste, needless rework, significant expense, occasionally harm, and often lost profits. Quality leaders such as Deming, Crosby, and Juran recognized the value of addressing processes, manpower training, and other factors that ultimately accounted for 80% of the errors in manufacturing.

In the 1990s, health care leaders such as Don Berwick began to focus the country's attention on similar factors affecting health care quality and safety. Although his message did not fall on totally deaf ears, it would take almost a decade for a series of national reports quantifying the loss of life and related harm to patients due to medical errors, to bring the nation's attention to the issue. Of equal or greater historical significance to health care quality is the work of Donabedian, a physician and health services researcher who proposed a framework for evaluating health services and care quality as early as 1966. Understanding Donabedian's framework of structure, process, and outcome measures as a way of viewing quality improvement is critical for all health providers. This framework has been the accepted methodology for examining and influencing the issues surrounding health care quality and remains as the primary model utilized in health care-related discussions (Donabedian, 2005).

In Donabedian's framework, *structure* describes the context in which care is delivered, including the workforce needed, the setting of care and the facilities, and the financial and equipment resources. *Process* represents the activities, interactions, and decisions that occur among health professionals, patients, and the health care system in the delivery of health care. *Outcomes* are the resulting impact of health care processes and structure on the health status of individual patients and populations. For example, when a patient falls there are *structural* factors that may impact the likelihood of the fall, for example, slippery floors or insufficient staff to respond to patients who need assistance to the bathroom. There are *processes* in hospitals for assessing and managing patients who are at risk for falling, as well as tactics that nurses might employ, such as hourly rounding on patients, special bracelets and identification bracelets, and signs to warn others that certain patients are a higher risk for injury. The *outcome* of interest is a reduction in the actual number and severity of falls to patients. In other words, an outcome measure for reducing falls with injury would look at the total number of falls occurring to patients, along with the total number of patients on that clinical unit, how many patients were injured, and how severely they were injured. As of this writing, in most quality discussions, outcome measures are the most highly valued measures of quality care.

DRIVING FORCES FOR QUALITY AND SAFETY

The efforts to address medical errors, patient harm, and climbing health care costs have been national in scope. The last decade or more has seen the advent of several major national quality initiatives. The first and most sustainable of these has been the National

Quality Forum (NQF). Begun as a private, not-for-profit entity, it has become central to the establishment of standards and policy relative to health care quality. Although it has not taken on the role of developing measures of quality, it has created the standards that all measures must meet in order to be NQF-endorsed. It is in the enviable position of having Congressional support in that the CMS must stipulate NQF-endorsed measures in its reimbursement strategy or answer to Congress as to why not. The NQF model has generated a collective effort of over 1,000 entities who participate as organizational members. The members represent health professional groups, consumers, pharmaceuticals, business groups with a focus on health, and many others. This membership body represents a significant policy setting effort around quality.

As of the writing of this chapter, there are over 700 health care quality measures that have been NQF-endorsed, many of which have been maintained or modified to stay current over time, a requirement for their continued use. NQF has formed within its structure the Measure Application Partnership (MAP) to attempt to better sort out and align the measures in each area, for example, care coordination measures, to reduce conflicting or confusing measures and data collection burdens. Although nursing and other professions have developed measures to evaluate many aspects of care, unless they are broadly applicable and NQF-endorsed, they are neither likely to be drivers of reimbursement activity nor will they be publicly reported.

The implication for APRNs and for nursing is that relatively few measures reflect the impact on patient outcomes of nurses specifically and those that measure the practice of APRNs, regardless of role, are virtually all physician-oriented measures. As a result, the measures may not represent the best that APRNs uniquely have to offer to patients. APRNs have a significant leadership opportunity, regardless of role, to develop endorsable nondisease-specific measures that reflect the quality of care APRNs and other providers can deliver, to change the dialogue around the measurement of quality.

NURSING ALLIANCE ADDS VOICE TO IMPROVEMENT OF QUALITY AND SAFETY

Although NQF may represent the largest collective effort, health care quality and policy have likewise been the focus of a number of alliances, such as the Hospital Quality Alliance, the Ambulatory Care Alliance, the Pediatric Quality Alliance, the Pharmacy Quality Alliance, and others. All of these were included in a collective effort called the Quality Alliance Steering Committee (QASC). In 2008, the Robert Wood Johnson Foundation (RWJF) engaged the George Washington University School of Nursing to create and implement a Nursing Alliance for Quality Care (NAQC) in order to provide a voice at such tables as QASC, and to provide similar visibility and input into the national quality agenda. Nursing had been represented by the American Nurses Association on NQF's Board since the inception of NQF, but it took several years for a significant number of nursing organizations to likewise add their voices. The implementation of NAQC created a greater number of opportunities for nursing to be at national tables and to have a voice in the development and evaluation of measures, the quality agenda, and the priorities of the collective efforts of the health care industry. Of note during that time, the focus of many of the alliances was on the development of quality measures. Since 2010, the Hospital Quality Alliance (HQA) has disbanded, the Ambulatory Care Quality Alliance (AQA, now known as the AQA alliance) has evolved into a larger collective alliance not focused solely on ambulatory care, and all alliances have struggled to determine their future direction and level of sustainability. As of this writing, NAQC has approximately two dozen member organizations as members and has just transitioned from the GW School of Nursing to a more permanent home within the American Nurses Association.

In 2010, NAQC became a member of the National Priorities Partners (NPP), then a 30-member subset of NQF that advised federal agencies regarding the quality priorities for the nation. The creation of the NPP in 2008 provided an opportunity for nursing to advocate for those issues that were most sensitive to the skills of nurses. In 2011, the Department of Health and Human Services released a National Quality Strategy (NQS), largely informed by the work of the NPP. Subsequently, the Agency for Healthcare Research and Quality (AHRQ) was charged to drive the implementation of the NQS, and sought out the NPP to advise the best path forward. The diagram below depicts the current quality strategy which is now the main policy driver for improving and sustaining quality in the United States and as such it has major significance for APRNs. The goals of the NQS are to provide better care, more affordable care, and to improve the health of the population and communities. The priorities for achieving those goals, represented in green, provide ample opportunities to support the contributions of RNs and APRNs to the health and safety of patients (Advisory Council on Alzheimer's Research, Care, and Services, 2013).

The passage of the Affordable Care Act and its many provisions that support quality improvements have included new models of health care delivery (accountable care organizations and health care homes among them) and the CMS Innovation. One new initiative that has generated an amazing groundswell of action is Center for Medicare and Medicaid Innovation's (CMMI's) Partnership for Patients (P4P). Hospitals, community programs, national organizations, and networks have created P4P as a vehicle to disseminate good ideas, innovations, successes, and failures toward the goals of reducing harm to hospitalized patients by 40% and reducing hospital readmissions within 30 days by 20%. P4P has garnered institution and agency-level commitments from over 5,000 entities with amazing results on the ground in every state and jurisdiction. One such example is in the reduction of elective deliveries before 39 weeks gestation, an initiative that is succeeding with strong leadership from nurse midwives.

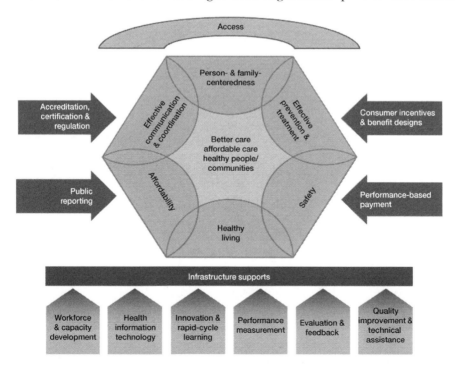

FIGURE 20.1 National Quality Forum Measure Applications Partnership (2011).

At a recent National Priorities Partnership meeting, it was shared that while much progress on the NQS has been made in some arenas through the P4P, there has been relatively little progress in the area of building healthier populations. This challenging area of health creates additional opportunities for APRNs to provide leadership and demonstrate success through expansion of APRN services in primary care, in nurse-led health care homes, and in conjunction with accountable care organizations.

THE LINK BETWEEN QUALITY AND SAFETY

Today, more than a decade after the Institute of Medicine (IOM) reports, data demonstrate that scant progress has been made to reduce adverse events, despite a national effort to keep patients safe. A large scale review of literature on adverse events summarized by Pham et al. (2012) describes the extent of the problem of adverse preventable events in a number of arenas, many of which APRNs must be aware, whether working in inpatient or ambulatory settings. The following represents a summary of those most pertinent to APRN practice.

- The IOM suggests that 1.5 million preventable drug events occur annually in the United States, with only 26% of them occurring in the inpatient sector. Reducing their frequency, particularly in ambulatory care and long-term care environments and other settings where APRNs provide increasing percentages of the care, must be a priority for all APRNs.
- Hospital HAIs, including urinary catheter-associated infections (CAUTI), central line-associated bloodstream infections (CLABSI), and wrong-site infections, are major sources of harm to patients. They require vigilance and dedicated follow-up, whether in the inpatient, outpatient, or home environment, as prolonged or unnecessary use and ineffective follow-up treatment can result in preventable deaths.
- Harm associated with poor communication via handoffs in care is a frequent occurrence when the continuity of care from one provider to another is broken. Although often thought to be about hospital handoffs, these gaps in communication (implicated in up to 70% of sentinel events) can and do lead to harm in and across all settings. Checklists, while helpful for performing "medication reconciliation" activities, do not substitute for critical questions about whether the right medications are being prescribed in the first place or whether their continuation is appropriate. Critical thinking skills are required for that.
- Diagnostic errors account for anywhere from 40,000 to 80,000 annual deaths in the United States. Diagnostic errors are the largest source of errors in emergency departments. With the advent of convenience care and urgent care centers, this risk of error extends to many more APRNs in nonacute care practice settings.

These examples of high-risk/high-volume negative patient events occur most often because of breakdowns in delivery of high standards of care. Breaks in quality occur because of a variety of factors, including but certainly not limited to: lack of or inconsistently applied processes, workforce shortages, workforce fatigue, frequent interruptions, lack of knowledge, or inadequate communications, to name a few. All health professionals must take responsibility for delivery of highly reliable care that prevents these factors from impacting patients. APRNs, both individually and in groups, must intervene to ensure that these factors are well controlled and eliminated from impacting quality of care and patient safety in the settings of care. Action may include interfacing with administration and other departments to eliminate staffing shortages, unsafe on-call expectations, insufficient, unsafe, or undocumented processes of care, and ineffective communication tactics. Patients' lives may depend on it.

LINKING TRANSPARENCY TO SAFETY AND QUALITY

Historically hospitals and other health care institutions have been reluctant to acknowledge their health care system's culpability when a patient has been harmed. Various states attempted in the early 1990s to employ state-level report cards for hospitals that identified adverse events. This approach was met by widespread resistance with many hospitals claiming that their patients were sicker than everyone else's and that such reporting was not equitable. After the IOM reports were released, it became clear that hospitals could no longer stand on this argument. Landmark cases in which children and prominent others died due to unsafe practices, poor processes, and immobilized providers occurred in some highly regarded institutions. Johns Hopkins' Josie King case (King, 2009), Dana Farber's Betsy Lehman case (Altman, 1995), and the Lewis Blackman case (Acquaviva, Haskell, & Johnson, 2013) represented preventable and needless tragedies. Such cases demonstrated that no one was immune from poor quality and unsafe practices.

A decade ago efforts to provide public reporting of numbers to represent quality was voluntary. With these cases hitting the media, it quickly became apparent that willingness to publicly report hospital level data in some way was necessary to regain the confidence of patients and providers alike. Willingness to step up and publicly acknowledge disasters like King's became acceptable, if not comfortable. In the decade since, several national consumer groups have arisen to push the public perspective for transparency and accountability. Parents who have lost children to medical error often articulate that it is most important that those responsible institutions acknowledge that they failed these children. They view this as a first step to the institution taking definitive and effective steps forward to prevent such disasters from occurring to others.

David Mayer, co-executive director for the University of Illinois at Chicago's Institute for Patient Safety Excellence, stated that although the terms are used interchangeably, there is a difference between transparency and disclosure. "Transparency is a part of a hospital's culture, meaning that every action flows from a shared belief in openness, honesty, and truth in the sharing of information. Disclosure is what happens after the fact. Something's occurred, and now you disclose or acknowledge it." Sandra Coletta, CEO and president of Kent Hospital, Warwick, Rhode Island, further stated that "transparency is about the willingness and ability of your staff to be honest with the organization about actions that may be putting patients at risk. That is where transparency makes so much more difference in terms of preventing future events" (Daughenbaugh & Martin, 2011).

Public reporting as a form of transparency has been strongly embraced by the Department of Health and Human Services, through agencies such as the CMS. Hospitalcompare.org, NursingHomecompare.org, and homehealthcompare.org are a few of the vehicles in which this has become the norm. Some states, such as Massachusetts, have created state-wide websites to disclose publicly the levels of nurse staffing available in every facility. Over the last decade, the Institute for Health Care Improvement conducted national campaigns, including the Saving 100,000

Lives Campaign and the Saving 500,000 Lives Campaign to encourage the collection and sharing of data on near misses. Although these data were not reported publicly, the data quantified the extent of the problems and how disclosure in some cases forced institutions to improve.

A group of 13 Rhode Island hospitals has been collaborating since 2010 to improve patients' safety through better reporting of data on adverse and near miss medical events (Daughenbaugh & Martin, 2011). In order to do this, the hospitals agreed to common reporting criteria and medical event reporting metrics. Equally essential, they joined a patient safety organization (PSO) that they use as a forum for sharing knowledge, best practices, and insights gained from the reported data. They believe that this forum approach leads to creating safer environments for their patients. This example begins to demonstrate the nature of learning health care systems as articulated by the IOM in its report, *Best Care at Lower Cost: The Path to Continuously Learning Health Care in America* (IOM, 2012b).

While all data are not being reported publicly, the willingness of hospitals and other institutions and agencies to own their health care system risks and failures has been a giant step toward identifying significant problems in providing care safely. Perhaps, the best example is that of wrong-site surgery in the operating room. Until there was nationwide reporting, there was no evidence to demonstrate the size of the problem. Although wrong-site surgery data may still under-represent the scope of the problem or be reported unevenly, the data have not only gotten the attention of hospitals and others, it has generated a series of widely used interventions to prevent events from occurring. Unfortunately, despite these interventions, estimates are that as many as 40 wrong site surgeries still occur in the United States weekly. Reporting has made it possible to know how far we still have to go. Although many APRNs are not directly involved in OR settings, it is critically important that all APRNs educate and emphasize to their patients who are contemplating surgical solutions, how they as patients have the right to advocate for and insist that all interventions be followed to prevent wrong-site surgery, as well as what those interventions should look like.

HEALTH CARE SYSTEMS THAT SUPPORT PATIENT SAFETY AND QUALITY

Although transparency may be important to patient safety, it is not so simple to achieve. There are numerous barriers to achieving transparency, which can include:

- Fear of retribution if they admit to either committing or witnessing an error
- Sense of apathy caused by lack of feedback about own performance and its impact on patients, either good or bad
- Feeling of isolation from consequences or solutions to improve quality or safety
- Lack of institutional leadership or establishment of active performance improvement initiatives when adverse events or safety risks occur
- Perceived lack of responsibility and accountability for the individuals in their care

Dr. Lucien Leape (2000) stated that the single greatest impediment to error prevention in the medical industry is that we punish people for making mistakes. Other industries, for example aviation, have recognized the value of allowing individuals to develop essential skills without negative consequences through the use of simulation laboratories. Such approaches, which require a minimum number of hours of practice in simulation environments, allow for both initial learning of necessary skills and ongoing recertification of essential high-risk skills to meet credentialing standards. For instance, nurse anesthetists acquire and maintain skills in intubation, administration of epidurals, spinals, and similar skills through high-fidelity simulation. Interprofessional crew resource management skills during situational crises and disasters are often best acquired through simulation, for example, rapid response teams.

Organizations willing to provide a safe environment for patients while their health professionals learn through repeated practice and preparation aid the process of transparency. Health system models of care supporting patient safety and quality share that philosophy. The following models portray similar concepts, whether they are (a) principles of a just culture, (b) principles of person-centered care, (c) principles of high-reliability organizations (HROs), (d) principles of health literate organizations, (e) principles of patient and family engagement, or (f) principles of learning health care systems. Many of the concepts are similar. What is critical is to appreciate that without embracing the concepts and principles described in these models, effective transparency that can lead to high levels of patient safety and quality is likely to remain unachievable.

- **Just Culture:** Organizations that embrace just culture agree that we are all accountable, across all departments, across all positions, and across all behaviors (Marx, 2009). These organizations subscribe to the belief that human error occurs and when it does, it is acknowledged. Furthermore, if a gap in knowledge caused the error, then that gap is filled or the individual is counseled in how to make a different decision in the future. Just culture organizations acknowledge that sometimes individuals unintentionally make choices that place patients at risk, requiring the individual's behavior to be addressed through counseling. However, just culture organizations also acknowledge that occasionally individuals intentionally choose reckless behaviors that place others at risk. In those cases, the individual may experience consequences up to and including termination.
- **HROs:** At the core of HROs are five key concepts that are essential for any improvement initiative to succeed (AHRQ, 2008) These concepts do not require a huge outlay of resources to achieve, but essential are leaders at all levels who are thinking about how the care their organizations provides can become better. Concepts include:
  - **Sensitivity to operations**, demonstrated by maintaining constant awareness by leaders and staff of the systems and processes that affect patient care, leading to noting risks and preventing them.
  - **Reluctance to simplify**, best explained by avoiding simple explanations for why things work or fail. The belief is that oversimplification leads to failing to understand the true reasons why patients have ended up at risk.
  - **Preoccupation with failure**, which emphasizes that near misses should be viewed as evidence that systems or processes need to be improved to reduce potential harm to patients, rather than accepted as proof that the system has effective safeguards in place.
  - **Deference to expertise**, which emphasizes the importance of leaders and supervisors being willing to listen and respond to the insights of staff who know how the processes really work and what risks patients really face.
  - **Resilience**, which demands that leaders and staff need to be trained and prepared to know how to respond when system failures occur.

- **Person-Centered Care:** Principles of person-centered care focus on the engagement of the person and their family as the center of all health care decisions and choices about care. Staff and leaders in organizations that embrace this model emphasize communication with the patient and family as key, along with all other members of the health care team. They engage in community outreach and involvement as an extension of the patient and family constellation. These organizations demonstrate consistent respect for the person's (patient's) preferences, values, and beliefs, such as all cultural attributes in every aspect of care. They focus on coordination and integration of care and emphasize holistic care that attends to comfort and supportive care as much as curative care (Gerteis, Edgman-Levitan, Daley, & Delbanco, 1993).
- **Health Literate Organizations:** Health literate organizations make it easier for people to navigate and understand the information and services that are available to take care of their health. This model casts a wide health care system net and requires that not only must providers embrace it, but all must subscribe, such as hospital staff, groups and teams, community health centers, pharmacies, insurers, and payers. Resources for becoming health literate organizations are available through AHRQ's Health Literacy Universal Precautions Tool Kit (AHRQ, 2010). The IOM (2012a) recently identified 10 attributes of health literate organizations. Those attributes state that the organization:

1. Has leadership that makes health literacy integral to its mission, structure, and operations;
2. Integrates health literacy into planning, evaluation, patient safety, and quality improvements;
3. Prepares the workforce to be health literate and monitors progress;
4. Includes populations being served in the design, implementation, and evaluation of information and services;
5. Meets needs of populations with a range of health literacy skills while avoiding stigmatization;
6. Uses health literacy strategies in interpersonal communications and confirms understanding at all points of contact;
7. Provides easy access to health information and services and navigation assistance;
8. Designs and distributes print, audiovisual, and social media content that is easy to understand and act on;
9. Addresses health literacy in high-risk situations, such as care transitions and communications about medications; and
10. Communicates clearly what health plans cover and what individuals will have to pay for services.

One could assume that such a list of attributes would not be difficult to achieve. But what must be understood in practical terms is that these attributes require development of educational materials, signage, forms and other aids, and communication pieces that are geared to no higher than a fifth-grade reading level, eliminate all jargon, and keep the amount of information in small chunks that can be easily and accurately retained and taught back to the provider by the patient or family members.

- **Patient Engagement:** Principles of patient engagement, identified by the NAQC (2013), rely on concepts of person-centered care, while incorporating many of the concepts of each of the other models above (Sofaer & Schumann, 2013). They are based on the philosophy that in every patient–provider encounter, there are two experts in the room and that each expert needs the other in order to be successful. One of those two experts is always the patient because the patient knows their preferences and values, their resources, and their own support system. Patient engagement is not about compliance and adherence. It is about (a) active partnership among the patient, the family, and the providers of the health care, and (b) a two-way exchange of information because patients are the best and ultimate source of information about their health status and retain the right to make their own decisions about care. The principles of patient engagement include:

  1. There must be an active partnership among patients, their families, and the providers of their health care.
  2. Patients are the best and ultimate source of information about their health status and retain the right to make their own decisions about care.
  3. In this relationship, there are shared responsibilities and accountabilities among the patient, the family, and clinicians that make it effective.
  4. While embracing partnerships, clinicians must nevertheless respect the boundaries of privacy, competent decision making, and ethical behavior in all their encounters and transactions with patients and families. These boundaries protect recipients as well as providers of care. This relationship is grounded in confidentiality, where the patient defines the scope of the confidentiality.
  5. This relationship is grounded in an appreciation of the patient's rights and expands on the rights to include mutuality. Mutuality includes sharing of information, creation of consensus, and shared decision making.
  6. Clinicians must recognize that the extent to which patients and family members are able to engage or choose to engage may vary greatly based on individual circumstances, cultural beliefs, and other factors.
  7. Advocacy for patients who are unable to participate fully is a fundamental nursing role. Patient advocacy is the demonstration of how all of the components of the relationship fit together.
  8. Acknowledgment and appreciation of culturally, racially, or ethnically diverse backgrounds are an essential part of the engagement process.
  9. Health care literacy and linguistically appropriate interactions are essential for patient, family, and clinicians to understand the components of patient engagement. Providers must maintain awareness of the language needs and health care literacy level of the patient and family and respond accordingly.

- **Learning Health Care Systems:** The IOM-sponsored Roundtable on Value and Science-Driven Health Care defines learning health care systems as those who generate and apply the best evidence for the collaborative health care choices of each patient and provider; drive the process of discovery as a natural outgrowth of patient care; and ensure innovation, quality, safety, and value in health care. In such systems, knowledge flows seamlessly between and among patients, providers, diagnostic facilities, and related community services. The best knowledge about treatments, diagnostics, and care delivery is naturally embedded in the delivery process and new knowledge is captured as an integral byproduct of the delivery experience (IOM, 2012b). The earlier cited IOM report on learning health care systems (IOM, 2012b) stated that the transition to a health care system characterized by continuous learning and improvement relies on public and private purchasers, health care organizations, clinicians, patients, and other stakeholders who focus their efforts on the foundational elements of a learning health care system. Those foundational elements include:

- Science and informatics—Real-time access to knowledge; digital capture of the care experience
- Patient–clinician partnerships—Engaged, empowered patients
- Incentives—Incentives aligned for value; full transparency
- Culture—Leadership-instilled culture of learning; supportive system competencies

All of the models described above demonstrate consistency with the priorities and infrastructures needed to achieve the goals of the NQS. These models are also internally consistent with each other. APRNs who are striving to deliver the highest levels of quality and patient safety will want to seek out organizations as partners or employers who embrace one or more of these models. Entrepreneurial APRNs who may own their own practices or participate in small group practices will want to consider how they can bring these principles and concepts forward to be embraced by their own teams. Individual APRN practice that is meeting the highest standards of quality will employ many and perhaps most of these concepts.

VALUE OF EVIDENCE-BASED PRACTICE TO DELIVERY OF QUALITY

The above delineation of continuously learning health care systems surfaces the importance of APRNs' use of evidence to support best practice and high quality. Although many APRNs are and will continue to practice at the master's level quite effectively, one of the cornerstones of the progression to doctor of nursing practice (DNP) programs includes gaining skill in the effective use of evidence. All providers of care, APRNs included, are being bombarded by more information, knowledge, and data than one provider can ever hope to retain. Learning how to sort through the plethora of material made available to providers can be overwhelming. Regardless of the level of education, APRNs must become proficient in critically analyzing studies in order to determine the strength and the level of evidence that supports or negates an expectation of practice. Amid all of the noise, APRNs will need to sift and winnow that which is the most compelling evidence. They must then be able to translate that evidence into improvements in their own practices and that of their colleagues. APRNs likewise need to share in the professional obligation of contributing to the profession's building of a solid evidence base to improve care. APRNs, as well as RNs, are good innovators; that innovation is important to the larger body of practice knowledge and APRNs will need to design methods to evaluate those innovations, write about their successes and failures, and disseminate that knowledge.

Patients and other stakeholders can readily access many if not all studies that are available to APRNs and other providers, if they choose to do so. They expect their APRNs and others to be prepared to carry on reasoned discussions about the pros and cons of current preference-sensitive approaches to care, including the facts that allow the patient to make appropriate choices. As patients become more activated and confident about shared health-related decision making, they not only will require these thoughtful discussions but need and expect the information to be presented in objective nonbiased terms, including using numbers about the odds of experiencing effective treatment that are meaningful for sound decisions. So it is not enough for the APRN to be well read; the APRN must also be effective in exchanging information that takes into account the health literacy of the patient and family, their cultural differences, and the linguistic skills. It is an intimidating responsibility to say the least. But it starts and ends with evidence.

DATA COLLECTION, MEANINGFUL USE, AND PUBLIC REPORTING CHALLENGES

As part of the evidence base critical to APRN practice, all APRNs need to be knowledgeable and well versed about the data that are available with regard to their practice, their setting of practice, their patient populations, and those with whom they might be compared. Until recently, providers managed the patients in their practice one patient at a time. Although a provider might have 50 patients with asthma in their practice, most providers would have found it impossible to provide a list of them and even less probable that they could identify which ones were doing well, what differences in treatment there might have been among them, and which treatment plans seemed to work best. Today, with wider adoption of electronic health records and databases, good systems include registry features that allow a provider to query the patient database in their office. Such queries can generate a list of patients with a particular disease process, determine how often each patient has been seen over the last year, identify what range of interventions were employed, and generate other meaningful data that might suggest best practice. These same registries might identify those needing updated vaccinations, those referred for specialist consultation, and those who have need of office follow-up.

APRNs need to go further to identify that meaningful data, which might be additionally collected in order to improve care or to study the outcomes of different approaches to the care of the patient populations they serve. The Office of the National Coordinator, who represents federal efforts to drive toward widespread adoption of electronic health records, has a multiphased approach to what is termed as Meaningful Use. The emphasis is on collecting those data that are specifically useful to making decisions about measuring or improving care, while being mindful of the burdens imposed on systems and providers that result from collecting data that may never be useful. The Consumer–Purchasers Disclosure Project (2011) has developed 10 criteria for meaningful and usable measures of performance that include important points relevant to APRNs who are providing data for any purpose. They include:

- Make consumer and purchaser needs a priority in performance measurement
- Use direct feedback from patients and their families to measure performance
- Build a comprehensive "dashboard" of measures that provides a complete picture of the care patients receive
- Focus measurement on areas of care where the potential to improve health outcomes and increase the effectiveness and efficiency of care is greatest
- Ensure that measures generate the most valuable information possible
- Require that all patients fitting appropriate clinical criteria be included in the measure population
- Assess whether treatment recommendations are followed
- De-emphasize documentation (check-the-box) measures
- Measure the performance of providers at all levels (e.g., individual physicians, medical groups, accountable care organizations [ACOs])
- Collect performance measurement data efficiently

As the above list highlights, any discussion of measures of performance must include the patient's view of the quality and safety of the care experience. For a decade or more, the health care industry collected patient satisfaction as a proxy for the quality of the patient experience. Patient satisfaction was not found to be a particularly useful measure of the quality or outcomes of care. This satisfaction tended to focus on tasks, for example, how long did you wait for your call light to be answered? More recently, patient experience of care measures have emerged as a better approach to getting at quality. Some of these have been considered for inclusion in meaningful use criteria, for example, patient access to online services, patient portals, clinical information, electronic health records, and so forth. The next evolution of patients' views of the quality of care will need to include measures of patient engagement, such as inclusion in the development of the care plan, shared decision making, and usefulness of the information provided to make choices about care, for example, decision aids. APRNs could have a significant role in providing leadership in this area given that APRNs are more comfortable interacting at this level with patients than many of their physician counterparts, whereas measures that reflect these experiences for patients have yet to be developed.

Although current public reporting of health care outcomes to consumers is limited to those federally sponsored programs and occasional state level initiatives, public reporting will be a key strategy of those competing in health care delivery. The transparency of the effectiveness of care, the number of complaints against established providers, the levels of staffing in health care facilities, and the frequency of adverse events will influence the consumer perspective at a greater level. Currently, accurate information on individual providers is challenging in many respects. For federal agencies, research is still determining what information is most useful to consumers and in what terminology is it most readily understood. AHRQ has created a template for web-based reporting that can be used by states or regions wanting to provide useful data to consumers about the outcomes of care (AHRQ, 2013). National databases that collect data regarding performance on physicians, nurses, dentists, and others, such as the National Practitioner Data Bank (NPDB), are not yet accessible to consumers. However, growing interest in transparency of data will demand it. Internet websites are proliferating rapidly in which consumers can identify (whether appropriately or not) their own views of particular providers and services (NPDB, 2013). These websites challenge the NPDB type databases to become consumer-friendly, in order that more accurate information about performance about individuals can be available.

PATIENT-CENTERED OUTCOMES RESEARCH INSTITUTE

This emphasis on patients and the knowledge they need to make sound decisions is further reinforced by a new federal initiative, PCORI. Consistent with the NQS, the Patient-Centered Outcomes Research Institute (PCORI) is authorized as one provision of the Affordable Care Act. The PCORI's purpose is to conduct research focused on how to provide information about the best available evidence to help patients and their health care providers make more informed decisions. Nursing experts have been included as part of the PCORI Research Methodology Advisory Board to identify the research priorities under which awarding of funds to entities would occur. To date, Congressional funding has allowed PCORI to grant awards to 51 projects, totaling more than $88 million, to focus on patient-centered comparative effectiveness research. PCORI's research is intended to result in giving patients a better understanding of the prevention, treatment, and care options available, and the science that supports those options. The PCORI (2012) Board offered the following definition of patient-centered outcomes research:

PCOR helps people and their caregivers communicate and make informed health care decisions, allowing their voices to be heard in assessing the value of health care options. This research answers patient-centered questions such as:

1. Given my personal characteristics, conditions, and preferences, what should I expect will happen to me?
2. What are my options and what are the potential benefits and harms of those options?
3. What can I do to improve the outcomes that are most important to me?
4. How can clinicians and the care delivery systems they work in help me make the best decisions about my health and health care?

APRNs are in a strong position to benefit from knowledge gained through PCORI, which can then be applied as an additional source of knowledge to benefit patients. APRNs would do well to stay alert for results of PCORI-funded projects as those results become available.

STRATEGIES FOR REDUCING ADVERSE EVENTS AND IMPROVING CARE

So how do health systems, and in particular, APRNs, succeed in driving down the numbers of adverse events while improving the quality of care for patients? Newly published, a 4-year evidence-based review of the literature supported by AHRQ (Shekelle et al., 2013) has analyzed the evidence regarding patient safety strategies. APRNs in many settings will find the following information very useful in improving patient safety. Based upon the strength and the quality of the evidence about effectiveness and implementation for each patient safety strategy, the authors concluded that the top patient safety strategies that ought to be *strongly encouraged* for adoption now include:

- Preoperative checklists and anesthesia checklists to prevent operative and postoperative events
- Bundles that include checklists to prevent central line-associated bloodstream infections
- Interventions to reduce urinary catheter use, such as catheter reminders, stop orders, or nurse-initiated removal protocols
- Bundles that include head-of-bed elevation, sedation vacations, oral care with chlorhexidine, and subglottic suctioning endotracheal tubes to prevent ventilator-associated pneumonia
- Hand hygiene
- The do-not-use list for hazardous abbreviations
- Multicomponent interventions to reduce pressure ulcers
- Barrier precautions to prevent health care-associated infections
- Use of real-time ultrasonography for central line placement
- Interventions to improve prophylaxis for venous thromboembolisms

Based on the evidence, the authors of the review also provided a list of patient safety strategies that should be *encouraged* for adoption, including:

- Multicomponent interventions to reduce falls
- Use of clinical pharmacists to reduce adverse drug events
- Documentation of patient preferences for life-sustaining treatment

- Obtaining informed consent to improve patients' understanding of the potential risks of procedures
- Team training
- Medication reconciliation
- Practices to reduce radiation exposure from fluoroscopy and CT
- Use of surgical outcome measures and report cards, such as those from American College of Surgeons National Surgical Quality Improvement Program (ACSNSQIP)
- Rapid-response systems
- Use of complementary methods for detecting adverse events or medical errors to monitor for patient safety problems
- Computerized provider order entry
- Use of simulation exercises in patient safety efforts

APRNs may view these strategies as something someone else should be responsible for initiating, for example, the institution, the practice manager, or the outpatient facility. But in reality, it is the provider, the APRN, who must voice the need to prevent harm and seek the support of others who can add their voices to drive the ongoing improvements in quality and safety of the patient. Quality and safety is everyone's business. Waiting for someone else to step up and insist that these strategies be initiated results in patients being harmed. Consumer groups who represent parents of children who have been harmed or who have lost their lives due to medical error, when asked about their experience, often say, "Where was the nurse? We recognized that the physician or the resident did not understand, but we counted on the nurse to be our ally, to echo the voice of the patient, and to be the safety net to keep our child from harm." As APRNs, you have the opportunity to be that voice and possess the added clout as a provider to drive safety and quality.

STRENGTHENING THE COMPETENCIES OF APRNs IN QUALITY AND SAFETY

So what is the solution to ensuring that every APRN and every student in an APRN program are competent to deliver safe, high-quality care? It is worth learning what has been done to imbue undergraduate nursing students with the knowledge and skills to employ principles of quality and safety. The nursing educational community in 2005 engaged in an initiative titled Quality and Safety Education for Nurses (QSEN). The focus of this work, supported by the RWJF, was to first identify those competencies that RNs must acquire in the areas of quality and safety. The competencies included five from the IOM—patient-centered care, teamwork and collaboration, evidence-based practice, quality improvement, and informatics. Patient safety was added to that list. In addition to these definitions, sets of knowledge, skills, and attitudes for each of the six competencies were created for use in nursing prelicensure programs. A second phase of the QSEN initiative identified pilot schools who would integrate the competencies into their nursing curricula. To support that integration, a website was developed and launched for the purpose of providing teaching strategies and resources around the competencies. Since then, pilot schools and others have developed methods for building the level of faculty expertise needed for nursing schools in the United States to teach these competencies in every program. Competencies have been institutionalized through inclusion in textbooks, standards of licensing, accreditation, and certification standards. This effort has now expanded to encourage faculty to develop innovation teaching strategies. Multiple national and regional workshops have been conducted to better prepare faculty to teach the quality and safety content implicit within the competencies. In 2012, leaders of the QSEN effort authored the text *Quality and Safety in Nursing: A Competency Approach to Improving Outcomes* (Sherwood & Barnsteiner, 2012). This book has quickly been adopted as a text for students and faculty as a source of further knowledge about quality and safety. For those APRNs who have not acquired basic competencies around quality and safety, that text is an important adjunct to this chapter.

In 2012, additional funding was received to extend the reach of the national QSEN initiative to graduate education programs. Graduate-level nursing competencies, building on the undergraduate competencies, were finalized in late 2012. This new funding provides educational resources and training to enhance the ability of faculty in master's and doctoral nursing programs to teach quality and safety competencies. The graduate-level competencies can be found at www.aacn.nche.edu /faculty/qsen/competencies.pdf (American Association of Colleges of Nursing, 2012).

CONCLUSION

This chapter described the legislation, regulation, and other policies implemented since 2010 to drive current safety and quality improvement efforts taking place across the country. Efforts to improve quality and safety are being measured by using the framework of structure, process, and outcomes. Outcome measures have become inextricably linked to new reimbursement strategies emerging from the CMS and private payers; these strategies have begun to force out fee for service approaches that have been in place for decades.

APRNs in any setting of care must acquire and effectively employ an understanding of how the measures are being used to quantify, publicly report, and reimburse their practices if they wish to survive financially. While some APRNs may not yet see visible evidence of the measurements being discussed, especially if working in large health systems, it may be because their numbers are being rolled in along with their physician counterparts. Every APRN should be seeking out information about how they are contributing to safe high-quality outcomes in order to both quantify their own successes and to understand how they are contributing to the bottom line.

In addition, this chapter provided numerous statistics to demonstrate the extent of the issues patients face relative to safety and quality when they seek care. To focus APRNs' attention on those aspects of care for which they have accountability for the patient's safety, the data described adverse events that included not only medication errors, but also errors of diagnosis, preventable infections, and wrong-site surgeries that lead to harm and even death. In addition to identifying barriers, this chapter focused on opportunities for APRNs to lead solutions focused on reducing preventable adverse events and even death. Central to all of these solutions is the importance of increasing transparency at all levels and among all providers in the health care delivery system. Work environments that emphasize transparency and public reporting, patient engagement, person-centered care, a just culture, continuous learning care organizations, health literate organizations, or HROs will most effectively support APRNs in preventing harm. What these work environments have in common are principles based on a belief that the patient and family are experts in their own right when it comes to health and health care decisions, and therefore must be at the core of care delivery and decision making. In addition, this chapter identified many strategies already proven to reduce errors and potential harm to patients that can and should be incorporated into the practice settings of APRNs.

Although APRNs must necessarily focus attention on the day-to-day activities of delivering patient care services that include diagnosis, assessment, and treatment, a focus on maintaining high-quality safe care must also be integrated into daily practice. Quality is not optional; little or no pay will occur for poor quality. Patients and their families expect to be full partners in every care encounter. This is the new world in which APRNs provide care. Policies have changed how that care will be provided, but it is the outcomes of the care APRNs provide that will be foremost in the minds of health care consumers.

DISCUSSION QUESTIONS

Assume you are setting up an independent group practice that subscribes to the safe environment philosophy outlined in this chapter. The practice will have two primary care nurse practitioners, a clinical nurse specialist in cardio-pulmonary, a certified diabetes educator (CDE), a medical technician, and a secretary. You anticipate a variety of patients, Spanish–English mix of 50–50, with about 20% families with school-age children, 50% working adults many from the local farm and meat packing industry, 20% from the over 55–70 population of retirees, and 10% over the age of 70. You have already set up a panel of referral physicians. Use this scenario to answer the questions below.

1. Select one of the following areas and develop an implementation plan for your practice showing how each of the members plays a part.
   a. Just culture
   b. Increased reliability
   c. Person centered care
2. Develop a plan for imbedding the concepts of health literacy and patient engagement into your practice. What barriers do you anticipate and how would you handle them?
3. How would you guarantee transparency in your practice setting?
4. What components of evidenced-based practice would be most pertinent to your practice?
5. What current health quality and safety regulations would impact your practice and how?
6. What components of the current health care and federal legislation might impact your practice and why?

REFERENCES

Acquaviva, K., Haskell, H., & Johnson, J. (2013). Human cognition and the dynamics of failure to rescue: The Lewis Blackman case. *Journal of Professional Nursing, 29*(2), 95–101.

Advisory Council on Alzheimer's Research, Care, and Services. (2013). *Inventories of federal efforts.* Retrieved from http://www.aspe.hhs.gov/daltcp/napa/092711/Mtg1-Slides2.pdf

Agency for Health Care Research and Quality (AHRQ). (2008). *Becoming a high reliability organization: Operational advice for hospital leaders.* Retrieved from http://www.ahrq.gov/professionals/quality-patient-safety/quality-resources/tools/hroadvice/hroadvice.pdf

AHRQ. (2010). *Health literacy universal precautions tool kit.* Retrieved from http://www.nchealthliteracy.org/toolkit/toolkit_w_appendix.pdf

AHRQ. (2013). *Downloading MONAHRQ® Software.* Retrieved from http://www.monahrq.ahrq.gov/monahrq_software.shtml

Altman, L. (1995). Big doses of chemotherapy drug killed patient, Hurt 2d. *The New York Times,* March 24, p. A18.

American Association of Colleges of Nursing. (2012). *Graduate-level QSEN competencies: Knowledge, skill and attitudes.* Retrieved from http://www.aacn.nche.edu/faculty/qsen/competencies.pdf

Consumer–Purchaser Disclosure Project. (2011). *Ten criteria for meaningful and usable measures of performance*. Retrieved from http://www.healthcaredisclosure.org/docs/files/CPDP_10_Measure_Criteria.pdf

Daughenbaugh, P., & Martin, K. (2011, November/December). The link between transparency and patient safety. Patient Safety and Quality Health Care. Retrieved from http://www.psqh.com/november-december-2011/1031-the-link-between-transparency-and-patient-safety.html

Deming, W. E. (1986). *Out of the crisis*. Cambridge, MA: MIT Press.

Donabedian, A. (2005). Evaluating the quality of medical care. *Milbank Quarterly, 83*(4), 691–729.

Gerteis, M., Edgman-Levitan, S., Daley, J., & Delbanco, T. L. (1993). *Through the patient's eyes: Understanding and promoting patient-centered care*. San Francisco, CA: Jossey-Bass.

Institute of Medicine (IOM). (1999). *To err is human: Building a safer health system*. Washington, DC: National Academy Press.

IOM. (2001). *Crossing the quality chasm: A new health system for the 21st century*. Washington, DC: National Academy Press.

IOM. (2012a). *Attributes of health literate organizations* (discussion paper). Washington, DC: National Academies Press.

IOM. (2012b). *Best care at lower cost: The path to continuously learning health care in America*. Washington, DC: National Academies Press.

King, S. (2009). *Josie's story*. New York, NY: Grove Press.

Leape, L. (2000). *Testimony before US Senate Subcommittee on Improving Health Care Safety*. Retrieved from http://articles.philly.com/2000-01-27/news/25598531_1_health-care-system-medical-errors-lucian-leape

Marx, D. (2009). *Whack-a-Mole*. Plano, TX: Your Side Studios.

National Committee on Quality Assurance (NCQA). (2013). *Quality compass*. Retrieved from http://www.ncqa.org/HEDISQualityMeasurement/QualityMeasurementProducts/QualityCompass.aspx

National Practitioner Data Bank (NPDB). (2013). *Health care organizations*. Retrieved from http://www.npdb-hipdb.hrsa.gov

Nursing Alliance for Quality Care (NAQC). (2013). *Fostering successful patient and family engagement: Nursing's critical role* (white paper). Retrieved from http://www.nursingAQC.org

Patient-Centered Outcomes Research Institute (PCORI). (2012). *Patient-centered outcomes research*. Retrieved from http://www.pcori.org/research-we-support/pcor

Pham, J., Aswani, M., Rosen, M., Lee, H., Huddle, M., Weeks, K., & Pronovost, P. (2012). Reducing medical errors and adverse events. *Annual Review of Medicine, 63*, 447–463.

Shekelle, P. G., Pronovost, P. J., Wachter, R. M., McDonald, K. M., Schoelles, K., Dy, S. M., … Walshe, K. (2013, March 5). The top patient safety strategies that can be encouraged for adoption now. *Annals of Internal Medicine, 158*, 365–368.

Sherwood, G., & Barnsteiner, J. (Eds.). (2012). *Quality and safety in nursing: A competency approach to improving outcomes*. West Sussex, United Kingdom: Wiley-Blackwell & Sons.

Sofaer, S., & Schumann, M. J. (March 15, 2013). Fostering successful patient and family engagement: Nursing's critical role. *Nursing alliance for quality care*. Washington, DC. Retrieved from http://www.naqc.org/WhitePaper-PatientEngagement

Moving Toward Accountable Care: A Policy Framework to Transform Health Care Delivery and Reimbursement

Susan M. Kendig

innovative reimbursement models

Fragmentation is a common denominator in the delivery of health care services in the United States, supported by the current fee for service system that rewards volume and intensity of services ahead of value and care coordination. Even when patients access health care services that meet high-quality standards, discontinuities in care coordination among multiple providers and sites fosters fragmentation and lack of accountability. The resulting "vacuum of accountability" leads to less than optimal patient outcomes and inefficient use of scarce health care resources (Guterman & Drake, 2010). Innovative reimbursement models designed to encourage providers to improve quality and value through care coordination are recognized as one mechanism with the potential to transform health care delivery.

The Patient Protection and Affordable Care Act of 2010 Pub. L. 111-148 ("PPACA" or "the Act") provides sweeping legislation that attempts to curb health care costs, improve health care quality, and increase access to care through affordable health insurance coverage. Titles III through VI, which make up over 50% of the bill, focus on improvements in quality and cost efficiency. Specifically, Title III focuses on linking payment to quality outcomes through the development of alternate care delivery models and payment structures (PPACA, 2010a).

In addition to introducing the "Medicare Shared Savings Program," which provides the framework for the Accountable Care Organization (ACO) model, the Act also authorizes the Secretary of the U.S. Department of Health and Human Services (the Secretary) to initiate programs and demonstration projects designed to control costs and improve the quality of care provided to Medicare, Medicaid, and CHIP beneficiaries. This chapter will provide an overview of the Act's ACO provisions and examples of PPACA's programs and demonstration projects that may inform ACO development. The Medicare Shared Savings Model's potential influence on private payer initiatives will be discussed.

accountable core organization

SETTING THE STAGE FOR ACOs: POLICY-DRIVEN ALTERNATE HEALTH CARE REIMBURSEMENT MODELS

Although PPACA has served to heighten interest in the development of alternate care delivery and payment models, Congress has passed prior legislation designed to move the Centers for Medicare and Medicaid Services (CMS) from a passive purchaser of volume-based health care to an active purchaser of value-based, high-quality health care. Earlier Medicare programs and demonstration projects authorized by Congress have targeted health care quality and efficiency improvements through payment reform. For example, the Medicare Prescription Drug and Modernization Act of 2003 (MMA), extended by the Deficit Reduction Act of 2005 (DRA), linked Medicare payments to hospital quality reporting. Under these statutes, hospitals reporting on specific quality measures received their full Medicare annual payment update; whereas those who failed to participate in the quality reporting initiative saw a 2% reduction in their annual payment update (MMA, 2003, Deficit Reduction Act of 2005, 2006a). Similarly, the Tax Relief and Health Care Act of 2006 (TRHCA, 2006a) and the Medicare Improvements Patients and Providers Act of 2008 (MIPPA, 2008) linked the Medicare value-based purchasing initiatives to physicians, providing bonuses to physicians reporting on specific quality measures. In 2009, the American Recovery and Reinvestment Act (ARRA, 2009) provided for financial incentives to providers that "meaningfully use" electronic health records as a quality improvement tool. These are but a few of the policy driven attempts to improve health care quality and efficiency that were underway well before PPACA's passage. *patient-population and services can act*

When PPACA became the law of the land in 2010, it authorized the Secretary to further explore provider reimbursement models aimed at driving down health care costs while maintaining or improving patient outcomes through quality and efficiency improvements. Under PPACA, new programs and demonstration projects were established, and current demonstration projects with implications for payment reform were extended. Some of these programs and demonstration projects created or extended by PPACA have significant implications for ACO development and implementation.

RELEVANT DEMONSTRATION PROJECTS AUTHORIZED BY PPACA

The National Pilot Program on Payment Bundling

The National Pilot Program on Payment Bundling is designed to develop and evaluate bundled payments for integrated care that includes acute, inpatient, and post-acute care for an episode of care beginning 3 days prior to hospital admission and continuing for 30 days postdischarge. The program goal is to improve coordination, quality, and efficiency of services around a hospitalization related to selected conditions (PPACA, 2010b).

The Independence at Home Demonstration Project

This initiative will test a payment incentive and service delivery model that utilizes physician and nurse practitioner-directed teams to deliver home-based primary care services to high-need Medicare beneficiaries. The teams will be available to provide care and home-based services 24 hours per day, 7 days per week. Participating independence at home medical practices teams will share in savings accomplished by reducing preventable hospitalizations and readmissions and other improvements in efficiencies of care and patient outcomes (PPACA, 2010c).

The Pediatric ACO Demonstration Project

In addition to the Medicare Shared Savings Program, PPACA provides for the development of Medicaid ACO models of care targeting the pediatric population. Under this provision, participating states may allow pediatric medical care providers who meet specific requirements to be recognized as an ACO. Such providers would be eligible to receive incentive payments in the same manner as a Medicare ACO, but for Medicaid and CHIP program savings (PPACA, 2010d).

Health Home for Medicaid and Medicare Beneficiaries With Chronic Disease

States, through a state plan amendment, may choose to provide medical care to Medicaid beneficiaries with chronic disease through a "health home," under different reimbursement models designed to promote quality and efficiency of care. Individuals eligible to participate in the health home include those who have two chronic conditions; those who have one chronic condition, and are at risk for developing a second chronic condition; or persons with one serious and persistent mental health condition. Health home services are comprehensive, timely services provided by a designated provider working within a health care team. Services are designed to include comprehensive care management, care coordination, health promotion, comprehensive transitional care, patient and family support, and referral to relevant community and social support services. Health information technology is used to link services, track data, and guide quality improvement (PPACA, 2010e).

Center for Medicare and Medicaid Innovation

This division of the CMS was created within the Act for the purpose of testing innovative payment and delivery models designed to improve quality and decrease costs. The models will address a defined population for which there are deficits in care leading to poor clinical outcomes or avoidable expenditures. The overall goal is to test innovative, comprehensive payment models that drive down health care costs through improved quality and efficiency (PPACA, 2010f).

Through PPACA, $10 billion was appropriated to the Center for Medicare and Medicaid Innovation (CMMI) to support innovation activities from 2011 through 2019. Since its inception, CMMI has been responsible for awarding funding to test innovations throughout the country. CMMI's portfolio includes Innovation Models in seven categories: accountable care, bundled payments for care improvement, primary care transformation, initiatives focused on the Medicaid and CHIP population, initiatives focused on Medicare–Medicaid enrollees, initiatives to accelerate development and testing of new payment and service delivery models, and initiatives to speed adoption of best practices. One example is the Pioneer ACO Model that awarded funding to 32 health care organizations and providers already experienced in patient care coordination across health care settings. The Pioneer ACO Program is designed to help these groups move more rapidly from a shared savings payment model to a population-based payment model on a track consistent with, but separate from, the Medicare Shared Services Program. The Pioneer ACO Program will provide more information about aligning accountable care processes with private payers to improve health and quality outcomes while driving down cost in both the public and private sector (CMMI, 2011).

Common throughout the PPACA initiatives is a theme of payment reform moving from a fee for service to payment for quality and value (CMMI, 2010). Given the significant amount of funding appropriated to and immediately available from CMMI, these funding opportunities have the potential to spark new collaborative efforts to achieve a cost and quality goals. Learnings from the demonstration projects enumerated in the statute and the CMMI initiatives will help to inform successful ACO models in both the public and private sectors.

THE ACCOUNTABLE CARE MODEL

ACOs are "provider groups that accept responsibility for the cost and quality of care delivered to a specific population of patients cared for by the groups' clinicians," and provide data to assess performance on cost and quality criteria (Shortell, Casalino, & Fisher, 2010). The organizational model has three features:

- local accountability for effective management of the full continuum of care;
- shared savings based on historical trends as adjusted for different populations; and
- performance measurement such as clinical outcomes, quality, and patient experience (Guterman & Drake, 2010).

Rather than focusing on providing singular care and billing for volume of services provided to an individual patient, the ACO model seeks to influence the health and wellness of a defined population, throughout the continuum of care. By accepting risk for a defined population, ACOs can receive a share of the savings accrued when efficiency of care is increased through quality and service delivery improvements. This is referred to as "upside" risk. Likewise, if such quality and cost benchmarks are not met, at a minimum the ACO receives no shared savings or may lose revenues through "downside" risk.

The ACO model may seem strikingly similar to the early Health Maintenance Organization (HMO) or Managed Care Organization (MCO) models that sought to drive down escalating health care costs by using financial incentives for managing populations in a less costly manner. However, accountable care models differ from the HMOs and MCOs of the past by assigning care management to a group of health care providers instead of payers, focusing on measurable outcomes, and leveraging technology advancements for risk adjustment, advanced analytics, and health data management (Muhlestein, Crowshaw, Merrill, Pena, & James, 2013). Rather than focusing on cost containment, the ACO is premised on health management that generates improved patient outcomes, which in turn will result in decreased cost.

TABLE 21.1 Comparison of Core Requirements of Traditional Versus Accountable Care

	TRADITIONAL CARE	ACCOUNTABLE CARE
Reimbursement model	Fee-for-service payment for individual visits, services, or procedures	Bear financial risk for a defined population
Patient care	Focus on individual patient at point of access to care	Coordinated, patient-focused system of clinical care for a defined population across the health care service continuum
Quality	Focus on individual patient- and/or site-specific outcomes. Cost and quality not linked	Provide measured outcomes related to both population health outcomes and cost efficiencies

The Medicare Shared Savings Model is built on earlier initiatives, including CMS's Physician Group Practice Demonstration (PGP). The PGP demonstration included 10 provider groups ranging from free standing physician group practices to integrated delivery systems. The groups continued to receive their usual fee-for service payments and also received bonuses for improving care through improved service delivery and care coordination, driven by quality and efficiency improvements. By year 3, all 10 sites had achieved success on most quality measures, with two groups meeting benchmarks on all 32 quality measures and five groups had achieved savings sufficient to trigger the shared savings bonus (CMS, 2009; McClellan, McKethan, Lewis, Roski, & Fisher, 2010). At the end of the fifth year, seven of the 10 groups had met benchmarks on all 32 quality measures and four met cost-efficiency benchmarks (CMS, 2011).

THE MEDICARE SHARED SAVINGS PROGRAM

In their 2009 Report to Congress, the Medicare Payment Advisory Commission (MedPAC) identified the ACO model as one tool for achieving payment and delivery system reform (MedPAC, 2009). Furthermore, MedPAC recommended that ACOs be compensated through a model that combines fee-for-service with financial incentives to reduce cost, improve quality, and achieve information transparency (MedPAC, 2009).

Consistent with the MedPAC recommendation, PPACA specifies a voluntary ACO program as a means to better align financial incentives with quality and cost goals. The Medicare Shared Savings Program is unique within PPACA. Unlike the National Pilot Program on Payment Bundling and other pilots and demonstration projects authorized under PPACA, the Medicare Shared Savings Program creates, in statute, a new clinical model and accompanying payment strategy premised on meeting quality and cost efficiency metrics.

The Act directed CMS to create the national voluntary program for ACOs by January, 2012, and to set forth eligibility requirements for ACO participation in the federal program (PPACA, 2010g). The ACO framework provided in PPACA §3022 outlines the eligibility criteria to participate as an ACO, required elements for ACO activities, reporting requirements, and a payment methodology. The following paragraphs provide a summary of key ACO requirements as presented in §3022.

ACO Providers

The following groups of service providers that have established a mechanism for shared governance are eligible to participate as an ACO:

- ACO professionals in group practice arrangements;
- Networks of individual practices of ACO professionals;
- Partnerships or joint venture arrangements between hospitals and ACO professionals;
- Hospitals employing ACO professionals; and
- Other groups as deemed appropriate by the Secretary.

PPACA defines ACO professionals according to XVIII of the Social Security Act (PPACA, 2010g). Under this definition, an ACO professional is defined as a physician, including a doctor of medicine or osteopathy, doctor of dental surgery or medicine, a podiatrist, optometrist, or chiropractor licensed by the state (U.S. Government

Printing Office, 2010a). Practitioners, defined as a physician assistant, nurse practitioner, clinical nurse specialist, certified registered nurse anesthetist, clinical social worker, clinical psychologist, or registered dietitian or nutrition professional, are also eligible to participate as ACO professionals (U.S. Government Printing Office, 2010b).

General Requirements

In order to qualify for recognition as a Medicare ACO, the Medicare Shared Savings provisions identify the following general requirements. The Medicare ACO must:

- be willing to be accountable for quality, cost, and overall care of their assigned Medicare fee-for-service beneficiaries
- agree to participate for 3 years
- have a formal legal structure to allow for receipt and distribution of shared savings payments
- include a sufficient number of ACO professionals to care for assigned Medicare beneficiaries
- have a minimum of 5,000 assigned Medicare beneficiaries
- have sufficient ACO professionals as determined necessary by the Secretary to support the assignment of Medicare fee-for-service beneficiaries and implementation of the quality and administrative requirements
- have in place a leadership and management structure that includes clinical and administrative systems
- have defined processes to promote evidence-based medicine and patient engagement, reporting on quality and cost measures, and care coordination
- meet patient-centeredness criteria as defined by the Secretary.

(U.S. Government Printing Office, 2010b)

Quality and Reporting Requirements

Participating ACOs are required to report data to CMS for the evaluation of the quality of care furnished by the ACO. Medicare ACOs are required to report on 33 quality measures, as well as a survey of patient experience of care. The quality measures are divided into four domains: patient/caregiver experience, care coordination/patient safety, preventive health, and at risk populations. The "At Risk Population" domain specifically targets metrics relevant to diabetes, hypertension, ischemic vascular disease, and coronary artery disease (Department of Health and Human Services, 2011). In order to be eligible for the shared savings, ACOs must meet minimum attainment levels in each domain. Failure to report quality data accurately, completely, and in a timely manner may result in the ACO's termination from the Medicare Shared Savings Program, and loss of financial incentives (U.S. Code of Federal Regulations, 2011a).

Payments and Treatment of Savings

At the start of each agreement period, the Secretary will set the ACO's established benchmark using the ACO's most recent available 3 years of per-beneficiary expenditures for Medicare Parts A and B services. Participating ACOs will be eligible to receive payment for shared savings if the ACO meets the established quality performance standards and their estimated average Medicare expenditure for each Medicare fee-for-service beneficiary for Medicare Part A and B services is at least the established percent below the established benchmark. If the ACO meets the accepted performance standards, a percent of the difference between the established benchmark and the average per capita annual Medicare expenditures may be paid to the ACO as shared savings.

APRNs WITHIN THE ACO FRAMEWORK

This discussion provides only a summary of the statutory provisions and the implementing regulations related to recognition as a Medicare ACO. Although the ACO general requirements described here appear to be fairly straightforward, over 500 pages of regulations and comments provide clarification and guidance to meeting the ACO's statutory provisions. Despite the vast amount of statutory and regulatory material related to ACOs, APRNs should be aware of key concepts and their potential impact on APRN practice and ACO success. Specifically, the requirements related to number of patients receiving care within the ACO, the ability to achieve quality and cost benchmarks, and patient-centeredness criteria may be influenced by the treatment of APRNs within the ACO provisions, as well as their utilization within the ACO itself.

Attribution of ACO Beneficiaries

Medicare beneficiaries are assigned, or "attributed to," a specific ACO based on a formula described in the ACO regulations. Despite the inclusion of APRNs within the definition of ACO professionals, the statute and its implementing regulations effectively limit APRN practices from joining or establishing ACOs within the Medicare Shared Savings Program by basing assignment of beneficiaries solely on primary care services provided by a physician (PPACA, 2010g). Although APRNs can participate in ACOs as ACO professionals, patients who choose an APRN as their primary care provider cannot be counted as beneficiaries for Medicare Shared Savings purposes. Because the statute explicitly defines "primary care services provided by a physician" as the sole predicate for beneficiary assignment to an ACO, the APRN's patients are precluded from being assigned to an ACO and any resulting benefits from ACO participation. CMS could not change this statutory language within the rulemaking process. However, recognizing that APRNs and other nonphysician health care providers can be significant assets to ACO success in achieving quality and cost-efficiency improvements, CMS sought a solution to this issue in the ACO rules through a stepwise approach to beneficiary assignment (Department of Health and Human Services, 2011). Under the final rule, beneficiaries are first assigned to an ACO if the allowable charges for primary services accessed by the patient were provided by a primary care physician within the ACO and if such charges were greater than the allowable charges for primary care services accessed through other ACOs or non-ACO providers. In Step 2, among the remainder of beneficiaries who have received at least one primary care physician service within the ACO and have not accessed other primary care services by any other primary care physician either within or outside of the ACO, the beneficiary will be assigned to the ACO if the allowable charges for primary care services by all ACO professionals who are providers (such as APRNs) within the ACO are greater than charges for such services by ACO professionals working in another ACO, or by physicians, nurse practitioners, and other nonphysician providers working in a non-ACO setting (U.S. Government, 2011b). Although an imperfect solution, this regulatory "fix" provides a mechanism for recognition of care by physician specialists, APRNs, and other nonphysician providers in driving assignment of beneficiaries to a specific ACO. In addition to placing an unnecessary barrier to patient participation in ACOs, the stepwise approach to assignment of beneficiaries may have implications for the ACO's overall success in meeting some of the general ACO requirements.

Attaining and Maintaining 5,000 Medicare Beneficiaries

The requirement that ACOs must have and maintain a minimum of 5,000 Medicare beneficiaries could also pose challenges to ACOs. Medicare fee-for-service beneficiaries are assigned to the ACOs, as described above, solely for the purpose of holding the ACO accountable for both the quality and cost of care to the beneficiary. The assigned beneficiary retains their "full rights as Medicare fee-for-service beneficiaries" to seek and receive care from their choice of health care providers who may not be part of their assigned ACO (Department of Health and Human Services, 2011). This means that ACO patients may seek care both within and outside of the ACO. If the ACO patient seeks care that is not recommended by the ACO professional, the patient's cost and quality metrics may be compromised, thus affecting the ACO's overall performance and ultimately access to shared savings. Likewise, if the ACO's assigned population drops below 5,000, the ACO's agreement can be terminated and the ACO will be ineligible to share in any savings (U.S. Government, 2011c). This means that ACOs must actively engage patients in their care, not only to improve their quality metrics, but also to maintain the required amount of beneficiaries necessary to maintain a viable ACO.

Patient Activation and Engagement

The Institute of Medicine (IOM) lists patient-centeredness as one of six aims for health care system improvement (Institute of Medicine, Committee on Quality of Health Care in America, 2001). In 2008, the National Priorities Partnership (NPP) identified patient and family engagement as one of six priorities with the most potential to reduce harm, eliminate disparities, decrease disease burden, and remove inefficiencies in health care delivery (National Priorities Partnership, 2008). Given the significance placed on patient-centeredness by these and other similar national recommendations, it is not surprising that ACOs are required to define processes to promote patient engagement and demonstrate that they meet patient-centeredness criteria (PPACA, 2010g).

Patient-centeredness means "providing care that is respectful of and responsive to individual patient preferences, needs, and values, and ensuring that patient values guide all clinical decisions" (Institute of Medicine, Committee on Quality of Health Care in America, 2001). The aim focuses on the patient's experience of illness and health care, and the effectiveness of health care delivery systems in meeting their individual needs. Patient-centeredness, as defined by the IOM, encompasses the qualities of compassion, empathy, and responsiveness to the patient's *expressed* needs and preferences related to the health care experience (Institute of Medicine, Committee on Quality of Health Care in America, 2001). Within the context of the ACO statute and regulations required to implement it, patient-centeredness criteria means that patient-centered care must be promoted by the ACO's governing body and integrated into practice by leadership and management working with the ACO's health care teams (Department of Health and Human Services, 2011).

Since inception of the term by the IOM, health care providers have struggled to identify, incorporate, and evaluate patient-centeredness in practice. Patient surveys of satisfaction with the health care experience are frequently used to evaluate patient-centered care (Davies et al., 2008). Criteria regarding ease of access to care, provider–patient communication, provider knowledge of the patient's history, responsiveness of office staff, care coordination, and general satisfaction with the health care provider and staff are examples of surrogates for patient-centered care (Davies, 2008; Rodriguez, 2009a). Consistent with these criteria, the ACO regulations cite eight elements as surrogates for proof of patient centeredness:

- A beneficiary experience of care survey with an accompanying quality improvement plan
- Patient involvement in ACO governance
- A culturally competent process and description of such process for evaluating the health needs of the assigned population
- Systems to identify high-risk individuals and processes to develop individualized care plans that integrate community resources for the targeted population
- Care coordination processes that include electronic technologies consistent with meaningful use criteria
- Health literacy processes to support communication of clinical knowledge to beneficiaries that allow for beneficiary engagement and shared decision making
- Written standards and a process for beneficiaries to access their medical records
- Internal processes to measure physician clinical or service performance across practices that are used to drive a quality improvement plan.

(U.S. Code of Federal Regulations, 2011d)

However, emerging evidence suggests that current team models may not meet some patient-centeredness measures. Approximately three-fourths of patients receiving team-based care in one large study rated the provider's communication skills and comprehensiveness of knowledge about the patient unfavorably. Patient satisfaction studies suggest that most primary care patients experience "invisible" team care, where the roles and identities of clinicians involved in their care, such as APRNs, are not clear to the patient (Safran, 2003). Visible teams (teams where the provider role is known to and understood by the patient) with a strong relationship focus (comprehensive care and coordination among all team members) are linked to higher quality primary care experiences (Rodriguez, 2009a).

Former CMS Director Berwick suggests that proper incorporation of patient-centeredness into new health care designs will "involve some radical, unfamiliar, and disruptive shifts in control and power, out of the hand of those who give care and into the hands of those who receive it" (Berwick, 2009). Although the new reimbursement models resulting from the Act support a team-based approach to care, the type of radical change Berwick describes as necessary to achieving patient-centeredness may be difficult to achieve if existing research on primary care structure and culture holds true. Evidence suggests that when practices attempt change, they often maintain existing structures without fundamentally evaluating and redefining team members' roles (Chesluck & Holmboe, 2010). Successful transition to a care model that utilizes each member to their full scope of practice and ability will require substantial communication, collaboration and flexibility among health care providers and staff, explicit communication with patients regarding team members' roles and responsibilities, and an organizational culture that fosters collaboration. Currently, primary care teams are used most often to create access. New care delivery models will require not only the physician, but each member of the health care team to create a sustained partnership with the patient (Chesluck & Holmboe, 2010).

Although "patient-centeredness" is only one of eight ACO requirements listed in the Act, it has the potential to significantly impact benchmarking criteria. Evidence suggests that emphasis on clinical quality and patient experience criteria, as opposed to productivity and efficiency, are associated with greater improvement in care coordination and office staff interaction (Rodriguez, 2009b). Attention to patient experience measures will be important in meeting ACO quality performance benchmarks.

Meeting Quality and Cost-Efficiency Measures

ACOs must meet quality benchmarks in four domains in order to qualify for shared savings. Poor care coordination and discretionary medical interventions contribute to inefficient utilization of health care resources and higher health care costs. Regional variations in health care spending are associated with variability in primary care provider discretionary decision making. Patients receive approximately half of the recommended processes for leading acute and chronic conditions (McGlynn et al., 2003). Care coordination and communication failures are linked to increased hospitalizations and readmission rates contributing to large Medicare expenditures (Jencks, 2009; Piekes, Chen, Schore, & Brown, 2009). APRNs consistently demonstrate positive rankings on overall levels of patient satisfaction, consultation time, and preventive screenings (Lenz, Mundinger, Kane, Hopkins, & Lin, 2004). It is likely that effective integration of APRNs into accountable care models will have a positive effect on cost and quality metrics.

Efficient, cost-effective care delivery requires access to patient information, decision support, and timely access to benchmarking data. The ACO serves as the information and data center for its population. Information technologies (IT) and analytical resources are necessary to achieve the level of clinical integration necessary to improve quality, reduce costs, and track performance against explicit quantitative benchmarking targets. Importantly, the Act authorizes the Secretary to determine each ACO's benchmarks for shared savings using the respective ACO's historical spending and utilization data (PPACA, 2010g). Accurate and complete ACO specific quality and cost information will be essential to maximizing the financial incentives. Appropriate IT systems and tools, such as disease registries that enable population-based decision making and predictive modeling to identify high-risk patients in need of care coordination, will be critical in facilitating the level of communication, data collection, monitoring, evaluation, and reporting activities necessary to fully support and capture the ACO's quality and cost improvements (Fields, Leshen, & Patel, 2010).

NON-MEDICARE SHARED SAVINGS PROGRAMS

Although the "accountable care" concept existed well before PPACA's passage in March 2010, the Act generated renewed interest in the ACO model. Two such accountable care-based models that preceded PPACA are the Group Health Cooperative of Puget Sound and Geisinger Health Systems' approach to integration.

The Group Health Cooperative of Puget Sound (Group Health) was founded in 1947. True to the founders' belief that "health was everybody's business and everybody's right," Group Health is one of only a few consumer-governed health plans in the United States. The majority of Group Health members receive care through the co-op's integrated network of primary care, specialty care, and hospital providers.

Consumer-based governance and reimbursement strategies that reward better care through quality and cost-efficiency improvements drive the innovation (Larson, 2009).

Geisinger is an integrated health system serving a large swath of central and northeastern Pennsylvania. This predominantly rural area is covered by Geisinger's employed primary care and specialty physicians, acute and specialty care hospitals, ambulatory surgery campuses, the Geisinger Health Plan (GHP), and other clinical and community-based outreach programs. The Geisinger Model is an organized system of care with many examples of clinical integration. Geisinger leverages the patients for whom Geisinger is both financially responsible, through their health plan (GHP), and clinically, through their care providers, to foster innovation (Paulus, Davis, & Steele, 2008). Geisinger's Proven Care model for managing acute episodes of care is looked to as a successful model of what application of evidence driven standardized care paths, aligned with significant financial incentives, can achieve.

The requirements for ACO participation as set forth in the Act create a broad framework for ACO implementation. As a result, several ACO models have been suggested, ranging from integrated delivery systems to "virtual ACOs" that encompass a wide range of small practices and providers in disparate locations. Despite variation in suggested organizational structures, the core concept of joint accountability for quality and cost improvement remains constant.

Although Medicare's version of ACOs has been formalized in statute and regulation, a variety of non-Medicare ACO models have emerged. In addition to the CMS recognized ACOs, private accountable care models sponsored by providers, such as hospital systems or independent provider associations, or insurance companies are present in the health care market. The majority of this first wave of ACOs is centered in areas with larger populations. Although hospital system-led ACOs remain as the majority model, physician group led models continue to grow (Muhlestein et al., 2013). While the framework for the Medicare ACOs is more proscriptive by virtue of the statutory and regulatory requirements, private models have more leeway to experiment with different approaches to population management and reimbursement.

CONCLUSION

As new accountable care models are developed in the private market, barriers to full utilization of APRNs must be identified and addressed. First, while the majority of both Medicare and non-Medicare ACOs currently reside in more densely populated areas and are hospital-led, as success is demonstrated in improved outcomes and cost efficiencies, it is likely that variations of the model will spread into more rural areas and to more vulnerable populations accessing care among safety net providers. Given current provider shortages and decreased access to care, APRNs provide a logical solution to expanding care in these areas.

Health care transformation to a quality and value-driven system, informed by best practices gleaned from evolving clinical integration demonstrations, has the potential to improve both individual and population health. Organizational structure, information technology capabilities, and strong quality improvement strategies are priorities in preparing for transition to an accountable care model. Practice patterns and patient factors are important considerations to inform the process. Evaluation of all of these factors and implementation of changes to support intra- and interpractice team collaboration and coordination is necessary to assure success in meeting quality and efficiency benchmarks, and ultimately transforming health care service delivery to a patient centric, value-driven model.

DISCUSSION QUESTIONS

1. The APRN skill set could be critical to the success of an ACO or clinical integration model. Consider the following:
   a. What types of unique skills does the APRN bring to the table that would significantly contribute to an ACO's successful achievement of quality and cost efficiency benchmarks?
   b. How can APRNs best articulate the necessity for their skill sets within the ACO team?
2. Consider the Medicare Shared Savings Program framework set forth in PPACA.
   a. Describe the points where APRNs seem to be most included in the framework.
   b. Discuss areas where APRNs could make the greatest impact within the framework.
   c. Discuss areas where APRNs are least included within the framework.
   d. With reference to areas that are less supportive of APRN inclusion, discuss how APRNs may affect policy change that is more favorable to APRN practice.
3. The ACO and ACO-like models are premised on the proposition that providers will access a share of "savings" that are directly attributable to meeting and exceeding quality and cost-benchmarks. Such models are often referred to as "provider incentives."
   a. If a practice is participating in a "shared savings model" how should APRNs be included?
   b. How could you broach the subject of APRN access to shared savings if you were employed by an ACO?
4. Access the CMMI website.
   a. Review a minimum of two payment/health care delivery models being tested.
   b. Identify any open requests for proposals.
   c. Discuss how an APRN-led model of care could be developed in response to one of these proposals.

REFERENCES

American Recovery and Reinvestment Act of 2009. Pub. L. 111-5.

Berwick, D. (2009). What patient-centered should mean: Confessions of an extremist. *Health Affairs, 28*(4), 555–565.

Chesluck, B., & Holmboe, E. S. (2010). How teams work—or don't—in primary care: A field study on internal medicine practices. *Health Affairs, 29*(5), 874–879.

Center for Medicare and Medicaid Innovation (CMMI). (2010). *The CMS Innovation Center.* Retrieved from http://www.innovation.cms.gov

CMMI. (2011). *Pioneer ACO Model.* Retrieved from http://www.innovation.cms.gov/initiatives /Pioneer-ACO-Model

Centers for Medicare and Medicaid Services (CMS). (2009). *Fact sheet: Medicare physician group demonstration—Physician groups continue to improve quality and generate savings under Medicare physician pay-for-performance demonstration.* Baltimore, MD: Author.

CMS. (2011, July). *Fact sheet: Medicare physician group demonstration—Physician groups continue to improve quality and generate savings under Medicare physician pay-for-performance demonstration.* Retrieved from http://www.cms.gov/Medicare/Demonstration-Projects/DemoProjectsEvalRpts/downloads /PGP_Fact_Sheet.pdf

Davies, E., Shaller, D., Edgman-Levitan, S., Safran, D. G., Oftedahl, G., Sakowski, H., & Cleary, P. D. (2008). Evaluating the use of a modified CAHPS survey to support improvements in patient-centered care: Lessons from a quality improvement collaborative. *Health Expectations, 11*, 160–176.

Deficit Reduction Act of 2005. Pub. L. 109-171, U.S.C. §5001(a).

Department of Health and Human Services. (2011, November 2). *Medicare program; Medicare shared savings program: Accountable Care Organizations* (Vol. 76, No. 212). Federal Register. Retrieved from http://www.gpo.gov/fdsys/pkg/FR-2011-11-02/pdf/2011-27461.pdf

Fields, D., Leshen, E., & Patel, K. (2010). Analysis and commentary: Driving quality gains and cost savings through adoption of medical homes. *Health Affairs, 29*(5), 819–826.

Guterman, S., & Drake, H. (2010). *Developing innovative payment approaches: Finding the path to high performance.* Washington, DC: Commonwealth Fund.

Institute of Medicine (IOM), Committee on Quality of Health Care in America. (2001). *Crossing the quality chasm: A new health system for the 21st century.* Washington, DC: National Academies Press.

Jencks, S. F., Williams, M. V., & Coleman, E. A. (2009). Rehospitalizations among patients in the Medicare fee-for-service program. *New England Journal of Medicine, 360*(14), 1418–1428.

Larson, E. B. (2009). Group Health Cooperative—One coverage and delivery model for accountable care. *New England Journal of Medicine, 36*(17), 1620–1622.

Lenz, E. R., Mundinger, M. O., Kane, R. L., Hopkins, S. C., & Lin, S. X. (2004). Primary care outcomes in patients treated by nurse practitioners or physicians: Two year follow-up. *Medical Care & Research Review, 61*(3), 332–351.

McClellan, M. M., McKethan, A. N., Lewis, J. L., Roski, J., & Fisher, E. S. (2010). A national strategy to put accountable care into practice. *Health Affairs, 29*(5), 982–990.

McGlynn, E. A., Asch, S. M., Adams, J., Keesey, J., Hicks, J., DeCristofaro, A., & Kerr, E. A. (2003). The quality of health care delivered to adults in the United States. *New England Journal of Medicine, 348*, 2635–2645.

MedPAC. (2009, June). *Report to Congress: Improving incentives in the Medicare program.* Retrieved from http://www.medpac.gov/documents/jun09_entirereport.pdf

MIPPA. (2008). Pub. L. 110-275, U.S.C. §131(b).

MMA. (2003). Pub. L. 108-73, U.S.C. §501(b).

Muhlestein, D. C., Crowshaw, A., Merrill, T., Pena, C., & James, B. (2013). *The Accountable Care Paradigm: More than just Managed Care 2.0.* Salt Lake City, UT: Leavitt Partners.

National Priorities Partnership (NPP). (2008). *National priorities and goals: Aligning our efforts to transform America's healthcare.* Washington, DC: National Quality Forum.

PPACA. (2010a). *(Pub. L. 111-148).*

PPACA. (2010b). *(Pub. L. 111-148) § 3023.*

PPACA. (2010c). *(Pub. L. 111-148) § 3024.*

PPACA. (2010d). *(Pub. L. 111-148) § 2706.*

PPACA. (2010e). *(Pub. L. 111-148) § 2703.*

PPACA. (2010f). *(Pub. L. 111-148) § 3021.*

PPACA. (2010g). *(Pub. L. 111-148) § 3022.*

Paulus, R. A., Davis, K., & Steele, G. D. (2008). Continuous innovation in health care: Implication of the Geisinger experience. *Health Affairs, 27*(5), 1235–1245.

Piekes, D. C., Chen, A., Schore, J., & Brown, R. (2009). Effects of care coordination on hospitalization, quality of care, and health expenditures among Medicare beneficiaries. *Journal of the American Medical Association, 301*(6), 603-618.

Rodriguez, H. P., von Glahn, T., Elliott, M. N., Rogers, W. H., & Safran, D. G. (2009a). The effect of performance-based incentives on improving patient care experiences: A statewide evaluation. *Journal of General Internal Medicine, 24*(12), 1281–1288.

Rodriguez, H. P., Scoggins, J. F., von Glahn, T., Zaslavsky, A. M., & Safran, D. G. (2009b). Attributing sources of variation in patients' experiences of ambulatory care. *Medical Care, 47*(8), 835–841.

Safran, D. G. (2003). Defining the future of primary care: What can we learn from patients? *Annals of Internal Medicine, 138*(3), 248–255.

Shortell, S. C., Casalino, L. P., & Fisher, E. S. (2010). How the Center for Medicare and Medicaid Innovation should test Accountable Care Organizations. *Health Affairs, 29*(7) 1293–1298.

Tax Relief and Health Care Act of 2006. Pub. L. 109-4332, Div. B, U.S.C. §101(b).

U.S. Code of Federal Regulations. (2010a). 42 U.S.C. § 1861(r)(l). Washington, DC: U.S. Government Printing Office.

U.S. Code of Federal Regulations. (2010b). 42 U.S.C. § 1842(b)(18)(C)(i). Washington, DC: U.S. Government Printing Office.

U.S. Code of Federal Regulations. (2011a). 42 CFR §425.502(d). Washington, DC: U.S. Government Printing Office.

U.S. Code of Federal Regulations. (2011b). 42 CFR § 425.402. *U.S. Code of Federal Regulations*. Washington, DC: U.S. Government Printing Office.

U.S. Code of Federal Regulations. (2011c). 42 CFR § 425.110. Washington, DC: U.S. Government Printing Office.

U.S. Code of Federal Regulations. (2011d). 42 CFR § 425.112(2). Washington, DC: U.S. Government Printing Office.

CHAPTER 22

A Systemic Approach to Containing Health Care Spending

*Ezekiel Emanuel, Neera Tanden, Stuart Altman, Scott Armstrong,
Donald Berwick, François de Brantes, Maura Calsyn, Michael Chernew,
John Colmers, David Cutler, Tom Daschle, Paul Egerman, Bob Kocher,
Arnold Milstein, Emily Oshima Lee, John D. Podesta, Uwe Reinhardt,
Meredith Rosenthal, Joshua Sharfstein, Stephen Shortell, Andrew Stern,
Peter R. Orszag, and Topher Spiro*

National health spending is projected to continue to grow faster than the economy, increasing from 18% to about 25% of the gross domestic product (GDP) by 2037 (Congressional Budget Office, 2012). Federal health spending is projected to increase from 25% to approximately 40% of total federal spending by 2037 (Congressional Budget Office, 2012). These trends could squeeze out critical investments in education and infrastructure, contribute to unsustainable debt levels, and constrain wage increases for the middle class (Emanuel, 2012; Emanuel & Fuchs, 2008).

Although the influx of baby boomers will increase the number of Medicare beneficiaries, growth in per capita health costs will increasingly drive growth in federal health spending over the long term (Congressional Budget Office, 2012). This means that health costs throughout the system drive federal health spending. Reforms that shift federal spending to individuals, employers, and states fail to address the problem. The only sustainable solution is to control overall growth in health costs.

Although the Affordable Care Act (ACA) will significantly reduce Medicare spending over the next decade (Sisko et al., 2010), health costs remain a major challenge. To effectively contain costs, solutions must target the drivers of both the level of costs and the growth in costs—and both medical prices and the quantity of services play important roles. Solutions will need to reduce costs not only for public payers but also for private payers. Finally, solutions will need to root out administrative costs that do not improve health status and outcomes.

The Center for American Progress convened leading health-policy experts with diverse perspectives to develop bold and innovative solutions that meet these criteria. Although these solutions are not intended to be exhaustive, they have the greatest probability of both being implemented and successfully controlling health costs. The following solutions could be implemented separately or, more effectively, integrated as a package.

PROMOTE PAYMENT RATES WITHIN GLOBAL TARGETS

Under our current fragmented payment system, providers can shift costs from public payers to private payers and from large insurers to small insurers (Reinhardt, 2011). Because each provider negotiates payment rates with multiple insurers, administrative costs are excessive. Moreover, continued consolidation of market power among providers will increase prices over time (Berenson, 2012). For all these reasons, the current system is not sustainable.

Under a model of self-regulation, public and private payers would negotiate payment rates with providers, and these rates would be binding on all payers and providers in a state. Providers could still offer rates below the negotiated rates.

The privately negotiated rates would have to adhere to a global spending target for both public and private payers in the state. After a transition, this target should limit growth in health spending per capita to the average growth in wages, which would combat wage stagnation and resonate with the public. We recommend that an independent council composed of providers, payers, businesses, consumers, and economists set and enforce the spending target.

We suggest that the federal government award grants to states to promote this self-regulation model. States could phase in this model, one sector (e.g., hospitals) at a time. To receive grants, states would need to publicly report measures of quality, access, and cost, and would receive bonus payments for high performance. For providers, the negotiated rates would be adjusted for performance on quality measures, which should be identical for public and private payers.

Funding for research, training, and uncompensated care—currently embedded in Medicare and Medicaid payments—should be separated out and increased with growth in the global spending target. These payments must be transparent and determined through negotiations or competitive bidding.

ACCELERATE USE OF ALTERNATIVES TO FEE-FOR-SERVICE PAYMENT

Fee-for-service payment encourages wasteful use of high-cost tests and procedures. Instead of paying a fee for each service, payers could pay a fixed amount to physicians and hospitals for a bundle of services (bundled payments) or for all the care that a patient needs (global payments).

Payers will need to accelerate the use of such alternative payment methods. As soon as possible, both public and private payers should adopt the bundles for 37 cardiac and orthopedic procedures used in the Medicare Acute Care Episode Program (Cutler & Ghosh, 2012; Mechanic, 2011). The bundles will also need to include rehabilitation and postacute care for 90 days after discharge. Within 5 years, Medicare should make bundled payments for at least two chronic conditions, such as cancer or coronary artery disease. Within 10 years, Medicare and Medicaid should base at least 75% of payments in every region on alternatives to fee-for-service payment.

Together, these policies would remove uncertainty about transitions from fee-for-service payment, allowing sufficient time for investment in infrastructure and technology by payers and providers.

USE COMPETITIVE BIDDING FOR ALL COMMODITIES

Evidence suggests that prices for many products, such as medical equipment and devices, are excessive (Government Accountability Office, 2012). Instead of the government setting prices, market forces should be used to allow manufacturers and suppliers to compete to offer the lowest price. In 2011, such competitive bidding reduced Medicare spending on medical equipment such as wheelchairs by more than 42% (Centers for Medicare and Medicaid Services, 2012). The ACA requires Medicare to expand competitive bidding for equipment, prosthetics, orthotics, and supplies to all regions by 2016 (The Patient Protection and Affordable Care Act, 2010).

We suggest that Medicare immediately expand the current program nationwide. As soon as possible, Medicare should extend competitive bidding to medical devices, laboratory tests, radiologic diagnostic services, and all other commodities (Office of Management and Budget, 2008). Medicare's competitively bid prices would then be extended to all federal health programs (Office of Management and Budget, 2011). To oversee the process, we recommend that Medicare establish a panel of business and academic experts. Finally, we recommend that exchanges—marketplaces for insurance starting in 2014—conduct competitive bidding for these items on behalf of private payers and state employee plans.

REQUIRE EXCHANGES TO OFFER TIERED PRODUCTS

The market dominance of select providers often drives substantial price variation (Commonwealth of Massachusetts, 2011a, 2011b). To address this problem, insurers can offer tiered plans. These insurance products designate a high-value tier of providers with high quality and low costs and reduce cost sharing for patients who obtain services from these providers. For instance, in Massachusetts, one tiered product lowers copayments by as much as $1,000 if patients choose from 53 high-value providers (Commonwealth of Massachusetts, 2011a, 2011b). We suggest that exchanges and state employee plans offer at least one tiered product at the bronze and silver levels of coverage. This requirement can be implemented by 2016 or sooner if feasible. To encourage participation in the tiered product, it must achieve a minimum premium discount. For instance, in Massachusetts, insurers must offer at least one tiered product with a premium that is at least 12% lower than the premium for a similar nontiered product (Commonwealth of Massachusetts, 2010).

Transparency and consumer education are essential (Sinaiko & Rosenthal, 2010). Quality and cost measures must be standardized and publicly disclosed, and standards must be set for how these measures are used to create tiers. Whenever possible, quality measures should use data from all payers. Finally, in contracts between insurers and providers, clauses that inhibit tiered products must be prohibited.

REQUIRE ALL EXCHANGES TO BE ACTIVE PURCHASERS

If exchanges passively offer any insurance product that meets minimal standards, an important opportunity will be lost. As soon as reliable quality-reporting systems exist and exchanges achieve the adequate scale, it is critical that federal and state exchanges engage in active purchasing—leveraging their bargaining power to secure the best premium rates and promote reforms in payment and delivery systems.

The ACA will provide bonus payments to Medicare Advantage plans with four- or five-star ratings on the basis of their performance on measures of clinical quality and patients' experience (The Health Care and Education Reconciliation Act, 2010). We recommend that exchanges adopt this or a similar pay-for-performance model for participating plans and award a gold star to plans that provide high quality at a low premium.

SIMPLIFY ADMINISTRATIVE SYSTEMS FOR ALL PAYERS AND PROVIDERS

The United States spends nearly $360 billion a year on administrative costs (Institute of Medicine, 2010), accounting for 14% of excessive health spending (Farrell et al., 2008). Section 1104 of the ACA requires uniform standards and operating rules for electronic transactions between health plans and providers (The Patient Protection and Affordable Care Act, 2010). Although plans must comply with these standards and rules, the law does not require providers to exchange information electronically.

First, we suggest that payers and providers electronically exchange eligibility, claims, and other administrative information as soon as possible. Second, public and private payers and providers should use a single, standardized physician credentialing system. Currently, physicians must submit their credentials to multiple payers and hospitals. Third, payers should provide monthly explanation-of-benefits statements electronically but allow patients to opt for paper statements. Fourth, electronic health records should integrate clinical and administrative functions—such as billing, prior authorization, and payments—over the next 5 years. For instance, ordering a clinical service for a patient could automatically bill the payer in one step.

Most important, we recommend that a task force consisting of payers, providers, and vendors set binding compliance targets, monitor use rates, and have broad authority to implement additional measures to achieve systemwide savings of $30 billion a year (U.S. Healthcare, 2010).

REQUIRE FULL TRANSPARENCY OF PRICES

Prices for the same services vary substantially within the same geographic area (Commonwealth of Massachusetts, 2011a, 2011b). Yet consumers almost never receive price information before treatment. Price transparency would allow consumers to plan ahead and choose lower-cost providers, which may lead high-cost providers to lower prices. Although price transparency could facilitate collusion, this risk could be addressed through aggressive enforcement of antitrust laws.

Moreover, both private and public models can achieve meaningful price transparency without leading to collusion (Government Accountability Office, 2011). Aetna provides the price it negotiated with a specific provider to members through an Internet website. Similarly, New Hampshire has a public website that provides the median price paid by an insurer to a specific provider on the basis of claims data.

It is important that all private insurers and states provide price information that reflects negotiated discounts with specific providers. The information should include one price that bundles together all costs associated with a service, individualized estimates of out-of-pocket costs at the point of care, and information on quality of care and volume of patients so that consumers can make informed decisions on the basis of value.

In contracts between insurers and providers, many providers prohibit insurers from releasing price information to their members (Government Accountability Office, 2011). These so-called gag clauses and other anticompetitive clauses must be prohibited. Finally, we recommend that state insurance commissioners and exchanges collect, audit, and publicly report data on prices and claims.

MAKE BETTER USE OF NONPHYSICIAN PROVIDERS

Restrictive state scope-of-practice laws prevent nonphysician providers from practicing to the full extent of their training. For instance, 34 states do not allow advanced-practice nurses to practice without physician supervision (Pittman & Williams, 2012). Making greater use of these providers would expand the workforce supply, which would increase competition and thereby lower prices.

We recommend that the federal government provide bonus payments to states that meet scope-of-practice standards delineated by the Institute of Medicine. Medicare and Medicaid payments to nonphysician providers should allow them to practice to the full extent permitted under state law.

EXPAND THE MEDICARE BAN ON PHYSICIAN SELF-REFERRALS

Many studies show that when physicians self-refer patients to facilities in which they have a financial interest, especially for imaging and pathology services, they drive up costs and may adversely affect the quality of care (Medicare Payment Advisory Commission, 2009; Mitchell, 2012). Under the so-called Stark law, physicians are prohibited from referring Medicare and Medicaid patients to facilities in which they have a financial interest. However, an exception allows physicians to provide "in-house ancillary services," such as diagnostic imaging, in their own offices (42 CFR § 411.355).

We believe that the Stark law should be expanded to prohibit physician self-referrals for services that are paid for by private insurers. In addition, the loopholes for in-office imaging, pathology laboratories, and radiation therapy should be closed. Physicians who use alternatives to fee-for-service payment should be exempted because these methods reduce incentives to increase volume.

LEVERAGE THE FEDERAL EMPLOYEES PROGRAM TO DRIVE REFORM

The Federal Employees Health Benefits Program (FEHBP) provides private health insurance to 8 million federal employees and their families. Although the FEHBP has encouraged various reforms to improve the quality of care (U.S. Office of Personnel Management, 2012), it could be much more innovative.

We recommend that the FEHBP align with Medicare by requiring plans to transition to alternative payment methods, reduce payments to hospitals with high rates of readmissions and hospital-acquired conditions, and adjust payments to hospitals and physicians on the basis of their performance on quality measures. In addition, the FEHBP should require carriers to offer tiered products and conduct competitive bidding on behalf of plans for all commodities. Finally, the FEHBP should require plans to provide price information to enrollees and prohibit gag clauses in plan contracts with providers.

REDUCE THE COSTS OF DEFENSIVE MEDICINE

More than 75% of physicians—and virtually all physicians in high-risk specialties—face a malpractice claim over the course of their career (Jena, 2011). Regardless of whether a claim results in liability, the risk of being sued may cause physicians to practice a type of defensive medicine that increases costs without improving the quality of care.

Strategies to control costs associated with medical malpractice and defensive medicine must be responsible and targeted. These strategies must not impose arbitrary caps on damages for patients who are injured as a result of malpractice. According to the Congressional Budget Office, arbitrary caps on damages would reduce national health spending by only 0.5% (Congressional Budget Office, 2009a, 2009b). But although such caps would have a barely measurable effect on costs, they might adversely affect health outcomes (Congressional Budget Office, 2009a, 2009b; Lakdawalla, 2009).

A more promising strategy would provide a so-called safe harbor, in which physicians would be presumed to have no liability if they used qualified health-information-technology systems and adhered to evidence-based clinical practice guidelines that did not reflect defensive medicine. Physicians could use clinical-decision-support systems that incorporate these guidelines.

Under such a system, the physician could use the safe harbor as an affirmative defense at an early stage in the litigation and could introduce guidelines into evidence to avoid a courtroom battle of the experts. The patient could still present evidence that the guidelines were not applicable to the particular situation, and the judge would still determine their applicability.

It is critical to develop guidelines with credibility. A promising step is an initiative called Choosing Wisely, in which leading physician groups released guidelines on 45 common tests and procedures that might be overused or unnecessary (Cassel, 2012). Given the important role of guidelines, physicians who participate in developing them must be free from financial conflicts of interest.

CONCLUSIONS

These are the types of large-scale solutions that are necessary to contain health costs. Although many in the health industry perceive that it is not in their interest to contain national health spending, it is a fact that what cannot continue will not continue.

Americans therefore face a choice. Payers could simply shift costs to individuals. As those costs become more and more unaffordable, people would severely restrict their consumption of health care and might forgo necessary care. Alternatively, governments could impose deep cuts in provider payments unrelated to value or the quality of care. Without an alternative innovative strategy, these options will become the default. They are not in the long-term interests of patients, employers, states, insurers, or providers.

We present alternative strategies to contain national health spending that allow Americans to access necessary care. Our approach addresses the system as a whole, not just Medicare and Medicaid. It is the path to rising wages, a sustainable federal budget, and the health system that all Americans deserve.

REFERENCES

42 CFR § 411.355.

Berenson, R. A., Ginsburg, P. B., Christianson, J. B., & Yee, T. (2012). The growing power of some providers to win steep payment increases from insurers suggests policy remedies may be needed. *Health Affairs, 31*, 973–981.

Cassel, C. K., & Guest, J. A. (2012). Choosing wisely: Helping physicians and patients make smart decisions about their care. *JAMA, 307*, 1801–1802.

Centers for Medicare and Medicaid Services. (2012). Competitive bidding update—one year implementation update. Retrieved from http://www.cms.gov/Medicare/Medicare-Fee-for-Service-Payment/DMEPOSCompetitiveBid/Downloads/Competitive-Bidding-Update-One-Year-Implementation.pdf

Commonwealth of Massachusetts. (2010). S.2585, an Act to promote cost containment, transparency and efficiency in the provision of quality health insurance for individuals and small businesses: Approved. Retrieved from http://www.malegislature.gov/Laws/SessionLaws/Acts/2010/Chapter288

Commonwealth of Massachusetts. (2011a). Office of Attorney General Martha Coakley. Examination of health care cost trends and cost drivers: Report for annual public hearing. Retrieved from http://www.mass.gov/ago/docs/healthcare/2011-hcctd.pdf

Commonwealth of Massachusetts. (2011b). Recommendations of the Special Commission on Provider Price Reform. Retrieved from http://www.mass.gov/eohhs/docs/dhcfp/g/p-r/special-commppr-report.pdf

Congressional Budget Office. (2009a). Letter to the Honorable John D. Rockefeller: Additional information on the effects of tort reform. Retrieved from http://www.cbo.gov/publication/41812

Congressional Budget Office. (2009b). Letter to the Honorable Orrin G. Hatch: CBO's analysis of the effects of proposals to limit costs related to medical malpractice ("tort reform"). Retrieved from http://www.cbo.gov/publication/41334

Congressional Budget Office. (2012). The 2012 long-term budget outlook. Retrieved from http://cbo.gov/publication/43288.

Cutler, D. M., & Ghosh, K. (2012). The potential for cost savings through bundled episode payments. *New England Journal of Medicine, 366*, 1075–1077.

Emanuel, E. J. (2012). What we give up for health care. *New York Times*. Retrieved from http://opinionator.blogs.nytimes.com/2012/01/21/what-we-give-up-for-health-care

Emanuel, E. J., & Fuchs, V. R. (2008). The perfect storm of overutilization. *JAMA, 299*, 2789–2791.

Farrell, D., Jensen, E., Kocher, B., Bradford, J. W., Knott, D. G., Levine, E. H., & Zemmel, R. N. (2008). Accounting for the cost of US health care: A new look at why Americans spend more. McKinsey Global Institute. Retrieved from http://www.mckinsey.com/insights/mgi/research/americas/accounting_for_the_cost_of_us_health_care

Government Accountability Office. (2011). Health care price transparency: Meaningful price information is difficult for consumers to obtain prior to receiving care. Retrieved from http://www.gao.gov/products/GAO-11-791

Government Accountability Office. (2012). Lack of price transparency may hamper hospitals' ability to be prudent purchasers of implantable medical devices. Retrieved from http://www.gao.gov/products/GAO-12-126

The Health Care and Education Reconciliation Act of 2010. (2010). Public Law 111–152. 111th Congress. Section 1102(c).

Institute of Medicine. (2010). *The healthcare imperative: Lowering costs and improving outcomes: Workshop series summary*. Washington, DC: National Academies Press.

Jena, A. B., Seabury, S., Lakdawalla, D., & Chandra, A. (2011). Malpractice risk according to physician specialty. *New England Journal of Medicine, 365*, 629–636.

Lakdawalla, D. N., & Seabury, S. A. (2009). *The welfare effects of medical malpractice liability*. Cambridge, MA: National Bureau of Economic Research (working paper wl5383). Retrieved from http://www.nber.org/papers/wl5383

Mechanic, R. E. (2011). Opportunities and challenges for episode-based payment. *New England Journal of Medicine, 365*, 777–779.

Medicare Payment Advisory Commission. (2009). Report to the Congress: Improving incentives in the Medicare program. Retrieved from http://www.medpac.gov/documents/jun09_entirereport.pdf

Mitchell, J. M. (2012). Urologists' self-referral for pathology of biopsy specimens linked to increased use and lower prostate cancer detection. *Health Affairs, 31*, 741–749.

Office of Management and Budget. (2008). Major savings and reforms in the President's 2009 budget. Retrieved from http://www.whitehouse.gov/sites/default/files/omb/assets/omb/budget/fy2009/savings_reform.html

Office of Management and Budget. (2011). Living within our means and investing in the future: The president's plan for economic growth and deficit reduction. Retrieved from http://www.whitehouse.gov/sites/default/files/omb/budget/fy2012/assets/jointcommitteereport.pdf

The Patient Protection and Affordable Care Act. (2010). Public Law 111–148, 111th Congress, Section 6410.

Pittman, P., & Williams, B. (2012). Physician wages in states with expanded APRN scope of practice. *Nursing Research and Practice, 2012,* 67197–67194.

Reinhardt, U. E. (2011). The many different prices paid to providers and the flawed theory of cost shifting: Is it time for a more rational all-payer system? *Health Affairs, 30,* 2125–2133.

Sinaiko, A. D., & Rosenthal, M. B. (2010). Consumer experience with a tiered physician network: Early evidence. *American Journal of Managed Care, 16,* 123–130.

Sisko, A. M., Truffer, C. J., Keehan, S. P., Poisal, J. A., Clemens, M. K., & Madison, A. J. (2010). National health spending projections: The estimated impact of reform through 2019. *Health Affairs, 29,* 1933–1941.

U.S. Healthcare. (2010). Efficiency index: national progress report on healthcare efficiency Retrieved from http://www.ushealthcareindex.org/ resources/USHEINationalProgressReport.pdf

U.S. Office of Personnel Management. (2012). FEHBP program carrier letter: Letter no. 2012-09, Retrieved from http://www.opm .gov/carrier/carrier_letters/2012/2012-09.pdf

EFFECTS OF THE SHIFTING SANDS OF POLICY ON NURSING ORGANIZATIONS

The Effects of Shifting Sands of Health Policy on Advanced Practice Nursing Organizations

Anita Finkelman

Health care delivery continues to undergo major changes and needs to make these changes based on current reports on quality (Institute of Medicine [IOM], 2001). This chapter addresses the critical issue of the role of professional nursing organizations in health policy development, implementation, and evaluation, particularly focusing on advanced practice registered nursing (APRN) organizations. Why is this important? "Full integration of the policy process becomes evident when professional nurses discern early the social implications of health problems, seize the opportunity to inform public officials with whom the nurses have credible relationships, provide objective data and subjective personal stories that help translate big problems down to a level of understanding, propose alternative solutions that acknowledge reality, and participate in the evaluation process to determine the effectiveness and efficiency of the outcomes" (Milstead, 2013, p. 276). APRN organizations can approach health policy from two perspectives as follows: (a) What is in it for the APRNs? and (b) How can the profession contribute to health policy such as health policy focused on quality care whether or not it has immediate benefits for APRNs? Both of these perspectives are important.

BACKGROUND AND SIGNIFICANCE

Professional Nursing Organizations and the Policy Process

"Advanced practice nurses became acutely aware of the critical importance of the role of political activist. Not only did APRNs need the basic knowledge, they understood the necessity of practicing the role, developing contacts, working with professional organizations, writing fact sheets, testifying at hearings, and maintaining the momentum to move an idea forward" (Milstead, 2013, p. 7). But is this enough? There needs to be better understanding and participation in the entire policy process where there are many opportunities for input and change. This is more than just how APRNs practice. Policy may be viewed as an entity—a product such as a piece of legislation and also as a process, the steps taken to reach a policy. This process requires a clear sense of direction or an agenda that focuses on a problem. The next step moves to the development of legislation and regulation, which could be at the local, state, or national level. This step is very complex. Once this is resolved, then implementation occurs and should be followed by evaluation. Evaluation may actually lead to other policy changes. APRN organizations can be involved in all these steps, though some are more involved than others.

It is critical that nursing as a profession is recognized as a source of expertise—do others think about asking nurses for their participation, even at the beginning step of agenda setting? This is the critical step, as it identifies the problem and the major issues around the problem. Are nurses of any type at the table when this is done? The legislative and regulatory step often now does include nursing input. This can be performed through political action groups of nursing organizations, letter writing or (as is more common today) through email contact with legislators and their staff and also agency staff who may be developing regulations to implement legislation, visiting legislators and their staff, and providing expert testimony. Many nursing organizations have staff lobbyists, who focus on this policy process as active representatives for the organization and its members.

How do professional nursing organizations ensure that organization members and the organization as a whole are active in health policy and assume an advocacy position?

Organizations address this issue from the top down and bottom up. The top-down approach comes from organization leadership identifying policy issues of interest to the organization and providing organization information and opinion to critical stakeholders in the policy process. They do this through the media, testifying to critical groups, publishing statements often referred to as white papers, and collaborating with leaders in other organizations, mostly other nursing organizations. The bottom-up approach encourages chapter- or state-level leaders to advocate for local and state issues, and widens the scope of membership participation to create a national advocacy plan that also draws in the members. Most professional organizations have adopted grassroots advocacy and do so by member awareness building, mobilization of the membership, and identification of policies of particular interest to support at the chapter, state, or national level. "Awareness building is an effective way to spread the message about an issue that APRNs should have the shared responsibility to resolve. Effective advocacy involves creating a blueprint to mobilize the membership to advocate for a specific issue. This mobilization should be done in such a way that the novice advocate can follow through and achieve success" (Sheehan, 2010, p. 280). The goal is power in numbers, but many nurse practitioners (NPs), as is true of nurses in general, are not comfortable with politics and advocacy (Taft & Nanna, 2008). Nursing education has been addressing this issue by providing more content and experiences related to political action for undergraduate and graduate students. Additional support for this approach is found later in this chapter. This type of approach should help to decrease the hesitancy that many nurses have in getting involved in health policy and political action.

"Creating opportunities for NPs to become familiar with advocacy and the political process in the safe environment of the professional nursing organizations will engage more NPs on a personal level" (Sheehan, 2010, p. 282). Professional organizations also provide their members with information and tools needed to navigate the policy process and political environment. Prior to the Internet, this was not as easy to do, but with the Internet quick access to information has become a part of

APRN ORGANIZATIONS: EXAMPLES OF HEALTH POLICY RESOURCES	BOX 23.1

- National Association of Clinical Nurse Specialists (NACNS)
  www.nacns.org/html/advocacy-policy.php
- National Association of Pediatric Nurse Practitioners (NAPNAP)
  www.napnap.org/NAPNAPAdvocacy.aspx
- National Organization of Nurse Practitioner Faculties (NONPF)
  www.nonpf.com/displaycommon.cfm?an=1&subarticlenbr=25
- American Association of Nurse Practitioners (AANP)
  www.aanp.org/legislation-regulation
- National Association of Nurse Practitioners in Women's Health (NPWH)
  www.npwh.org/i4a/pages/index.cfm?pageid=3299
- American Association of Nurse Anesthetists (AANA)
  www.aana.com/advocacy/Pages/default.aspx
- American College of Nurse-Midwives (ACNM)
  www.midwife.org/Advocacy---American-College-of-Nurse-Midwives

daily life and certainly has had an impact on what can be provided by professional organizations to their members, and this information is also often open to public access. Organization websites now typically include information about health policy and also political action or advocacy. See Box 23.1 identifying examples of websites that provide information for APRN members. This information is typically updated and in some cases one can find current information about legislation that would be of interest to APRNs. By using these resources, APRNs can participate actively in the political process in a timely fashion, for example, by contacting their congressional members or state legislative members, providing information to those developing health policy, participating early in the policy process to identify critical implications for health care and for APRN practice, and so on.

NURSING'S SOCIAL POLICY STATEMENT

The American Nurses Association (ANA) published the nursing professions' social policy statement in 1980, and today, we continue to maintain this statement, though there have been updates (2010). Why is this publication important to the topic of the role of APRN professional organizations in health policy? This statement identifies the profession's concerns, which then should become top priorities in the profession's involvement in health policy. This social policy statement applies to all nurses, including APRNs (ANA, 2010, pp. 4–5).

- **Organization, delivery, and financing of quality health care**
  Quality health care is a human right for all (ANA, 2008). To improve the quality of care, health care professionals must address these complex issues: increasing costs of care; health disparities; and the lack of safe, accessible, and available health care services and resources.
- **Provision for the public's health**
  Increasing responsibility for basic self-help measures by the individual, family, group, community, or population complements the use of health promotion, disease prevention, and environmental measures.

- **Expansion of nursing and health care knowledge and appropriate application of technology**
  Incorporation of research and evidence into practice helps to inform the selection, implementation, and evaluation processes associated with the generation and application of knowledge and technology to health care outcomes.
- **Expansion of health care resources and health policy**
  Expanded facilities and workforce capacity for personal care and community health services are needed to support and enhance the capacity for self-help and self-care of individuals, families, groups, communities, and populations.
- **Definitive planning for health policy and regulation**
  Collaborative planning is responsive to consumer needs and provides for best resource use in the provision of health care for all.
- **Duties under extreme conditions**
  Health professionals will weigh their duty to provide care with obligations to their own health and that of their families during disasters, pandemics, and other extreme emergencies.

These priorities are not "me" issues, focused only on what is relevant to the profession, but rather are concerned with society or community concerns and the connection of nurses and nursing to these concerns, whether it be through individual practice, participation in organizations that provide care, or in the development and implementation of health care policy to meet the needs of the society. The authority for nursing practice originates in social responsibility, as stated in the social policy statement and based on earlier work on professions done by Donabedian (1976). "There is a social contract between society and the profession. Under its terms, society grants the professions authority over functions vital to itself and permits them considerable autonomy in the conduct of their own affairs. In return, the professions are expected to act responsibly, always mindful of the public trust. Self-regulation to assure quality and performance is at the heart of this relationship. It is the authentic hallmark of the mature profession" (ANA, 2010, p. 5). The last two sentences in this statement are important in that they emphasize that nurses must pay attention to broader health care issues. This would also apply to APRNs.

ADVANCED PRACTICE NURSING ORGANIZATIONS AND POLICY INITIATIVES

Today, there are many nursing organizations and many of these organizations now focus on specialty nursing and also roles. For example, the American Psychiatric Nurses Association (APNA), American Association of Critical-Care Nurses (AACN), and the Oncology Nursing Society (ONS) are organizations that focus on a specialty area of nursing. Other organizations have developed that focus more on roles, though with a connection to a specialty area. The National Association for Clinical Nurse Specialists (NACNS) is an organization that has a role focus, the clinical nurse specialist (CNS) who may practice in a variety of specialty areas. These organizations as described here may have different purposes. The following are some of the APRN organizations:

- American Academy of Nurse Practitioners (AANP) (Now American Association of Nurse Pactitioners)
- American Association of Nurse Anesthetists (AANA)
- American College of Nurse-Midwives (ACNM)
- American College of Nurse Practitioners (ACNP) (Merged with the American Academy of Nurse Practitioners in January 2013—the new name is the American Association of Nurse Practitioners [AANP])

- Gerontological Advanced Practice Nurses of America (GAPNA)
- National Association of Clinical Nurse Specialists (NACNS)
- National Association of Nurse Practitioners in Women's Health (NPWH)
- National Association of Pediatric Nurse Practitioners (NAPNAP)
- National Organization of Nurse Practitioner Faculties (NONPF)

There are also initiatives to consolidate NP organizations and thus gain more strength and increase membership. An example of this approach was the merger of the ACNP and the American Academy of Nurse Practitioners (AANP) to form a single organization. The purposes of this consolidation were to (AANP, 2012):

- Capitalize on growth in the demand for NPs as primary, specialty, and acute care providers
- Shape and direct NP policy and legislative priorities
- Achieve the goals and objectives of NPs
- Provide resources for grant writing, education, and research
- Increase public awareness about issues faced by NPs
- Secure international growth opportunities

These purposes focus on APRN professional issues and do not directly address the important APRN responsibilities for participating in health policy development, implementation, and evaluation as it pertains to broader health care issues.

With the increasing nursing recognition of the importance of health policy, other organizations have been created to focus on health policy and nursing. An example is the NP round table. This organization includes a number of advanced practice nursing organizations as its members such as the former ACNP, AANP, NAPNAP, NOPF, GAPNA, and NPWH. As a collaborative organization, the round table represents more than 140,000 APRNs. Its purpose is to advocate in Washington, DC, for APRNs. This is a critical need; however, how does this then relate to participation in health policy in general, not just when a policy impacts APRNs?

APRN EDUCATION REQUIREMENTS AND COMPETENCIES RELATED TO HEALTH POLICY?

The *Essentials of Master's Education in Nursing* (American Association of Colleges of Nursing, 2011) includes requirements for master's graduates to be prepared in health policy. This document states "policy shapes health care systems, influences social determinants of health, and therefore determines accessibility, accountability, and affordability of health care. Health policy creates conditions that promote or impede equity in access to care and health outcomes. Implementing strategies that address health disparities serves as a prelude to influencing policy formation" (American Association of Colleges of Nursing, 2011, p. 21). In addition, the *Essentials* document also supports the need for master's graduates to be prepared in quality improvement. APRNs need to assume active roles in all levels of health policy development, implementation, and evaluation—not just for the needs of the APRN such as greater reimbursement, expansion of role, and other professional concerns. APRNs need to assume their critical role as health care professionals adding their knowledge and expertise to the health care process.

Other organizations have established competencies for APRNs. One of the NACNS competencies relates to health policy. The competency is: "Ethical Decision Making, Moral Agency and Advocacy Competency: Identifying, articulating, and taking action on ethical concerns at the patient, family, health care provider, system, community, and public policy levels" (2010, p. 25). The CNS advocates for equitable patient care by participating in organizational, local, state, national, or international level of policy-making activities for issues related to their expertise and evaluating the impact of legislative and regulatory policies as they apply to nursing practice and patient or population outcomes. This competency is a clear statement of need for CNSs to participate in health policy from a broader perspective rather than only from the perspective of APRN professional concerns. The competency recognizes that CNSs have knowledge and expertise that can benefit the health policy dialogue. The National Task Force on Quality Nurse Practitioner Education (2012) identifies criteria to evaluate NP programs, though the criteria do not specifically mention curriculum content such as health policy. This document refers to the need to meet national APRN standards in curricula, and the major source would be the *Essentials of Master's Education in Nursing* (American Association of Colleges of Nursing, 2011), which does include health policy.

WHAT IS IN IT FOR APRNs?

Health policy provides many opportunities for APRNs to become involved in developing a health care environment in which there is more effective use of APRNs (Naylor & Kurtzman, 2010). Getting APRNs involved in policy analysis as well as the development of policy through APRN professional organizations can impact some critical APRN concerns listed as follows (Naylor & Kurtzman, 2010):

- Remove unwarranted restrictions to practice and standardize nurse practice acts so that there is no variation in practice restrictions
- Equalize payment by Medicare with comparable payment regardless of the practitioner type
- Increase nurses' accountability by, for example, including information about APRN performance in the Agency for Healthcare Research and Quality (AHRQ) Health Care Quality Report Card Compendium
- Expanding nurse-managed centers
- Addressing professional tensions between professions such as nurses and physicians
- Fund pipeline expansions to increase the number of APRNs
- Pursue further study to better understand roles and outcomes

MOVEMENT AWAY FROM THE "ME" APPROACH TO BROADER HEALTH POLICY ISSUES

Slowly, more APRN professional organizations are expanding their perspective of involvement in health policy. This includes greater recognition of the second health policy perspective to improve care. This change moves the APRN organizations to less focus on what is in it for "me" or "us" from the perspective of APRN roles to inclusion of more activities that impact health care from the perspective of care as a whole, whether or not APRNs are involved. This gives APRNs greater voice in the dialogue about the need to improve care and how to improve care effectively (Finkelman, 2012, 2013). Early in their existence, it was natural for APRN organizations to first focus on professional issues as the organizations became involved in health policy. The organizations primarily asked "how does this policy impact what we do and how we are paid?" These are not questions that should be ignored, as they are still very relevant, but this approach to health policy analysis and response does little to support the need for nursing as a health care profession to be active in major health policy decisions. "Nurses' involvement in policy debates brings our professional values to bear on the process" (Warner, 2003). "Master's-prepared nurses will use their political efficacy and competence to improve the health outcomes of populations and improve the quality of the health care delivery system" (American Association of Colleges of Nursing, 2011, p. 20).

As APRN organizations move more toward a mixed perspective of their connection to health policy, this requires the ability to gather data, analyze it, and arrive at possible solutions that may or may not be positive for APRNs, but may be best for health care as a whole. This is a professional organization maturity level that requires the ability to step back from always saying first, "How will this benefit me or benefit APRNs?" For example, prior to the merger with AANP, the ACNP Political Action Committee for Nurse Practitioners, ACNP-PAC stated, "As we celebrate the 10th anniversary of our PAC in 2012, we remain committed to the mission of uniting and advocating for NPs as well as promoting quality health care for individuals and families" (ACNP, 2012). This statement goes on to encourage members to donate to the PAC because the PAC work will impact NP reimbursement. There is nothing wrong with saying this and providing examples to support how the members can work to improve APRN reimbursement, but there are no examples about how the PAC might work to improve care that may or may not help APRNs directly. The intent here is not to say that it is unimportant for APRN professional organizations to work for policies that positively impact APRNs in areas of role, reimbursement, and so on, but rather to point out that if the organizations do only this, then their level of health policy involvement is limited. In addition, this has an impact on how others view APRN organization involvement. If the view is that these organizations are only interested in themselves—in what they can get out of policy to benefit their members—then these organizations may find it difficult to build coalitions with others and work to improve health care as a whole. For example, the NONPF identifies the key issues for NPs in health reform (2012):

- Full recognition and utilization of NPs as primary care providers in all health care systems/models.
- Full recognition of NP practices in coordinated care models such as Medical/Health Homes.
- Full participation of NPs and NP practices in Accountable Care Organizations (ACOs).
- Full participation of NPs and NP practices in chronic care and transitional care models included in the legislation.
- Maintenance of the nondiscrimination language contained in the Senate Finance Bill.
- Maintenance of the funding stream for Nurse-Managed Clinics in the HELP bill.
- Maintenance of the Graduate Nurse Education Funding Stream as proposed in the Senate Finance Bill.
- Authorization of NPs to certify patients eligible for home health care services.

All of these issues are very important, but one might ask why there is no key issue that focuses on quality care and improvement, recognizing that this is a critical need that APRNs support and will work toward whether it be in their own practice, as team member regardless if they are the team leader, or that they will participate in broader health care professional perspective such as organization-wide or within their communities. Yes, one can say this may be implied in this list of issues, but why

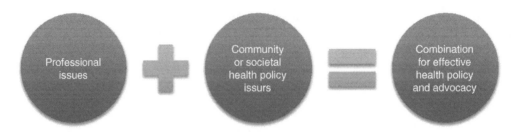

FIGURE 23.1 APRN Organizations Health Policy Perspectives.

is it not stated? APRNs as nurses and members of the nursing profession have vast clinical experience and should use this in the dialogue and development of strategies to improve care, as should any member of the health care team (Finkelman, 2012, 2013). Figure 23.1 illustrates the key focus health policy perspectives that APRN organizations might assume.

The ACNP was involved in health policy for its members prior to the merger. Its 2012 health policy agenda included (2012):

- Acknowledge the central role of NPs in the design and implementation of an optimal U.S. health care delivery system and incorporate the NP perspective in national health care reform strategy
- Ensure that reimbursement is based on outcomes and aligned with services provided and not based on the type of provider
- Include provider-neutral language in all federal legislation, regulation, and other policies
- Recognize the NP's authority to order home health and hospice services and to admit patients to skilled nursing facilities and reverse recent regulations that now preclude NPs from directly ordering durable medical equipment
- Support policies that recognize NPs as primary care providers and enable them to fully participate in all settings including medical homes and ACOs
- Preserve and, where possible, increase federal funding for nursing faculty, advanced practice nursing and basic nursing education and research
- Support development of a national NP database and tracking mechanism
- Ensure inclusion of NPs in the development of health IT policy and system infrastructure

This agenda also focuses more on the needs of APRNs and less on broader health care concerns, though one could say that the broader concerns of health care are implied. On February 24–26, 2013, the "new" AANP held the 2013 National Nurse Practitioner Health Policy Conference in Washington DC, a conference previously convened by ACNP yearly. There were over 200 persons in attendance. "The high-energy gathering was a great beginning for the "new" AANP and set the pace for future participation by NPs as true advocates both for their role as providers of high-quality health care and for their patients" (http://www.aanp.org/conferences /health-policy-conference).

The NACNS not only includes a number of items focused on the role of the CNS, but also includes the need to "advocate for and support programs and initiatives that will ensure a safe and quality driven environment for patients and patient care providers" (NACNS, 2012). This is a direct call for CNS involvement in health policy.

Nursing organizations have a long history of increasing their involvement in policy making in Washington, DC. In the fall of 2012, a meeting was held at the White House. Nursing leaders were invited to discuss health care quality improvement and patient health. Staff from President Obama's administration and also from the Department of Health and Human Services were part of the discussion. The major goal for the meeting was to discuss delivery system transformation and how the Affordable Care Act can support efforts to provide high-quality care to patients. Challenges and opportunities faced in clinics, hospitals, and communities were discussed. Approximately 60 nursing leaders attended. The president of the NACNS commented that the message she walked away with "is that the CNS needs to continue to share how we bring value to the health care system, whether the value be meeting the needs of the public, implementing processes that improve outcomes, cost savings that we bring to organizations, and how we improve patient safety" (Moody, 2012, p. 231). There is no doubt that APRN professional issues were discussed; however, if the leaders of the APRN organizations had gone to the meeting with only this as their agenda item, they would not have been effective leaders. First, there were leaders from many types of nursing groups and organizations, and not all were directly committed to improving advanced practice nursing. Secondly, the White House and the Department of Health and Human Services have multiple concerns and goals, and these are not just focused on the role of the APRN. This is a good example of when it is important to collaborate and work together toward common health care concerns, such as the goal for this meeting, improving care and health of patients.

Exemplar: IOM Quality Chasm Series of Report

The Institute of Medicine (IOM) is a nonprofit organization, located in Washington, DC, that provides services to examine health policy issues and makes recommendations. The IOM cannot make laws or regulations; however, its reports and recommendations are influential in health policy. Legislators and their staff, government agency staff, health professionals and their organizations, and professional education look to the IOM for advice. In 1999, the IOM published the first in its *Quality Chasm* series of reports on the U.S. health care delivery system, followed by a number of significant reports highlighted here. Box 23.2 provides a list of the core reports.

THE INITIAL REPORTS IN THE IOM QUALITY CHASM SERIES   **BOX 23.2**

- *To Err Is Human* (1999)
- *Crossing the Quality Chasm* (2001)
- *Envisioning the National Healthcare Quality Report* (2001)
- *Unequal Treatment* (2002)
- *Guidance for the National Healthcare Disparities Report* (2002)
- *Priority Areas of Care* (2003)
- *Health Professions Education: A Bridge to Quality* (2003)
- *Health Literacy* (2004)
- *Keeping Patients Safe: Transforming the Work Environment of Nurses* (2004)

All reports can be accessed at www.iom.edu

- *To Err Is Human* (1999)

  This report focused on errors in the health care delivery system. The results indicated that there was a high rate of errors in the system. In addition, the climate in health care organizations was one of blame and punishment of staff involved in errors, and there was limited consideration of the impact of the system on errors. Recommendations focused on the need to change this climate and also a need for national monitoring of patient safety and development of strategies to reduce errors. Since this report was published, many changes have occurred; however, errors continue. This type of report has great significance for nursing, but at the time of publication limited notice was made by nursing organizations.

- *Crossing the Quality Chasm* (2001)

  Because of the high rate of errors from the 1999 report, which focused only on one segment of quality, errors, the IOM continued to examine the quality of health care. The conclusions from this report were that health care is fragmented and poorly organized and required fundamental change and improvement. The report emphasized the need to focus on six goals. Health care should be (a) safe, (b) effective, (c) patient-centered, (d) timely, (e) efficient, and (f) equitable. Nursing professional organizations and APRNs did not get very involved in this issue at the time the report was published.

- *Envisioning the National Healthcare Quality Report* (2001)

  This IOM report described the framework that would be used to monitor health care on a national basis. As a result of the report, the United States now has an annual report describing health care status and a companion report on disparities reports. The AHRQ manages this monitoring and publishes the report online (www.ahrq.gov/qual/qrdr10.htm). This annual monitoring report has relevance to better understanding health care and needs for improvement, and thus impacts health policy.

- *Unequal Treatment* (2002) and *Guidance for the National Healthcare Disparities Report* (2002)

  Unequal Treatment addressed the problem of disparities in health care. Earlier IOM reports had indicated that there could be a major problem but more examination of the issue was required. This report confirmed that there were extensive disparities in health care and recommended that disparities should be monitored separately from the national health care quality report. *Guidance for the National Healthcare Disparities Report* described the framework for this monitoring. Health care disparities are now critical health policy issues and are also monitored by AHRQ.

- *Priority Areas of Care* (2003)

  This report provided the initial description of what areas would be monitored in the annual health care quality report. It was recognized that the monitoring could not be performed on all areas of health care and also that the system would have to allow for change as problems improved and new problems arose.

- *Health Professions Education: A Bridge to Quality* (2003)

  As it became clearer that the U.S. health care system was in need of major improvement and quality was weak, the IOM looked to addressing the preparation of health care professionals, focusing on the need for core competencies that all health care professionals should meet. The five health care professions core competencies are: (a) provide patient-centered care, (b) work in interprofessional teams, (c) employ evidence-based practice, (d) apply quality improvement, and (e) use informatics. All of these apply to all nurses, including all APRNs.

- *Health Literacy* (2004)
  This report is a companion report to the other reports on health care diversity and disparities. It noted the importance of health literacy in health care such as its impact on errors and on patient outcomes. There is greater need to prepare health care providers in this area and to develop strategies to improve health literacy.
- *Keeping Patients Safe: Transforming the Work Environment of Nurses* (2004)
  This report is highly significant for nursing though it was not noticed much when published (Finkelman & Kenner, 2012). It provided an extensive review of nursing in acute care and the needs of staff nurses, who provide most of the nursing care in the United States. The conclusions emphasized that nurses are the critical element in the system and need a work environment in which they can provide quality care. Nurse should assume leadership in quality but are not prepared to do so. This report was published in 2004 and yet was not recognized much. The *Future of Nursing* (IOM, 2011) report highlights some of the same areas but not in the depth of the 2004 report. The 2004 report was far ahead of the *Future* report in examining the need for nursing leadership and quality improvement, plus many other critical concerns of nursing.

The IOM quality reports are highly significant to nursing and as such are important to APRNs. APRN organizations need to pay attention to these types of reports from organizations that have major impact on health policy. As more and more attention is paid to quality care concerns, there is need for nursing input and expertise. APRN organizations can best participate in health policy by an awareness of critical reports, seeking opportunities to have direct input into analysis of health care issues and strategies to improve or address problems, whether or not this has direct impact on APRN professional issues.

LEADERSHIP REQUIRED FOR EFFECTIVE PARTICIPATION IN POLICY

The Future of Nursing: Leading Change, Advancing Health (IOM, 2011), a report from the IOM, is based on the early work done by the IOM on health care quality (IOM *Quality Chasm* series of reports). Some of these key reports have been discussed in this chapter. However, at the time of the publication of most of the quality reports, nursing took limited interest in them. However, when the *Future of Nursing* report was published in 2011, nursing as a profession took notice of this report with limited understanding of the background behind the report, such as the 2004 report on nursing and all the reports on quality. This notice mostly came from nursing leaders, nurse administrators, and APRNs. The majority of nurses who provide most of the nursing care are not part of this movement to focus on the *Future* report unless their managers have shared information about the report with them. For the most part, it is not something most nurses view as relating directly to them unless they are being told by management to complete a RN-BSN program. Both undergraduate and graduate students are more aware of the report due to its influence on nursing education. The following are the eight recommendations made in the report. It is from reports like this that policy is developed. This report has influenced policy both on the legislative side and in nursing education. Consider each of the recommendations and how they might influence health policy (IOM, 2011, pp. 278–283).

- *Recommendation 1:* **Remove scope-of-practice barriers**. APRNs should be able to practice to the full extent of their education and training.

- *Recommendation* 2: **Expand opportunities for nurses to lead and diffuse collaborative improvement efforts**. Private and public funders, health care organizations, nursing education programs, and nursing associations should expand opportunities for nurses to lead and manage collaborative efforts with physicians and other members of the health care team to conduct research and to redesign and improve practice environments and health systems. These entities should also provide opportunities for nurses to diffuse successful practices.
- *Recommendation* 3: **Implement nurse residency programs**. State boards of nursing, accrediting bodies, the federal government, and health care organizations should take actions to support nurses' completion of a transition-to-practice program (nurse residency) after they have completed a prelicensure or advanced practice degree program or when they are transitioning into new clinical practice areas.
- *Recommendation* 4: **Increase the proportion of nurses with a baccalaureate degree to 80% by 2020**. Academic nurse leaders across all schools of nursing should work together to increase the proportion of nurses with a baccalaureate degree from 50% to 80% by 2020. These leaders should partner with education accrediting bodies, private and public funders, and employers to ensure funding, monitor progress, and increase the diversity of students to create a workforce prepared to meet the demands of diverse populations across the life span.
- *Recommendation* 5: **Double the number of nurses with a doctorate by 2020**. Schools of nursing, with support from private and public funders, academic administrators and university trustees, and accrediting bodies, should double the number of nurses with a doctorate by 2020 to add to the cadre of nurse faculty and researchers, with attention to increasing diversity.
- *Recommendation* 6: **Ensure that nurses engage in life-long learning**. Accrediting bodies, schools of nursing, health care organizations, and continuing competency educators from multiple health professions should collaborate to ensure that nurses and nursing students and faculty continue their education and engage in life-long learning to gain the competencies needed to provide care for diverse populations across the life span.
- *Recommendation* 7: **Prepare and enable nurses to lead change to advance health**. Nurses, nursing education programs, and nursing associations should prepare the nursing workforce to assume leadership positions across all levels, while public, private, and governmental health care decision makers should ensure that leadership positions are available to and be filled by nurses.
- *Recommendation* 8: **Build an infrastructure for the collection and analysis of interprofessional health care workforce data**. The National Health Care Workforce Commission, with oversight from the Government Accountability Office and the Health Resources and Services Administration, should lead a collaborative effort to improve research and the collection and analysis of data on health care workforce requirements. The Workforce Commission and the Health Resources and Services Administration should collaborate with state licensing boards, state nursing workforce centers, and the Department of Labor in this effort to ensure that the data are timely and publicly accessible.

Leadership is a critical part of the APRN role and leadership is also needed in health policy—APRNs need to use leadership to effectively influence health policy.

Working with their APRN professional organizations, APRNs can strengthen their influence and develop their leadership in the health policy arena. This need has even been recognized by addressing methods to develop leadership in health policy for graduate students. In August 2012, the American Association of Colleges of Nursing launched a Graduate Nursing Student Academy (GNSA) for students in masters and doctoral programs that will assist in the development of leadership development and other topics such as career pathways, advance practice role exploration, grant research funding and grant writing, and success in teaching positions. This type of initiative is connected to recommendations from *The Future of Nursing* (IOM, 2011) report as well as earlier IOM reports that encourage more nursing leadership. Learning more about political advocacy and policy will be of benefit to APRNs and also provide greater support to the need to emphasize not only APRN professional concerns in health policy but also the contributions that APRNs can make to many health policy concerns.

CONCLUSION

This chapter has discussed the role of nursing professional organizations, particularly APRN organizations, in health policy. These organizations may focus on the needs of the profession and/or health policy issues that pertain to broader health care issues that may or may not have a direct impact on APRNs. Ideally, both should be the focus of these organizations.

SYNTHESIS EXERCISES

1. In a classroom debate, address the following question: Should APRN professional organizations only focus on health policy "me" issues? Students participating should assume either the supportive stance or the nonsupportive stance.
2. Discuss the relevance of the IOM reports to health policy.
3. Why do you think it took a long time for the nursing profession and for APRNs to recognize the value of the IOM reports on quality?
4. What can be done now by APRN professional organizations to respond to the IOM *Quality Chasm* series of reports? Provide a specific plan for recommendations from these reports for APRNs and a specific APRN organization.
5. Select one of the APRN organizations listed in Box 23.2 and examine what is found on its website related to health policy.
6. Search for two current bills in Congress or in your state legislature that relate to APRN professional concerns, health care delivery from a broader perspective, or both. Discuss the intent of the legislation and how you think your APRN organization should respond to the bill, both its content/message and methods you would use to participate in policy development, implementation, and evaluation.
7. Take one of the eight recommendations from *The Future of Nursing* report and discuss how it might impact health policy in general and how your APRN organization might respond to it. Search for examples of health policy that have been influenced by the recommendation. Examples may also relate to nursing education.

REFERENCES

American Academy of Nurse Practitioners (AANP). (2012). *Countdown to consolidation.* Retrieved from www.aanp.org/about-aanp/aanp-acnp-merger

American Association of Colleges of Nursing. (2011). *Essentials of master's education in nursing.* Washington, DC: Author.

American Association of Colleges of Nursing. (2012). *Graduate nursing student academy.* Retrieved November 10, 2012, from www.aacn.nche.edu/students/gnsa

American College of Nurse Practitioners (ACNP). (2012). 2012 ACNP health policy agenda. Retrieved from www.acnpweb.org (redirects to AANP website).

American College of Nurse Practitioners (ACNP). (2012, October 18). *Political action committee for nurse practitioners.* Retrieved from www.acnpweb.org/acnp-pac (to AANP website).

American Nurses Association (ANA). (2008). ANA's health system reform agenda. Retrieved from www.nursingworld.org/healthreformagenda

American Nurses Association (ANA). (2010). *Nursing's social policy statement: The essence of the profession.* Silver Spring, MD: Author.

Donabedian, A. (1976). *Forward.* In M. Phaneuf (Ed.), *The nursing audit: Self-regulation in nursing practice* (2nd ed., p. 8). New York: Appleton-Century Crofts.

Finkelman, A. (2012). The movement to improve care: Institute of Medicine quality reports and implications for advanced practice nurse. *Nursing Clinics of North America, 47*(2), 251–260.

Finkelman, A. (2013). The clinical nurse specialist: Leadership in quality improvement. *Clinical Nurse Specialist, 27*(1), 31–35.

Finkelman, A., & Kenner, C. (2012). *Teaching IOM: Implications of the Institute of Medicine reports for nursing education* (3rd ed.). Silver Spring, MD: American Nurses Association.

Institute of Medicine (IOM). (1999). *To err is human.* Washington, DC: National Academies Press.

IOM. (2001). *Crossing the quality chasm.* Washington, DC: National Academies Press.

IOM. (2004). *Keeping patients safe: Transforming the work environment for nurses.* Washington, DC: National Academies Press.

IOM. (2011). *The future of nursing: Leading change, advancing health.* Washington, DC: National Academies Press.

Milstead, J. (2012). Advanced practice nurses and public policy, naturally. In S. Denisco & A. Barker (Eds.), *Advanced practice nursing: Evolving roles for the transformation of the profession* (2012) (2nd ed.). Boston, MA: Jones & Bartlett Learning.

Moody, R. (2012). NACNS newsletter column: President's message. *Clinical Nurse Specialist, 26*(5), 231–233.

National Association of Clinical Nurse Specialists (NACNS). (2012). *National Association of Clinical Nurse Specialists 2011–2012 legislative and regulatory agenda.* Retrieved from www.nacns.org/html/advocacy-policy.php

National CNS Competency Task Force. (2010). *Clinical nurse specialist competencies: Executive summary 2006–2008.* Philadelphia, PA: National Association for Clinical Nurse Specialists.

National Organization of Nurse Practitioner Faculties (NONPF). (2012). *Health policy.* Retrieved November 10, 2012 from www.nonpf.org/displaycommon.cfm?an=1&subarticlenbr=25

National Task Force on Quality Nurse Practitioner Education. (2012). *Criteria for evaluation of nurse practitioner programs.* Washington, DC: National Organization of Nurse Practitioner Faculties.

Naylor, M., & Kurtzman, E. (2010). The role of nurse practitioners in reinventing primary care. *Health Affairs, 29*(5), 893–899.

Sheehan, A. (2010). The value of health care advocacy for nurse practitioners. *Journal of Pediatric Health Care, 24*(4), 280–282.

Taft, S., & Nanna, K. (2008). What are the sources of health policy that influence nursing practice? *Policy, Politics, & Nursing Practice, 9*(4), 274–287.

Warner, J. R. (2003). A phenomenological approach to political competence: Stories of nurse activities. *Policy, Politics, & Nursing Practice, 4*(2), 135–143.

CHAPTER 24

The American Nurses Association

Cindy Balkstra and Andrea Brassard

The American Nurses Association (ANA), the only full-service nursing organization representing all of nursing, has been in existence since 1896. It was first conceived by a group of 10 alumnae associations who met near New York City to discuss the feasibility of a national nursing association. In 1898, the nurses-associated alumnae of the United States and Canada, which was originally a part of the group, held their first convention. When the group was incorporated in the state of New York in 1901, Canada had to be dropped from the name. Individual states also started organizing at this time to begin regulating nursing; North Carolina was the first state to do so, along with New York, New Jersey, and Virginia. It was in 1911 that the Alumnae changed their name to the ANA. The ANA was responsible for the first census of nursing resources in the country in 1918 and, over the years, has been instrumental in many other efforts that support nursing practice and welfare that nurses still benefit from today.

ANA AND ADVANCED PRACTICE REGISTERED NURSES

ANA believes strongly in the value of advanced practice registered nurses (APRNs) and their contribution to improving access to health care services. ANA represents the interests of all APRNs: certified nurse practitioners (CNPs), certified registered nurse anesthetists (CRNAs), clinical nurse specialists (CNSs), and certified nurse midwives (CNMs). ANA, together with constituent member (State) Associations, is working to remove geographic and practice setting limitations for APRNs, seeking fair and consistent practice authority and direct reimbursement across the country.

ANA's Early Involvement With the APRN Movement

CNSs and nurse practitioners were the two APRN roles that were the focus of ANA's early involvement with the APRN movement. Nurse anesthetists had already organized as early as 1931 into the American Association of Nurse Anesthetists and the nurse midwives followed in 1955 as the American College of Nurse Midwives. In the 1960s, the term "nurse practitioner" was defined by ANA's Committee on Education as "any person prepared and authorized by law to practice nursing and therefore, deemed competent to render safe nursing care" (ANA, 1965, p. 106). Following the advent of the first pediatric practitioner program at the University of Colorado, the term "nurse practitioner" took on its expanded meaning.

ANA's Commission on Nursing Education developed a definition of nurse practitioner for use in interpreting the federal Nurse Training Act of 1971. A nurse practitioner "has completed a program of study in an expanded role whose responsibility encompasses:

1. Obtaining a health history
2. Assessing health-illness status
3. Entering a person into the health care system
4. Sustaining and supporting persons who are impaired, infirm, ill, and during programs of diagnosis and therapy
5. Managing a medical care regimen for acute and chronically ill patients within established standing orders
6. Aiding in restoring persons to wellness and maximum function
7. Teaching and counseling persons about health and illness
8. Supervising and managing care regimens of normal pregnant women
9. Helping parents in guidance of children with a view to their optimal physical and emotional development
10. Counseling and supporting persons with regard to the aging process
11. Aiding people and their survivors during the dying process
12. Supervising assistants to nurses"

(ANA, 1971)

Building on the above list of nurse practitioner responsibilities, ANA's Congress for Nursing Practice provided definitions for nurse practitioner, nurse clinician, and CNS, stating that "[u]nfortunately, rather than clarifying nursing practice, all these terms and definitions have had a tendency to confuse levels of practice within the nursing professions as well as for other professions and consumers" (ANA, 1974). As cited in this study, nurse practitioners learned history taking and physical examination through continuing education or in a baccalaureate nursing program. Nurse clinicians were also baccalaureate prepared, but CNSs held a master's degree in nursing.

ANA collaborated with other professional organizations, including the American Academy of Pediatrics and the American School Health Association, in the 1970s to issue position statements on pediatric nurse practitioners, school nurse practitioners, and geriatric nurse practitioners. ANA also accredited continuing education programs for nurse practitioners and developed certification exams for nurse practitioners and CNSs. ANA operationally defined CNSs both as expert practitioners in a specific area of clinical nursing who provides direct patient care and as change agents within the health care system (ANA, 1976, cited by Hamric & Spross, 1983).

ANA Certifies CNSs and NPs

Although specialty certification was conceived by ANA in the mid-1950s, the ANA certification program was not established until 1973 (Johnson, Dawson, & Brassard, 2010). ANA's first advanced practice certification exams were the pediatric nurse practitioner and the psychiatric mental health clinical nurse specialist exams issued in 1974, followed by the adult, geriatric, and family nurse practitioner exams. ANA added more certification exams for nursing administration and other nursing specialties and in 1990 created the American Nurses Credentialing Center (ANCC). Today,

ANCC provides 22 advanced practice exams and two advanced practice credentials through a portfolio mechanism. In addition to ANCC's credentialing programs, ANCC recognizes health care organizations that promote nursing excellence and quality patient outcomes, while providing safe, positive work environments (Magnet Recognition Program® and Pathways to Excellence Program®). ANCC also accredits health care organizations that provide and approve continuing nursing education as well as offering educational materials to support nurses and organizations.

As implementation of the APRN Consensus Model progresses, ANCC is updating certifications to more closely reflect the roles and populations in the model. New certifications will be offered, names of a couple of existing certifications will change, and a few certification exams will be retired. Most notably, there will be three adult-gerontology APRN certifications: adult-gerontology acute care nurse practitioner, adult-gerontology primary care nurse practitioner, and adult-gerontology CNS. The CNS certification will include content from wellness through acute care and is slated for a 2014 launch. Refer to the ANCC website for more details http://www.nursecredentialing.org/APRN-FAQ.aspx

ANA'S NURSE PRACTITIONER COUNCILS AND THE COUNCIL OF CNSs

Returning to ANA's early involvement with APRNs, ANA sponsored conferences, councils, and papers. ANA held a national conference on nurse practitioner education in 1974, with keynote speaker Loretta Ford, noted for founding the first nurse practitioner role (the pediatric nurse practitioner), and sponsored by ANA's two nurse practitioner councils: the Council of Nurse Practitioners in Nursing of Children and the Council of Family Nurse Practitioners and Clinicians. These two ANA councils merged to become the Council of Primary Health Care Nurse Practitioners later in the decade. ANA released a position paper pamphlet, "Scope of Primary Nursing Practice for Adults and Families," in 1976, which included definitions, scope, and professional responsibilities. "Family health care is a team effort. The composition of this team may include nurses, social workers, physicians, therapists, and others. It is imperative that there be mutual recognition of each profession's unique expertise." The 1976 statement foreshadows the patient-centered team idea much talked about now by including the phrase "the consumers' involvement in decisions that affect their health care is paramount."

Primary care was explored further in a monograph written by the American Academy of Nursing and published by ANA (1977). Physical assessment skills were viewed as key to primary care services. Consumer choice of primary care provider was raised as an issue, as was direct reimbursement of nursing services. The monograph cites Barbara Bates, legendary physical assessment textbook author, who wrote "the successful nurse practitioner will integrate her new medical role with her earlier nursing role, achieving a new and balanced professional approach" (p. 23). The monograph also points out the distinction between nurses and physician assistants. "The PA is a physician extender who does not have an identity of his own. If the physician leaves the practice, the PA is out of a job. The nurse has her own identity, is licensed in her own right, accountable for her practice, and is in command of a separate body of knowledge" (p. 31). Claire Fagan's wise words regarding scope of practice continue to resonate:

> The internal professional struggles about scope are probably as serious as the external. For example, how many nurse writers have described functions as dependent? Responsibility for one's own actions and accountability to the consumer in no way

permit the notion of dependent functions for the professional in primary care. To some extent, we have been willing to narrow our scope of practice by getting rid of washing floors and dishes, but we have been more tentative about expanding it. It seems to me that the scope of nursing practice is defined by what nurses are willing to be accountable for, based on their knowledge, skill, and experiential success. I believe that the scope of nursing practice is more limited by nurses' unwillingness to assume the authority that goes with responsibility (i.e., accountability) than by any other single factor. We must confront this problem, since it is clear that the scope of nursing as a professional discipline can meet most of what have been identified as primary care needs. (p. 41)

In addition to fear of accountability, Fagan lists four other factors that limited scope of practice in the 1970s and continue today: legal limits, educational factors, political factors, and economic factors.

ANA's Council of CNSs conducted a national survey of CNSs who were the members of state nurses associations within ANA. More than 3000 CNSs were surveyed; response rate was 74%. The vast majority of respondents, 98%, held master's degrees. The most common specialty area was psychiatric and mental health adult nursing (32%). Most of the respondents were employed by hospitals (55%); about 10% worked in private practice. The Council of CNSs published *The Role of the Clinical Nurse Specialist* (ANA, 1986).

CHANGING POLICIES ON ADVANCED EDUCATION AND LICENSURE

ANA's (1980) positions on APRN education and practice evolved. The Council on Primary Health Care Nurse Practitioners' 1980 position statement encouraged graduate preparation of nurse practitioners, and according to the ANA (1984a) House of Delegates, all nurse practitioners must be prepared at the graduate level by 1990. Regarding APRN practice, ANA discouraged listing nurse practitioner tasks or functions in policy or regulation "since it is inflexible and limiting to the judgment of the professional practitioner. The nurse is accountable for her practice and utilizes the breadth and depth of her educational preparation" (Waddle, 1981). ANA took a broader perspective, publishing *Scope of Practice of the Primary Health Care Nurse Practitioner* in 1986, followed by *Standards of Practice for the Primary Health Care Nurse Practitioner* in 1987.

Also, ANA (1984b) published *Issues in Professional Nursing Practice*. Part 1 Nursing: Legal Authority for Practice described ANA policy on specialty and advanced nursing practice. Thirty years earlier, in 1954, ANA had the misguided recommendation that states insert a disclaimer at the end of the definition of nursing practice stating that "the foregoing shall not be deemed to include acts of diagnosis or prescription of therapeutic or corrective measures." This recommendation (which was removed from official ANA policy in 1965) became a statutory barrier to advanced nursing practice in many states. In 1985, ANA's position was that professional organizations should establish the scope and standards of advanced or specialty nursing practice. ANA advised against state regulation of advanced or specialty nurse practice in the 1970s and 1980s, fearing that additional clauses in nurse practice acts that authorized state boards of nursing to regulate specialty or advanced nursing practice would increase physician involvement in nursing laws and regulations. *Issues in Professional Nursing Practice* listed state examples of physician involvement, including joint protocols, written agreements, and the regulation of advanced practice nursing by joint boards of medicine and nursing. ANA warned that "this kind of physician involvement relinquishes part of the legal control of nursing practice to another profession and results in a superordinate–subordinate relationship …. The degree of specificity of the [scope of practice] rules … is restrictive and harmful" to expansion of advanced practice.

A NATIONAL ALLIANCE OF NURSE PRACTITIONERS

Perhaps in response to the promulgation of restrictive laws and regulations, in 1983, a NP survey conducted by *The Nurse Practitioner* journal found that the NP respondents expressed the need for a strong organized voice for NPs. Fifty-five percent of the NP respondents looked "to organize forces under the auspices of the ANA" (Harper & Billingsley, 1983, p. 24). In response, ANA convened a meeting of six existing national nurse practitioner groups: ANA's Council of Primary Health Care Nurse Practitioners, the Association of Faculties of Pediatric Nurse Practitioner and Associates Programs, the National Association of Nurse Practitioners in Family Planning, the National Association of Pediatric Nurse Associates and Practitioners, the National Organization of Nurse Practitioner Faculties, and the Nurses' Association of the American College of Obstetricians and Gynecologists. These six organizations agreed to form a national coalition of nurse practitioner organizations "to promote the visibility, viability, and unity of nurse practitioners to improve the health of the nation through primary care." Coalition priorities included legislative and political action, marketing of the nurse practitioner as a provider of health care, and communication among all participants in the coalition. The National Alliance of Nurse Practitioners was short lived. At the 1985 national conference, ANA did not answer the call to house the National Alliance, and the formation of a new NP organization, the American Academy of Nurse Practitioners, was announced (Medscape, 2000).

ANA'S FEDERAL WORK

ANA has a long history of advocating for patients, registered nurses, and APRNs. ANA was the first association to endorse the creation of the Medicare program in 1965. In 1977, ANA lobbied for the introduction of a health services bill to expand primary care services, encouraging utilization of nurse practitioners. In the 1980s, ANA responded decisively to an APRN malpractice insurance crisis. ANA had sponsored malpractice insurance for nurses at the rate of $58 per year for coverage of $1,000,000 per occurrence and $3,000,000 in the aggregate per year. In 1987, Fireman's Fund, the last insurance company in the country that accepted all types of nurse practitioner applicants, notified ANA that it would not continue coverage. Following discussions and pressure, it agreed to cover for one additional year those nurse practitioners who were currently covered. Fireman's Fund, however, increased the premium from $58 to $1500 per year. ANA worked to find other insurance carriers, writing letters to Congress and testifying before the National Association of Insurance Commissioners (ANA, 1989).

The 1980s ended with landmark federal legislation that allowed pediatric and family nurse practitioners to be paid directly for the Medicaid services they provide. Additionally, nurse practitioners and CNSs, working in collaboration with a physician, were now permitted under Medicare to certify and recertify a patient's need for skilled nursing care in a nursing home.

Between 1992 and 1996, the Agency for Health Care Policy and Research (now the Agency for Healthcare Research and Quality) sponsored a series of clinical practice guidelines. ANA was asked to review *Clinical Practice Guideline for Depression* and expressed concern about the absence of psychiatric and mental health CNSs as providers of mental health services. Unfortunately, the final version did not mention nurses at all and ANA did not endorse the guideline (Betts, 1992).

APRN reimbursement has been and continues to be an ANA priority. ANA lobbied effectively for direct payment to nurse practitioners, nurse midwives, and CNSs under the federal employees health benefits plan (FEHBP). ANA advocates for "same payment for same service"; nurses should not be paid less for providing health care services, and it took exception to Medicare's "incident to" payment. Although Medicare has paid for "incident to" services since its inception, "[i]ncident to was designed to reimburse physicians for the services of their employees, not to recognize the services of autonomous professionals" (ANA, 1996).

For decades, ANA has been advocating for health care reforms that would guarantee access to high-quality health care for all. In the 1990s, ANA collaborated with the nursing community to develop *Nursing's Agenda for Health Care Reform* (Betts, 1996). With the passage of the Patient Protection and Affordable Care Act (PPACA) in 2010, millions of Americans will have health insurance and access to health care services. ANA is committed to informing nurses and the public about health care reform, now and in the future (www.ana.nursingworld.org/MainMenuCategories /HealthcareandPolicyIssues/HealthSystemReform.aspx).

COLLABORATION

Collaboration has always been and continues to be a hot-button issue. In 1993, ANA testified before the Physician Payment Review Commission to express its concerns about statutory requirements for collaboration:

> Advanced practice nurses are, as are all registered nurses, independently licensed and accountable for their actions. [They are] ... able to deliver ... services independent of their relationship with physicians or other health care providers .... Collaborating with and referring to other health providers is a matter of good professional practice .... Regardless of practice setting or supervision requirements, advanced practice nurses, like most health professionals, generally maintain a network for referral to and collaboration with other professionals and maintain a means to access emergency back-up.
>
> *ANA (1998, p. 4)*

ANA leaders met with leaders of the American Medical Association in 1993–1994 to discuss collaboration issues. After much discussion and negotiation, the following definition was proposed:

> Collaboration is the process whereby physicians and nurses plan and practice together as colleagues, working interdependently within the boundaries of their scopes of practice with shared values and mutual acknowledgment and respect for each other's contribution to care for individuals, their families, and their communities.
>
> *ANA (1998, p. 6)*

The above definition of collaboration was adopted by the ANA Board of Directors in 1994; the American Medical Association took no further action.

Almost 20 years later, after the release of the Institute of Medicine's (2011) report *The Future of Nursing: Leading Change, Advancing Health*, 12 physician and nurse leaders, including ANA, met to produce a document on interprofessional collaboration. This more recent effort failed following the leak of a confidential draft document and objections from organized medicine (Jablow, 2013).

CONSTITUENT AND STATE NURSES ASSOCIATIONS AND APRNs

The constituent and state nurses associations (C/SNAs) have been instrumental in working with licensing boards, legislatures, and regulatory agencies to bring quality, affordable, and accessible care to the public through the full utilization of APRNs. This work has been going on for decades and continues today, as the goal of independent practice for APRNs still remains in the future for many. The examples given in this review are not meant to be inclusive but to provide an understanding of the nature of this important work as it is conducted throughout the country.

Frequently, the struggle to achieve independence has resulted in C/SNAs' building coalitions to ensure strong connections within and external to the advanced practice community. Nurse practitioners, nurse anesthetists, nurse leaders/executives, CNSs, and nurse midwives have often joined the respective C/SNA individually or collaboratively in order to speak with one influential voice when addressing regulatory issues. For example, the Utah Nurses Association (UNA), the Utah Nurse Practitioner Association (UNPA), and the Utah Association of Nurse Anesthetists (UANA) chose to work together during the 2013 legislative session to monitor bills related to nursing and were successful in replacing negative language for nurse practitioners (i.e., physician extenders) with appropriate terminology (i.e., NP and APRN). Language is often an issue with legislation; identifying this prior to any enactment is crucial to ensuring inclusion of APRNs. Whereas these collaborations were not formalized, the Utah Action Coalition was; currently it consists of the UNA, the UNPA, the Utah Organization of Nurse Leaders, and other professional groups. Together, they are encouraging the director of the Utah Medicaid Office to expand reimbursement for all advanced practice registered nurses.

In a similar effort five years ago, ANA/California and the California Association of Psychiatric Mental Health Nurses in Advanced Practice (CAPNAP), an affiliate of ANA/California, convened the state's first APRN Summit at West Coast University. Nearly 60 APRN representatives from the California Nurse Midwives Association, the California Association for Nurse Practitioners, the California Association of Nurse Anesthetists, the California Association of Clinical Nurse Specialists, the California chapter of the American Psychiatric Nurses Association, and the California School Nurses Organization, along with the faculty from APRN programs and members of the Board of Registered Nursing, attended this historic event. A second summit was held in May 2013 under a new name, the California Action Coalition. Their work continues today (a white paper is in progress) as they move toward prescriptive authority and licensed independent practitioner status for all California APRNs.

When it is possible, partnering with physician legislative colleagues can yield significant results. The Oregon Nurses Association (ONA) chose a physician legislator to sponsor a bill (HB2902 B) that would establish payment parity with commercial insurance carriers for APRNs. The bill met serious opposition and was not successful until the third attempt, but did pass both the Oregon House and Senate in 2013. In addition to parity, the bill authorizes a task force to study the reimbursement practices of commercial insurance carriers for primary care services.

Similar yet different is the idea of establishing a network of providers in order to hire an independent party to negotiate with insurance carriers for better fee schedules. The ONA is in the exploratory phase of this project, working with nurse practitioners in Oregon. Called an IPA or Independent Provider Association, the Psychiatric/ Mental Health Nurse Practitioners already have such a group in this state.

Another way that C/SNAs have worked together is through a shared lobbyist, ensuring consistency of the message. This happened in Vermont during the 1990s when the Vermont State Nurses Association led the charge for independent practice.

At times, APRN councils of C/SNAs have become autonomous in order to devote all of their resources to overcoming APRN barriers. For example, the Maryland Nurses Association (MNA) represented nurse practitioners, who served on their Primary Care Special Interest Council, during the first 20 years of the role in this state. While continuing a positive working relationship with MNA, the Nurse Practitioner Association of Maryland became an independent organization in 1992.

Sometimes advancement in one state can be the catalyst for movement in another, as it has been for the state of West Virginia (WV). In 2012, the WV Nurses Association (WVNA) was successful with Senate Resolution 93, mandating a study of APRNs. This resolution cited the increase in expansion of APRNs' scope of practice in the border state of Maryland as one of several reasons for the state to consider similar legislation, lest it lose the best APRNs to another state. As part of the study, the Federal Trade Commission staff testified in front of a legislative panel recommending removal of the collaborative agreement required for APRN prescriptive authority in WV. With this introduction, WVNA is submitting a sunrise application in 2013 to expand prescriptive authority for APRNs, remove the requirement for written collaborative agreements, and provide global signature allowance of documents. The Nebraska Nurses Association is also moving in this direction but plans to submit legislation in 2014. They are currently working with the Nebraska Nurse Practitioner group by providing testimony and support for the credentialing review process, a prerequisite for legislative action.

Without a white paper or archived documents, it is difficult to retrieve all the work that has been done by the C/SNAs. Recently, the Missouri Nurses Association (MONA) convened a task force to author a white paper entitled "A Template for Change in the State of Missouri." This document covers the state of health care in Missouri (MO), defines APRNs and their role in health care, describes barriers and recommends removal of such to support full scope of practice. It is updated regularly so it can be used to guide legislators and others who have the opportunity to make changes. In 2013, one small step forward came with the allowance of a waiver to the required physician on-site supervision in the collaborative practice agreement for rural health clinics. Similarly, in South Carolina (SC), the Board of Nursing compiled a white paper in 2011 that concluded with a list of suggestions to bring the state into compliance with the APRN Consensus Model. The document was endorsed by the South Carolina Nurses Association in addition to other professional organizations. Unfortunately, the SC Board of Nursing declined to move forward with the proposals. Other state nurses associations that have assisted with the development of white papers include those in California, Florida, Indiana, Michigan, Nebraska, New Jersey, and West Virginia.

Indeed, the integration of the APRN Consensus Model is another area where C/SNAs have been hard at work. Although many continue to pursue this endeavor, WVNA and more recently the Arizona and North Dakota Nurses Associations have been successful in getting the recommendations placed into state code. WVNA's partnership with the WV Board of Nursing resulted in alignment of state rules and regulations with the consensus model in 2012. Furthermore, in June 2013, the Rhode Island Nurses Association witnessed the governor of Rhode Island signing HB 5656A, which recognized all four categories of APRNs, thus bridging the gap between existing statute and the consensus model in that state.

In keeping with the APRN Consensus Model, CNSs have needed to establish themselves as APRNs in some states. In Georgia, for example, the Georgia Nurses Association (GNA) along with the Atlanta and Southeast Affiliates of the National Association of Clinical Nurse Specialists (NACNS) petitioned the Board of Nursing to make a rule change rather than open the Nurse Practice Act during a legislative session. In the fall of 2011, the rule change was made after much debate with a new board-appointed Advanced Practice Committee. Unfortunately, the board declined grandfathering; thus, the final requirements essentially preclude most of the state's CNSs who have practiced as such for years from being recognized as APRNs.

For all of the challenges that APRNs face, significant milestones continue. On Friday, May 31, 2013, the Iowa Nurses Association won a state Supreme Court decision when it recognized the Iowa Board of Nursing as the agency that defines the scope of nursing practice, including that of APRNs. The case involved CRNAs and other APRNs and the use of radiologic techniques in the provision of care. The ANA Office of General Counsel assisted in this matter.

ORGANIZATIONAL AFFILIATES

ANA's affiliates are nursing organizations that belong to ANA as organizations. Working together, ANA and these organizations seek to share information and collaborate in finding solutions to issues that face the nursing profession, regardless of specialty. While each organization maintains its own autonomy, the nursing profession and health care consumers benefit from opportunities to speak with aligned voices as a result of the collaboration that occurs between ANA and our affiliates. Three national APRN organizations are affiliated with ANA: the American Association of Nurse Anesthetists, the American College of Nurse Midwives, and the National Association of Clinical Nurse Specialists. The American College of Nurse Practitioners (ACNP) was an organizational affiliate of ANA until ACNP merged with the American Academy of Nurse Practitioners to become the American Association of Nurse Practitioners.

ANA'S POLICY PRIORITIES: APRNs

With a limited number of seats at many policy tables, ANA is often the sole voice of nursing. This position has become increasingly crucial, yet sensitive, with the growth of nursing specialties and the increasing importance of varied nursing roles. As a historical convener of the larger nursing community, ANA seeks to fully and accurately represent the nursing community. ANA's work on "APRN issues" is wide ranging and, given the nature of policy work, evolving. ANA has dedicated a full-time senior policy fellow to address APRN issues. Lisa Summers, DrPH, CNM, originated this role in 2009; Andrea Brassard, PhD, FNP, FAANP, took over this position in 2013.

The following list is a brief overview of ANA's current APRN policy priorities. Each of these objectives is prefaced with "work with other organizations representing APRNs and key stakeholders to…"

- Ensure that the role of the APRN is recognized and included in regulatory language, policy documents, data collection tools, etc., especially as related to health system reform.
- Ensure the ability of APRNs to practice to the full extent of their education and training. ANA's policy work in this area is through the Coalition for Patients'

Rights (www.patientsrightscoalition.org) and also through state nurses associations, which is supported by Janet Haebler, MSN, RN, Associate Director, ANA State Government Affairs.

- Implement the APRN Consensus Model.
- Provide a legal challenge to arbitrary practice restrictions in the form of laws, regulations, policies, or guidelines. ANA's Office of General Counsel has filed numerous amicus briefs in support of APRNs and responds to concerns about anticompetitive behavior.
- Gather and disseminate workforce and payment data that will better demonstrate the economic value of nursing, including APRNs. Health economist Peter McMenamin, PhD, leads this work at ANA.
- Achieve equitable reimbursement for APRNs. ANA supports initiatives at the federal and state level, aimed at both public and private payers, to remove barriers to direct and equitable reimbursement, including eliminating physician oversight requirements. ANA represents the entire nursing profession of the American Medical Association's Relative Value Scale Update Committee (RUC) and Current Procedural Terminology (CPT) Committee, which formulate reimbursement policy for Medicare and private payers.
- Facilitate the ability of APRNs to be licensed as independent providers in institutions. ANA sits at a number of professional and technical advisory committees (PTACs) of the Joint Commission and ensures that the needs of APRNs as well as staff nurses are represented in that work.
- Ensure that nurses are involved in the design, development, and implementation of health information technology (HIT) systems, and that APRNs are eligible for funding to enhance adoption of HIT.
- Ensure that ANA's expansive work in the national quality enterprise (providing leadership and a strong voice for nursing in the Hospital Quality Alliance, the National Priorities Partnership, and the National Quality Forum, among others) and the growth of the National Database of Nursing Quality Indicators® is in concert with APRNs' efforts to be included in national performance measurement programs currently designed for physicians.
- Advocate for increased funding for APRN education, including expansion of the graduate nurse education (GNE) demonstration project (ANA's Policy Priorities, 2012, June).

To keep abreast of ANA's policy and advocacy work on behalf of APRNs, visit the Advanced Practice Nurse webpage on *Nursing World* (www.nursingworld.org/EspeciallyForYou/AdvancedPracticeNurses), read the "APRN Focus" column in *The American Nurse* (www.theamericannurse.org/?cat=20), and sign up for the ANA blog, *One Strong Voice* (www.nursingworld.org/HomepageCategory/NursingInsider/Archive_1/2012-NI/Apr-2012-NI/Welcome-to-One-Strong-Voice.html).

DISCUSSION QUESTIONS

1. Are you or have you ever been a member of ANA and/or your state nurses association? Are you a member of an APRN organization? Is there current and future need for joint efforts of ANA and APRN organizations? Why or why not?
2. Visit *The American Nurse* website and view past "APRN Focus" columns (www.theamericannurse.org/?cat=20). What issues should be addressed in future columns?

REFERENCES

American Nurses Association (ANA). (1965). American Nurses Association's first education. *American Journal of Nursing, 65*(12), 106–111.

ANA Commission on Nursing Education. (1971, December). *Definition of the term Nurse Practitioner.* ANA Archives. Howard Gotlieb Archival Research Center, Boston, MA: Boston University.

ANA Congress for Nursing Practice. (1974, May 8). *Definition: Nurse practitioner, nurse clinician and clinical nurse specialist.* ANA Archives. Howard Gotlieb Archival Research Center, Boston, MA: Boston University.

ANA Council of Family Nurse Practitioners and Clinicians. (1976, May). *Scope of primary nursing practice for adults and families.* ANA Archives. Howard Gotlieb Archival Research Center, Boston, MA: Boston University.

ANA Council of Primary Health Care Nurse Practitioners. (1980, May). *The primary health care nurse practitioner.* ANA Archives. Howard Gotlieb Archival Research Center, Boston, MA: Boston University.

ANA House of Delegates. (1984a). *Implementation standards for advanced nursing practice as a nurse practitioner.* ANA Archives. Howard Gotlieb Archival Research Center, Boston, MA: Boston University.

ANA. (1977). *Primary care by nurses: Sphere of responsibility and accountability, american academy of nursing monograph, 1977.* ANA Archives. Howard Gotlieb Archival Research Center, Boston, MA: Boston University.

ANA. (1984b). *Issues in professional nursing practice, Volume 1. Nursing: Legal authority for practice.* ANA Archives. Howard Gotlieb Archival Research Center, Boston, MA: Boston University.

ANA. (1984c). *Statement on the nurse practitioner and clinical nurse specialist, prepared for the September 1984 ANA/AMA leadership conference.* ANA Archives. Howard Gotlieb Archival Research Center, Boston, MA: Boston University.

ANA. (1986). *The role of the clinical nurse specialist.* Council of Clinical Nurse Specialists.

ANA. (1989, March 2). *Press release.* ANA Archives. Howard Gotlieb Archival Research Center, Boston, MA: Boston University.

ANA. (1996, September). Nursing Reimbursement under Medicare and Medicaid. *Nursing Trends & Issues, 1*(3), 4–5.

ANA. (1998, May). Collaboration and Independent Practice: Ongoing Issues for Nursing. *Nursing Trends & Issues, 3*(5), 1–9.

ANA. (2013). Health system reform webpage. *Nursing World.* Retrieved from http://www.nursingworld.org/MainMenuCategories/Policy-Advocacy/HealthSystemReform

American Nurses Credentialing Center (ANCC). (2013). *FAQ: Consensus Model for APRN Regulation webpage.* Retrieved from http://www.nursecredentialing.org/APRN-FAQ.aspx

Betts, V. T. (1992, November 25). [Letter to J. Jarrett Clinton]. American Nurses Association Archive, Silver Spring, MD.

Betts, V. T. (1996). Nursing's agenda for health care reform: Policy, politics, and power through professional leadership. *Nursing Administration Quarterly, 20*(3), 1–8.

Hamric, A. B., & Spross, J. (1983). *The clinical nurse specialist in theory and practice.* New York: Grune & Stratton.

Harper, D. C., & Billingsley, M. C. (1983, July–August). Organizing for power. *Nurse Practitioner, 8*(7), 24–33.

Institute of Medicine (IOM). (2011). *The future of nursing: Leading change, advancing health.* Washington, DC: National Academies Press (prepublication copy). Retrieved from http://www.nap.edu/catalog/12956.html

Jablow, P. (2013, January 9). *How to foster interprofessional collaboration between physicians and nurses?* Retrieved from www.rwjf.org/en/research-publications/find-rwjf-research/2013/01/how-to-foster-interprofessional-collaboration-between-physicians.html

Johnson, J., Dawson, E., & Brassard, A. (2010). Consensus model for advanced-practice nurse regulation: A new approach. In E. M. Sullivan-Marx, D. O. McGivern, J. A. Fairman, & A. S. Greenberg (Eds.), *Nurse practitioners: The evolution and future of advanced practice* (pp. 125–142). New York: Springer.

Medscape. (2000, January 4). *Nurse practitioners: Remembering the past, planning the future.* Retrieved from www.medscape.com/viewarticle/408388

Waddle, F. I. (1981, October 6). [Letter to Jean R.H. Dickson]. American Nurses Association Archive, Silver Spring, MD.

CHAPTER 25

State Implementation of the APRN Consensus Model

Tracy Klein

The *Consensus Model for APRN Regulation: Licensure, Accreditation, Certification and Education* (APRN Joint Dialogue, 2008) is a significant step toward consistency in how advanced practice registered nurses (APRNs) are prepared and recognized for practice. Although the document itself does not hold the force of law, the model has been endorsed by 44 nursing organizations with the authority to implement it (American Nurses Association [ANA], 2009). A primary stakeholder in the development was the National Council of State Boards of Nursing (NCSBN), which is a national membership organization for state boards of nursing. The final document represents a process that was initially contentious and generated from reaction to an original document authored by NCSBN titled *Vision Paper: The Future Regulation of Advanced Practice Nursing* in 2006 (Chan & Hackenschmidt, 2006; NCSBN, 2006). *The Vision Paper*, as it came to be known, was never released beyond draft form due to the substantial comments received from nursing stakeholders. For the purpose of this discussion, the final *Consensus Model for APRN Regulation: Licensure, Accreditation, Certification and Education* (APRN Joint Dialogue, 2008) will be referred to by the term *Consensus Model*.

The purpose of this chapter is to identify and discuss policy principles and concepts applicable to assessing and evaluating the process of state-based regulatory implementation of *Consensus Model* recommendations.

DEFINITIONS

Two definitions from the *Consensus Model* frame the implementation of the recommendations to stakeholders. The first is the term *APRN*, which stands for advanced practice registered nurse. For legal and policy purposes, APRN is defined in the *Consensus Model* as a restricted and ultimately statutorily protected term that cannot be used by just any nurse with advanced nursing training or education. As defined in the *Consensus Model*, APRN specifically refers to four nursing roles that include practice beyond the scope of the basic registered nurse license: certified nurse practitioner

(CNP), certified nurse midwife (CNM), clinical nurse specialist (CNS), and certified registered nurse anesthetist (CRNA). APRNs have preparation to prescribe, practice autonomously, and manage individual patients in defined populations such as family, pediatrics, or adult/geriatrics. APRNs are nationally certified after graduate education at the master's or doctoral level that prepares them for their unique scope of practice (SOP) (APRN Joint Dialogue, 2008). APRN as a term does not refer to nurses with advanced degrees in education, informatics, community health, or policy, as examples, unless those degrees also include specific clinical and didactic preparation for national certification as a CNP, CNM, CNS, or CRNA. The adoption of this definition of APRN into state law has implications for grandfathering those already practicing or licensed under the title who may not meet the requirements of the *Consensus Model*. Ultimately, the term *APRN* is projected to replace multiple terms currently written in statute and regulation, which describe nurses practicing in an advanced role, including advanced practice nurse (APN) and advanced registered nurse practitioner (ARNP).

The term *consensus* does not imply uniform agreement. Stakeholders involved in the *Consensus Model* used a 66% majority process to identify final recommendations. Although consensus implies generalized endorsement of terms found in the *Consensus Model*, several stakeholders continue to dialogue regarding implementation strategies or timelines. This chapter will highlight a few of the relevant controversies that have potential impact on the actual implementation of the model at a state level.

APRN CONSENSUS MODEL VERSUS MODEL ACT AND RULES

The *Consensus Model* (APRN Joint Dialogue, 2008) serves as an organizing document that helps define terms, state relationships, and provide guiding principles for institutional implementation. As noted, however, the model does not have the force of law. In order to implement the *Consensus Model*, regulatory bodies such as the state boards of nursing will need to use the political process on a state basis to adopt final statutes and rules. States may, but are not required to, use language developed and adopted by the NCSBN to implement changes in the *Consensus Model*. In order to facilitate use of the model act and rules, which are revised and adopted through a voting delegate assembly at the NCSBN annual meetings, NCSBN launched its Campaign for APRN Consensus in 2011. NCSBN (NCSBN, 2013a) provides maps that regularly update the public regarding state-based legislative changes moving each state closer to the requirements of the *Consensus Model*. The current model act and rules may be freely downloaded and distributed for use in evaluating and modifying existing state Nurse Practice Acts (NCSBN, 2013b).

POLICY CONCEPTS

The APRN *Consensus Model* implementation process illustrates several policy concepts. Framers of the *Consensus Model* emphasized its social benefits to nurse stakeholders, including autonomous practice, state-to-state mobility, and enhanced title recognition. Constraints that slowed or blocked implementation include (a) opposition to social construction of underlying principles, (b) inability of stakeholder to embrace uniform social identity, and (c) political preference for incremental rather than comprehensive legislative change.

Social Construction and Policy Design

The *Consensus Model* is an exemplar of social construction impacting specific target populations. Social construction is an explanatory theory used to identify and consciously build a group through policy design. Policy design selects a target population that will receive benefits in exchange for some perceived burdens (Ingram, Schnieder, & deLeon, 2006). The group, in this case APRNs, develops and implicitly endorses stated goals to be achieved, tools intended to change behavior, rules for inclusion or exclusion, a rationale for the policy change, and an implementation structure (Ingram, Schnieder, & deLeon, 2006, p. 95). The success of social construction depends on the ability of its assumptions to be legitimized in authoritative policy. In the exemplar of the *Consensus Model*, successful legitimization requires adoption of regulatory changes by a majority of states, as well as congruent policy changes in accreditation, certification, and education of APRNs in the future. Burdens include changes that will eliminate certain previously legitimized roles such as the geriatric or oncology nurse practitioner (NP), which were deemed too narrow for cross-state autonomous practice goals and legally defensible board certification testing. Other burdens include ineffectively defined mechanisms for previously legally grandfathered APRNs, such as CNSs, to continue to practice (NACNS, 2012). Distribution of burden must be perceived as lesser than the benefits of becoming an advantaged group, in order to gain political power and capital through greater numbers of participants in the socially constructed role.

Social Identity Theory

The *Consensus Model* defines APRNs as inclusive of CNSs, CNPs, CRNAs, and CNMs. Its framework presumes a high degree of group identity for each of the four roles and emphasizes their similarities rather than differences. However, current practice status for the four roles emphasizes their unique rather than uniform properties. Uniqueness is communicated to the public in several ways by professional groups, who obtained their professionalism status by emphasizing unique skills, educational preparation, and SOP. This unique status has been codified into law across the United States, as demonstrated through rights to prescribe, practice autonomously, admit patients, and order durable goods or equipment. These rights are currently assigned to certain APRNs (primarily CNPs) and not others. Unique status is also represented by distinct oversight for educational preparation, such as the program level accreditation required for CNM and CRNA education in addition to national or regional educational accreditation.

The *Consensus Model* as a policy document proposes two new identities: an individual titled APRN and an institution called "LACE." The latter serves as a mechanism for members of four groups who license, accredit, certify, and educate APRNs to engage in goal setting toward a common identity and set of professional benefits. Dimaggio and Powell (1983) identify steps toward institutional maturation that include *isomorphic* changes where organizations become more similar as they try to generate change. These similarities allow participants to deal rationally with uncertainty, change, and growth. The emergence of the LACE process suggests maturation of the professional identity of the APRN.

Conflict between the APRN group members and their stakeholders initially represented barriers to implementation of the *Consensus Model*, as target populations struggled with their social identity. Brewer (1991) developed optimal distinctiveness theory to explain the alliance formed by groups, such as APRNs, who must balance fundamental needs for assimilation and differentiation when form-ing a social identity. Exemplars of group conflict related to social identity will be discussed further in an overview of controversies during implementation of the *Consensus Model.*

In addition to individual social identity, group membership conveys other types of social identity, including geographic identity. Tajfel and Turner (1986) identify mul-tiple conditions under which diverse groups will favor their own above a compari-son group, particularly when outcomes are not clearly defined and benefits are not readily visible. Early adapters of the *Consensus Model* were therefore not states that already had autonomous APRN practice, such as Oregon and Washington. Multistate licensure agreements for APRNs were adopted by Texas, Iowa, and Utah before the *Consensus Model* was implemented. However, they were never implemented due to lack of uniformity of APRN practice across states and inability to resolve differences in prescriptive authority (NCSBN, 2012c). New revisions are being adopted that pro-pose a multistate compact for APRNs consistent with the *Consensus Model* (APRN Joint Dialogue, 2008; NCSBN, 2012c), involving executive officers and legal counsel from Arizona, Iowa, Idaho, Texas, and Utah. Current dialogue recognizes state pref-erences for historical licensure requirements (NCSBN, 2012c).

Incrementalism

The diversity of regulations governing APRN practice, as well as the uneven adop-tion of scope, educational, and role changes in regulation, are examples of incre-mentalism in policy implementation. Incrementalism involves making small rather than large changes in policy to minimize risk and unanticipated outcomes. Initial adoption of the APRN role, particularly those of the CRNA and CNP, often involved state-mandated physician collaboration or supervision in return for recognition of the role in statute. Negotiated authority is historically particularly common with pre-scribing (Keely, 2007). Examples include restrictions on prescriptive authority such as formularies or standards and protocols in return for expanded nursing authority. Charles Lindblom (1959, 1970) is credited with identification and analysis of the use of incrementalism in public policy, which he termed "muddling through." Benefits of incrementalism include the ability to limit issues and discussion to immediate problems that can gain consensus in a more expedient manner. However, there are many drawbacks to using incrementalism as a strategy for APRNs. Diver (1981) identifies three characteristics of incrementalism in policy making: (a) piecemeal and tightly restricted in scope to the exclusion of remote or uncertain consequences, (b) dynamic and remedial resulting in a policy of fixing errors rather than long-range goal strategies, and (c) decentralization that favors policy making to fit local conditions rather than national functions and needs. The resultant patchwork of state law related to APRN practice to date has therefore been a barrier to wide-spread policy initiatives. The legislative consequence of incremental policy making requires each state to individually change SOP laws that restrict APRN mobility and practice. Publication of the *Consensus Model* provided a road map for strategic planning and change. Complementary documents published by both the American Nurses Association (ANA, 2009) and NCSBN (2012a, 2012b) include model legis-lation, rules, talking points, and implementation strategies, which can be used to impact long-term comprehensive change in state law. The shift from an incremental strategy to a global strategy reflects maturation of the professional role (Dimaggio & Powell, 1983) as well as a change in policymaking strategy. Diver (1981) calls this process "comprehensive rationality" and identifies its characteristics in stark contrast to the muddling through of incrementalism. Comprehensive rationality includes a deliberative analysis of goals, alternatives, effective mechanisms, and evaluation of outcomes. Modern policy makers who implement the *Consensus Model* are therefore using contemporary methods such as evidence-based practice and research data analysis to achieve their policy goals. While some states still incorporate degrees of the incremental strategy, such as adopting scope changes but not title changes, others have implemented the *Consensus Model* recommendations with sweeping legislation that changed titles, practice, and functions for all four APRN roles.

CONTROVERSIES

In order to successfully implement the *Consensus Model*, individuals, groups, and state policy makers needed to identify and mitigate barriers to consensus. Failures to identify and strategize around areas of policy resistance are likely to result in incremental rather than comprehensive policy making. Failure to address concerns about social construction, social identity, or policy style can also result in lack of ability to implement change to the status quo for APRN practice. The immediate years leading up to and following the 2008 publication of the *Consensus Model* reflect the negotiation of multiple controversies by stakeholders. The following discussion highlights some of the controversies documented in national dialogue about the *Consensus Model*.

Social Construction and Social Identity

Titles

Individual identity during the process of consensus was important to nursing groups. The construction of a consensus-based identity of APRN required specific inclusion of the roles CNP, CNM, CRNA, and CNS. One process of constructing group identity involves forming a title that is unifying and recognizable by the public. APRNs to date had been primarily identified by their specialty (CNM or nurse midwife, FNP or family nurse practitioner, and AOCNS or oncology CNS as examples) rather than a generalist title similar to the RN or MD. State law adopted and protected titles incrementally from 1977 onward, resulting in geographic disparity. Lack of uniform titling provided several disadvantages to APRNs who are required to use state-protected titles in business communications, particularly when practice is located across state lines. The following example (see Box 25.1) illustrates how titles for a single APRN could differ in one geographic region, resulting in public confusion and potential legal risk if titles are misused or confused in practice.

Despite the political and social advantages of having a uniform title recognized by the public, there were initial objections to the use of the descriptor "APRN" to refer to four distinct roles of practice. As an example, the American College of Nurse Midwives (ACNM, 2009) initially advocated for continued use of the title "CNM" by nurse midwives in state and national policy making. However, the ACNM dropped its initial objections to the use of the term APRN for nurse midwives after a legal analysis revealed that using a national certification title (CNM) for state licensure "was problematic and not recommended" (ACNM, 2008). The American Nurses Association (ANA, 2007) linked uniform titling and second licensure for APRNs to concerns about interstate compact formation among states that could impede the

TITLES OF APRNs IN OREGON, ALASKA, IDAHO, WASHINGTON, AND MONTANA (2012)	BOX 25.1

Alaska
ANP (advanced nurse practitioner, includes nurse midwives)
CRNA (certified registered nurse anesthetist)
CNS—no recognition

Idaho
APPN (advanced practice professional nurse, includes all roles)
APRN (advanced practice registered nurse, includes all roles) (after July 1, 2013)

Oregon
NP (includes nurse midwives, further differentiated in title by population such as FNP for family nurse practitioner, NMNP for nurse midwife nurse practitioner)
CNS (generalist title, clinical nurse specialist)
CRNA (generalist title, certified registered nurse anesthetist)

Montana
CNS-APRN (generalist; however, only CNS in psychiatric mental health is eligible for prescriptive authority)
CNM-APRN
CRNA-APRN
NP-APRN

Washington
ARNP (advanced registered nurse practitioner, generalist title for NP, CNM, and CRNA, does not include CNS as of 2013)

state's constitutional right to govern nursing practice parameters and requirements. Despite initial concerns, both organizations endorsed the *Consensus Model* by the time it was published and have continued to support its implementation by individual states.

Roles

The initial model for future APRN regulation proposed by the NCSBN was described in its *Vision Paper* (2006). Although controversial due to its exclusion of the CNS role as an APRN role, the *Vision Paper* (2006) started the joint dialogue process among regulators, educators, and certifiers that resulted in the *Consensus Model*. From 2006 to 2008, nursing groups struggled with the identification and differentiation of APRNs as distinct from nurses with advanced education, skills, or expertise. One vocal group ultimately excluded from the definition of APRN was the public health nurse. Public health nurses, unlike other registered nurses, historically were educated at the baccalaureate level and above for a community-based autonomous role, which sometimes included expanded SOP such as diagnosis and providing medications before this was legally codified for NPs (ACHNE, 2007; Keeling, 2007). Some states also license public health nurses as a unique category of nurses with additional education and qualifications, and restrict hiring in the area of public health to those duly licensed by the board of nursing (California, 2012). Advanced certification and the title of advanced practice public health nurse have been promoted by the profession as a distinct role (ACHNE, 2007). The Quad Council's Competencies for Public Health Nurses (2011) identifies three levels of practice: generalist, programmatic, and systemwide. However, the *Consensus Model* did not accept prior differentiation by education, licensure, or certification as a priori identifiers of advanced nursing practice, and grandfathering of prior recognized roles continues to be an area of controversy and disagreement. Instead, the primary differentiating factors between APRNs and nurses with advanced education and certification continue to be direct clinical practice with individuals that includes diagnosing and prescribing, according to the *Consensus Model*. Advanced practice public health nurses, who primarily practice population-based care, were therefore not identified as practicing outside of the basic RN scope and requiring APRN recognition.

Clinical nurse specialists were ultimately included in the *Consensus Model* definition of APRN, implying general consensus with the uniform educational standards, prescriptive authority, and second licensure issues, which had previously divided the profession. The model requires that all four APRN roles be nationally certified in a population-based focus. Goudreau (2011) identified the advantages of CNS recognition as APRNs, but also the challenge of national certification exams that would need to change to incorporate the CNS role as population focused. The CNS role before the implementation of the *Consensus Model* was primarily recognized and certified at the specialty level. Grandfathering of CNSs who do not meet the *Consensus Model* population-focused role, and are not eligible for a current nationally based certification exam, remains a significant issue for state licensure and mobility from state to state. The National Association of Clinical Nurse Specialists (NACNS, 2012) identifies the primary challenges to widespread implementation of the APRN *Consensus Model* for CNSs as being:

- Variability in state title protection of the CNS
- Inconsistency of state adoption of grandfathering of the CNS
- Lack of a regulatory approach to accepting grandfathered CNSs to practice in other states
- CNSs losing jobs based on misperception of the model
- Certifiers that have not developed population-based CNS examinations for all populations, resulting in limited certification exams for the CNS
- Accreditors establishing changes with limited time for schools to respond
- Curriculum challenges

Scope

The *Consensus Model* (APRN Joint Dialogue, 2008) represented the status quo for few states and APRN roles at the time it was published. Autonomous SOP existed for 13 states and the District of Columbia, and primarily for one role, NP (Pearson, 2008; NCSBN Member Boards, 2008). Nurse midwives, while practicing autonomously in many states, were subject to scope restrictions by hospital bylaws governed by physician-controlled bodies. States such as Oregon had implemented legislation in the mid-1990s which allowed midwives broad privileges to practice in the hospital setting through recognition as NPs, including admitting privileges. However, the bylaw restrictions (ORS 441.064) continued to allow hospitals to require physician supervision and oversight of SOP, despite fully autonomous legal status.

Washington State, while enjoying broad autonomous practice for APRNs, was not successful in implementing prescriptive authority for controlled substances until it agreed to a collaborative practice requirement limited to prescribing this class of drugs only. Between 1979 and 2001, CNPs had independent legal authority for all legend drugs and Schedule V (Kaplan et al., 2006). Legislation passed in 2000 was an incremental step to full autonomous practice that allowed further research into CNP practice norms and barriers, including identifying internal barriers to expanding practice (Kaplan et al., 2006). The requirement was removed in 2005 after CNPs increasingly obtained the new scope and successfully used it to manage their patients.

Incremental strategies for implementation of the *Consensus Model* often focused on expansion of prescriptive authority with some type of limitation such as collaboration, formularies, or practice-based authority, even though the *Consensus Model* did not advocate such intermediary strategies. There were significant limitations to changing from a normative to a data-driven policy strategy when attempting to change SOP. APRNs were defined and titled differently from state to state. "Autonomy" was measured differently in several studies of state regulation (Lugo et al., 2007; NCSBN, 2012a; Pearson, 2008; Pittman & Williams, 2012). As an example, use of the national provider identifier (NPI) number as a tracking mechanism for autonomous APRN practice was researched by Skillman et al. (2012). Although providing useful information to compare rural and urban practice patterns, there are significant limitations to the use of this data set, including its poor representation of CNSs and CNMs (Skillman et al., 2012). Difficulties in providing evidence-based data on APRN practice patterns were criticized by opponents such as the American Medical Association (2009) when legislative change was sought to implement the *Consensus Model* recommendations to expand scope autonomy. States that had accepted previous restrictions to SOP, with the hope that they could be incrementally removed, faced challenges to "prove" their ability to practice in a new scope (Kaplan et al., 2006).

CRNA SOP was historically well defined related to the provision of anesthesia services in an in-patient setting. However, as CRNAs became more prevalent and practice expanded to community-based settings, new areas of practice such as pain management became a scope question. In 2011, a major regional Medicare carrier stopped paying for pain management services provided by CRNAs unless they were provided incident to a physician's supervision, regardless of whether or not a state's practice act allowed it to be done autonomously. In 2012, the Centers for Medicare and Medicaid Services (CMS) nationally reversed the decision of the regional carrier to allow for provision of pain management by CRNAs under independent medical privileges as provided by state law. This decision was anticipated to further influence changes in scope related to physician supervision and collaboration in state law, which the American Association of Nurse Anesthetists (AANA) framed as codifying the scope that already exists for provision of care (AANA, 2012). The previous example illustrates the linkage among state law, autonomy, and reimbursement for services.

Other scope issues that surfaced during the implementation of the *Consensus Model* included the merging of several discrete CNP and CNS specialties into population-based roles; the preparation, certification, and licensure for acute versus primary care (NONPF, 2011/2012); and the requirement for preparation to prescribe articulated in the *Consensus Model*, which influenced curriculum and state regulation requirements.

SUCCESSFUL STRATEGIES

States hoping to implement the roles and scope outlined in the *Consensus Model* were required to make a series of policy decisions on whether to seek incremental or comprehensive change to state law. Rapid change in state law could result in several negative outcomes for already practicing APRNs, including the inability to be grandfathered, or ineligibility for licensure from state to state. Several states were able to make changes to their laws from 2008 to 2012 that expanded scope and potentially increased access to APRNs.

Pearson (2012) noted change in scope of CNP practice in 2009 in Alabama, Alaska, Arizona, California, Colorado, Florida, Georgia, Hawaii, Idaho, Kentucky, Louisiana, Maine, Mississippi, Montana, New Hampshire, New Jersey, New Mexico, New York, North Dakota, Ohio, Oklahoma, Oregon, Pennsylvania, Rhode Island, South Dakota, Tennessee, Texas, Utah, Virginia, Washington, and West Virginia. Some states implemented the recommendations of the *Consensus Model* partially; others changed all aspects of their practice act including titling. By 2012 (NCSBN, 2012a), six states had implemented legislative changes to APRN scope and practice (Arizona, Idaho, Massachusetts, Maryland, West Virginia, and Virginia), and nine more states had legislative changes pending.

Successful implementation of the *Consensus Model* goals on a state level relies on learning from mistakes of the past, such as the failed implementation of the baccalaureate degree for entry into nursing practice (Smith, 2010). It also requires keeping a vision of the future of nursing, most recently articulated in the Institute of Medicine's (IOM) *Future of Nursing* (2011). Many states reported that use of the IOM (2011) document was helpful to illustrate to legislators the need for practice at the top level of licensure, and IOM (2011) sponsorship was seen as a neutral endorsement of expanded nursing practice. Other documents used by states to advocate for expanded or codification of scope as explained in the *Consensus Model* were the findings of the Josiah Macy Jr. Foundation's multidisciplinary conference on primary care, which advocated for the removal of regulatory barriers to APRN practice (Cronenwett & Dzau, 2010). Madler, Kalanek, and Rising (2012) reported that all three policy documents were very influential in the ability to move North Dakota's APRNs to autonomous practice related to prescriptive authority.

Pearson (2012) published yearly detailed surveys of state regulation, though her reports were limited to CNP scope and practice changes. A comprehensive overview of scope changes from 2008, when the *Consensus Model* was published, to 2012 noted rapid expansion of autonomy, particularly in the removal of mandated collaboration or supervision language (Pearson, 2012). In 2009, 31 states reported some degree of an expanded legislative or regulatory CNP SOP. This number increased from 22 states that expanded their CNP SOP in 2008 and 19 states that did so in 2007 (Pearson, 2012). Pearson (2012) noted that other strategies for scope change included alliances in Texas between the business interests of owners of retail health clinics staffed by NPs and medical organizations.

Despite its previously discussed limitations, successful strategies on a state level for implementation of the *Consensus Model* sometimes involved incrementalism. State lobbyists were able to use data gleaned under more restrictive statutes to successfully demonstrate safe practice when driving expansion of APRN practice (Kaplan et al., 2008; Madler et al., 2012). The NCSBN, ANA, and NACNS published talking points and toolboxes for legislative action.

Alliances were formed with several national organizations outside of nursing to promote access to APRN care. Restrictions to practice in regulation were consistently framed by policy makers as denying choice or access to patients for their chosen provider. This strategy was successful in providing support for nursing that focused on patients rather than professional promotion. Organizations active in promoting regulatory change for APRN consistent with the *Consensus Model* included the AARP, the Robert Wood Johnson Foundation, and the Federal Trade Commission (FTC). The latter wrote a letter of support for legislation in Kentucky to remove requirements for APRNs to have a signed agreement with a physician to prescribe noncontrolled drugs such as antibiotics (Federal Trade Commission, 2012). The FTC also provided written testimony to promote change in state law regarding APRN practice in West Virginia, Texas, and Louisiana. Other state alliances included rural health associations, workforce institutes, and community care organizations.

EVALUATION AND APPLICATION TO PRACTICE

The primary application to practice of the *Consensus Model* is portability of practice across state lines and settings, recognition of all four APRN roles in statute and practice, and consistency of curricular design and practice preparation (ANA, 2009; Goudreau, 2011; NCSBN, 2012a). Entities charged with national accreditation or privileging of APRNs, such as the Veterans Administration, the CMS, and the Drug Enforcement Administration, are changing policy to reflect more consistent practice from state to state to the benefit of APRNs. As an example, CMS (2012) changed its requirements to permit hospitals to credential APRNs as members of medical staff with full privileges. Congruency between state and national policies will not only help consumers attain care but will also allow for continuous evaluation of best practice for APRNs through research and data collection.

Despite previously identified limitations in national data sets due to past inconsistent regulation of APRNs, new data reflect successful implementation of the *Consensus Model*. Outcomes of success in regulatory implementation of the model are tracked by NCSBN based on changes in state law regarding autonomy, prescriptive practice, and titling (NCSBN, 2012a). Studies have also been published which refute negative impact to physician economic status by increased APRN autonomy (Pittman & Williams, 2012) and support enhanced or analogous patient outcomes when care is provided by CNSs, CRNAs, CNMs, or CNPs (Newhouse et al., 2011).

Changes in state practice law require education of licensees and other stakeholders regarding practice expansion. Not all APRNs take advantage of scope expansion, due to lack of knowledge, concern about liability, or institutional refusal to privilege the new scope (Kaplan et al., 2006; Klein, 2012; Redmond, Palumbo, & Rambur, 2012). Evaluation strategies should include periodic assessment of barriers to full implementation of changes in state law.

DISCUSSION QUESTIONS

1. Identify several ways to evaluate successful outcomes in APRN state law change related to recommendations in the *Consensus Model*.
   a. Patient based
   b. System based
   c. Policy based

2. Using your state as an example, name four key *non-nursing* stakeholders that could form a coalition with APRNs interested in changing state law to enhance the APRN scope of practice. Why would their help be useful and what would be their focus of interest in APRN practice?

ANALYSIS AND SYNTHESIS EXERCISES

1. Your state legislator is on a committee that will vote on removing mandatory supervision of CRNAs by physicians. Write a one-page summary (talking points) with scholarly citations to provide your legislator information on why he or she should support this change.
2. Attend a state board of nursing meeting or committee meeting that has at least one agenda item related to APRN practice. Write a summary of the issue with the supporting and opposing views expressed, and provide your conclusion of support or opposition.

CLINICAL APPLICATION CONSIDERATIONS

1. Propose a model for grandfathering APRNs who practice in your state and are not eligible for national certification as proposed by the *Consensus Model*.
2. Your state law allows CNSs to be credentialed and privileged as APRNs in a hospital setting. You have just been hired as a CNS in the cardiology ICU. Physicians, nurses, and physician's assistants primarily staff the unit and the medical staff has no familiarity with CNS practice and scope. Write a three- to four-page document that could be used to obtain privileges, utilizing CNS core competencies (2011) and other appropriate documents.

REFERENCES

American Association of Nurse Anesthetists. (2012). *Fact sheet on Medicare coverage of chronic pain management provided by certified registered nurse anesthetists.* Retrieved from 20121112_Fact_Sheet_2pgr_on _Medicare_CRNA_Pain_Mgt_Final_Rule.pdf

American College of Nurse Midwives. (2009). *Dear ACNM member.* Retrieved from http://www.midwife .org/ACNM/files/ccLibraryFiles/Filename/000000001770/ACNM_to_Members_on_LACE.pdf

American Medical Association. (2009). *AMA scope of practice data series: Nurse practitioners.* Chicago, IL: Author.

American Nurses Association. (2007). *The nurse interstate licensure compact talking points.* Retrieved from http://www.midwife.org/ACNM/files/ccLibraryFiles/Filename/000000001770/ACNM_to _Members_on_LACE.pdf

American Nurses Association. (2009). *ANA issue brief: Consensus model for APRN regulation: Licensure, accreditation, certification and education.* Retrieved from http://www.nursingworld.org/consensus modeltoolkit

Association of Community Health Nurse Educators. (2007). Graduate education for advanced practice public health nursing: At the crossroads. Retrieved from http://www.achne.org/files/public /GraduateEducationDocument.pdf

APRN Joint Dialogue Group. (2008). *Consensus model for APRN licensure, accreditation, certification and education.* Retrieved from https://www.ncsbn.org/7_23_08_Consensue_APRN_Final.pdf.

Brewer, M. (1991). The social self: On being the same and different at the same time. *Personality and Social Psychology Bulletin, 17,* 475–482.

California State Board of Nursing. (2012). Public health nurse licensure application. Retrieved from http://www.rn.ca.gov/pdfs/applicants/phn-app.pdf

Centers for Medicare and Medicaid Services. (2012). Medicare and Medicaid programs: Reform of hospital and critical access hospital conditions of participation (CMS-3244-F). Retrieved from www .cms.gov

Chan, G., & Hackenschmidt, A. (2006). Understanding the influences that determine nursing practice and the opportunities for involvement: A study of the NCSBN vision paper. *Journal of Emergency Nursing, 32*(4), 350–354.

Cronenwett, L., & Dzau, V. J. (2010). Co-chairs' summary of the conference: Who will provide primary care and how will they be trained? Josiah Macy Jr. Foundation. Retrieved from www.macyfoundation .org/docs/macy_pubs/jmF_ChairSumConf_Jan2010.pdf

Dimaggio, P., & Powell, W. (1983). The iron cage revisited: Institutional isomorphism and collective rationality in organizational fields. *American Sociological Review, 48*(2), 147–160.

Diver, C. (1981). Policymaking paradigms in administrative law. *Harvard Law Review, 95*(2), 393–434.

Federal Trade Commission. (2012). FTC staff letter to the honorable Paul Hornback, Senator, Commonwealth of Kentucky State Senate concerning Kentucky SB 187 and the regulation of advanced practice registered nurses. Retrieved from http://www.ftc.gov/os/2012/03/120326ky _staffletter.pdf

Goudreau, K. (2011). LACE, APRN consensus . . . and WIIFM (What's in it for me?). *Clinical Nurse Specialist, 25*(1), 5–7. doi:10.1097/NUR.0b013e3182036221

Ingram, H., Schneider, A. L., & deLeon, P. (2007). Social construction and policy design. In P. A. Sabatier (Ed.), *Theories of the policy process* (pp. 93–126). Boulder, CO: Westview Press.

Institute of Medicine. (2011). *The future of nursing: Leading change, advancing health.* Washington, DC: National Academies Press.

Kaplan, L., Brown, M. A., Andrilla, H., & Hart, L. G. (2006). Barriers to autonomous practice. *The Nurse Practitioner, 31*(1), 57–63.

Keeling, A. (2007). *Nursing and the privilege of prescription, 1893–2000.* Columbus, OH: Ohio State University Press.

Klein, T. A. (2012). Implementing autonomous clinical nurse specialist prescriptive authority: A competency-based transition model. *Clinical Nurse Specialist, 26*(5), 254–262.

Lancaster, J. (2006). Letter from the American Association of Colleges of Nursing to the National Council of State Boards of Nursing (NCSBN) regarding the NCSBN's vision paper. *Journal of Professional Nursing, 22*(3), 145–149.

Lindblom, C. (1959). The science of "muddling through." *Public Administration Review, 19*, 79–88.

Lindblom, C. (1970). Still muddling, not yet through. *Public Administration Review, 39*, 517–526.

Lugo, N., O'Grady, E., Hodnicki, D., & Hanson, C. (2007). Ranking state NP regulation: Practice environment and consumer healthcare choice. *American Journal for Nurse Practitioners, 11*(4), 8–24.

Madler, B., Kalanek, C., & Rising, C. (2012). An incremental regulatory approach to implementing the APRN consensus model. *Journal of Nursing Regulation, 3*(2), 11–15.

National Association of Clinical Nurse Specialists. (2012). *National Association of Clinical Nurse Specialists's statement on the APRN consensus model implementation.* Retrieved from http://www.nacns.org /docs/NACNSConsensusModel.pdf

National Council of State Boards of Nursing. (2006). *Draft: Vision paper: The future regulation of advanced practice nursing.* Retrieved from https://www.ncsbn.org/Draft_APRN_Vision_Paper.pdf

National Council of State Boards of Nursing. (2008). *Member board profiles.* Chicago, IL: Author.

National Council of State Boards of Nursing. (2012a). *APRN consensus model legislation.* Retrieved from https://www.ncsbn.org/aprn.htm

National Council of State Boards of Nursing. (2012b). *Model act and rules.* Retrieved from https://www .ncsbn.org/1455.htm

National Council of State Boards of Nursing. (2012c). *APRN compact model draft revisions.* Retrieved from https://www.ncsbn.org/Agenda_item_6_APRN_Compact_Model.pdf

National Organization of Nurse Practitioner Faculty. (2011/2012). Statement on acute care and primary care practice. Retrieved from http://www.nonpf.org/associations/10789/files/ACPCStatement FinalJune2012.pdf

Newhouse, R., Stanik-Hutt, J., White, K., Johantgen, M., Bass, E., … Weiner, J. (2011). Advanced practice nursing outcomes (1990-2008): A systematic review. *Nursing Economics, 29*(5). Retrieved from http://www.nursingeconomics.net/ce/2013/article3001021.pdf

Oregon Revised Statutes. (2012). ORS 441.064. Retrieved from www.oregon/gov

Pearson, L. (2008). The Pearson report. *American Journal for Nurse Practitioners, 13*(2).

Pearson, L. (2012). A national overview of nurse practitioner legislation and healthcare issues. Retrieved from http://www.pearsonreport.com/overview

Pittman, P., & Williams, B. (2012). Physician wages in states with expanded APRN scope of practice. *Nursing Research and Practice,* 2012. doi:10.1155/2012/671974

Quad Council Public Health Nursing Competencies. (2011). Retrieved from http://www.achne.org /files/Quad%20Council/QuadCouncilCompetenciesforPublicHealthNurses.pdf

Redmond, T., Palumbo, M., & Rambur, B. (2012). Certified nurse practitioner awareness of regulatory changes in Vermont. *Journal of Nursing Regulation, 3*(3), 13–18.

Skillman, S., Kaplan, L., Fordyce, M., & Mcmenamin, P. (2012). Understanding advanced practice registered nurse distribution in urban and rural areas of the United States using national provider identifier data. WAAMI Rural Health Research Center. Retrieved from http://depts.washington.edu /uwrhrc/uploads/RHRC_FR137_Skillman.pdf

Smith, T. (October 5, 2009). A policy perspective on the entry into practice issue. *OJIN: The Online Journal of Issues in Nursing, 15*(1). doi:10.3912/OJIN.Vol15No01PPT01

Tajfel, H., & Turner, J. C. (1986). The social identity theory of inter-group behavior. In S. Worchel & L. W. Austin (Eds.), *Psychology of intergroup relations* (pp. 7–24). Chicago, IL: Nelson-Hall.

CHAPTER 26

Advanced Practice Registered Nursing: The Global Perspective

Judith Shamian and Moriah Ellen

The roles of advanced practice registered nurses (APRNs) have been in existence globally and under discussion in many countries for several decades. While developed countries like the United States, Canada, and others have made progress in introducing the roles through legislation, regulation, and education, in many countries the roles of advanced practice nurses (APNs) and nurse midwives have not been formalized. The roles have not been developed to the level that the nursing community thinks will best serve global health and the citizens of the world.

This chapter describes some of the background work in this area by the International Council of Nurses (ICN), the World Health Organization (WHO), and others. Furthermore, this chapter discusses some of the efforts that have to be undertaken to build a universal recognition and implementation of the role for the benefit of both nursing and the public.

GLOBAL CONTEXT

What does "advanced practice registered nursing" mean in the global community? International Council of Nurses (ICN, 2008):

> A Nurse Practitioner/Advanced Practice Nurse is a Registered nurse who has acquired the expert knowledge base, complex decision-making skills and clinical competencies for expanded practice, the characteristics of which are shaped by the context and/or country in which s/he is credentialed to practice. A Master's degree is recommended for entry level.
>
> *International Nurse Practitioner/Advanced Practice Nursing Network,*
> *Definition and Characteristics of the Role, ICN (2001)*

In recognition of the growing need for advanced nursing practice (ANP) and the emergence of the APRN in various forms, ICN started the global discussions in 1992, and a formal network for APNs was created in 2000 under the ICN umbrella. The aims and objectives of the International Nurse Practitioner/Advanced Practice Nursing Network (INP/APNN) are:

> to become an international resource for nurses practising in nursing practitioner (NP) or advanced nursing practice (ANP) roles, and interested others (e.g., policymakers, educators, regulators, health planners) by:
>
> 1. Making relevant and timely information about practice, education, role development, research, policy and regulatory developments, and appropriate events widely available;
> 2. Providing a forum for sharing and exchange of knowledge expertise and experience;
> 3. Supporting nurses and countries who are in the process of introducing or developing NP or ANP roles and practice;
> 4. Accessing international resources that are pertinent to this field.
>
> *INP/APNN website (2013); International Nurse Practitioner/Advanced Practice Nursing Network, "Definition and Characteristics of the Role," ICN (2001)*

The APRN can take on multiple roles in the global community. Most commonly they are called advanced practice nurses (APN) or nurse practitioners (NPs) and these terms will be used interchangeably for the remainder of the chapter. Although the evolution of APN roles in acute care is relatively recent, the roles of clinical nurse specialists (CNSs) and APNs in primary health care (PHC) have been in existence for many decades with or without independent legislation or/and regulations. In many countries nurses practice advanced roles either without any legislative frame or under medically delegated acts. The CNS role in many countries is expected to support nursing practice of nurses and not to provide advanced clinical care. One of the roles of APN which has been in existence for many decades is that of the nurse midwife. Worldwide and especially in the low middle income countries (LMIC), the independent practice of nurse midwives has been in place for decades.

While the development of the APN concept and the evolution of the role started at a country level over the last few decades, both ICN and WHO have developed several documents that are meant to guide and support the thinking and development of the NP role on an international basis. It is important, however, to distinguish between the ICN and WHO focuses. ICN's focus is on the APN role and its multiple facets from acute to CNS. The WHO's main focus is in the context of PHC (WHO, 2008) and its emphasis on "Health for All" through the Millennium Development Goals (MDGs) (WHO, 2011) and Non-Communicable Diseases (NCDs) (WHO, 2010).

It is important to note that the nurse anesthetist APRN role is seen within both Canada and the United States and several other countries globally. The role exists in other countries but not necessarily at the APRN level. For example, in Africa, nurse anesthetists can be found in Democratic Republic of Congo, in Tunisia, and more. In Asia, the role is in place in Taiwan, Cambodia, and a few other countries. In the Caribbean countries, the role exists in Jamaica and some other countries in the region. In 1989, the International Federation of Nurse Anaesthetists was formed and currently 41 countries are members (www.ifna-int.org).

ICN AND WHO: A PERSPECTIVE ON THE APRN ROLES

The International Council of Nurses: APN Network (ICN-APNETWORK)

Over the last few decades, ICN has recognized the need to have a global nursing voice and shared agreement among the nursing community to articulate the elements associated with the APN role. ICN has established a formal network for APNs, which can be found at the following URL: www.icn-apnetwork.org.

Although the concept of nurse midwives has been in existence for a long time, with or without the APN designation, in many countries the concept of a community-based NP, acute care NP, CNS, and APN in anesthesiology is virtually unknown. Furthermore, although in many countries nurses prescribe and do other forms of clinical care that often are in the realm of an APN in developed countries, there is no regulatory or educational infrastructure in place to recognize the role as an advanced role that builds on the role of the registered nurse (RN). The work of the ICN's NP/APN Network (INP/APNN) offers the information and tools that go beyond one country's experience and helps nurses, nursing organizations, policy makers, and others in each country to benefit from the richness of knowledge and information of other country-level policies and practices.

Among the world nations, it is common for similar terms to be used for different purposes. It is important to clarify the meaning of a term. For example, in some countries the reference to CNS is about an individual who has private clients, and who can prescribe and diagnose. In other countries, the very same term means a nurse with advanced preparation who provides professional support to practicing clinical nurses. Also, in other countries the two definitions above are blended so that the CNS could have private clients, prescribe, diagnose, and the same time address nursing and system-level issues so that quality and safety are maximized. As you can see, these are seemingly divergent definitions and practices.

The work that ICN has undertaken helps with understanding the role of APNs, regardless of what they are called. This is achieved through clarifying the scope, competencies, roles, and responsibilities of an APN on an international level.

The ICN (2005) defines the APN scope of practice as:

> the cognitive, integrative and technical abilities of the qualified nurse to put into practice ethical and culturally safe acts, procedures, protocols and practice guidelines. The clinical practice of the APN is scientifically based and applicable to health care practice in primary, secondary and tertiary settings in all urban and rural communities. The role also encompasses the dimensions of patient and peer education, mentorship, leadership, management and includes the responsibility to translate, utilize and undertake meaningful research to advance and improve nursing practice. (p. 3)

Furthermore, the document created by the ICN (2005) outlines what the APN can do. The activities that an APN can undertake include diagnosis, prescribing, initiating treatment, and more. What is essential to understand is that the APN can do all of these within the independent scope of practice. In many of the countries that do not have a legal, regulatory, and educational framework, nurses can often be found who engage in similar activities, but they do it under medical delegation or without any legal and/or professional authority. Some countries do not yet have a basic "nursing act" to govern the practice and the title protection of a nurse. In those countries, the practice is carried out by individuals who are considered nurses in those countries, while some have had only some academic preparation or on-the-job training.

In an effort to increase the quality and standard expectations for APN practice, the ICN documents also clearly articulate that competencies of APNs are built on the RN competencies and must be within a regulatory framework. Again the challenge in the majority of developing countries and some of the developed countries are that there are no regulatory frameworks in place for APN practice and no standards or competencies defined in regulation. Furthermore, in some countries the registration as a nurse happens at the government level and often happens once in a lifetime and is not renewed on a regular basis. This brings into question the ongoing competence of the nurse. In a growing number of countries, there are efforts under way to establish an independent, regulatory body whose mandate is to regulate nurses and where the licensing and regulation of APNs should happen.

The educational preparation of APNs internationally varies significantly and can be grouped under several categories. The first category consists of those countries that have legislation in place to govern APN practice and have a regulatory body to designate the title, to qualify individuals, and to establish clear standards that govern the educational programs that lead to APN licensing. The second category consists of countries that do not have the formal structure described and can fall into different subcategories. For example, a number of countries have "academies" and/or "specialty interest groups," with some of these countries having formal educational programs. For example, they have educational preparation to become a nurse midwife, a community nurse, and perhaps more. The final category is where the functions and the advanced role that nurses assume is a result of necessity in the field and is self-taught knowledge or on-the-job training. In most developed and developing countries, there are an insufficient number of APNs prepared at the graduate level to meet the standards described by ICN as the desired level of educational preparation.

Having the ICN documents that outline the competencies, standards, roles, and expectations of APNs is extremely important and helps nurses and the governments of countries to know how to move forward if there is the political and the professional will to do so. The standards and core competencies are expected to provide a foundation and broad guidelines for APNs and contributing authorities all over the world. The expectation is that they will then develop this role within their own country while meeting the established professional, authorized, and regulatory frameworks and requirements.

World Health Organization (WHO): Primary Health Care

As stated at the beginning of this chapter, the main focus of WHO in relation to the APRN is linked to the focus on PHC. In 2008, the WHO celebrated its 60th anniversary and the 30th anniversary of the Declaration of Alma Ata on PHC (WHO, 2008). The principles underlying the declaration are still relevant today, and there is wide recognition that the principles can provide the basis for health care policy reform in many countries for the coming years. The intent and the spirit of the Alma Alta Declaration were to have global access to primary care for *all* by the year 2000. That goal was not attained, but there was significant progress in many countries. WHO and the international community reaffirmed that PHC services are essential in building healthy and productive societies.

Nurses and midwives embraced the Alma Ata Declaration of 1978 and have been strong proponents of the principles that guide it, as evidenced by the rapid reorientation of professional training and transformation of nursing and midwifery practice to support PHC. With the renewed emphasis on PHC, the Office of the Nurse Scientist at WHO, together with the WHO Global Advisory Group (GAG) have renewed their efforts to accelerate nursing's involvement in and contribution to PHC. The compendium of case studies illustrating successful PHC initiatives, *Now, More than Ever: Nursing and Midwifery Contribute to Primary Health Care* (WHO, 2009a), gathered by the Office of Nursing and Midwifery at the WHO, illuminates that the contribution of nurses and midwives to PHC is substantial and their experience is valuable. Examples from the compendium illustrate how nurses and midwives have contributed in all the new reform areas. The case studies can be located at the following URL: www.who.int/hrh/nursing_midwifery/documents/en/index.html (WHO, 2009b).

WHO and many other organizations, including ICN, recognized that the way to global health is through PHC. The reality hit when the year 2000 came and went, and the goal of "Health for ALL by 2000" (HFA, 2000) was not accomplished. Several global meetings were held to review accomplishments and revitalize efforts to accelerate the efforts to build comprehensive global PHC. The 2008 WHO report (WHO, 2008) dealt with the renewal of PHC and why it has not been achieved. The WHO Global Advisory Group (GAG) was established in the 1990s to make recommendations to the DG of WHO on nursing and midwifery issues. The group also studied how nursing can accelerate its contribution to global PHC. GAG fully embraced the PHC renewal and, under the leadership of Dr. Jean Yang, the Chief Nurse Scientist of the time, undertook a tremendous amount of work to demonstrate the role and contribution that nurses generally, and nurse practitioners in particular, can make to PHC.

The MDGs (WHO, 2011) call for the attainment of nine focused goals by 2015. Among the nine were goals to reduce infant and maternal mortality and the strengthening of health systems through renewed PHC. It is clear that PHC systems have become critical on a global scale. Many agree with the DG of the WHO in stating that the MDGs can only be reached with the renewal of the PHC principles.

Examining the WHO website will provide the reader with some major documents that have been published through the last couple of decades. One of the two major WHO reports worth examining further is the WHO Commission on Social Determinants of Health (SDH), *Closing the Gap in a Generation* (WHO, 2008), which describes how social factors such as poverty have an impact on the health of a population. The document identifies how new knowledge and understanding of the interrelationship of many societal variables have been observed, and health is seen partly as a product of societal situations.

The consistent theme that emerges in evaluating the global challenges when dealing with health issues is that policy makers failed to put in place the required policies. The report urges policy makers, in health and other areas, to rise to the challenge of improving social conditions instrumental in securing health. Placing the responsibility for lack of success squarely on the shoulders of policy makers, the Commission of Social Determinants of Health champions PHC as a model that acts on the underlying social, political, and economic causes of ill health. APNs could contribute to a lot of these issues, as their proposed competencies address their abilities to do community assessment, planning, and interventions.

The second important document is the WHO report *Primary Health Care: Now More than Ever* (WHO, 2008), which revisits the 1978 Alma Ata Declaration principles of PHC and considers the revision of the principles in light of new knowledge and 30 years of experience. In the report, new observations and learning since Alma Ata are incorporated into the new reforms, particularly knowledge based on the social determinants of health and the MDGs.

The WHO report (2008) maintains that as societies modernize, people increasingly want to have a say in important decisions that affect their lives, including issues such as allocation of resources and organization and regulation of care.

THE ROLE OF NURSES AND MIDWIVES IN THE ALMA ATA RENEWAL

In 1992, the World Health Assembly adopted resolution WHA45.5 on "Strengthening Nursing and Midwifery in Support of Strategies for Health for All," urging the DG to establish an advisory group, which he did in 1992. The Global Advisory Group of Nursing and Midwifery (GAGNM) is thus an advisory group responsible for advising the DG on policies supporting nursing and midwifery development in WHO member states.

The DG, at a meeting with GAGNM in March 2009, stated that the challenge of "PHC/Health for All" was that key stakeholders were not involved early enough, resulting in multiple definitions of the concepts, especially by professionals. For this renewal, nursing and midwifery and other health professionals should be involved.

The GAG communicated to the WHO Director General that GAGNM recognizes the importance of WHO regional nursing and midwifery programs that support progress toward the achievement of health-related MDGs, particularly through improving the quality of nurse and midwife education postqualification level. Furthermore, WHO should support countries in maximizing/expanding the scope of practice of nurses and midwives. This could lead to the establishment of APN roles using legislation, education, and regulation.

Continued international efforts and commitments being made toward improving global nursing and midwifery workforce strategies are important. The *Kampala Declaration and Agenda for Global Action* (2008) and the *WHO Regional Office for the Western Pacific Strategic Plan for Strengthening Health Systems* (2008) both call for greater government commitment to improving the health care workforce, and enhancing the collection and use of reliable Human Resources for Health (HRH) data in making informed policy decisions. With continued global backing for the improvement of the health care workforce, it is hoped that international health outcomes will improve and global health targets will be met.

The 2008 "Chaing Mai declaration" was made by over 700 health care professionals, including nurses, doctors, midwives, and other interested stakeholders, from 33 countries from all of the six regions of WHO. The participants were at the International Conference on *New Frontiers in Primary Health Care: Role of Nursing and Other Professions.* An excerpt of the declaration is provided below:

We declare that:

> Nursing and Midwifery is a vital component of the health workforce and are acknowledged professionals who contribute significantly to the achievements of PHC and the MDGs.
>
> Nurses and midwives can successfully lead health teams that are essential for successful PHC to achieve MDGs.
>
> PHC and the MDGs will not be fully achieved if the nursing and midwifery workforce continues to be neglected.
>
> Key PHC policy decisions, at all levels, must involve nursing and midwifery leaders for effective and informed decision-making.
>
> *(WHO, 2008b)*

The recommendations of this declaration call on policy makers to recognize and include nurses in decision making and planning for PHC. It also calls for legislation and educational systems to be put in place to prepare the necessary health care professionals.

THE REALITY ON THE GROUND

The role and the concept of APNs in the PHC setting are several decades old. In some of the developed countries, which will be referred to as the Organization for Economic Co-operation and Development (OECD), like the United States and Canada, the role, scope, regulation, education, and practice are established but continuously evolving. The establishment of these roles came about through much research and advocacy. The same advocacy and policy push by the nursing community existed and continues to exist in several of the OECD countries to introduce and/or increase the use and availability of APNs.

The concept of an APN for PHC is extremely important in the low and middle-income countries (LMC), but takes on a different meaning. In the LMC countries outside of the urban setting, far too often the nurse is the primary clinician and for periods of time the only clinician. Often he or she is the nurse, the midwife, the generalist, the specialist, and the maker of clinical decisions. So he or she prescribes, orders tests, sutures, delivers babies, comforts those who are in need, and much more. In these circumstances, the notion that there is room for a different class of practitioners on top of the nurse is great but not realistic. The key challenge for policy makers, educators, providers of fiscal resources, and the health care community, including nursing leadership, is to identify in a comprehensive manner how capacity can be built to provide the nurse with APN knowledge and/or access to APNs virtually.

This issue is a serious one that raises significant debates within the nursing community. Some are of the opinion that we need to advocate for the same Western-OECD level of health care, roles, and functions because everyone should have the right to the same health care. Philosophically and ideally, the ICN is in full support of these ideas. The reality is that most maternal child deaths, much of the infectious diseases, and a growing number of NCDs (non-communicable diseases and chronic diseases) can be found in much higher proportion in the LMIC than in the OECD countries. Therefore we need to improve the health of the population as quickly as possible while attending to raising the scope, role, education, and research levels of health professionals and nurses in the LMC.

So What Is the Reality on the Ground?

The reality is that many RNs who work in rural communities work in the capacity of APN without the regulatory designation and often without the desired knowledge and tools. In some countries, the front-line "nurse" is not an RN but has some other designation and education level. Although that is not the desired reality, they still are the front-line people who deal with clinical emergencies, and often, they are the only one in the field. The more common reality is that there are RNs and some are RN midwives who have gone through additional training to enhance their midwifery skills but do not have the APN designation and level of knowledge and competencies of an APN.

The OECD conducted a survey regarding APN roles in 2009 (Delamaire & Lafratune, 2010). The countries that participated were organized under two groups. The first group consisted of countries with experience with APN, including

Australia, Canada, Finland, Ireland, United Kingdom, and the United States. These countries have led the charge in building the APN roles and getting the required infrastructure, and continue to be at the forefront in pushing the boundaries and challenging the possibilities and opportunities for the roles. The second group had less experience with the APN roles; this group included Belgium, Cyprus, Czech Republic, France, Japan, and Poland. These countries are distributed among three continents. The interest in the APN role goes beyond the North American and European regions; furthermore, while all these countries are members of OECD, there are different levels of country development. Countries like Poland and the Czech Republic are more recent members of OECD versus countries like Ireland, the United States, Canada, and others, which have been considered to be "developed countries" for a while. The survey results found that APNs do two broad types of activities (OECD Survey, 2009):

1. *Substitution:* services formerly provided by doctors, reduce workload of doctors, improve access to care, and reduce cost
2. *Supplementation:* new services (e.g., quality improvement), CNSs with the main aims—improve services/quality of care

The survey findings indicate that the greatest impact on patient care made by APRNs was in the areas of access to care and quality of care by doing some primary care as first contact for minor illnesses, and that patients were as satisfied with the APRN care or more satisfied than the care by physicians.

APPLICATION OF APRN PRACTICE: COUNTRY-LEVEL EXAMPLES AND DISCUSSION

Each country's experience in establishing the role of APRN is different; often countries need to make compromises to start the role and then continue to advance the role to the optimal level of education, funding, practice, and legislation. To demonstrate this point, let us explore the experience in Jamaica and the Caribbean.

The APRN role which is called APN started in Jamaica in 1977 with a certificate jointly approved by the Ministry of Health and the Faculty of Medical Sciences (FMS), University of the West Indies (UWI). From the inception of the program, the UWI School of Nursing, Mona (formerly Advanced Nursing Education Unit, UWI) has been responsible for curriculum development, monitoring, selection of entrants for the program, and the examination process. The Dean of FMS and the Permanent Secretary, Ministry of Health, jointly signed the certificates for graduates.

In 2002, the program was fully transferred to the UWI with the support of the Government of Jamaica. The existing certificate curriculum was upgraded and approved to a master degree status, reflecting global trends in ANP. The Master of Science in Nursing (MScN) for APN is offered over five semesters. It is offered full-time and part-time.

Family Nurse Practitioner (Delivered at UWI)

The credit load for the family nurse practitioner is 45 credits. Applicants must be an RN and midwife, and have at least five years current clinical practice. Applicants must have three years post-RN licensure/registration for nursing administration, nursing education, and CNS, and five years post-RN licensure/registration clinical practice as an RN in an approved recognized agency, institution, or organization where primary, secondary, tertiary, or extended health care services are offered. In 2009, a new track was introduced in gerontological nursing.

Clinical Nurse Specialist—Gerontology Track

This new track produces a cadre of nurses prepared at the advanced clinical level to provide evidence-based care to elderly persons along the wellness illness continuum at the primary, secondary, and tertiary levels of care. They will be prepared to deliver advanced nursing care in the clinical and functional areas of nursing practice. At this time (2013), only graduates from Barbados have been employed as CNS.

Nurse practitioners practice in the following countries in the Caribbean region: Antigua, Bahamas, Barbados, Dominica, Jamaica, St. Kitts, St. Lucia, Montserrat, St. Vincent, and the Grenadines. They are employed in various settings such as government services, health centers and clinics, accident and emergency units, army, private practice, and school health (personal communication with Drs. Whinney-Dehaney & Hewitt, June, 2013; Seivwright, 1982a, 1982b).

Another example that demonstrates the effectiveness of the APN role is outlined by some comments from the government chief nurse in Zimbabwe, Mrs. Cynthia MZ Chasokela. During a meeting hosted by the WHO in Kenya in 2009, Mrs. Chasokela identified that she has been very successful in moving forward the health care and nursing agenda in her country. She described the role of nurses in PHC as: community education and training in use of appropriate technology; early detection and correct diagnosis of illness and disability; effective treatment and management of conditions; routine health care work, including data collection, processing, and its use for planning and decision making at the level of collection; and more many of the responsibilities often identified as part of the competencies of APN. She was referring to individuals with the preparation and designation of APN as defined and recognized in some of the countries like the United States and Canada that have the education, legislation, and regulatory framework for APNs. Although many of the countries recognize the need for more advance preparation and the need for APNs, there is no political climate that will allow for it to happen. These two examples clearly demonstrate the different ways that the nursing community and others advance the APRN role for the benefit of the population and the advancement of the profession.

The other area of evolution that has taken shape over the last decade and accelerated with the MDGs is the role of midwives. Historically in many countries, primarily the former British colonies, RNs went through a 12 to 18 months' specialty training to become nurse midwives. In the United States, the nurse midwifery designation is considered to be at the APN level. This is not the case in other countries. Nurses in some countries, like the UK, can be licensed both as nurses and midwives under two separate regulatory bodies, and they do not have to keep their nursing license in order to maintain their midwifery license. The more recent trend and pressure by the International Council of Midwives (ICM) is to build direct entry programs to midwifery without having a nursing designation. This issue creates a lot of international controversy and is not supported by many in the nursing community. There is no debate about whether midwifery is an advanced role; rather, the disputed issue is whether it is a separate profession or is part of the nursing APN role.

To understand the issues and impact of country-specific needs for APNs, one needs to understand the country context, regulation, role of government, role of other non-nursing organizations, the education system, and the overall environment. The readiness of the population to consider these roles is also an essential element. This is at varying levels globally and it may be a significant amount of time before we can globally claim a common understanding of the APN roles.

BARRIERS TO APRN ROLES

Although the contribution APRNs make to the health of the population and the positive impact they have is clear and well documented, the existence of the role is not widespread, and even for those countries that have achieved the legislation, funding, and preparation of the APRN roles, it came through many years of struggle and political activism. The question to be asked is why are there so many barriers to establish and implement a role that can be so useful to the health of people? The barriers mostly relate to the traditional tension between the medical and nursing professions, and lack of role clarity as to the different roles of APRNs and others. For example, the likelihood that the South American countries and some of the Middle Eastern countries will have a strong presence of APRNs is limited because of the high ratio of physicians per population. Until recently there were two to three doctors per nurse. Current policies are in development that are trying to even out the doctor–nurse distribution. Although the APRN role is different than an MD role, the overlap is perceived to be sufficient to pose a threat to the medical profession. Politicians are reluctant to embrace an agenda that will meet stiff opposition from any major interest group. Physicians are globally considered a very strong interest group (Delamaire & Lafratune, 2010; Pulcini, Gul, & Loke, 2010).

Furthermore, funding is another barrier to the establishment of APRN roles. Governments, insurance companies, and other funders are hesitant to add new categories of professionals that can charge for services. National human resource plans often do not include a national plan for APRNs. Lack of educational funding and dedicated faculty to establish APRN programs are additional barriers.

The biggest barriers are often the lack of advocacy by the nursing community, and the lack of efforts by the organized nursing community to educate the public of the value and importance of the APRN role to advance the health of the nation. The health care provider community has been engaged primarily in a discussion of the importance of team work and collaboration among nurses, APRNs, and doctors; it is believed that more emphasis on this interprofessional cooperation might lead to better appreciation of the different roles and removal of some of the resistance to the APRN roles.

To resolve and/or minimize these barriers, nursing groups, health care groups, the public, and government should work together. Strengthening the concept of a team education of health care professionals and team practice is one way to help future health care professionals to gain role clarity and respect for each other's work. In the LMC, where there are too few nurses, midwives, doctors, and others, the ability to bring APRN roles to communities can make a very strong impact on the health of the community. Governments should accelerate the passing of legislative and regulatory frameworks to facilitate the APRN roles and provide the funding frameworks for both education and practice.

CONCLUSION

The need for APRNs is global. One can argue that the current reality is the inverse. In those countries where there are tremendous health care needs, like in the LMIC and in high-risk communities and population, the need for qualified well-prepared APRNs is tremendous, but the current reality is that those countries are most likely to require infrastructure, education, and regulation that allow and encourage the creation of APRN roles. Most often, APRNs, the needed infrastructure, education, regulation, and positions can be found in the OECD countries where the burden of disease is lower.

At the same time, there are insufficient resources (both financial and human) to build an APRN system similar to those that currently exist in the OECD countries. All countries could benefit from a well-established APRN community. It is important to have a global image, plan, advocacy agenda, and more to achieve the desired availability of APRNs, but there also needs to be a recognition that there are skills and competencies that reside in the APRN roles at some of the OECD countries that are urgently needed in the LMIC. That is the challenge, and the international community and the international nursing and health organizations, like ICN, WHO, International Monetary Fund (IMF), and more, must support the development of the roles and services.

DISCUSSION QUESTIONS, ANALYSIS AND SYNTHESIS EXERCISES, AND CLINICAL APPLICATION CONSIDERATION

1. Should APRNs practice under legislation and regulations that are unique and focused on the APRN role?
2. What should be the role of international nursing organizations in advancing the uptake of the APRN role?
3. What should be the role of global organizations like WHO and others in advancing the role of APN?
4. Why is the APRN role more formalized in the developed countries?
5. What can be done to remove barriers to the APRN role internationally?
6. What contribution can the APRN role make to the health of international communities in need?

Disclaimer: The information, views, and opinions contained in this chapter are those of the authors alone and were developed prior to Dr. Shamian's election as president of the International Council of Nurses (ICN). They do not necessarily reflect the views and opinions of the ICN.

REFERENCES

Clinical Nurse Specialists. (2009). *Position statement*. Canadian Nurses Association.

Delamaire, M. L., & Lafrotune, G. (2010). Nurses advanced roles: A description and evaluation of experiences in 12 developed countries. OECD Health Working Paper No. 54.

International Council of Nurses. (2005). *Scope of practice and standards for advanced practice nurses*. Retrieved from http://international.aanp.org/HealthPolicy.htm on July 4, 2013.

International Conference Dedicated to the 30th anniversary of the Alma-Ata Declaration on Primary Health Care–Almaty, Kazakhstan, 16–17 October 2008. *Conference conclusions and recommendations*.

Pulcini, J., JelicRaisaGul, M., & Yuen Loke, A. (2010). An international survey on advanced practice nursing education, practice, and regulation. *Journal of Nursing Scholarship*. Retrieved from http://onlinelibrary.wiley.com/doi/10.1111/j.1547-5069.2009.01322.x/abstract

Seivwright, M. (1982a). Nurse practitioners in primary health care: The Jamaican experience, Part 1. *International Nursing Review, 29*(1), 22–24.

Seivwright, M. (1982b). Nurse practitioners in primary health care: The Jamaican experience, Part 2. *International Nursing Review, 29*(2), 51–59.

World Health Organization. (2008a). The world health report 2008: Primary health care (now more than ever). Retrieved on October 30, 2013 from http://www.who.int/whr/2008/en

World Health Organization. (2008b). The Chaing Mai declaration: Nursing and midwifery for primary health care. Retrieved on October 30, 2013 from http://www.who.int/hrh/nursing_midwifery/chiang_mai_declaration.pdf

World Health Organization. (2009a). *Now, more than ever: Nursing and midwifery contribute to primary health care.* Compendium of Primary Case studies.

World Health Organization. (2009b). *A compendium of primary health care studies.* Geneva: World Health Organization.

World Health Organization. (2010). Global status report on noncommunicable diseases 2010. Retrieved on October 30, 2013 from http://www.who.int/nmh/publications/ncd_report2010/en

World Health Organization, Commission on Social Determinants of Health. (2008). *Closing the gap in a generation: Health equity through action on the social determinants of health.* Geneva: World Health Organization.

CHAPTER 27

Credentialing Across the Globe: Approaches and Applications

Frances Hughes and Catherine Coates

A combination of factors—globalization, deregulation, privatization, health care restructuring, and nursing shortages—have all led to an increase in focus on systems and processes, which serves to promote and validate the quality of nursing and health care globally. Credentialing is being increasingly recognized as offering an opportunity to apply formal processes to verify qualifications, experience, professional standing, and other relevant professional attributes to assess competence, performance, and professional suitability to provide a safe, high-quality health care service within specific environments.

Health care has come to value accreditation in general and valuing excellence—individual excellence, organizational excellence, and educational excellence—is part of the credentialing process, and is becoming increasingly important on an international scale.

The term "credentialing" has various definitions internationally, but for the purpose of this chapter, credentialing refers to a process used to assign specific clinical responsibilities to health practitioners on the basis of their education. It commences on employment, and continues for the period of employment.

AN INTERNATIONAL APPROACH TO THE APPLICATION OF CREDENTIALING TO NURSING

Credentialing is a core component of clinical and professional governance or self-regulation where members of a profession set standards for practice and competence within their specialist domain beyond entry to practice. Although there is a worldwide shortage of nurses, "there is an increasing demand for nurses with enhanced skills who manage a more diverse, complex, and acutely ill patient population than ever before" (Duffield, Gardner, Chang, & Catling-Paull, 2009).

Internationally we have guidance on the positive impact of credentialing from multiple sources. We also have opportunities to learn from the experience (both good and not so good) of other countries in introducing credentialing. Evidence-based, consensus standards and principles are important for the overarching framework for all countries. Professional nursing organizations have developed these over time but often without the accompanying ability to ensure compliance and mandate requirements. As a result, we have variability in the structure, uptake, and impact of credentialing across the globe, which may reduce its effectiveness. For example, the International Council of Nurses (ICN), through its advanced practice network, has developed policies and standards on advanced practice, which are outlined later in the text, but member countries have varying ability to mandate them.

ICN is a pillar for the global introduction of credentialing in nursing. In 2000, it established a Credentialing and Regulators Forum with the purpose of serving as a mechanism for countries with an interest in developing "dynamic regulatory processes and credentialing programs to communicate, consult and collaborate with one another on trends, problems, solutions, etc." (ICN, 2013). This forum also provides an opportunity to promote and enable nursing's role at the forefront of health care and the development of contemporary regulatory and credentialing systems, and to advise ICN on developments and needs in regulation, credentialing, and quality assurance.

The United States and the United Kingdom both have well-developed credentialing processes and systems. The American Nurses Credentialing Center (ANCC), which is a subsidiary of the American Nurses Association, aims to promote excellence in nursing and health care globally through credentialing programs (ANCC, 2013). It is the most significant nurse credentialing organization in the United States.

ANCC has established internationally renowned credentialing programs, which certify and recognize individual nurses in specialty areas. The organization also recognizes health care organizations for promoting safe and positive work environments, and accredits continuing nursing education organizations. Under the umbrella of ANCC, a range of programs are offered:

- Accreditation program—This recognizes the importance of high-quality nursing education and skills-based competency programs. ANCC accredits organizations internationally; these organizations provide nurses with the knowledge and skills to improve care and patient outcomes.
- Certification program—This enables nurses to demonstrate their specialty expertise and validate their knowledge to employers and patients. Targeted exams incorporate the latest nursing practice standards and ANCC certification empowers nurses with pride and professional satisfaction.
- Magnet® recognition program—Organizations that achieve Magnet® recognition have demonstrated nursing excellence and quality patient outcomes.

In the UK, the Royal College of Nursing (RCN) accredits a range of training programs and providers, while the Nursing and Midwifery Council sets the standards for nursing, midwifery, and health visiting care. The RCN follows a detailed process of accreditation, which includes systems for recruiting applicants to programs; registering and tracking applicants; and the collection and verification of evidence. The accreditation process involves peer review by expert representatives drawn from clinical, management, and educational fields of practice who have the appropriate professional background and experience (Coates, 2010). Examples of the programs accredited by the RCN include:

- Clinical leadership program
- Expertise and practice

- Accredited facilitator
- Mental health
- Emergency nursing
- Workplace accreditation
- Standards for higher-level practice for consultant nurses
- Nursing and midwifery council practitioner programs

There is considerable diversity in approaches toward credentialing internationally. Many countries are currently working actively on continuing education and credentialing of nurse practitioners (NPs) and nurses in specialist or advanced practice. It appears to be becoming increasingly common for national nursing organizations to collaborate with other associations and regulatory bodies or multidisciplinary agencies in relation to credentialing. The number and variety of agencies involved in the credentialing process appear to vary depending on the country.

Despite country variations in process and procedures, credentialing appears to be becoming increasingly accepted as a mechanism to formally recognize expertise and specific skill sets in registered nurses (Cioffi et al., 2003). Countries with substantive well-established bodies are increasingly assisting others, which is important for countries with fewer resources. The international network of professional nursing bodies is crucial in maintaining professional standards and reflecting these in an overarching credentialing framework. Stronger emphasis may now be needed to galvanize this network into working on strategies for compliance, to reduce variability across the globe. Professional specialist/advanced practice membership is key to achieving this compliance and reducing variability, although we must recognize that individual countries need to work within their own legislation, professional structures, and cultural and social dynamics (Newton, Pillay, & Higginbottom, 2012).

The following two case studies are examples of professional mental health nursing organizations developing and applying processes of credentialing, using the term differently for different purposes.

CASE STUDY 1—CREDENTIALING OF REGISTERED NURSES DELIVERING MENTAL HEALTH CARE WITHIN PRIMARY HEALTH CARE SETTINGS IN NEW ZEALAND

In New Zealand, the first step toward mental health credentialing for nurses was introduced in 2011; this section describes the process used to assign specific clinical responsibilities to health practitioners on the basis of their education. A credential in mental health nursing refers to registered nurses who undertake activities in mental health but who are not specialist mental health nurses. Mental health nurses, on the other hand, are registered nurses with specific education and training in the specialty area of mental health.

Te Rau Hinegaro (Oakley-Brown, Wells, & Scott, 2006) was the first national mental health survey conducted in New Zealand and identified that people with mental health issues, including substance use, do not necessarily visit a primary health care practitioner in relation to mental health concerns. Approximately 58% of people with a serious disorder, 37% with a moderate disorder, and 19% with a mild disorder present to a health service to discuss their mental health concerns. In addition, it is well recognized that people with mental health issues are vulnerable to a wide range of other health and social problems.

Although an international evidence base demonstrating these findings was well established, this was the first study specific to New Zealand to support these international findings. At the same time, it was becoming clear that the present system was not offering nurses, employers, or consumers any certainty about the knowledge and skills required by registered nurses in order to competently and confidently provide a primary care response for people who have mental health and/or substance use issues. Clarity and consistency were required about the level of knowledge and skill needed by registered nurses working in the primary health sector in order to ensure competence and safety for people with mental health and substance use problems.

The responsibility of credentialing in New Zealand is delegated to professional bodies. In the specialty area of mental health, any registered nurse working in a primary health care service who has the knowledge, skills enhancement, and experience to apply mental health and addiction assessment, referral, and interventions in a primary care setting may apply to Te Ao Māramatanga (the New Zealand College of Mental Health Nurses) to become credentialed.

Credentialing commences on appointment and continues for the period of employment. The process is peer led and requires periodic recredentialing in order to maintain the credential. It recognizes the competence of an individual to perform agreed clinical activities within a designated environment. A credential complements a nurse's existing performance review by confirming the current credentialed status of the nurse (Te Ao Māramatanga, 2013).

Applicants must complete an evidence-based record (EBR) in order to be considered for becoming credentialed in mental health nursing in primary care settings. The EBR is a record of the applicant's learning and education or training activity. Education and training are based on evidence-based New Zealand tools and guidelines (where possible) and include:

- Identifying common presenting issues
- Principles of motivating behavior change
- Screening and health promotion—for example, recognizing people who are at risk of developing moderate to severe mental illness and addiction
- Brief assessment skills
- Brief intervention skills
- Knowledge of commonly prescribed medications and their side effects
- Knowledge of community resources
- Referral and consultation pathways
- Working in shared care arrangements with specialist mental health and addiction treatment nurses/services
- Continuing management (follow-up) of people with chronic conditions, inclusive of enduring mental health illness and addictions
- Familiarity with web-based primary care packages

The EBR is then submitted to Te Ao Māramatanga's Credentialing Review Panel with the initial application and then again when recredentialing is required three years later. A credential awarded by Te Ao Māramatanga is valid for three years from the date of issue. The successful applicant receives a certificate, which is designed with space on the back to place an updated recredentialed sticker for every successful reapplication received.

The credential means that the nurse has specific skills in mental health and addiction assessment intervention in the primary health environment, but not to the level required for mental health nursing.

A credential from Te Ao Māramatanga in mental health benefits the individual nurse by ensuring that the nurse's skills in mental health and addiction meet certain standards and that the nurse will be supported to maintain and extend his or her skills. Credentialed registered nurses then become associate members of Te Ao Māramatanga (New Zealand College of Mental Health Nurses). This provides access to a website with regular updates, journal articles, and other relevant information, and provides a forum to engage with other credentialed primary care nurses.

Employers of credentialed nurses are expected to support those nurses in the development of the knowledge and skills required to main their credentialed status. This can include, for example, enabling access to relevant training and information; providing the opportunity for registered nurses to use their credentialed skills in everyday practice; and ensuring access to relevant clinical supervision and peer support, as well as review forums.

For specialist mental health nurses in New Zealand, Te Ao Māramatanga uses the term "certified" meaning they meet a set of standards in mental health nursing to hold themselves out to be recognized as a mental health nurse. Te Ao Māramatanga is working on a process to introduce certification which will provide formal recognition that a registered nurse has met the professional standards for mental health nursing set by Te Ao Māramatanga, and so will then be called a certified mental health nurse. It is proposed that new graduate registered nurses will be eligible to seek certification as a mental health nurse after completing a mental health new graduate program and working an additional 12 months in mental health. Existing registered nurses could follow a number of pathways, including having completed the mental health entry-to-specialty-practice program, or having completed a postgraduate qualification or equivalent with a mental health focus and working for three years or more as a registered nurse in mental health.

CASE STUDY 2: CREDENTIALING OF NURSES WITHIN AUSTRALIA'S HEALTH CARE SYSTEM

Unlike New Zealand, Australia's health care system is managed at the federal level and overseen by federal governments in each of Australia's six states and two territories.

The Royal College of Nursing Australia (RCNA) has actively promoted credentialing via a range of initiatives, including establishing a national center for nurse credentialing (Royal College of Nursing Australia, 2011).

Four specialty organizations offer a credentialing service: the Australian College of Critical Care Nurses; the Australian College of Mental Health Nurses; PapScreen Victoria and Western Australia; and the Gastroenterological Nurses College of Australia. In order to compare and contrast the specific systems used in New Zealand and Australia, the example of credentialing mental health nurses in Australia is used as a case study.

The Australian College of Mental Health Nurses (ACMHN) is the body responsible for the credentialing of nurses in mental health. The ACMHN Credential for Practice Program (CPP) was launched nationally in October 2004, and since then over 1100 registered nurses have been recognized as specialist mental health nurses through this program (Gendek, 2011). The ACMHN CPP is the only national credentialing program currently implemented within Australia, and it recognizes the skills, expertise, and experience of nurses who are practicing as specialist mental health nurses. The credential demonstrates to employers, professional colleagues, patients, and carers that an individual nurse has achieved the professional standard for practice in mental health nursing, as well as recognizing the contribution mental health nurses make to the mental health of the community (Royal Australian College of Mental Health Nurses, 2011).

In Australia, credentialing is a core component of clinical and professional governance or self-regulation. Members of the profession set the standards for practice and establish a minimum requirement for entry, continuing professional development, endorsement, and recognition.

In order to apply to become a credentialed mental health nurse in Australia, applicants must demonstrate that they:

- Hold a current license to practice as a registered nurse within Australia
- Hold a recognized specialist/postgraduate mental health nursing qualification
- Have at least 12 months of experience since completing specialist/postgraduate qualification or have three years of experience as a registered nurse in mental health
- Have been practicing within the last three years
- Have acquired minimum continuing professional development points for education and practice
- Are supported by two professional referees
- Have completed a professional declaration agreeing to uphold the standards of the profession

Applicants are required to complete an EBR detailing professional activities undertaken as part of continuing professional education and continuing practice development as a mental health nurse.

AN OPPORTUNITY FOR GLOBAL PROCESSES AND PROCEDURES

Increasing debate is taking place about the feasibility of globally accepted competencies and education standards that remain locally responsive and achievable. Some commentators argue that there is a need to make transparent, standardize, and harmonize existing credentialing processes to ensure that migrating registered nurses can apply their skills and expertise more broadly than within their own country of education (Singh & Sochan, 2010).

The feasibility of applying consistent credentialing processes globally needs to be examined both from a professional and a practical point of view. Education is linked to practice and the planning and delivery of care; in the case of nursing, the body of knowledge is continually growing and scopes of practice expanding. The health care system itself is complex and technology, medicines, and demands continue to change rapidly. At the core, confidence in a high-quality health care workforce that continues to be able to keep up with a fast-moving professional world, and to provide leadership within that world, is paramount.

The two case studies illustrated that even between two countries with many similarities that are close in geographic proximity, there are demonstrable differences, which could challenge any ability to apply consistent systems and processes with regard to credentialing. At a basic level, terminology differs between countries, and is not well understood, with the terms "accreditation,"[1] "credentialing," and "certification"[2] used interchangeably in the international scene (Coates, 2010).

In the examples of Australia and New Zealand mental health nurse credentialing, Australia's use of the term *credentialing* equates to New Zealand's term *certification*. Neither the Australian nor New Zealand example refers to an advanced level of practice; rather, they refer to the recognition of the specialist practice of experts. Confusion over terminology as well as over roles, scopes of practice, and professional boundaries of nurses in an international context has emerged in the literature (Duffield et al., 2009).

Both New Zealand and Australia have experienced changes over the last decade in their national registration processes. This has had a particular impact on mental health nurses, as up until these changes occurred, separate registrations were in situ for psychiatric nurses and they were deemed to be a nursing specialty by the fact of registration. Since 2003 in New Zealand and 2010 in Australia, these registrations have no longer been in place; thus, it became increasingly difficult to define and determine who was a mental health nurse, and confusion therefore occurred. Credentialing (Australia), and potentially, certification (New Zealand) are increasingly being seen as a way of determining who is a specialist mental health nurse.

The provision of services that are responsive to local needs is vitally important to ensure the highest level of patient care. Providing services that ensure cultural needs and specificities are met is equally important, and it therefore becomes difficult to balance consistent processes while ensuring that services are responsive to local needs.

The application of any process or system needs also to be examined in practical terms, including legal considerations; international processes; costs; economic and political forces; marketing; minimum acceptable standards; stakeholder input; monitoring standards; and the feasibility of maintaining local, national, and global databases. An examination of international experience of credentialing enables an opportunity to establish that many of these issues exist, not only at a global level, but also within individual countries where different jurisdictions within a country have their own regional or state regulations and transferability between regions and states becomes problematic.

Any attempts, therefore, to introduce a consistent transferrable credentialing process on an international platform could ultimately result in slowing down workforce mobility rather than enhancing it.

ADVANCED PRACTICE VERSUS SPECIALIZATION

The issue of advanced practice versus specialization is increasingly emerging as an issue. As described, in New Zealand and Australia, credentialing recognizes the specialist expertise of registered nurses, but does not, however, refer to an advanced level of practice. Differentiation should occur between those registered nurses who are required to complete postgraduate programs in order to meet credential requirements. This level of educational preparation constitutes an advanced level of practice. The International Council of Nurses (ICN) network for advanced practice has been tackling these issues for many years through working with member countries. This process has facilitated an ongoing exchange of resources and information and helps ensure that ICN has the appropriate specialist advice.

DEFINITION

A Nurse Practitioner/Advanced Practice Nurse is a registered nurse who has acquired the expert knowledge base, complex decision-making skills and clinical competencies for expanded practice, the characteristics of which are shaped by the context and/or country in which s/he is credentialed to practice. A Masters degree is recommended for entry level.

(ICN, approved 2002)

Characteristics

Educational Preparation

- Educational preparation at advanced level
- Formal recognition of educational programs preparing nurse practitioners/advanced nursing practice roles accredited or approved.
- Formal system of licensure, registration, certification and credentialing.

Nature of Practice

- Integrates research, education, practice and management.
- High degree of professional autonomy and independent practice.
- Case Management/own caseload
- Advanced health assessment skills, decision-making skills and diagnostic reasoning skills.
- Recognized advanced clinical competencies.
- Provision of consultant services to health providers.
- Plans, implements and evaluates programs.
- Recognized first point of contact for clients.

Regulatory Mechanisms—Country Specific Regulations Underpin NP/APN Practice

- Right to diagnose.
- Authority to prescribe medication.
- Authority to prescribe treatment.
- Authority to refer clients to other professionals.
- Authority to admit patients to hospital.
- Legislation to confer and protect the title "Nurse Practitioner/Advanced Practice Nurse"
- Legislation or some other form of regulatory mechanism specific to advanced practice nurses.
- Officially recognized titles for nurses working in advanced practice roles.

(ICN, approved 2002)

WHOSE ROLE TO ADMINISTER—REGULATORS OR THE PROFESSION?

A further emerging issue is the increasing debate regarding definitions and applications of "advanced practice" and "credentialing," and whether processes should be administered by regulatory organizations or by professional bodies.

> Understanding the balance between internal and external regulation is important for professionals because their regulatory systems are based on a subtle balance between these systems of control. The purpose of internal regulation (within the profession) is to ensure the advancement of nursing while serving the public interest: external regulation (outside the profession) exists chiefly to protect the public.
>
> *(Joel 2003, p. 392)*

Credentialing can then play a part in internal regulation, as it is based on expert peer opinion, knowledge, and processes. In the United States, the lines do become blurred as the regulatory bodies (nursing boards) use credentialing (certification exams) as a requirement or proxy for advanced practice licensure. Thus, in the United States, advanced practice certification would be viewed as a mechanism for "public protection."

International trends show a changing emphasis in the roles of regulatory bodies. They are having an increased role in standard setting and competency assurance, but some jurisdictions are reducing their focus on advocacy and enhancement of the profession. Regulatory bodies are also experiencing a reduced role in the accreditation of nursing programs.

CONCLUSION

Credentialing is an important tool, which offers an opportunity to formally recognize that a practitioner is providing a safe, high-quality health care service within specific environments. It builds on the regulatory bodies' requirements for registration, and thus provides a more specific context of practice for specialty areas. This clarity for both employers and consumers is important, as our health care environments are more mobile and more complex, and more specialized nursing skills are being demanded on an international platform.

It is important that professional organizations in nursing be the bodies to provide the platform for credentialing. Many multinational organizations provide credentialing/accreditation/certification services, and nurses are rightly wary of being incorporated into processes that create profit for multinational groups or are equated to the same processes used in product industries. For smaller countries, we need to reach across the globe to nursing organizations that can assist and provide services to others. This then can enable nursing to provide wider, stronger networks across the globe, and nurses can become a true borderless workforce within a credentialed framework.

Today the same challenges still exist that were highlighted by Styles (Styles & Affara, 1997). Terminology and processes need to be consistent, credible, and culturally appropriate and have integrity and cultural nuances, and issues need to be addressed into any processes.

DISCUSSION QUESTIONS

1. What do you see as the benefits for your practice in being credentialed?
2. Is credentialing just about advanced practice?
3. Why is there still difficultly in defining advanced practice?
4. What else is needed in the policy and regulatory environment to assist the development of credentialing?

NOTES

1. Accreditation = the process for formally recognizing services and providers by meeting a set of standards.
2. Certification = the formal recognition that an individual meets set standards established by a professional body.

REFERENCES

American Nurses Credentialing Center. (2013). *American nurses credentialing center.* Retrieved from www .nursecredentialing.org (accessed 5 February 2013).

Australian College of Mental Health Nurses. (2011). *What is credentialing?* Retrieved from www.acmhn .org/credentialing/what-is-credentialing.html (accessed 31 January 2013).

Cioffi, J. P., Lichtveld, M. Y., Thielen, L., & Miner, K. (2003). Credentialing the public health workforce: An idea whose time has come. *Journal of Public Health Management and Practice, 9*(6), 451–458.

Coates, C. (2010). *Accreditation, certification and credentialing in mental health nursing: A review of selected literature*. Report prepared for the Ministry of Health and the New Zealand College of Mental Health Nurses Te Ao Māramatanga.

Duffield, C., Gardner, G., Chang, A. M., & Catling-Paull, C. (2009). Advanced nursing practice: A global perspective. *Collegion: The Australian Journal of Nursing Practice, Scholarship and Research*, 16(2), 55–62.

Gendek, M. (2011). *Recognising specialist mental health nurses–A national success*. Retrieved from www.acmhn.org/credentialing/what-is-credentialing.html (accessed 31 January 2013).

International Council of Nurses. (2013). *The credentialing and regulators forum*. Retrieved from www.icn.ch/pillarsprograms/the-credentialing-forum/ (accessed 31 January 2013).

Joel, L. (2003). *Kelly's dimensions of professional nursing*. New York: McGraw-Hill.

Newton, S., Pillay, J., & Higginbottom, G. (2012). The migration and transitioning experiences of internationally educated nurses: A global perspective. *Journal of Nursing Management*, 20(4), 534–550.

Oakley-Brown, M. A., Wells, J. E., & Scott, K. M. (Eds). (2006). *Te Rau Hinegaro: The New Zealand mental health survey*. Wellington: Ministry of Health.

Royal College of Nursing Australia. (2011). *International council of nurses credentialling forum 2011. Country Paper: Australia*. Retrieved from www.rcna.org.au (accessed 31 January 2013).

Singh, M. D., & Sochan, A. (2010). Voices of internationally educated nurses: Policy recommendations for credentialing. *International Nursing Review*, 57(1), 56–63.

Styles, M. M., & Affara, F. A. (1997). *ICN on regulation: Towards 21st century models*. ICN: Geneva.

Te Ao Māramatanga, New Zealand College of Mental Health Nurses. (2013). *Credentialing*. Retrieved from www.nzcmhn.org.nz/Credentialing (accessed 27 January 2013).

WHAT DOES THE FUTURE HOLD FOR ADVANCED PRACTICE REGISTERED NURSE PRACTICE AND HEALTH CARE POLICY

Health Policy for Advanced Practice Registered Nurses: An International Perspective

Madrean M. Schober

Nursing is at a crossroads worldwide, as key decision makers increasingly recognize that achieving successful health care systems for the future rests on the future of nursing. The growing presence of advanced practice registered nurses (APRNs) suggests that nurses in these roles will provide leadership in achieving accessible, high-quality care and expertise. The success of these endeavors will, for the large part, depend on the development of supportive health policies, relevant policy processes, and promotional campaigns. This chapter focuses on events or policies that have impacted the development of APRN roles internationally and aims to demonstrate the complex nature of health policy and various courses of action that have influenced role development worldwide. It begins by providing an international contextual background for advanced practice nursing. Subsequent sections describe specific health policies or actions that have supported or impeded APRN practice. Illustrations of actions in specific countries or regions of the world provide examples of the effects health policy has on role development.

BACKGROUND: THE INTERNATIONAL CONTEXT

Although the United States has defined four categories of the "APRN," this title and the same delineation of advanced nursing practice are not found in other countries. The literature (DiCenso et al., 2010; Gardner et al., 2004; Schober & Affara, 2006) indicates that there is an awareness of advanced practice role development in the United States; however, titles, role definitions, and scopes of practice are specific to the country in which the role is developing or emerging. To promote an understanding of these differences and enhance an understanding of relevant policy directives, this section provides an overview of the international context.

The difficulty in trying to portray advanced practice nursing from an international point of view is that there is no international consensus on what this actually means. Unfortunately, confusion and lack of clarity surround any attempt to define these roles from a global perspective. An international survey (Pulcini et al., 2010) representing responses from over 30 countries indicated that 14 different titles were used to refer to "advanced practice nursing." In addition, from country to country and within institutions in the same country, there are inconsistencies in role definitions, scopes of practice, educational preparation, and regulations, making it difficult to clearly understand international development. For the purposes of this chapter, the term *advanced practice nurse (APN)* will be used as an umbrella term even though, depending on the country, titles such as nurse practitioner (NP), clinical nurse specialist, or nurse specialist are used. When providing specific country illustrations, the title used within the country will be referred to.

International surveys conducted from 2001 to 2010 estimated that anywhere from 30 to 60 countries were in various stages of exploring the potential for APN roles (ICN, 2001; Pulcini et al., 2010; Roodbol, 2004). In August 2012, the International Council of Nurses (ICN) noted an increase in these numbers and announced that 78 countries had indicated an interest through membership in the ICN International Nurse Practitioner/Advanced Practice Nursing Network. Most of these countries were noted to be in exploratory or early stages of role development. The International Council of Nurses had been following worldwide development since 1994 and noted the variations in referring to an APN. To guide countries in various stages of development, ICN suggested a definition that could be referred to and used to assist health care planners and key decision makers. The International Council of Nurses defines an APN as:

> a registered nurse who has acquired the expert knowledge base, complex decision-making skills and clinical competencies for expanded practice, the characteristics of which are shaped by the context and/or country in which s/he is credentialed to practice. A master's degree is recommended for entry level.
>
> *(ICN, 2002)*

To provide further guidance for these developing nursing roles, ICN, in its ICN Regulation Series, provided *The Scope of Practice, Standards and Competencies of the Advanced Practice Nurse* (ICN, 2008), and the *ICN Framework of Competencies for the Nurse Specialist* (ICN, 2009). Both publications attempted to provide clarity to the debate over the extension of traditional nursing practice by providing frameworks for consideration. In addition to country variations in attempts to define the APN role, key institutions, agencies, or individuals in pivotal positions of authority influence health policy impacting role development. These levels of influence differ from country to country.

Pivotal individuals in positions of influence and their associated decision-making networks impact the initiation and development of APN roles in various ways. The following sections discuss ways health policy and policy decisions have affected the launching or authorization of the APN role.

AUTHORIZATION: LEGITIMIZING THE ROLE

In principle, as countries consider launching an APN initiative, it would seem ideal to have a health policy in place to lend support for role development and implementation. However, multiple agencies and decision makers with various opinions and interpretations of what an APN is or what a person in this role should do are in positions to define and shape a profile for this role. These varied ideas do not easily translate into policy-driven support for a new category of health care professionals; instead, they often can impede progress. Although the full influence internationally of models in the United States is not known, representatives of countries seeking a successful APN campaign often strive to emulate this country's achievements. However, from country to country, health systems vary and policy resulting in laws or legislation has a significantly different dynamic compared to what is familiar in the United States.

Who Has the Authority to Develop Health Policy Relevant to the APN?

Patterned on the success in the United States, representatives of other countries appear to embrace this accomplishment with enthusiasm and good intentions. However, an eager approach to the APN concept may fail to fully understand the policy processes and/or institutional structures along with the complexities of policy decisions that must be navigated to legitimize this new nursing role. In addition, the establishment of law and legislation may lag behind the actual momentum that led to the introduction of the APN into the health care workforce.

Oman

For example, since 2006 the Directorate of Nursing and Midwifery Affairs under the auspices of the Minister of Health for the Sultanate of Oman, with support from the World Health Organization—EMRO (Eastern Mediterranean Region), has been exploring APN roles, especially for primary health care. As of April 2013, even though positive sentiments continue for this change, differences of opinion among government officials and health professionals have faced a policy system slow to respond to this heightened interest. This dissension has impeded the official launching of the APN role. In principle, a National Task Force continues to promote the APN and plans to move forward with an education plan while waiting for official policies that would authorize and legitimize the role (personal communication, Majid Al-Maqbali, March 13, 2013).

France

Similarly, France has been investigating the APN role for a number of years by conducting pilot projects. Although progress has been slow, the first education program for APNs was launched in 2009. Several key institutions and agencies have the authority to influence APN policy. They include:

- Ministère de la santé (Ministry of Health)
- Haute autorité de santé (HAS) (High Authority of Health)
- Fédération hospitalière de France (Federation of Hospitals in France)

Two health policy documents influenced APN development in France even though there is not yet official authorization for the role: La coopération entre les professionnels de santé (Co-operation between health professionals) and Protocole de coopération entre professionnels de santé: Mode d'emploi (Protocol of co-operation between health professionals: Directions for use) (retrieved April 2, 2013, from www .hassante.fr/portail/jcms/c_978700/protocole-de-cooperation-entre-professionnels -de-sante-mode-d-emploi and www.sante.gouv.fr/la-cooperation-entre-les-profess ionnels-de-sante.html).

The law HPST (Article 51) 2009 provided a countrywide agenda in France resulting in the beginnings of supportive legislation for APNs, including a practice act. However, this category of nurse still does not have title protection and faces diverse obstacles in working to integrate mainly hospital-based specialty roles into the health care workforce (personal communication, Debout, March 29, 2013).

Singapore

The introduction of APNs in Singapore provides an example of the lag that can occur between the initiation of role preparation and the official provision of legislation for the role. The National University of Singapore developed an APN program following discussions among key representatives of the Ministry of Health and the university. The first group of students began their education in 2003 and completed the 18-month program in 2004. Although the policies developed through the ministry are specific in protecting the title, defining an APN, and identifying punitive actions for persons misrepresenting themselves as an APN without the required qualifications, these policies were not announced until 2006. This resulted in the initial graduates returning to their practice sites with only a vague notion of what was expected of them and no supportive health policies. Lack of role clarity among the APNs and relevant managers, along with a lack of fundamental policies at the time, led to an environment of confusion and conflict in the early stages of role implementation (Schober, on site 2007 to 2012).

Ireland

Health policy in Ireland took a different turn with the establishment of advanced nurse practitioner (ANP) and advanced midwife practitioner (AMP) policies. In 2013, the National Council for the Professional Development of Nursing and Midwifery (referred to here as The National Council) released the fourth edition of the *Framework for the Establishment of Advanced Nurse Practitioner and Advanced Midwife Posts.* The development of a career pathway by the Commission on Nursing (Government of Ireland, 1998) was created to retain expert nurses in direct patient care and served to develop clinical nursing and midwifery expertise. The establishment of the clinical pathway was a function vested in The National Council that in turn developed a definition, core concept, and competencies for the role of the ANP/AMP. In addition, this agency determined the requirements for nurses and midwives to be accredited as an ANP/AMP, as well as giving official approval for the post (employment position) where the ANP or AMP would practice. The development of ANP/AMP roles and services was part of the strategic development of the overall health service reform in the country (Department of Health and Children, 2001; Department of Health and Children, 2003). The comprehensive nature of the Irish plan provides an illustration of how ANP/AMP role development became a subset of a national health care approach and related policies.

Australia

The first NP in Australia was endorsed/authorized in the year 2000 following 20 years of exploring this option for provision of health care services in the country. Australia had six state and two territory governments with differing requirements for endorsement until July 2010, when national registration for nurses and other health professionals was implemented with the creation of the Australian Health Practitioner Regulatory Agency (AHPRA) and the Nurse and Midwifery Board of Australia (NMBA). As of April 2013, there were 788 NPs qualified to practice in Australia with authorization now through the Nursing and Midwifery Board (www .nursingmidwiferyboard.gov.au). In some ways, the original approach of health policy impacting NPs was similar to the United States in that authority and jurisdiction had been mainly under the separate states. With this unification, there is an effort to reevaluate and provide universal NP competency standards for the country (retrieved March 21, 2013, from www.icn-apnetwork.org).

Republic of South Africa

The state of affairs for nursing in general in a country can dictate whether health policy will embrace the concept of advanced practice nursing. South Africa provides an example of how an attempt to rejuvenate the health care system and thus health policy affects all of nursing, including APNs. The Minister of Health in South Africa introduced a number of policies to revitalize the health system in the country. This approach included the following:

- Reengineering the primary health care system
- Introducing a National Health Insurance that will be piloted at first and implemented over 14 years, each with its impact on nursing

The revised health strategy highlights the South African nurse-based health system and suggests that there is a great need for specialist nurses with advanced skills, as seen in some of the teams proposed in these policies. This highlights the need of the country for APNs. The policy change to allow nurses to initiate antiretroviral treatment (ART) is likely the policy that brought about the largest amount of support for the APN role in the country. From 2010 to 2012, the persons who could initiate ART increased from 250 to 10,000. This has increased the life expectancy of South Africans over a period of three years (personal communication, Geyer, March 22, 2013). Refer to the subsequent section on education for discussion on how health policy influenced relevant standards for nursing education, including APNs, in South Africa.

Saudi Arabia

Saudi Arabia provides another example of how health policy relevant to nursing in general impacts the development of APN roles. The kingdom of Saudi Arabia has had established nurse training programs for around 40 years, with movement away from hospital-based education to university baccalaureate and master's-level programs. Although the Saudi Commission for Health Specialties (SCFHS) registers all nurses working within the kingdom, nursing as a profession still has a long way to go. The World Health Organization has recognized the need for APNs within the Middle East including Saudi Arabia; however, there is as yet no postgraduate university education aimed at developing APNs (clinical nurse specialist or nurse practitioner programs). The SCFHS has recently accredited a 12-month, full-time, hospital-based Enterostomal Therapy Education Program (wound, ostomy, and continence) aimed at developing nursing expertise to an advanced level within this specialist field. Additionally, Saudi nurses are encouraged to avail themselves of scholarship opportunities internationally, sponsored by the Saudi government, in order to gain advanced clinical practice qualifications in countries such as the United Kingdom and the United States. However, to date very few APNs are in clinical practice within the kingdom of Saudi Arabia (personal communication, Green, March 10, 2013).

Israel

Israel provides an example of how authority for APN-like roles is granted by institutions employing these nurses while they work in this advanced capacity without national health policy or legislation supportive of the role. Like other western countries, advances in technology and the increasing aging of the population have led to increased specialization within the health care system, including the need for nurses to specialize. In addition, health services have been shown to be more limited in the peripheral regions of the country. These trends have been linked to the grassroots development of advanced practice-like roles. For example, many hospitals have positions, similar to those of the clinical nurse specialist or the nurse specialist, for nurses to serve as clinical consultants or experts in roles such as pain nurse, stoma nurse, and infection control nurse. In the community, nurses who work in outpatient clinics, especially in the periphery, may practice in roles that are similar to the NP; however, their practice is very structured and they work within very defined and prescribed medical protocols. These nurses are given the authority to perform these roles by their institutions rather than a countrywide policy. Although they have advanced clinical knowledge and basically function as APNs, these nurses do not have the legal title or authority to practice over and above any other registered nurse. They also do not have the autonomy, independence, or legal liability to practice as specialists. Most of the nurses who pioneered these roles were taught as apprentices to physicians and some were trained by attending courses and/or conferences outside of the country (retrieved April 3, 2013, from www.icn-apnetwork.org).

HEALTH POLICY THAT INFLUENCES APN EDUCATION

In addition to acknowledging or authorizing the presence of APNs in health care systems worldwide, health policies often establish education requirements for the qualified APN prior to the presence of supportive health policies for the role. This section provides country-specific examples and illustrations of how governmental agencies or professional bodies have made decisions or developed policy that affects educational standards.

Republic of South Africa

In South Africa, in addition to the Ministry of Health developing new policies for health care in the country, the South African Nursing Council (SANC) has played a major role in the development of regulations for the APN role. In view of the changing health care needs of the country, there was a need to revise the scope of practice and educational preparation of nurses to fulfill these needs. This led to the development of a revised qualification framework (see Table 28.1) for nursing in the country, which for the first time established the position of APN (in this framework, the title used is Advanced Specialist Nurse) in the hierarchy of qualifications (the breakdown of credits is 120 per academic year).

TABLE 28.1 Revised Qualification Framework for Nursing in South Africa

NQF	QUALIFICATIONS	CREDITS	CATEGORY OF NURSE
10	Doctoral degree	360 credits at level 10	Advanced specialist nurse
9	Master's degree	180 credits at level 9	
8	Postgraduate diploma Bachelor's honours degree (professional degree)	120 credits at level 8 480 credits at level 8 and 96 at level 6	Specialist nurse Registered professional nurse
7	Bachelor's degree Advanced diploma	360 credits at level 7 and 96 at level 5 120 credits	Registered staff nurse
6	Diploma	360 credits with minimum 60 at level 7 and maximum 120 at level 5	Registered auxiliary nurse
5	Higher certificate	120 credits	

In addition, the Department of Higher Education in South Africa has had an important influence on the direction of nursing education policy. The Higher Education Act (Act 101 of 1997) amended definition (www.che.ac.za/documents /d000004/Higher_Education_Act.pdf) of *higher education programs* included nursing programs, and as such all nursing programs from 2015 will be at a higher education level, which will include both university and nursing college programs. This also means that nursing programs will be accredited by the Council of Higher Education, not only SANC. With the newly devised qualification framework for nursing, the SANC has initiated the development of competencies and scopes of practice for specialist and advance practice category of nurses. Nursing professionals in the relevant fields have been participating in the exercise that would finally result in regulations under the Nursing Act, which will formalize the position of the APN (personal communication, Geyer, March 22, 2013).

Ireland

Advanced nursing practice in Ireland as a clinical career pathway for registered nurses was formalized under a recommendation of the Commission on Nursing Report (1998). Following the release of this report, a statutory body, the National Council for the Professional Development of Nursing and Midwifery (NCNM), was established with the responsibility for setting the parameters of educational preparation and accreditation. Advanced nurse practitioners/advanced midwife practitioners (ANP/AMPs) in Ireland are expected to demonstrate "exemplary" theoretical and practical knowledge as well as "exemplary" critical thinking skills. The minimum educational requirement for an ANP/AMP in Ireland is a master's-level degree relevant to the ANP/AMP practice area. Any education taken should include a major clinical component. ANP/AMPs also need to have a minimum of 7 years postregistration experience with a minumum of 5 years in their specialty practice area before they can register to practice in Ireland.

Israel

The advanced practice role exists in Israel mostly at the grassroots level; however, more recent developments and health policies have been promoting the legal authority for this role. In 2009, the first advanced practice role was approved by the Ministry of Health: the Nurse Specialist in Palliative Care. The legal authority for this role was given by executive order by the Director General of the Ministry of Health. Prior to this, the only formal advanced training for nurses was provided in post-basic certification courses in specific clinical areas such as critical care, oncology, geriatrics, midwifery, and dialysis. Nurses complete a theoretical and clinical program mandated by the Nursing Division within the Ministry of Health. These courses range from several months to 1.5 years in length. At the end of this period, nurses take a national licensing specialization exam. The Nursing Division in the Ministry of Health determines the curriculum of the programs and administers these licensure exams. Those who receive post-basic licensure are entitled to perform certain procedures that are considered to be delegated to them from medical practice that are beyond the scope of practice of the generalist registered nurse. These programs were often taught within schools of nursing; however, they are not within an academic framework and no degree is offered to the graduates of these programs. However, approximately 50% of registered nurses have some type of post-basic certification. This high percentage is most probably due to the significant increase in salary above that of the generalist registered nurse for those who obtain post-basic certification and to the Ministry of Health requirement that certain specialty areas such as critical care units hire nurses with post-basic certification. Four universities offer master's degrees in nursing. One program focuses only on nursing research, and another on nursing education and administration with some clinical component. The third program contains theoretical courses of a clinical nature but does not include any clinical experiences. Only one university offers a master's degree in advanced nursing practice where students are taught both theoretical and clinical advanced practice skills within the same program. When countries lack policies or legislation providing specific support or governance for the APN scope of practice, professional organizations and governmental bodies initiate nonlegislative actions to more clearly delineate this level of nursing. The next section describes this approach.

SCOPE OF PRACTICE: NATURE OF THE ROLE AND RESPONSIBILITIES

Ideally, health policies for APNs should promote full practice authority without placing undue restrictions on full and direct access for consultation, care coordination, and referral. Although new initiatives debate the ability of the APN to make a diagnosis of a presenting concern or manage a full caseload, the more contentious issues emerge around prescriptive authority, reimbursement, and establishment of autonomous practice. In the event that health policy is absent, countries develop innovative approaches to promote and support the role.

Republic of South Africa

The challenge in South Africa remains one of designated clinical practice and prescribing by APNs. Authorization to prescribe remains a special concession and then can only be exercised if a nurse works in the public sector. A few nurses in the private sector do have prescribing authority. This includes midwives working for themselves and nurses working in occupational health care services (occupational health is a designated service as determined by section 56 of the Nursing Act, 2005) (www.sanc .co.za/publications.htm). Reimbursement is selectively done for self-employed nurses working in the private sector, although many medical aids (insurance schemes) do not provide any member benefit coverage for nursing/midwifery services. Self-employed wound care specialist nurses are a new group that functions as independent practitioners, and they are consulted by other practitioners, including medical practitioners (personal communication, Geyer, March 22, 2013).

The Netherlands

In the initial stage of development, the most important driver for the establishment of the nurse practitioner (NP) (now titled nurse specialist) position was the shortage of physicians. In addition, there was a desire to diminish the dominant position and power of the physicians in the political arena. In this context, the key entities influencing health policy for the APNs are the general professional nursing organization, as well as the professional APN organization, the national registration committee for the APN, the Minister of Health, the universities of applied science, and insurance companies. The countrywide agenda has been in the hands of the general nursing organization, with a pivotal one-person campaign led in the early stages by Dr. Petrie Roodbol. Supported by international colleagues and under nursing leadership, all practice acts including prescribing have been developed and implemented. However, the current problem in 2013 is reimbursement, which is especially a problem for the psychiatric NP. The insurance companies have refused reimbursement because they find the number and kind of "helpers" in psychiatric care complex enough without including the NP. With this kind of policy directive from insurance companies, the NPs in this field are losing their jobs (personal communication, P. Roodbol, March 17, 2013).

United Kingdom

Discussions in the UK on advanced nursing practice have been long and complex, because many roles have evolved in an unregulated and unplanned manner. Barton et al. (2010) indicated that the ad hoc development of advanced nursing roles, the random use of titles that imply levels of clinical expertise that cannot be verified, and varied educational development all point to the need to govern advanced nursing practice at the employer level. In addition, because of the lack of health policies governing all four countries in the UK, representatives of Scotland and Wales have worked to develop guidelines, frameworks, and toolkits to support APN roles (National Leadership and Innovation Agency for Health Care, 2010; Scottish Government, 2008; Welsh Assembly Government, 2010).

Barton et al. (2012) suggested that good governance regarding role development and implementation must be based on consistent expectations of the level of practice required to deliver the service, and that this is best achieved through nationally agreed standards and processes. However, the UK has not been able to establish health policy through its Nursing and Midwifery Council that provides acceptable and universal governance; thus, individual countries have established their own frameworks. Discussions in the UK on advanced nursing practice have been long and complex, spanning over 20 years since the late 1980s and early 1990s as service and strategic interest in advanced nurse roles grew (Fulbrook, 1995; Kaufman, 1996; Stilwell, 1988). Despite extensive strategic intent since then, title protection and legislation governing the profession have not been achieved. Barton et al. (2012) noted that the

> Council for Healthcare Regulatory Excellence (2008) outlined the complexity of professional regulatory issues and made it clear that, in its view, the code of professional conduct (Nursing and Midwifery Council, 2008) encompasses advanced practitioner practice, negating any need for additional formal regulation. That view led indirectly to the development of the Advanced Practice Toolkit (Scottish Government, 2008) under the auspices of Modernising Nursing Careers (Department of Health, 2006). This provided some national conformity and guidance to employers, practitioners and educators. More recently, two documents looked to governance as a mechanism of employer-led local regulation—the DH's [Department of Health] (2010) position statement on advanced practice and the Welsh framework for advanced practice.
>
> *National Leadership and Innovation Agency for Health Care (2010, p. 2)*

As of 2013, it appears that there is no perceived need for centrally focused health policies for APNs in the UK. In this environment, employer-led frameworks of governance that could guide the country-specific National Health Services have been proposed to fill this need.

New Zealand

A task force established by the Government of New Zealand in 1998 recognized that nurses were already providing some services at an advanced level and decided to identify obstacles that might be preventing nurses from improving health care services to patients (NCNZ, 2002). This task force studied strategies to remove barriers that limited the full potential for nursing practice. The government adopted the task-force recommendations. Critical to the success for promotion of the possibility for the NP role in New Zealand was the presence of a supportive Chief Nursing Advisor at the Ministry of Health. The presence of a person in a position of authority achieved government recognition that formal recognition and employment of NPs would improve health outcomes for the population. The Nursing Council of New Zealand (NCNZ, 2002) along with the Ministry of Health defined two clear areas of work:

- Consultation and policy development around the title, education standards and competencies
- Policy development around prescribing, including mechanisms to regulate prescribing, establish education standards, curricula and competencies.

Schober and Affara (2006, p. 57)

Action was taken by the Ministry of Health to remove barriers to NP practice, including enacting necessary legislative changes to allow prescribing. Currently the Nursing Council of New Zealand (www.nursingcouncil.org.nz) and the Association of Nurse Practitioners for New Zealand (www.nurse.org.nz/npnz-nurse-practitioners -nz.html) offer information about becoming an NP (now the legally protected title).

CONCLUSION

International momentum for APN roles continues to grow. Enthusiasm for this nursing role is often based on observed successes in the United States and other countries with histories of experience in development. At times, eagerness to introduce APNs into health care systems is based on a limited understanding of the complexities of the development of health policy and policy processes. This chapter has sought to portray the international differences in approaching the concept of advanced practice nursing and the variety of factors that influence policy that impacts APN role development and sustainability. It was not intended that the content of this chapter should provide a comprehensive view of all health policy initiatives worldwide relevant to APNs, but rather that it should provide snapshots and illustrations showing how the variance in how health policy directives from a wide variety of government agencies, professional organizations, and other institutions influence role development. Knowledge of the complexities of health policies affecting APNs and the pivotal interactions that occur among key stakeholders can provide insight into the dynamics underlying any APN initiative.

REFERENCES

Barton, T. D., Bevan, L., & Mooney, G. (2012). Advanced nursing 2: A governance framework for advanced nursing. *Nursing Times, 108*(25), 22–24.

Department of Health. (2006). *Modernizing nursing careers: Setting the direction.* Edinburgh: Scottish Executive. Retrieved August 2006 from http://www.scotland.gov.uk/Resource/Doc/146433 /0038313.pdf

Department of Health. (2010). *Advanced level nursing: A position statement.* UK: DOH Publications. Retrieved from http://www.gov.uk/government/uploads/system/uploads/attachment_data /file/215935/dh_121738.pdf

DiCenso, A., & Bryant-Lukosius, D. (2010). *Role of clinical nurse specialists and nurse practitioners in Canada: A decision support synthesis.* Canadian Health Services Research Foundation.

Fulbrook, P. (1995). What is advanced practice? *Intensive and Critical Care Nursing, 11*(1), 53.

Gardner, G., Carryer, J., Dunn, S., & Gardner, A. (2004). *Nurse practitioner standards project.* Report to the Australian Nursing Council: Author.

Government of Ireland. (1998). *Report of the commission on nursing: A blueprint for the future.* Dublin: Stationery Office.

International Council of Nurses. (2001). Update: *International survey of nurse practitioner/advanced practice nursing roles.* Retrieved from http://www.icn-apnetwork.org

International Council of Nurses. (2002). *Definition and characteristics of the role.* Retrieved from http://www.icn-apnetwork.org

International Council of Nurses. (2008). *The scope of practice, standards and competencies of the advanced practice nurse* (The ICN Regulation Series). Geneva: Author.

International Council of Nurses. (2009). *ICN framework of competencies for the nurse specialist* (The ICN Regulation Series). Geneva: Author.

Kaufman, G. (1996). Nurse practitioners in general practice: An expanding role. *Nursing Standard, 11*(8), 44–47.

National Council for the Professional Development of Nursing and Midwifery. (2005). *A preliminary evaluation of the role of the advanced nurse practitioner.* Dublin: NCNM.

National Council for the Professional Development of Nursing and Midwifery. (2013). *Framework for the establishment of advanced nurse practitioner and advanced midwife posts* (4th ed.). Dublin: NCNM.

National Leadership and Innovation Agency for Health Care. (2010). *Framework for advanced nursing, midwifery and allied health professional practice in Wales.* Lianharan, Wales: Innovation House.

Nursing Council of New Zealand. (2002). *The nurse practitioner: Responding to health needs in New Zealand* (3rd ed.). Wellington: Author.

Nursing and Midwifery Council. (2008). *The Code: Standards of conduct, performance and ethics for nurses and midwives.* London: NMC.

Pulcini, J., Jelic, M., Gul, R., & Loke, A. I. (2010). An international survey on advanced practice nursing education, practice and regulation. *Journal of Nursing Scholarship, 42*(1), 31–39.

Roodbol, P. (2004). *Survey carried out prior to the 3rd ICN-International Nurse Practitioner/Advanced Practice Nursing Network Conference.* Groningen, The Netherlands.

Schober, M., & Affara, F. (2006). *Advanced nursing practice.* Oxford, UK: Blackwell.

Scottish Government. (2008). *Supporting the development of advanced nursing practice—A toolkit approach.* CNO directorate, Scottish Government.

Stilwell, B. (1988). Patients' attitudes to a highly developed extended role: The nurse practitioner. *Recent Advances in Nursing, 21,* 82–100.

Welsh Assembly Government. (2009). Post registration career framework for nurses in Wales. Retrieved from http://www.wales.nhs.uk/sites3/docmetadata.cfm?orgid=580&id=148258

Welsh Assembly Government. (2010). Delivering a five year service, workforce and financial strategic framework for NHS Wales. Retrieved from www.wales.nhs.uk/documents/Framework-five-year.pdf

CHAPTER 29

The Future for Nurse Practitioners

Jan Towers

Nurse practitioners have been around for only a little over 45 years. In essence, they are the "babies" of the health professionals. Yet they have come far, and accomplished much in that short period of time. It is clear that there was a need for nurse practitioners and that they have filled a gap in the health care world. That gap has continued to grow, and so has the need for nurse practitioners.

HISTORY

In the 1960s, a projected shortage of primary care providers (physicians) stimulated a search for alternative paths for providing primary care services to the citizens of the United States. That, combined with a proliferation of medics returning from the Vietnam War, stimulated an effort to expand the training of people other than physicians for the provision of primary care services. Coupled with this innovative thinking was the increasing awareness that the contribution of primary prevention, wellness programs, and a focus on patient-centered care could improve the health of the country. Looking at the opportunities these conditions provided, it became clear that nurses could make a major contribution to meeting this need by expanding the scope of health care to the preventive domain. As a result, in a number of states such as North Carolina and Maryland, public health nurses began to physically assess patients coming into their well-baby and women's health clinics.

Recognizing the tremendous need and the opportunity for nurses to make a contribution in this scenario, Loretta Ford and Henry Silva, both faculty at the University of Colorado, entered into a cooperative partnership to provide primary care to children by preparing nurses to provide primary care services to pediatric patients in Colorado. The program graduated its first class of pediatric nurse practitioners in 1965 (AAN, 1999). The program was a success and the role of the nurse practitioner began to expand to include women's health, followed by family, adult, and geriatric care, all with great success.

Initially, certificate programs were developed through a variety of entities, including continuing education programs from schools of nursing and medicine, hospitals, and other continuing education venues. As the idea of nurses providing these essential primary care services expanded, the federal government became interested in supporting the preparation of nurse practitioners and began to provide grants for the development of formal nurse practitioner educational programs within the academic framework of graduate nurse education. With the provision of financial support, universities became interested in opening formal programs of study, and nursing education undertook the formalization of graduate educational programs to prepare nurse practitioners, first at the master's level and now at the doctoral level.

This was not undertaken without controversy. The nursing community did not endorse the "expanded" role initially, and worried that nurses would once again become the "handmaidens" of physicians as they took on "traditional medical activities" such as diagnosing and treating illnesses. Opposing articles were written in the major nursing journals, and nurse practitioners were often not supported by nurses in the workplace. Interestingly, the physician community was more supportive, and actively participated in the early educational endeavors to prepare nurse practitioners. It was not until after the late 1990s, when nurse practitioners were authorized to provide and be paid for Medicare services, that organized medicine began to resist the contributions nurse practitioners could make to the provision of health care in this country.

THE CURRENT SITUATION

Now we have entered another period when a monumental shortage of health care providers is evident. With the passage of the Patient Protection and Affordable Care Act (PPACA) (legislation requiring health insurance for everyone in the country), it is projected that another 40,000,000 people will be required to have health care insurance coverage in the very near future—and these people will be seeking care from a limited supply of health care providers. Nurse practitioners are ready to contribute to the reduction of that shortage and are working diligently to remove barriers that prevent them from doing so.

The barriers that exist at the time of writing include outdated scope of practice laws in some states, and obsolete payment barriers at the state and federal levels. Historically, state governments control the scope of professional practice. The federal government, states, and, to a certain extent, commercial insurance carriers control payment for medical/health care services.

Scope of practice laws, more commonly known as practice acts, are based in state statute and regulation. They are the basis for licensure of members of the health care professions such as medicine and nursing, as well as attorneys and other service providers such as beauticians and funeral directors. Changes in scope of practice require the amending of scope of practice laws within each state. As a result, change in nurse practitioner scope of practice has occurred state by state over the years. Efforts to build consistency from state to state, as well as to implement scope of practice laws that authorize nurse practitioners to practice to the full extent of their education and clinical preparation, have led to the development of a stakeholder consensus document and model practice act that describes the educational preparation, national certification, and scope of practice for all APRNs, including nurse practitioners. This document has served as the basis for consistent change, recognition, and authorization of nurse practitioner practice.

At the time of writing, a third of the states have achieved plenary (full practice) authority, authorizing nurse practitioners to assess, diagnose, and treat (including prescribing medication) without the supervision of another health care provider

(AANP, 2013). The remainder of the states authorize nurse practitioners to assess, diagnose, and treat with some kind of collaborative or supervisory relationship with physicians. Nurse practitioners' diagnosis and treatment include the prescription of legend drugs in all 50 states and the prescription of controlled/schedule drugs in 49 states and the District of Columbia. With the exception of seven states (Arkansas, Florida, Georgia, Louisiana, Oklahoma, South Carolina, and West Virginia) (AANP, 2012), nurse practitioners are authorized to independently prescribe Schedule II–V DEA-controlled drugs that require federal authorization to prescribe. Six of these seven states authorize nurse practitioners to independently prescribe Schedule III–V. Only Florida limits nurse practitioners to prescribing legend drugs (DEA, 2013). Nurse practitioners are educationally prepared and able to provide the full range of primary care services to their patients.

Obsolete statutes and regulations in the reimbursement realm create access problems for patients. Considering certain provisions in Medicare law alone, the inability for nurse practitioners to order home health, supervise cardiac and pulmonary rehabilitation, admit patients to skilled nursing facilities (SNFs), and order certain types of durable medical equipment, to name a few examples, creates problems for safe, high-quality, patient care. Removal of those barriers alone would facilitate prompt care, reduce secondary complications, and actually stretch the dollars available for Medicare services.

Likewise, obsolete statutory and regulatory language, limiting a variety of services within the scope of nurse practitioner practice to physician-only performance, creates unnecessary barriers to the fulfillment of a variety of services, form as simple as required physical examinations, to the ordering and coverage of services associated with chronic diseases such as chronic obstructive pulmonary disease (COPD) and diabetes—all well within the scope of practice for nurse practitioners. Although nurse practitioners have been able to surmount a vast number of hurdles, lifting these additional barriers will significantly improve the profession's ability to provide needed care.

THE FUTURE

Nurse practitioners have a long history of documented high-quality, cost-effective care, despite the barriers still to be overcome. In less than 50 years, they have moved from a small group of pediatric nurse practitioners to more than 167,000 individuals (88% of whom are primary care providers) and growing (AANP, 2012b; Goolsby, 2011). Their rate of growth is exceeding that of primary care physicians. Their acceptance among patient populations has grown by leaps and bounds (AANP, 2012a, 2012b; Newhouse et al., 2012a). Increasingly, policy experts have recognized the contribution nurse practitioners can make to the health and well-being of the public, and interestingly, the media is reinforcing that worth and value.

So what should the future bring? As further steps are taken to implement the PPACA, the need for health care providers will expand. This applies to primary as well as specialty care. Nurse practitioners have been the underpinnings of primary care services to the underserved in rural and urban communities for years; their skill in providing care to the elderly and the chronically ill has been well documented. As our population grows and becomes older, the need for their services in this realm will increase significantly.

As new models of care develop, nurse practitioners will have extensive opportunity to provide leadership in their development and implementation. Their nursing and primary care roots provide them with the skills that can make the new models work as they are implemented.

NEW MODELS

Medical Home

The "Medical Home Model" is the traditional framework for nurse practitioner practice. Accessible, holistic, safe, high-quality personalized care—the hallmarks of the medical home—have always been the basis of nurse practitioner practice. Nurse practitioner practices should be the cornerstone of this model, giving guidance to the health care community in its development. This model has, at the behest of the physician community, become certifiable. Entities such as the National Committee for Quality Assurance (NCQA, 2013) and The Joint Commission (Joint Commission, 2013) have developed standards for the recognition of medical home practices. These standards are used to certify the eligibility of primary care practices for recognition and reimbursement in a variety of programs, including Medicare and Medicaid. Nurse practitioner practices are eligible for recognition under these standards as medical homes (Joint Commission, 2013; NCQA, 2013; URAC, 2013). As the requirements for this model of care become the basis for inclusion and reimbursement in health care programs (public and private), it will be important for nurse practitioners to be sure that their practices, wherever they are, meet these standards and are recognized as medical homes.

Accountable Care Organizations (ACOs)

The growth of ACOs spurs incentives for the provision of high-quality, cost-effective care. Through the practice of shared facilities, service, and communication, the goals of ACOs are best met through the inclusion of nurse practitioners who have already demonstrated their worth in the realm of providing high-quality, cost-effective care. Studies of healthcare effectiveness data and information set (HEDIS) reports, use of quality indicators, and other outcome studies all demonstrate that nurse practitioners will be an asset in ACOs, whether as a clinician in a member practice or clinic, a nurse practitioner practice, or a nurse practitioner-owned and/or led ACO (AANP, 2012a).

Transitional and Coordinated Care

Studies have demonstrated that care coordination and follow-up care after hospitalization reduce the number of hospital admissions. The utilization of nurse practitioners in the provision of these services elevates the quality of these fundamental nursing activities with significant results. Nurse practitioners should be expected to serve as clinicians as well as practice owners and managers in the provision of both transitional and coordinated care in the community. They are well prepared to provide these services with a high level of knowledge and expertise (Naylor et al., 2004).

Long-Term Skilled Nursing Care and Home Care Nursing Services

Nurse practitioners are particularly well qualified to provide primary care services and medical oversight in SNFs, nursing facilities (NFs), and home nursing care programs. Their knowledge regarding the diagnosis and management of chronic illness, as well as acute disease, prepares them well to treat and keep patients out of hospitals, avoid complications, and maintain the quality of life for patients in these settings. The holistic approach to care provided by nurse practitioners is key to the well-being of patients under their care in both long-term NFs and home health care services (AANP, 2012b; Newhouse et al., 2012).

It is clear that nurse practitioners are the primary care stars of the future. Their combination of nursing and medical knowledge and expertise, and their ability to integrate the two into the care they provide, as well as their expertise in the areas of health promotion and disease prevention, make them the ideal provider for the management of both acute and chronic diseases and the maintenance of health in patients of all ages and walks of life.

As their numbers grow, nurse practitioners will continue to provide high-quality care in ever-expanding settings. They have grown from a small number of clinicians providing care for children to experts in providing care to all ages and types of patients (Goolsby, 2011). They are the primary care providers of the future. As today's barriers are further removed, they will be even better able to share their skills in the communities where they reside. Currently over 75% of nurse practitioners practice in primary care and over 6,000 nurse practitioners report that they have their own practices (AANP, 2012b).

Will nurse practitioners expand their settings to include hospitals and specialty care settings? There is already evidence of the successful utilization of nurse practitioners in these areas (Kleinpell & Goolsby, 2012). As models of care continue to develop, it is projected that nurse practitioners will provide increased leadership and service in these settings as well.

CONCLUSION

It will be important for nurse practitioners to be at the table as new models of health care are developed, to serve as leaders in the exploration and development models that can keep the nation and the world healthier and active. It has taken a relatively short time for nurse practitioners to demonstrate their ability and their worth. If we are to have a high-level system of health care, it will be important for them to take a leadership role in the development of a safe, high-level health care system for the future. The abilities are there, and a bright future is waiting for them in both primary and acute care, but they must stay active and involved not just in the provision of care coming to them in their practices, but in the development of health care policy for the future.

REFERENCES

AAN. (1999). *Living legends*. Retrieved from http//www.aan.org/living legends

AANP. (2012). *Nurse practitioner prescriptive authority (map)*. Austin, TX: AANP.

AANP. (2012a). *Position statement: Quality of nurse practitioner practice*. Austin, TX: AANP. Retrieved from http//www.AANP.org/publications

AANP. (2012b). *Position statement: Nurse practitioners in primary care*. Austin, TX: AANP. Retrieved from http//www.AANP.org/publications

DEA. (2013). Retrieved from http://www.justice.gov/dea/druginfo/ds.shtml

Goolsby, M. J. (2011). 2009–2010 AANP national practitioner sample survey: An overview. *Journal of the American Academy of Nurse Practitioners, 23*(5), 266–268.

Joint Commission. (2013). Retrieved from http//www.JointCommission.org/accreditation/pchi/aspx

Kleinpell, R. M., & Goolsby, M. J. (2012). American Academy of Nurse Practitioners national nurse practitioner sample survey: Focus on acute care. *Journal of the American Academy of Nurse Practitioners, 24*(12), 690–694.

National Committee for Quality Assurance (NCQA). (2013). Retrieved from http//www.ncqa.org/programs/recognition/patient centered medical home

Naylor M. D., Brooten, D. A., Campbell, R. L., Maislin, G., McCauley, K. M., & Schwartz, J. S. (2004). Transitional care of older adults hospitalized with heart failure. *Journal of the American Geriatric Society, 52*, 675–684.

Newhouse, R. P., Stanik-Hutt, J., White, K. M., Johantgen, M., Bass, E. B., Zangaro, G., … Weiner, J. P. (2011, September–October). Advanced practice nurse outcomes 1990–2008: A systematic review. *Nursing Economics, 29*(5).

Newhouse, R. P., Weiner, J. P., Stanick-Hutt, J., White, K. M., Johantgen, M., Steinwachs, D., & Bass, E. B. (2012). Policy implications for optimizing advanced practice registered nurse use nationally. *Policy, Politics & Nursing Practice, 13*. Retrieved on August 31, 2012 from http//ppn.sagepub.com /content/early/2012/08/29/1527154412456299

URAC. (2013). Retrieved from http//www.URAC.org/pchch

CHAPTER 30

What the Future Holds for Clinical Nurse Specialist Practice and Health Policy

Rachel Moody

The landscape of health policy is ever changing and recently shifted significantly in relation to the Affordable Care Act (ACA). The ACA is actually two acts: the Patient Protection and Affordable Care Act and the Healthcare and Education Reconciliation Act. Both of these acts were passed in March 2010 (Cady, 2012). According to policies within the ACA, the following are the two main goals: make health care more affordable and improve the safety and quality of care for patients. The Department of Health and Human Services (HHS) states that the overarching goal of these policies is to assist the physicians, hospital/organizations, and other health care professions by focusing on the needs of the patients, aligning payments to outcomes (HHS, 2011). Affordable care is cost-effective, safe, and improves quality of care. Achieving affordable care can be done through value-based purchasing, quality reporting, improving performance, and increasing the incentives for quality and outcomes (Cady, 2012).

The National Quality Strategy was announced by HHS in March 2011. This strategy is a tool that will assist public and private partners in better coordinating quality initiatives (HHS, 2011). A new Center for Medicare and Medicaid Innovation (CMMI) was initiated through the Affordable Care Act. The goal of this center is to establish and test innovative care and health care delivery models (HHS, 2011).

Advanced practice registered nurses (APRNs) will have opportunities in the future based on the implementation of the ACA and future health policy development. The language used to describe the health care practitioner in the ACA was "practitioners" and "providers" rather than "physician," so APRNs can be recognized as an important part of the health care team. It will be up to each individual state to determine the scope within which an APRN will be able to practice (Henderson, Princell, & Martin, 2012).

Accountable care organizations (ACOs) were developed as a provision in the ACA to improve the quality of health care (HHS, 2011). An ACO is a group of health care providers working to better coordinate patient care. When care is better coordinated, it results in reduced health care costs and higher quality, patient-centered care. ACOs have an incentive payment based on shared savings that aligns quality performance to the payment received. Health care providers will need to work together to coordinate care across multiple settings for patients (Cady 2012; Henderson et al., 2012). These settings can range from offices and hospitals to long-term care facilities (HHS, 2011). Five areas that affect patient care are the proposed quality measures. These measures are "patient/caregiver experience of care, care coordination, patient safety, preventative health, and at-risk population/frail and elderly health" (HHS, 2011). The impact that the clinical nurse specialist (CNS) can have on health care reform is based on the long-standing focus CNSs have always had on patient safety, quality of care, and cost-effectiveness, which makes this a perfect place for the CNS to flourish.

APPLICATION/EVALUATION/DISCUSSION

The Affordable Care Act has implications for the future for CNSs and future development of health policy. CNSs are ready to meet these challenges in health policy, through leadership, cost savings, and a focus on outcomes, chronic disease management, transitions in care, and inclusion/participation/support of health policy development.

Health policy is built on research, evidence-based practice, guidelines, and innovation. Health policy encourages input of the different disciplines of health care, government, and the public. The health policy landscape and structure are being laid based on the impact from many quality and patient safety initiatives. Clinical nurse specialists are well suited to influence health policy due to their work and focus on quality, safety, and outcomes (patient, nursing, and organizational); see Figure 30.1.

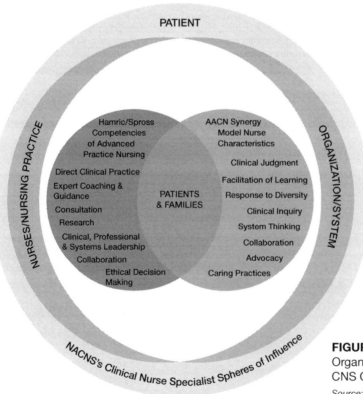

FIGURE 30.1 Model Depicting Organizational Framework for CNS Core Competencies.

Source: NACNS (2010).

The foundation for CNS practice is within the three spheres of influence defined by the National Association of Clinical Nurse Specialists (NACNS, 2010) (Patient, Nurse/Nursing Practice, and Organization/System). CNSs utilize this foundation in their practice.

Health care today is rapidly evolving and CNSs need to be involved in health policy in order for their value and contribution to health care to be known, integrated, and supported. Support can be accomplished in many ways: through legislation that defines the scope of CNS practice in a favorable manner, inclusion of CNSs in reimbursement, and inclusion in federal and state health care exchanges. CNSs historically have been involved in shaping the quality and patient safety initiatives of health care and thus are well positioned to shape health policy. One of the barriers that CNSs encounter is that at times their involvement has been too silent. Now is the time for CNSs to share their value and contributions to the health care systems and demonstrate how they positively impact delivery of care to the public.

Many agencies are currently involved or have been involved in setting the tone for health policy development, such as the Alliance for Health Policy Systems Research, American Health Quality Association, Medicare Payment Advisory Commission, National Academy for State Health Policy, National Academy of Social Insurance, National Quality Forum, and many others (National Library of Medicine, 2013). CNSs are also responsible as a profession within nursing to help set this tone as well. It is important to note that CNSs have been meeting the needs of the public for specialty nursing for more than 50 years (Fulton, Lyon, & Goudreau, 2010; NACNS, 2004).

The future for CNSs is to meet the new demands of a reformed health care system. The CNS needs to lead organizations in innovative ways to reduce readmissions, improve quality and safety, and continue to meet the needs of the public. Johnson, Smith, and Mastro (2012) state that health care organizations need to look at ways to be more efficient to meet these demands of health care reform. This is the work that CNSs have been doing and now is the time to let others know. The value to the health care organizations lies in decreasing waste and costs by utilizing lean principles while improving quality and productivity (Johnson, Smith, & Mastro, 2012). In 2012, the National Association of Clinical Nurse Specialists (NACNS) shared ways in which the CNS meets the new demand, in a press release. Box 30.1 is a summary of these central themes in which CNSs can meet the demands.

SUMMARY OF THE CENTRAL THEMES IN WHICH CNSS CAN MEET NEW DEMANDS (NACNS, 2012)	BOX 30.1

CNSs can meet the need to:

- Increase the effectiveness of transitioning care from hospital to home and prevent readmissions
- Improve the quality and safety of care and reduce health care costs
- Educate, train, and increase the nursing workforce needed for an improved health system
- Increase access to community-based care
- Increase the availability of effective care for those with chronic illness
- Improve access to wellness and preventative care

TRANSITIONS IN CARE

The CNS plays an important role in assisting patients in their transitions in care. "Care transitions describes a continuous process in which a patient's care shifts from being provided in one setting of care to another, such as from a hospital to a patient's home or to a skilled nursing facility and sometimes back to the hospital" (Burton, 2012, p. 1). Others describe transitions as "handoffs," which are the points when chronically ill patients transition or move to another location of care, whether it be home, hospital, home care, nursing home, and so on (Naylor et al., 2011). Transitions in care also include the goal of the most optimal placement of the patient based on his or her care needs. The dangers with these transitions in care are in gaps in quality, safety, and communication (Laker, 2011; Naylor et al., 2011). Coordination of care is integral in managing effective transitions in care, redesigning discharge from the hospital, and ultimately improved planning and communication among all care providers along the continuum of care for the patient (Laker, 2011). Currently, many programs for transitions in care have been developed under the Affordable Care Act of 2010; these were designed to help manage chronically ill patients in the safest, most cost-effective manner without compromise of quality of care (Naylor et al., 2011). Effective transitions in care may help reduce health care expenditures, improve patient outcomes, increase patient satisfaction, and decrease readmissions to the hospital (Burton, 2012). CNSs have been providing transitions in care for patients with chronic diseases. When transitions in care are managed, the outcome for patients is improved quality of life, better patient outcomes, and ultimately decreased readmissions (Naylor et al., 2004; Ryan, 2009). This management of transitions in care is a perfect match for the CNS. One way CNSs can develop a comprehensive discharge planning process is based on their specialty (e.g., heart failure, chronic obstructive pulmonary disease [COPD], asthma, epilepsy, and diabetes); through these plans, CNSs follow patient posthospital discharge in management of patients' symptoms, lifestyle, and other care aspects to prevent readmission to the hospital. A study conducted by Naylor et al. in 2004 found that when an APRN directed discharge planning and follow-up at home, there was a reduction in readmissions, lower mean total health care costs, and short-term improvement in quality of life and patient satisfaction. The study conducted by Ryan (2009) looked at the impact of a coordinated health care team which included CNSs, nurse manager, and nursing staff. The results of this study identified that there were reduced readmissions for a heart failure patient population when coordinated care was provided. Moore and McQuestion (2012) shared how to get involved with transitions by providing follow-up with discharged chronically ill patients, which can be implemented as a simple phone call, other support, and monitoring. Chronically ill populations that were provided transitions in care that assisted in promotion of self-care and a reduction in health care expenditures were asthma, heart failure, chronic pulmonary disease, and epilepsy patients (DeJong & Veltman, 2004; Horner, 2008; Naylor et al., 2004; Naylor & Keating, 2008; Naylor et al., 2011; Naylor, 2012; Ryan, 2009).

Implications for CNS Practice

CNSs must become involved with the initiatives surrounding transitions in care, as this relates directly to each of the CNS core competencies. Transitions in care are the work of the CNSs as identified in the CNS core competencies: direct care, consultation, systems leadership, collaboration, coaching, and ethical decision making. CNSs need to be involved as health policy evolves regarding transitions in care, whether this is through development and participation of the models or sharing with policy makers the impact that transitions in care have on patients, families, organizations, and overall health care spending. CNSs need to implement innovative mechanisms for improving transitions in care, such as improved communication with patients and caregivers. Communication has been noted to be at the root of many events or problems on many levels. When looking at transitions in care, CNSs need to utilize evidence-based tools and educate nursing personnel staff on how to use the tools; for example, the "Teach Back" method, which the health care provider educates the patient and/or family and the patient and/or family will then "teach back" the health care provider the information they learned or even demonstrate the skill learned (IHI, 2006). Moore and McQuestion (2012) emphasized that the CNS delivers care that is cost-effective and of high quality to patients and/or families. This is done through education, support, advocacy, and coordination of care, all of which directly correlate with the CNS core competencies.

IMPROVE QUALITY AND SAFETY OF CARE AND REDUCE HEALTH CARE COSTS

Improving clinical outcomes for patients and families is, and has been, the work of the CNS. CNSs provide innovative, evidence-based, quality nursing care within their specialty. The CNS provides the leadership in assessment, development, implementation, and evaluation of programs that focus on care of a specialty population (Finkelman, 2013; NACNS, 2004). Ellerbe and Regen (2012) stated that in today's environment of rapidly changing regulatory requirements, quality initiatives, and customer expectations, the health care organizations need to adapt and change to be fiscally responsible and remain in a competitive market. Not only are cost-effectiveness, quality, and patient safety looked at as an outcome in health care, but so is patient satisfaction. This is also known as *value-based purchasing*. These are all central components of the core competencies held by the CNS. CNSs can assist through their leadership and knowledge of outcomes and patient-centered care. The leadership of the CNS is seen in leading the health care team, implementing evidence-based changes to reduce complications (Murray & Goodyear-Bush, 2007). CNSs are able to set and achieve best practices, improve patient and/organization outcomes, and decrease health care costs (Vollman, 2006). CNS practice reduces health care cost through many avenues, for example, through reducing length of stay, reducing frequency of emergency room visits, increasing patient satisfaction, and reducing complications of hospitalized patients (Murray & Goodyear-Bush, 2007; Richardson & Tjoelker, 2012; Vollman, 2006). CNSs who practice within intensive care units (ICUs) have been able to reduce length of stay in the ICU, and prevent or reduce hospital acquired conditions (e.g., ventilator associated pneumonia [VAP], central line associated bloodstream infections, pressure ulcers, and so on) (Murray & Goodyear-Bush, 2007; Richardson & Tjoelker, 2012; Vollman, 2006).

CNS work is also accomplished through system redesign in relation to quality and patient safety. IHI's *Leadership Guide to Patient Safety* (2006) discusses redesigned systems and improved reliability as a couple of its steps to attaining patient safety. This is truly the work of the CNS through systems leadership; consultation; coaching; collaboration; interpretation, translation, and use of evidence; and evaluation of clinical practice. IHI describes redesigning care processes to increase reliability of outcomes. IHI suggests that a way to accomplish this is to "[i]ncrease standardization, include redundancies, and take advantage of human factors engineering (i.e.

understanding the interactions of people and equipment), all key principles in creating safer systems" (IHI, 2006). IHI noted work for sepsis, VAP, and central line bundles (IHI, 2012) as meeting this need for standardization, redundancies, and improved human factors engineering.

System redesign is accomplished through change, implementation of evidence-based practice, and utilization of synthesized research. CNSs are clinical expert leaders of change within organizations. They facilitate quality and safety in many ways, and design and implement evidence-based programs. The programs CNSs are involved in are to prevent avoidable complications, improve the quality of care, improve safety, prevent readmission to the hospital, reduce the length of stay, increase patient satisfaction, improve patient outcomes, and reduce health care costs (NACNS, 2012). IHI (2012) discusses the utilization of care bundles to improve care and save health care expenses by implementing an "all or none" philosophy. The study conducted by Murray and Goodyear-Bruch (2007) found that when bundled strategies were implemented, VAP rates declined. The study conducted by Vollman (2006) found that a program on pressure ulcer reduction developed and directed by a CNS reduced pressure ulcer prevalence by 50% to 80%. CNSs need to share their innovations and tools that improve quality and patient safety with the community at large, not just within their discipline. The types of programs and initiatives that CNSs implement can help shape health policy, set standards and guidelines, and assist in meeting the needs of patients, nursing, and organizations.

Discussion and Implications for the CNS

A couple of the recommended steps that organizations need to take in regard to patient safety were outlined in IHI's *Leadership Guide to Patient Safety* (2006). These recommendations are to address strategic priorities, culture, and infrastructure; utilize safety briefings; and provide support to the patients and staff who may have been involved in a near miss or error. CNSs are leaders who can assist health care organizations in creating cultures that support patient safety. One way that the CNS can accomplish this is through full implementation of the core competencies of consultation, direct care, systems leadership, collaboration, coaching, research, and ethical decision making. CNSs need to be involved in patient safety initiatives, coalitions, and centers—at local, regional, state, and national levels. CNSs need to become members of patient safety initiatives and/or centers within their own health care organizations, regions, and states.

Another recommendation from IHI (2006) was to utilize safety briefings. Safety briefings are a way to communicate and build awareness surrounding safety within health care organizations. These safety briefings should be done by the CNS. CNSs, for example, help create staff awareness in relation to safety issues/concerns (falls, medication errors, and so on), educate staff, integrate evidence-based information, and share unit data surrounding patient safety. CNS can run the safety briefings and then over time assist the nursing personnel in running them by themselves. An important follow-up as a CNS would be to assist with evidence-based practice changes to the safety briefing and evaluation of clinical practice.

Leadership of Patient Safety (2006), which is part of the Institute for Healthcare Improvement Innovation series, sets out methods and models for improvement (IHI, 2006). Utilizing these methods and models provides another avenue for the CNS to work on innovative strategies and lead patient safety initiatives. The leading of patient safety initiatives is another hallmark of the CNS, which they need to disseminate to others. It is important that leader CNSs know the methods, models, and tools that are available so that they can implement change and assist others in implementing change. CNSs as leaders can also provide support to staff and patients who were involved in errors and harm.

CNSs need to assist the organizations they work within, or develop their own consulting companies to assist organizations, in adapting to meet the rapidly moving and changing regulatory landscape, regulatory requirements, quality improvement initiatives, patient safety initiatives, and customer satisfaction and expectations. Health care organizations must be able to adapt to this rapid movement in health policy; otherwise they may not survive, remain competitive, and stay fiscally responsible (Ellerbe & Regen, 2012). CNSs must assist in these efforts. CNSs should also think about how they can integrate the utilization of technology when they are transforming health care systems and environments. Ellerbe and Reagen (2012) noted that the use of technology is needed in order to transform nursing and improve processes that impact the delivery of safe quality care.

In the IOM 2004 report, *Keeping Patients Safe: Transforming the Work Environment of Nurses*, one of the salient points is on transformational leadership. Transforming work environments is another area that the CNS can impact. Finkelman (2013) stated that it was this report that sparked the initiative Transforming Care at the Bedside (TCAB). The TCAB initiative involved the work of the CNS realizing the impact on patient outcomes due to a greater emphasis and focus on nursing surveillance. CNSs have always been involved in patient outcomes, which translate into safety and quality initiatives.

EDUCATE, TRAIN, AND INCREASE THE NURSING WORKFORCE NEEDED FOR AN IMPROVED HEALTH SYSTEM

Role modeling, consultation, and education to improve nursing practice are areas in which the CNS can have an impact (NACNS, 2004). This can be done through supporting nursing in their delivery of care, that is, supporting safe and quality care that is evidence based. Nurses today should be graduating from nursing programs that implement the Quality and Safety Education for Nurses (QSEN) competencies.

Discussion and Implications for the CNS

CNSs will be working with nursing personnel who may not have had the education or training or other exposure to know the QSEN competencies. This national initiative was funded by the Robert Wood Johnson Foundation (RWJF) (Cronenwett et al., 2007, 2009). The overarching goal of QSEN was to transform nursing education by embedding quality and safety competencies within the curriculum. The quality and safety competencies were drawn from the 2003 Institute of Medicine (IOM) report, *Health Professions Education*.

QSEN competencies directly relate to the CNS core competencies as well. Finkelman (2013) compared CNS core competencies to the IOM competencies for health care professionals. See Table 30.1 for the similarities across the competencies, which demonstrate that CNSs are well aligned for future health care in relation to competencies.

The IOM (2010) published a Robert Wood Johnson Foundation report, *The Future of Nursing: Leading Change, Advancing Health*, which emphasized that "[n]urses should practice to the full extent of their education and training . . . . [N]urses should be full partners, with physicians and other health care professionals, in redesigning health care . . . . Effective workforce planning and policy making require better data collection

TABLE 30.1 Comparing CNS Core Competencies, QSEN Competencies, and IOM Health Professional Competencies

CNS CORE COMPETENCIES NACNS	QSEN COMPETENCIES CRONENWETT ET AL. (2007)	IOM HEALTH CARE PROFESSIONAL COMPETENCIES*
Direct care	Patient-centered care Evidence-based practice Safety Informatics	Provide patient-centered care Utilize informatics
Consultation	Patient-centered care Team work and collaboration Quality improvement Safety	Provide patient-centered care Work in interprofessional teams Apply quality improvement
Systems leadership	Team work and collaboration Evidence-based practice Quality improvement Safety Informatics	Work in interprofessional teams Apply quality improvement Utilize informatics
Collaboration	Team work and collaboration	Work in interprofessional teams
Coaching	Team work and collaboration Quality improvement Safety	Apply quality improvement Work in interprofessional teams
Research: 1. Interpretation, translation, and use of evidence 2. Evaluation of clinical practice 3. Conduct of research	Evidence-based practice Quality improvement Safety Informatics	Employ evidence-based practice Utilize informatics Apply quality improvement
Ethical decision making	Patient-centered care Team work and collaboration	Provide patient-centered care Work in interprofessional teams

*Finkelman (2013).

and information infrastructure" (IOM, 2010, s-3). Organizations are currently conceptualizing these priorities and utilizing "advanced practice nurse[s to] play an important role to mentor the nursing staff and promote interdisciplinary, collaborative relationship between all health care disciplines and community support programs" (Ellerbe & Regen, 2012, p. 124). CNSs need to be involved in their own organizations to ensure that they are able to practice to their full scope of education and training, according to their state practice act. In addition to practicing to their full scope, CNSs must educate others regarding their role. CNSs should also take it a step beyond education and develop a template to share with others as to the work they do and the outcomes of their work, and try to quantify this in relation to health care dollars saved. This report should be widely shared with others in the organization (e.g., chief nursing officer, chief financial officer, quality committee, patient safety committee, risk managers, and so on). The organization needs to know and be able to speak to the benefit of having a CNS. It is the responsibility of the CNS to ensure that this happens.

INCREASE ACCESS TO COMMUNITY-BASED CARE

CNS practice focuses on wellness and preventative care to populations at risk for chronic diseases. Currently, more than 40 specialty areas of CNS practice have been identified. Specialties arise as a result of meeting the public's need for advanced nursing practice. CNSs practice in many settings. Examples of these settings that apply to community-based care are outpatient offices and community clinics (NACNS, 2004). CNSs practice within the community to meet the needs of the public. Health policy should include access to CNSs in the community setting in order to meet these needs. The DeJong et al. (2004) study looked at a community program for patients with COPD that was led by a CNS. The study found that 47% of subjects who were contacted postscreening indicated that they had stopped smoking, were in the process of quitting, or were seriously considering quitting.

CNSs need to be sharing the innovative ways in which they are providing access and services to the community. CNSs need to be advocating for reimbursement for these services and getting involved in sharing with legislators the work that they are doing and the outcomes of their work.

INCREASE THE AVAILABILITY OF EFFECTIVE CARE FOR THOSE WITH CHRONIC ILLNESS

CNSs work with and provide effective care to patients with chronic illness. The practice focuses on both wellness and preventative care for the patient population that is at risk for development of chronic illnesses. CNS practice assists with managing symptoms, improving quality of life (as defined by the patient), and improving the functional status of the patient. Through this practice, patients are able to improve patient outcomes, reduce health care costs, and increase patient satisfaction. Moore and McQuestion (2012) did a review of the literature on CNSs and chronic diseases, intending to find a way to better define the work of the CNS with the patient population with multiple chronic diseases (cardiovascular and oncology). Moore and McQuestion (2012) found in their review that CNSs had a positive impact on this patient population. Key themes that these researchers found in outcomes included improvement in quality of life, more patient and health provider satisfaction, fewer and shorter rehospitalizations, and lower costs of care (Moore & McQuestion, 2013).

The HHS administration (2011) noted that multiple chronic conditions are present in one of every four Americans today. CNSs should be involved with the development of outcome measures for patients with multiple chronic diseases. The National Quality Forum (2012) Multiple Chronic Conditions Measurement Framework committee developed a document discussing concepts that could be leveraged for patients with multiple chronic diseases. One of these concepts is on transitions of care between multiple providers and practice settings.

Another opportunity for CNSs is with patient-centered care. The Partnership to Fight Chronic Diseases publication, *Needs Great, Evidence Lacking for People with Multiple Chronic Conditions* (2012), found that there are gaps and barriers to providing patient-centered care today to patients with multiple chronic diseases. A couple of the barriers noted in relation to patients with multiple chronic diseases are lack of guidelines, quality measures, and outcomes.

When clinical practice guidelines for a single chronic disease are applied to patients with multiple chronic diseases, the single-condition guidelines potentially can conflict with guidelines for the other chronic diseases present in the patient. CNSs need to be involved in initiatives to reduce such problems, through direct care, consultation, systems leadership, collaboration, coaching, research, and ethical decision making. CNSs can assist in the development of tools that can be utilized for patient-centered care of patients with multiple chronic diseases/conditions. Current quality guidelines, when applied to patients with multiple chronic diseases, can overlook many potential vulnerabilities, potentially harmful care, harmful interactions, and overutilization of health care due to the complications/side effects (Partnership to Fight Chronic Diseases, 2012).

Needs Great, Evidence Lacking for People with Multiple Chronic Conditions (Partnership to Fight Chronic Diseases, 2012), also discussed other challenges in relation to patients with multiple chronic diseases/conditions, such as the need to enhance care quality and measure outcomes. CNSs are leaders in quality and outcomes and can assist in the development of performance and outcomes guidelines and measures for these patient populations. The Partnership to Fight Chronic Diseases (2012) notes that there needs to be thoughtful and deliberate consideration for the future of how quality will be measured and evaluated, because currently outcome measures/performance measures are only focused on one chronic disease.

Discussion and Implications for the CNS

The CNS must get involved now and be a part of the teams and initiatives that are defining multiple chronic disease guidelines and outcome measures. Once guidelines and outcome measures have been developed and accepted by the health care community, these measures will become part of health policy. Another avenue for policy involvement would be in meeting the needs of the public with multiple chronic diseases and working on prevention and management of the multiple chronic conditions (e.g., diabetes, COPD, and heart failure). Policy implications need to emphasize how quality of care can be improved in the population with multiple chronic conditions, due to the current lack of evidence-based standards for this population (Partnership to Fight Chronic Diseases, 2012).

The National Quality Forum (2012) did publish a measurement framework looking at multiple chronic diseases. The goal of the framework was to guide development, evaluation, and establishment of performance measures. There are synergies between the U.S. Department of Health and Human Services funded work and the NQF's Multiple Chronic Conditions Strategic Framework. There are limited resources within the literature regarding patients with multiple chronic diseases. The CNS must work with coordinated, interprofessional care teams to address these gaps in the literature, in addition to assisting in developing evidence-based practice/clinical guidelines for this patient population. The Patient Centered Outcomes Research Institute (PCORI) identified multiple chronic diseases as research priorities on their national research agenda. Some of the areas highlighted were improvement of care and outcomes, investigation of other models of care, and coordination of care/transitions in care for the multiple chronic condition population (PCORI, 2012).

CNSs need to be aware of other organizations' policy agendas; this drives research priorities and health policy development. The NACNS *Public Policy Agenda* is accessible through the website www.nacns.org/docs/2009PublicPolicyAgenda .pdf

Patients with chronic disease(s) usually receive care from multiple providers; if we fail to coordinate their care, it can result in higher costs and worse care. Uncoordinated care leads to lack of appropriate care, duplicative care, and an increased risk of errors (HHS, 2001). CNSs must be engaged in care coordination and be part of the interprofessional teams. When coordinated care is provided to patients with chronic diseases, both patients and organizations benefit, through improved quality of care and reduced overall health care cost.

IMPROVE ACCESS TO WELLNESS AND PREVENTATIVE CARE

CNSs can improve access to wellness and preventative care to populations at risk; for example, populations that are at risk for development of chronic diseases such as heart failure and diabetes. In addition, CNSs provide wellness care through employer companies with the goal of providing ongoing care to keep the employees healthy. The employer can expect its employees to be healthier and see an overall decrease in health care costs.

The CNS can identify patients at risk for chronic diseases through wellness and/or prevention screenings. CNSs can be innovative and develop their own company that would provide services of wellness and prevention to others (e.g., employers, government agencies, etc.).

CONCLUSION

Quality and safety in health care are major concerns to consumers, providers, governments, and so on. Health policy will be driving the consumer's decisions, health care dollars, research, and much more. CNSs must be part of the solution. CNSs must demonstrate their contributions in improving care, and this can be done through documenting, publishing, or presenting their work. CNSs need to be involved in research and evidence-based decisions, and they should know what the various research agendas are in relation to health policy. Moore and McQuestion (2012) state that there is a need within research literature for CNSs to study the outcomes of the various CNS roles, initiatives that they implement, interprofessional work, and impact on patients and families in all settings (e.g., community, hospital, offices, clinics, schools, correctional facilities, and so on) and throughout the health continuum through support of transitions in care, wellness and prevention, and chronic disease management (inclusive of multiple chronic disease management). In addition to research and publication, there is a need to share successes with health-related professionals outside of nursing, for example, at the CMS Innovation Center (www .innovations.cms.gov); see Figure 30.2. Best practice sharing is a must for CNSs so that others can learn from the outcomes that CNSs are able to attain.

CNSs must get involved! CNSs need to get involved within their organizations, communities, states, and on a national level. NACNS has resources that were put together to assist in advocating for key issues on the state and federal levels. The *Starter Kit for Impacting Change at the Government Level: How to Work with Your State Legislators and Regulators* is available through the NACNS website (http://nacns.org/html/toolkit.php).

For example here is one of the items that have been funded: "Indiana University will implement an intervention in 20 nursing facilities in the Indianapolis region of Indiana. This organization has created a program called "OPTIMISTIC" ("Optimizing Patient Transfers, Impacting Medical quality, and Improving Symptoms: Transforming Institutional Care") which includes the deployment of RNs and advanced practice nurses (APNs) to be on-site at the nursing facilities, allowing for enhanced recognition and management of acute change in medical conditions. RNs and APNs will coordinate with nursing facility staff and residents' primary care providers. In addition to employing INTERACT tools, this enhanced staffing model will adapt and apply other evidence-based models which have proven to reduce hospitalizations in other settings."

http://www.innovations.cms.gov/initiatives/rahnfr/index.html

FIGURE 30.2. OPTIMISTIC Innovations.

CNSs need to become involved on many levels to make sure that CNS practice is an accepted part of health care policies. Finkelman (2013) cites that it is critical for CNSs to get involved in policy making and to demonstrate the leadership role that CNSs take with improving patient care. CNSs need to share their work with more than their peers. Sharing can be done with employers, government officials, health care professionals outside of nursing, nurse educators, and nursing professional organizations (Finkelman, 2013). Henderson et al. (2012) discuss how nurses need to advocate for change in health policy. This can be done by participating in health policy through self-education, supporting the current initiatives (e.g., ACOs, patient-centered medical homes, and so on), participating in legislative activities (voting and running for office), supporting nursing organizations that are pursuing health policy changes, and educating others in health care and outside health care (Henderson, 2012).

CNSs must get involved in their own states with health policy and involvement, through state boards of nursing. If we do not have CNSs at the table, this may result in barriers to practice for CNSs. These barriers to practice ultimately reduce the CNS's ability to meet the needs of the public. CNSs need to know their resources, use them, and direct others to them. One such document for CNSs is *The Starter Kit for Impacting Change at the Government Level*; this and other documents are provided by NACNS on the website www.cns.org. Barriers for APRNs still exist, more in some states than others. CNSs from varying states have been challenged with being able to practice to their full scope of education and training, as some are not currently recognized by their state as an advanced practice nurse or even recognized as a clinical nurse specialist through title protection. The future of the CNS can be changed on the basis of individual states implementation of legislation and language in the nurse practice act. Our future depends on it, so get involved in your state legislature to ensure that this occurs.

REFERENCES

Agency for Healthcare Research and Quality (AHRQ). *Patient safety tools: Improving safety at the point of care.* Rockville, MD: Author. Retrieved from http://www.ahrq.gov/qual/pips

APRN Consensus Work Group & the National Council of State Boards of Nursing APRN Advisory Committee. (2008). Consensus model for APRN regulation: Licensure, accreditation, certification & education. Retrieved from https://www.ncsbn.org

Burton, R. (2012). Health policy brief: Care transitions. *Health Affairs*, September 13, 2012. Retrieved from http://www.healthaffairs.org/healthpolicybriefs/brief.php?brief_id=76

Cady, R. F. (2012). Healthcare reform after the supreme court ruling: Implications for nurse executives. *JONA's Healthcare Law, Ethics, and Regulation, 14*(3), 81–84.

Cronenwett, L., Sherwood, G., Barnsteiner, J., Disch, J., Johnsons, J., Mitchell, P., … Warren, J. (2007). Quality and safety education for nurses. *Nursing Outlook, 55*(3), 122–131.

DeJong, S., & Veltman, R. H. (2004). The effectiveness of CNS-led community based COPD/screening and intervention program. *Clinical Nurse Specialist, 18*(2), 72–79.

Ellerbe, S., & Regen, D. (2012). Responding to health care reform by addressing the Institute of Medicine report on the future of nursing. *Nursing Administration Quarterly, 36*(3), 210–216.

Finkelman, A. (2013). The clinical nurse specialist: Leadership in quality improvement. *Clinical Nurse Specialist, 27*(1), 31–35.

Fulton, J. S., Lyon, B. L., & Goudreau, K. A. (Eds.). (2010). *Foundations of clinical nurse specialist practice.* New York, NY: Springer Publishers.

Henderson, S., Princell, C. O., & Martin, S. D. (2012). The patient-centered medical home: This primary care model offers RNs new practice—and reimbursement—opportunities. *American Journal of Nursing, 112*(12), 54–59.

Horner, S. D. (2008). Childhood asthma in a rural environment: Implications for clinical nurse specialist practice. *Clinical Nurse Specialist, 22*(4), 192–198.

Institute of Medicine. (1999). To err is human: Building a safer health system. Retrieved from http://www.nap.edu/catalog/9728.html

Institute of Medicine. (2001). Crossing the quality chasm: A new health system for the 21st century. Retrieved from http://www.nap.edu/catalog/10027.html

Institute of Medicine. (2003). Health professions education: A bridge to quality. Retrieved from http://nap.edu/catalog/10681.html

Institute of Medicine. (2004). Keeping patients safe: Transforming the work environment of nurses. Retrieved from http://www.nap.edu/catalog/10851.html

Johnson, J. E., Smith, A. L., & Mastro, K. A. (2012). From Toyota to the bedside: Nurses can lead the lean way in health care reform. *Nursing Administration Quarterly, 36*(3), 234–242.

Laker, C. (2011). Decreasing 30-day readmission rates. *American Journal of Nursing, 111*(11), 65–69.

Moore, J., & McQuestion, M. (2012). The clinical nurse specialist in chronic diseases. *Clinical Nurse Specialist, 26*(3), 149–163.

Murray, T., & Goodyear-Bruch, C. (2007). Ventilator-associated pneumonia improvement program. *AACN Advanced Critical Care, 18*(2), 190–192.

National Association of Clinical Nurse Specialists. (2004). *Statement on clinical nurse specialist practice and education* (2nd ed.). Harrisburg, PA: Author.

National Association of Clinical Nurse Specialists. (2009). *Public policy agenda*. Retrieved from http://www.nacns.org/docs/2009PublicPolicyAgenda.pdf

National Association of Clinical Nurse Specialists. (2010). Clinical nurse specialist core competencies: Executive summary 2006–2008. Retrieved from http://nacns.org/html/competencies.php

National Association of Clinical Nurse Specialists. (2012). Clinical nurse specialist. Retrieved from http://www.nacns.org/docs/CNSOnePager.pdf

National Association of Clinical Nurse Specialists. (2012). NACNS Position Paper: National Association of Clinical Nurse Specialists statement on the APRN consensus model implementation. *Clinical Nurse Specialist, 26*(3), 185–189.

National Association of Clinical Nurse Specialists. (2012). The National Association of Clinical Nurse Specialists response to the Institute of Medicine's *The Future of Nursing* report. *Clinical Nurse Specialist, 26*(4), 205–211.

National Library of Medicine. Health policy key organizations. Retrieved from http://www.nlm.nih.gov/hsrinfo/health_economics.html#511Health Policy Key Organizations.

National Quality Forum. (2012). Multiple chronic conditions measurement framework. Retrieved from http://www.qualityforum.org/Publications/2012/05/MCC_Measurement_Framework_Final_Report.aspx

Naylor, M. D. (2012). Advancing high value transitional care: The central role of nursing and its leadership. *Nursing Administration Quarterly, 36*(2), 115–126.

Naylor, M. D., Aiken, L. H., Kurtzman, E. T., Olds, D. M., & Hirshman, K. B. (2011). The importance of transitional care in achieving health reform. *Health Affairs, 30*(4), 746–754.

Naylor, M., Brooten, D., Campbell, R., Maislin, G., McCauley, K., & Schwartz, J. (2004). Transitional care for older adults hospitalized with heart failure: A randomized, controlled trial. *Journal of the American Geriatrics Society, 52*(5), 675–684.

Naylor, M., & Keating, S. A. (2008). Transitional care: Moving patients from one care setting to another. *American Journal of Nursing, 108*(9), 58–63.

Partnership to Fight Chronic Disease. (2012). Needs great, evidence lacking for people with multiple chronic conditions. Retrieved from http://www.fightchronicdisease.org/media-center/resources/needs-great-evidence-lacking-people-multiple-chronic-conditions

Patient-Centered Outcomes Research Institute (PCORI). (2012). National priorities for research and research agenda. Retrieved from http://www.pcori.org/assets/PCORI-National-Priorities-and-Research-Agenda-2012-05-21-FINAL.pdf

Richardson, J., & Tjoelker, R. (2012). Beyond the central line associated bloodstream infection bundle: The value of the clinical nurse specialist in continuing evidence-based practice changes. *Clinical Nurse Specialist, 26*(4), 205–211.

Ryan, M. (2009). Improving self-management and reducing readmissions in heart failure patients. *Clinical Nurse Specialist, 23*(4), 216–221.

Stiefel, M., & Nolan, K. (2012). *A guide to measuring the triple aim: Population health, experience of care, and per capita cost* (IHI Innovation Series white paper). Cambridge, MA: Institute for Healthcare Improvement. Retrieved from www.IHI.org

U.S. Department of Health and Human Services (HHS). (2011). Accountable care organizations: Improving care coordination for people with Medicare. Retrieved from http://www.healthcare.gov/news/factsheets/2011/03/accountablecare03312011a.html

Vollman, K. (2006). Ventilator-associated pneumonia and pressure ulcer prevention targets for quality improvement in the ICU. *Critical Care Nursing Clinics of North America, 18*(4), 453–467.

CHAPTER 31

Health Policy and Special Needs Populations: Advanced Nursing Practice in Low-Income Countries

Patricia L. Riley, Jessica M. Gross, Carey F. McCarthy,
Andre R. Verani, and Alexandra Zuber

Although efforts to identify educational standards and competencies for the clinical advanced practice registered nurse (APRN) have been under way since 2006, a similar discussion pertaining to APRNs specializing in global health has yet to occur (National CNS Competency Task Force, 2010). Most recently, courses that provide an introduction to primary care in low-income settings as well as an overview of relevant epidemiology, pathophysiology, management of infectious and parasitic diseases, and maternal–child health have been available for nursing faculty and students working (or planning to work) in low-resource settings (University of Alabama at Birmingham, 2013; Global Health Delivery Online, 2012). However, APRNs interested in global health leadership also require orientation to health policy, program development, and evaluation—focal areas distinct from those previously identified. Additionally, there is a corresponding need for professional consensus regarding specific competencies in these areas so that the training for global advanced practice registered nursing is consistent, adequate, and harmonized across multiple universities and training centers.

This chapter aims to describe advanced nursing practice in low-income countries and identify issues affecting nursing and health service delivery, as well as the professional competencies essential for a career in global nursing. The chapter's specific learning objectives include:

- Providing an overview of health systems and human resources for health (HRH)—cross-cutting issues impacting global health
- Identifying competencies essential for APRNs within these areas
- Presenting a case study that incorporates a conceptual framework for strengthening nursing and midwifery regulation in the east, central, and southern Africa regions

This case also demonstrates how APRNs can evaluate change, identify legal considerations impacting health services and health practitioners, and create an evidence base in global nursing.

HEALTH SYSTEMS AND HUMAN RESOURCES FOR HEALTH

Regardless of their clinical focus or programmatic area of engagement, global APRNs must be familiar with the cross-cutting issues of health systems and HRH. Both are essential for advancing a variety of interventions promoting health (The Global Challenge of HIV/AIDS, Tuberculosis, and Malaria, 2011; Institute of Medicine [IOM], 2010a, 2010b; Joint Learning Initiative, 2004; Reich et al., 2008).

Health Systems

The World Health Organization (WHO) defines *health systems* as the embodiment of organizations, people, and actions whose primary intent is to promote, restore, or maintain health (2007). This definition encompasses the determinants of health as well as the broader definition of health-improving activities related to public health and government-endorsed health protections and policies. The overall goals of health systems are to improve health and health equity for a national population and present the best and most efficient use of available resources. As illustrated in WHO's *Framework for Action* (2007), health system components are discrete building blocks (Figure 31.1). Together, they constitute a complete health system, and when functional, result in achievement of the overall goals of improved health and demonstration of responsiveness to a community's health needs.

Due to weakened health infrastructure resulting from decades of neglect and insufficient investment, progress toward reaching the United Nations Millennium Development Goals (MDGs) for health has been compromised in most low-income countries (World Health Organization Maximizing Positive Synergies Collaborative Group, 2009). Reasons for inadequate health systems in many of these settings relate to economic crises and political unrest followed by conditional debt repayment and reduced investment in public health spending. Collectively, these events have negatively affected health service delivery and have resulted in the out-migration of highly skilled, yet poorly paid health care providers. These factors contributed, in part, to many low-income countries' inability to effectively respond to the global HIV epidemic early in the crisis. Furthering global health requires an awareness of health systems concepts (WHO, 2007), including health care delivery, health systems information, and knowledge capacity within that system (DeSavigny & Adam, 2009).

Human Resources for Health

Although global policies and resolutions in the early 2000s brought increased attention to the need for strengthening HRH capacity and HRH information systems in low-income countries (WHO, 2001, 2004), the first analysis of how health workforce shortages (e.g., nurses, midwives, and doctors) affect health services and health outcomes was reported by the Joint Learning Initiative (JLI)—a consortium of more than 100 global health leaders launched by the Rockefeller Foundation with a supported secretariat at Harvard University's Global Equity Initiative (Joint Learning Initiative, 2004). As illustrated in Figures 31.2 and 31.3, JLI's findings document that workforce density makes a critical difference regarding mortality rates of vulnerable

SYSTEM BUILDING BLOCKS   **OVERALL GOALS/OUTCOMES**

| SERVICE DELIVERY |
| HEALTH WORKFORCE |
| SERVICE DELIVERY |
| INFORMATION |
| MEDICAL PRODUCTS, VACCINES & TECHNOLOGIES |
| LEADERSHIP/GOVERNANCE |

ACCESS
COVERAGE

QUALITY
SAFETY

| IMPROVED HEALTH (LEVEL AND EQUITY) |
| RESPONSIVENESS |
| SOCIAL AND FINANCIAL RISK PROTECTION |
| IMPROVED EFFICIENCY |

THE SIX BUILDING BLOCKS OF A HEALTH SYSTEM: AIMS AND DESIRABLE ATTRIBUTES

Good health services are those which deliver effective, safe, quality personal and non-personal health interventions to those who need them, when and where needed, with minimum waste of resources.

A well-performing health workforce is one which works in ways that are responsive, fair and efficient to achieve the best health outcomes possible, given available resources and circumstances. I.e., There are sufficient numbers and mix of staff, fairly distributed; they are competent, responsive and productive.

A well-functioning health information system is one that ensures the production, analysis, dissemination and use of reliable and timely information on health determinants, health systems performance and health status.

A well-functioning health system ensures equitable access to essential medical products, vaccines and technologies of assured quality, safety, efficacy and cost-effectiveness, and their scientifically sound and cost-effective use.

A good health financing system raises adequate funds for health, in ways that ensure people can use needed services, and are protected from financial catastrophe or impoverishment associated with having to pay for them.

Leadership and governance involves ensuring strategic policy frameworks exist and are combined with effective oversight, coalitionbuilding, the provision of appropriate regulations and incentives, attention to system-design, and accountability.

FIGURE 31.1 The Six Building Blocks of a Health System: Aims and Desirable Attributes.
Adapted from WHO Health System Framework (World Health Organization, 2007).

populations, such as mothers, infants, and children. A similar association was noted with regard to workforce density and health services coverage (Chen et al., 2004).

Although host countries and donor organizations have begun addressing provider shortages with pre-service investments (i.e., formal training prior to graduation), resolving the provider imbalance in low-income countries will require years of sustained support (Kinfu et al., 2009; Willis-Shattuck et al., 2008). Some of the HRH issues affecting health services include professional out-migration, workforce retention, and maldistribution of health care providers (Gross et al., 2010). More recently, a variety of interventions designed to offset these shortages have been introduced to

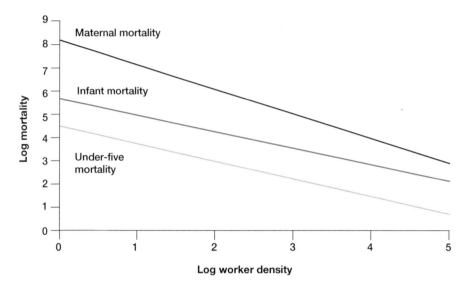

FIGURE 31.2 Association Between Worker Density and Mortality Rates.

Source: Chen et al. (2004).

sub-Saharan Africa. The Nurse Education Partnership Initiative (NEPI), for example, targets nursing and midwifery education in sub-Saharan Africa. In addition to training investments, other examples of HRH interventions include task shifting—recently renamed task sharing (Institute of Medicine, 2010b)—and emergency hire initiatives. Each is briefly described below.

Educational Investments

Launched in 2009, NEPI is a five-year initiative supported by the Health Resources and Services Administration of the Department of Health and Human Services, with funding from the U.S. President's Emergency Fund for AIDS Relief (PEPFAR) and implemented by Columbia University (www.pepfar.gov/partnerships/initiatives

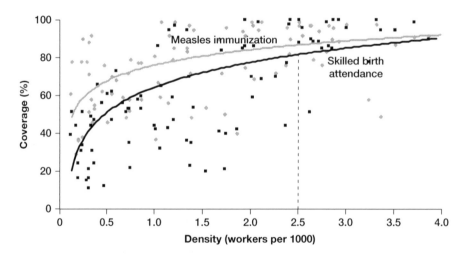

FIGURE 31.3 Association Between Worker Density and Service Coverage.

Source: Chen et al. (2004).

/nepi/index.htm). NEPI's objectives include increasing nursing and midwifery capacity by strengthening education programs in both pre-service and in-service settings. Currently operational in eight countries (Democratic Republic of Congo, Ethiopia, Ivory Coast, Kenya, Malawi, Swaziland, Republic of South Africa, and Zambia), additional components of this initiative include developing educational strategies that transform and enhance nursing and midwifery capacity. Although seen as an important contribution for strengthening Africa's nursing educational infrastructure, a recent analysis of current numbers of health workers and professional training program outputs suggests that pre-service support (along with other workforce incentives) needs to be significantly expanded in order to improve health worker inflow and offset out-migration (Kinfu et al., 2009). Short- and long-term impact from these kinds of investments requires program monitoring and evaluation—skills for which the global APRN must be equipped.

Task Sharing

In 2007, WHO, in collaboration with PEPFAR and UNAIDS, introduced the concept of task shifting, defined as the process whereby certain clinical skills are delegated from doctors to nurses (or from nurses to other, less-specialized health workers). WHO initially proposed task shifting as a workforce option for countries needing to reach the United Nation's goal of universal access to HIV prevention, care, and treatment (Samb et al., 2007; WHO, 2007). Recent studies have shown that appropriate delegation of HIV management, such as nurse-initiated and managed antiretroviral therapy (NIMART), can produce health outcomes comparable to physician-initiated and prescribed HIV treatment in certain settings (Callaghan, Ford, & Schneider, 2008; Morris, et al., 2009; Sanne et al., 2010). Based on these findings, NIMART is now considered an important clinical and policy component for reaching PEPFAR's most recent AIDS-free generation targets (PEPFAR Blueprint: Creating an AIDS-Free Generation, 2012). In their 2010 report, *Envisioning a Strategy for the Long-Term Burden of HIV/AIDS: African Needs and US Interests*, the Institute of Medicine (IOM) redefined this type of task delegation as "task sharing," thereby emphasizing team collaboration and partnership in the delivery of health interventions (IOM, 2010b). As task sharing takes hold in sub-Saharan Africa, there will be a need to assess its impact and ensure that adequate, updated nursing regulations are in place; these functions represent the skills APRNs need in order to provide leadership to issues impacting global nursing practice.

Emergency Hire Initiatives

A number of donors and global initiatives have invested in emergency hire programs (EHPs) (Adano, 2008). In Kenya, EHPs were financed by a variety of global initiatives and non-governmental organizations (Gross et al., 2010). EHPs represent a fast-track hiring and deployment intervention designed to augment the ability of ministries of health to scale up workforce staffing within government health facilities. Whereas Gross documented that EHPs resulted in increased hiring of nurses and the reopening of health facilities previously closed due to staffing shortages, there has been minimal research evaluating the longer-term effects of this intervention on core health services at the local level (Vindigni et al., 2013).

The following pages present a case study regarding the African Health Professions Regulatory Collaborative for Nurses and Midwives (ARC)—a four-year PEPFAR-supported nursing and midwifery initiative. ARC provides an example of how APRNs can develop, implement, and evaluate interventions designed to strengthen nursing and midwifery regulatory practices and policy in low-resource settings. The case study highlights competencies necessary for bolstering the professional infrastructure governing nurses and midwives and demonstrates how well-conceived interventions can influence funding priorities, policy, and ultimately nursing and midwifery practice in global settings.

CASE STUDY: THE AFRICAN HEALTH PROFESSION REGULATORY COLLABORATIVE FOR NURSES AND MIDWIVES

In sub-Saharan Africa, nurses and midwives frequently experience variance between professional regulation and the clinical practice environment (IOM, 2010). For example, although some ministries of health endorse task sharing—which enables nurses to provide antiretroviral therapy (ART), thereby increasing access to HIV services (Fairall et al., 2012; Sanne et al., 2010)—nursing education and their regulatory policies are not always aligned with expanded practice. This incongruence can create situations whereby nurses are required to practice beyond their clinical competencies or outside their professional regulatory environment (IOM, 2010). Although professional regulatory bodies, such as nursing and midwifery councils, have a mandate to govern professional practice (including the provision of ART), when new health initiatives are introduced in a country, involvement of these councils is frequently overlooked (McCarthy & Riley, 2012). Despite this occurrence, nursing regulations pertaining to professional scopes of practice, licensure, and training accreditation are essential for ensuring that nurses and midwives are adequately trained and competent to deliver health services (ICN, 2009). The ARC initiative specifically addresses this shortcoming by targeting nursing regulatory bodies and enabling their leadership to update and reform national regulatory frameworks (McCarthy & Riley, 2012).

ARC Overview

Conceived as a regional initiative serving countries in east, central, and southern Africa (ECSA), ARC's mandate is to strengthen nursing and midwifery regulation in 17 countries (Figure 31.4). Funded by PEPFAR through the U.S. Centers for Disease Control and Prevention (CDC) and implemented by the Lillian Carter Center for Global Health and Social Responsibility at the Emory University, ARC's partnerships also include the Commonwealth Nurses Federation (www.commonwealthnurses .org), the Commonwealth Secretariat (www.thecommonwealth.org), and the East, Central, and Southern Africa Health Community (ECSA-HC) (www.ecsahc.org), and most recently, the WHO. ARC's core objectives include supporting national nursing and midwifery leadership teams in the ECSA region to:

1. Sustain the scale up of HIV services through strengthened nursing and midwifery regulatory frameworks
2. Align accreditation, licensing, continuing education, and scopes of practice among other key regulatory functions with global guidelines and regional standards
3. Review legislation and regulation to strengthen the alignment of policy and practice for nurses and midwives
4. Enhance the capacity and collaboration of national organizations to perform key regulatory functions and mobilize resources, and
5. Foster a sustained regional network of nursing and midwifery regulatory leaders to facilitate the exchange of best practices.

ARC's overarching mission is to strengthen and synergize nursing and midwifery regulatory practices through peer-led learning and ARC-convened meetings

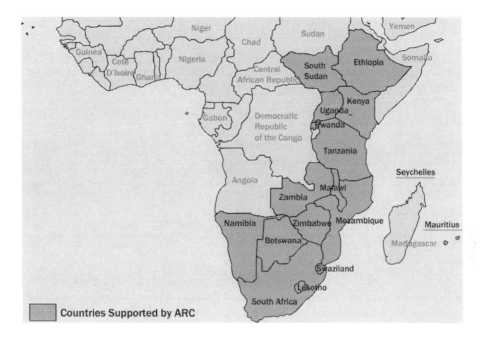

FIGURE 31.4 Countries Receiving ARC Support.

of national nursing and midwifery leadership teams. These teams (referred to as "the quad") comprise the chief nursing officer within the ministry of health, the registrar of the nursing/midwifery regulatory council, the president of the national nurses association, and an academic representative from a pre-service training institution. Together these positions represent the four main pillars of nursing and midwifery practice: government health ministries, professional regulatory bodies, professional associations, and academic institutions. With assistance from ARC, each team works toward identifying national regulatory priorities that they will address through locally designed solutions.

The ARC conceptual framework is based on the Institute for Healthcare Improvement's model for "breakthrough change" (IHI, 2003) and represents a col-laborative model that promotes rapid improvement in an identified priority area of regulation. The process by which change occurs includes country team participation in alternating series of "learning sessions" in which teams of national nursing leaders convene, share experiences, and participate in peer-led mentoring; this is followed by "action periods" whereby country quads work within their teams toward resolv-ing their respective regulatory issue (Figure 31.5). ARC also convenes an annual summative congress, which is used to communicate the direction and plans for the forthcoming year. Key components of ARC's breakthrough model include formation of the national quad, identification of a regulatory topic needing improvement, and recruitment of ARC faculty (or technical advisors) to assist with their regulatory pri-ority. While ARC promotes south-to-south (country to county) collaboration, it also convenes global, regional, and national leaders in nursing and midwifery regulation to assist in providing technical assistance.

Each year ARC awards regulatory improvement grants of up to $10,000 to coun-try team proposals to address their identified regulatory priority. These grant requests are developed and submitted by the respective country quad teams. ARC awards these funds based on the quality and feasibility of each proposal. Each country team

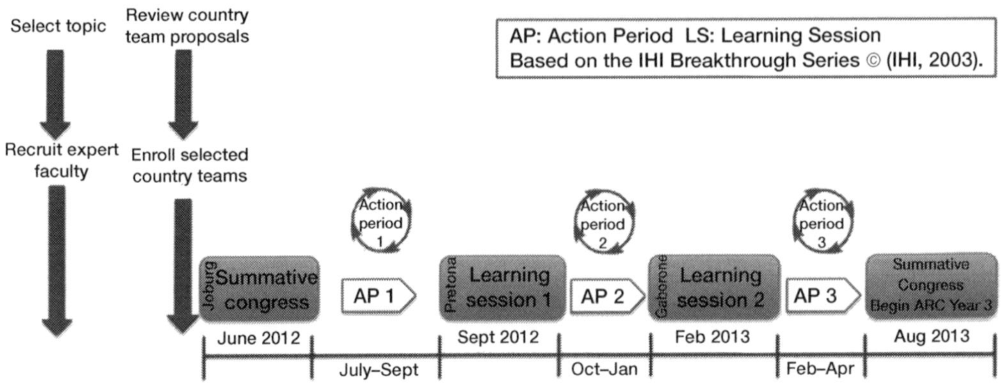

FIGURE 31.5 ARC Year 2 Model for Collaborative Regulatory Improvement.

receiving an ARC grant is invited to participate in ARC-convened learning sessions over a 12-month period. At the end of a funding cycle, awardees present their final reports, key results, and lessons learned during ARC's annual summative congress.

Regulatory Improvement Grants

ARC's regulatory improvement grants are designed to stimulate country quad discussion, consensus, and identification of short-term "winnable battles" in nursing and midwifery regulation. During the inaugural 2011 Summative Congress, participating country teams identified a variety of national regulatory priorities, such as reviewing and revising national nursing acts; developing and strengthening continuing professional development (CPD) programs; aligning national scopes of practice with population health needs; and enhancing nursing councils' regulatory information systems. Between 2011 and 2013, the ARC awards supported proposals from Botswana, Kenya, Lesotho, Malawi, Mauritius, Seychelles, Swaziland, Tanzania, Uganda, and Zimbabwe. These locally conceived regulatory proposals encompassed the following areas:

- Developing and strengthening national CPD programs
- Initiating nursing legislative reform
- Updating national nursing acts in order to elevate the profile of nurse educators and strengthen the professional regulatory council
- Revising professional scopes of practice—including reviewing and updating scopes of practice for nurses and midwives
- Decentralizing regulatory services to four pilot zonal offices, thereby making the process of licensure renewal more accessible to nurses assigned to rural posts

In addition to receiving fiscal support, each country team is assigned a dedicated ARC faculty member (from the participating organizations) who provides mentorship and project facilitation during the funding cycle. In this way, ARC supports country-driven initiatives that address nationally identified priorities in nursing and midwifery regulation.

Providing Targeted Technical Assistance

Although funding is not sufficient to provide grants to all countries, ARC has advanced unfunded country submissions through the provision of targeted technical assistance (TA). In 2011, Tanzania and Uganda received TA to support the development and implementation of their regulatory priority. Mozambique received global nursing and midwifery guidelines translated into Portuguese. In 2012, South Africa and Zambia received TA to advance their respective CPD programs. South Sudan also received TA with regard to developing their health professional examination and licensure board for their nascent government. In Mozambique, assistance included a review of a draft bill that would establish a national nursing regulatory council.

Regional Harmonization of Nursing Practice

Similar to the *Consensus Model for APRN Regulation* (American Nurses Association, 2009), the ARC initiative promotes harmonization of accreditation, education, certification, and licensure standards among ECSA countries. This approach is especially beneficial in low-income settings, where nurses and midwives routinely confront ethical challenges in which client health needs exceed nurse training and professional scopes of practice. By supporting nursing leaders to address these regulatory challenges and by creating opportunities in which they are able to share experiences and problem-solving approaches, ARC is helping to ensure congruence between regulatory policies and a demanding and frequently changing clinical practice environment.

Evaluating ARC

The ARC case study underscores the value of a well-conceived and conscientiously implemented initiative. Even the most thoughtfully designed projects must be evaluated for effectiveness in achieving their objectives and to ascertain whether further support is warranted. As stated previously, included among the ARC's objectives are the alignment of accreditation, licensing, continuing education, scopes of practice with global guidelines and regional standards, and reviewing (and revising) legislation and regulation to strengthen the alignment of policy and practice for nurses and midwives. Thus, a central component of ARC has been measuring and evaluating the impact of this initiative on nursing and midwifery regulations and standards, at both the regional and national levels. This section provides an example of an evaluation framework that an advanced global health nurse practitioner could design and use to assess the impact of an intervention such as ARC.

Establishing a Baseline

ARC's evaluation activities began with an initial baseline survey of nursing and midwifery regulation in all 14 countries present at the inaugural meeting in Nairobi, Kenya (McCarthy et al., 2013). Data from this survey provided a cross-sectional snapshot of what regulations countries did and did not have in place. Survey findings indicated that countries varied with regard to what regulations were in place (Table 31.1). These findings indicated that countries are at different points in terms of the regulations established and suggested that countries are not yet implementing regulations that meet globally recognized standards, such as those set by the International Council of Nurses (ICN), the International Confederation of Midwives (ICM), the World Health Organization (WHO), and the East, Central, and Southern African College of Nursing (ECSACON).

TABLE 31.1 Selected Country Status on Licensure, CPD, and Education Accreditation

COUNTRY	LICENSURE		CONTINUING PROFESSIONAL DEVELOPMENT (CPD)		PRE-SERVICE EDUCATION ACCREDITATION	
	LICENSES ARE ISSUED TO NURSES AND MIDWIVES	LICENSURE EXAM REQUIRED FOR NURSES AND MIDWIVES	CPD PROGRAM IN PLACE	CPD REQUIRED FOR LICENSE RENEWAL	DOES THE COUNCIL ACCREDIT PRE-SERVICE EDUCATION?	RENEWAL OF ACCREDITATION STATUS
Botswana	Yes	No	In design	N/A	No response provided	No response provided
Lesotho	Yes	Yes	In design	N/A	Yes	Every 2 years
Mozambique	No	N/A	No	N/A	No (Ministry of Education; Ministry of Health)	"Regularly"
Namibia	Yes	Yes	Yes	Planned	No (National Qualification Authority)	Requirement not established
Swaziland	Yes	No	In design	N/A	Yes	No response provided
Tanzania	Yes	No	No	N/A	No (National Council of Technical Education)	Every 2 years
Uganda	Yes	Yes	Yes	Planned	Yes	Requirement not established
Zambia	Yes	No	Yes	No	Yes	Requirement not established

Data excerpted from McCarthy, Voss, Verani, et al. (2013).

Identifying a Measurement Approach

In order to assess whether ARC is effective in helping countries strengthen regulations, an evaluation tool would need to capture the initial degree of regulatory activity for each country as well as measure progress in improving regulations against their baseline. Design of the ARC evaluation tool has been descirbed elsewhere (McCarthy et al., 2014). A Capability Maturity Model (CMM) is a tool to assess the ability of an organization to perform its core functions and to document the organization's advancements in performing those functions (Paulk et al., 1994). The most well-known CMM was designed by Carnegie Mellon University's Software Engineering Institute (SEI) to assess capability in software design organizations (Table 31.2). CMMs contain two components: a list of key functions an organization must carry out and a description of a stepwise path to improving the performance of each key function (Humphrey, 1987). The stepwise path is comprised of five sequential stages, beginning from an "initial" stage where performance is low to an "optimized" stage where performance is very high. Each stage describes a discrete level of capability, characterized by certain elements that must be in place before advancing to the next stage (Strutt, Sharp, Terry, & Miles, 2006). The stages in a CMM are sequential; advancement from one stage to the next represents a meaningful improvement in organizational functioning (Figure 31.6) (Humphrey, 1987). Together, the five stages outline an ordinal scale for assessing capacity and measuring advancement in key organizational functions.

Adapting a CMM to Nursing and Midwifery Regulation

The first step in designing a CMM is deciding the critical functions an organization must perform to meet its objectives. To identify the core functions of a nursing and midwifery regulatory body, a literature search of peer-reviewed articles, grey literature, and websites pertaining to nursing and midwifery regulation was conducted. Based on the available literature, seven essential regulatory functions were identified: registration

TABLE 31.2 Five Stages in the Software Design Capability Maturity Model (Paulk et al., 1994; Strutt et al., 2006).

STAGE	NAME	DESCRIPTION OF STAGE
1	Initial	The organization typically operates without formalized policies or processes; project activities are reactive rather than proactive or planned; achievements are usually the result of exceptional efforts by individuals.
2	Repeatable	Organizational policies and processes guide project management; basic project data is collected; there is a reasonable measure of commitment or control in projects; early successes can be repeated; new challenges are frequently encountered.
3	Defined	The organization has achieved the foundation for major and continuing progress; project management processes are documented, standardized, and integrated; technical data on projects is tracked.
4	Managed	Organizational processes are well-defined, predictable, and quantifiable; expanded data collection methods indicate that project performance consistently falls within acceptable quantified boundaries.
5	Optimized	The organization is now focused on continuously improving processes; data is used to identify the weakest elements in a process and improve it; improvements are incremental and incorporate new technologies and innovations.

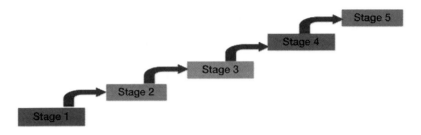

FIGURE 31.6 Stepwise Progression of CMMs.
Adapted from Paulk et al. (1994).

and data collection, licensure, scope of practice, continuing professional development, accreditation of pre-service institutions, professional conduct and discipline, and influencing the revision of nursing and midwifery legislation, such as nurse practice acts (Buchan & Dal, 2003; ICM, 2011; ICN, 2009a, 2009b, 2011; Munjanja, Kibuka, & Dovlo, 2005; UNFPA, 2011; Walshe, 2003; WHO, 2009, 2011; WHO-EMRO, 2002).

The second step in designing a CMM is to describe an evolutionary path of improvement in each core function from an early capability level to a level of high capability. Examples of various stages of nursing and midwifery regulations, such as registration, scopes of practice, disciplinary procedures, accrediting nursing programs, and revising legislation were found in the literature (Dohrn, Nzama, & Murrman, 2009; Feeley & O'Hanlon, 2007; Miles et al., 2007; Miles, Seitio, & McGilvray, 2006; Philips, Zachariah, & Venis, 2008; Plager & Razaonandrianina, 2007; Rajaraman & Palmer, 2008; Rakoum, 2010; Riley et al., 2007; Seloilwe, 2001; USAID, 2010; WHO, 2006, 2011; WHO/PEPFAR/UNAIDS, 2008; Zachariah et al., 2009). Using these examples in conjunction with the SEI principles for characterizing discrete stages of capability, five sequential levels of regulation implementation were drafted. Global guidelines and standards for key nursing and midwifery regulations from ECSACON, ICM, ICN, and WHO were used as end points for the highest level of performance, stage 5.

Validation and Pilot Testing

The draft nursing and midwifery regulation CMM was presented to country leadership teams and global regulation experts attending an ARC learning session. Each country team was asked to review the seven functions and consider whether they appropriately reflected the key functions of their nursing and midwifery regulatory council. Small-group discussions were held with each team to note their feedback. In a large-group session, country teams and global experts reviewed and revised the five stages of CPD regulation and revision of national nursing and midwifery law. These two functions were then used as templates on which to base descriptions of five-step capability paths for the remaining five functions. The completed draft CMM for documenting and evaluating progress in nursing and midwifery regulation in the ECSA region was named the Regulatory Function Framework (RFF).

At a subsequent learning session, the RFF was pilot tested for contextual and descriptive accuracy by three country teams implementing ARC regulation improvement grants. Each country team was given the RFF to review and asked to select the stage (1–5) that best characterized the state of regulation in their country at the beginning of ARC (February 2011). If a stage did not adequately reflect a country's stage with regard to a regulation, they were instructed not to select a stage for that function. All three countries reported that they were able to select a stage that accurately captured their capability for that regulation. Each team was also asked to look specifically at the regulatory function for which they were receiving ARC funding and indicate two stages for that function—the stage of the regulation at the beginning of ARC (February 2011) and the stage that best characterized the regulation at that moment (October 2011). As seen in the following figures, two countries progressed at least one stage over the course of time examined; one country did not quite advance to the next stage. The results from the three countries are listed in Figures 31.7–31.9.

The Importance of Evaluating Impact

The RFF developed for ARC is a regionally relevant and stakeholder-vetted framework for assessing a stepwise progression of improvements in nursing and midwifery regulation. This framework will allow for documenting each country's baseline stage

Country A	Planning (Stage 1)	Developing (Stage 2)	Defining (Stage 3)	Managing (Stage 4)	Optimizing (Stage 5)
Continuing Professional Development (CPD)	MoH policy requiring CPD for health professionals is in place. Nursing and midwifery CPD framework in planning stages.	National nursing and midwifery CPD framework developed. Implementation of CPD in pilot or early stages. CPD not yet required for re-licensure.	National CPD program is in place. CPD is required in legislation for re-licensure. CPD tracking system not yet developed.	Electronic tracking of CPD undertaken by nurses and midwives is in place. A system to monitor compliance is in place together with penalties for noncompliance.	Multiple types of CPD are available, including web-based models. CPD content aligns with regional standards or global guidelines.

FIGURE 31.7 Progress in CPD Regulation by Country A Between February and October 2011.

Country A	Planning (Stage 1)	Developing (Stage 2)	Defining (Stage 3)	Managing (Stage 4)	Optimizing (Stage 5)
Continuing Professional Development (CPD)	MoH policy requiring CPD for health professionals is in place. Nursing and midwifery CPD framework in planning stages.	National nursing and midwifery CPD framework developed. Implementation of CPD in pilot or early stages. CPD not yet required for re-licensure.	National CPD program is in place. CPD is required in legislation for re-licensure. CPD tracking system not yet developed.	Electronic tracking of CPD undertaken by nurses and midwives is in place. A system to monitor compliance is in place together with penalties for noncompliance.	Multiple types of CPD are available, including web-based models. CPD content aligns with regional standards or global guidelines.

FIGURE 31.8 Progress in CPD Regulation by Country B Between February and October 2011.

Country C	Planning (Stage 1)	Developing (Stage 2)	Defining (Stage 3)	Managing (Stage 4)	Optimizing (Stage 5)
Revisions to Nursing and Midwifery Law	There is consensus among key stakeholders on issue(s) to be reformed in legislation.	Draft of legislative change(s) has been approved by stakeholders. MoH supports and approves proposed legislative change.	MoH fully engages, supports, advances, and represents updated draft of legislation.	Draft referred to legislative body for induction and passage. Act promulgated, published, and commenced.	Implementation in nursing and midwifery practice environments. Compliance and impact monitored.

FIGURE 31.9 Progress in Revising Nursing and Midwifery Law by Country C Between February and October 2011.

of regulation, assessing yearly progress in updating and strengthening regulation, and tracking the overall impact of ARC's national and regional regulation-strengthening efforts. The responses on the RFF permit cross-country comparisons to gain an understanding of the strengths and gaps in nursing and midwifery regulations in the ECSA region. The evidence of varying stages of regulations in the region indicates that improvement goals are not identical for all countries. However, the RFF helps set a common pathway for improvement, and documents progress—not only if regulations reach stage 5, but also through meaningful incremental achievements. By capturing smaller-scale achievements, the RFF is a valuable instrument to measure the impact of ARC support for professional councils and regulatory reform.

USING RESEARCH TO DRIVE SYSTEMS-LEVEL CHANGES TO NURSING PRACTICE

One of the key spheres of influence for APRNs includes the "system," the overarching health care organization that supports nursing practice (National CNS Competency Taskforce, 2010). In global health, driving improvements to the nursing system in countries includes improving policies, administrative practices, decision making, regulation, and standards that ensure quality, cost-effective health outcomes of nursing practice. A key way to influence this sphere is through the practice of research, which is a standard competency for APRNs (The National CNS Competency Taskforce, 2006–2008). Examples of global nursing research include: evaluating programs to improve nursing practice; conducting literature reviews to document evidence-based nursing practice; administering key informant surveys to ascertain nursing preferences; and even conducting studies with experimental designs to assess the impact of changes to nursing practice on service delivery.

Research in global nursing is growing, as can be seen in a wide range of international, peer-reviewed nursing journals, such as *International Journal of Nursing Studies*, *International Nursing Review*, and the *African Journal of Midwifery and Women's Health*. Global nursing research topics can also be found in a wide range of other nursing and non-nursing journals, including *Journal of Nursing Quality Care*, *Research in Nursing and Health*, *Journal of Advanced Nursing*, *Nursing Research*, *Applied Nursing Research*, *Journal of Clinical Nursing*, *Journal of the Association of Nurses in AIDS Care*, *Human Resources for Health Online*, *Health Policy and Planning*, and the *Bulletin of the World Health Organization*. Conducting and publishing research through these vehicles, and helping translate this research into systems-level changes through advocacy, collaboration, consultation, and systems leadership, is an essential skill set in global health nursing (*The National CNS Competency Taskforce*, 2006–2008). The following case study demonstrates how advancing a particular study around nursing regulation is being used to drive systems-level changes in global nursing practice for HIV/AIDS.

RESEARCHING NURSE-INITIATED AND MANAGED HIV TREATMENT, IN PRACTICE, POLICY, REGULATION, AND TRAINING, IN EAST AND SOUTHERN AFRICA

In early 2012, experts from the CDC identified a systems-level challenge in the nursing practice of several sub-Saharan African countries. Through the course of their global health work, they had observed the broad scale-up of nurse-initiated and managed antiretroviral therapy (NIMART) in the practice setting of many African countries, without the requisite attention to establishing enabling nursing policy, regulation, and quality assurance for the practice, in line with WHO guidelines (WHO, 2008).[1] The CDC staff became concerned that nurses were not, in some settings, adequately trained or regulated for NIMART practice, a scenario that posed worrisome risks in terms of patient safety, health outcomes, and nurses' own medical liability. The staff saw this as a strategic issue for the PEPFAR initiative as a whole, as scaling up high-quality nurse-led HIV treatment services is vital to expanding HIV treatment coverage in Africa—a region that has the highest HIV burden in the world, and the lowest health workforce densities, especially among physicians (Kinfu, 2009; Van Damme, 2008; WHO, 2006; Zachariah, 2009).

The CDC staff determined that a research study was needed to objectively and systematically document the implementation of NIMART in the practice, policy and regulation, and education and training settings in the Africa region. The aim of the study was to inform PEPFAR and the global health community of the strengths and weaknesses of NIMART implementation, to recommend systems-level changes that would improve the delivery of nurse-led HIV/AIDS services across Africa, and thereby enhance the quality and coverage of HIV treatment in the region.

Establishing a Collaboration of Coauthors

The first step to conducting this study was for the principal investigator (P.I.) to establish research collaboration among four experts in policy, legislation, nursing practice, and HIV care and treatment in Africa, all of whom worked under the PEPFAR initiative. These experts included a PhD nurse researcher, a public health lawyer, a senior HIV/AIDS care and treatment advisor, and a senior nursing leader (and former Nursing Council Registrar) from Zambia who had special insight into nursing issues in Africa. The coauthors then pursued the key steps in research implementation outlined in the *Clinical Nurse Specialist Core Competencies* for the conduct of research (National CNS Competency Taskforce, 2010), featured below.

Identify Questions for Inquiry

The research team first outlined the major domains of inquiry that the study would address: characteristics of NIMART implementation pertaining to (a) nursing practice, (b) policy and regulation, and (c) education and training within the sub-Saharan Africa region.

Conduct Literature Reviews

The research team then conducted a literature review of NIMART to determine whether this study was novel and contributed to the existing evidence-base. Using the research database PubMed, as well as the Internet search engine "Google," the team searched for articles with key search terms, including "task-shifting and HIV/AIDS," "task-shifting and nurses," "nurse-led HIV treatment," and "nurse-initiated and managed ART." The team also used a snowball method of obtaining articles, by using the reference sections of the articles retrieved to identify new articles of possible interest. The P.I. drafted an annotated bibliography of the most relevant documents, which documented each relevant article retrieved and summarized the key and relevant findings of that article. This document was a useful tool for the coauthors to establish a shared understanding of the study context.

Study Design and Implementation

As the next step, the research team designed the research methodology. The team determined that the ARC Summative Congress, which convenes the senior nursing leadership of 17 countries in the east, central, and southern Africa region, would represent a useful opportunity to survey a convenience sample of authoritative key informants. The research methods were to administer a group survey to each nursing leadership team from 17 countries. The survey instrument was a structured questionnaire, containing multiple choice and open-ended questions on the implementation of NIMART in the practice setting, in national policy and nursing regulation and legislation, and in pre-service and in-service training in the country.

The team drafted a protocol, which is a document that summarizes the rationale for the study; the methods for data collection, storage, and analysis; and the risks and protection for the people participating in the study (the "human subjects"). After submitting this protocol to the CDC Associate Director for Science and receiving scientific approval to conduct the study, the team then conducted validity testing of the questionnaire, by having an individual who was representative of the survey respondents take the questionnaire to ensure that the questions would be interpreted in the intended manner and solicit accurate responses from survey respondents.

Data Collection

The team presented a summary of the research aims and methods to the ARC Summative Congress participants, and asked for verbal consent to participate in the research. The team conducted the survey over a 45-minute period and collected the written surveys. The team then entered survey findings into a Microsoft Excel database, and had a research assistant conduct data cleaning and validation to ensure that there were no mistakes in the data collection and entry.

Data Analysis

Using the Excel database, the team conducted basic frequencies, or tallying of the frequencies of particular survey responses. The team also conducted thematic analysis of the open-ended questions, by categorizing responses by key concepts (e.g., "training") and tallying the number of responses that fell in that category.

Dissemination of Findings

The authors wrote up the findings in a 3,000-word manuscript, organized into introduction, methodology, results, and discussion sections. This manuscript was submitted to be published in a peer-reviewed publication. The team then developed a plan for disseminating the findings and advocating for programmatic changes to NIMART in the region. First, the research team presented the findings at the subsequent ARC Summative Congress, to facilitate discussion among nursing leadership teams in the region on the policy, regulation, and legislative changes needed to improve nursing practice of NIMART. The team also presented the findings in several subsequent meetings with CDC HIV Treatment experts to plan how the PEPFAR initiative can advance systematic changes to support NIMART globally. From the findings, the team additionally identified two countries that were in special need of systems-level changes to advance the practice, policy, and training for NIMART- Mozambique and Tanzania- and worked with U.S. government and MOH leadership in both countries to advance discussion and investment in NIMART. Once the findings are published, the team will also circulate the final manuscript to additional global stakeholders working with nursing and HIV service delivery, to further advocate for more comprehensive investment in policy, regulation, and training for NIMART globally.

ADVANCING GLOBAL NURSING AND MIDWIFERY PRACTICE THROUGH LAW AND REGULATION

Another facet of the ARC collaborative is to reduce the burden of HIV and AIDS by improving global public health competencies for law, regulation, and policy as they relate to nursing in the ECSA region. Public health competencies or action areas that public health professionals should be expected to engage in include law, regulation, and policy (PAHO/WHO, 2007). *Public health*, in turn, has been defined as "the practice of preventing disease and promoting good health within groups of people, from small communities to entire countries" (APHA, 2013). Therefore, when engaged in public health nursing, nurses' clients include not only individual patients but also their families, communities, and societies.

Before delving into the subject matter of advancing APRN globally through law, a few terms should be defined. *Law*, as used here, is understood to be a system of social rules created, instituted, and enforced through and by governments. Citizens or residents of countries may influence the law through their governments, although ultimately it is the government that passes and enforces the law. *Legislation* is a specific type of law passed by the legislative branch of government (i.e., an act or statute). A common piece of legislation found in east, central, and southern Africa is a nursing act, which among other things creates a nursing council to regulate the profession. *Regulation* is a type of law, more specific than, following from, and subsidiary to legislation. For example, a nursing council established by a nursing act can be empowered in that piece of legislation to issue regulations that are more detailed and specific than the act.

But why worry about laws and regulations if your primary concern involves the clinical aspects of advanced practice registered nursing? Whether in Africa, Asia, Australia, Europe, North America, or South America, the nursing profession is governed by laws. Though these laws vary substantially across and even within countries, they also have much in common. Laws serve to create nursing professional regulatory bodies (i.e., nursing councils), shape who governs such bodies, and provide their mandates. Laws and regulations affect APRNs in myriad other ways.

Think of your own path to becoming an APRN. Although one may not always be aware of it, the law structures the educational and professional path by requiring certain actions, prohibiting others, and providing discretion to persons and organizations that regulate nurses. For example, your educational degree program may be accredited as required by certain laws or regulations. *Accreditation* is a means of achieving and certifying minimum quality or standards, whether in nursing education or other areas (International Council of Nurses, 2009). Law can require accreditation, specify standards to be attained, and determine which organization(s) will serve as accrediting entities. Such is the case in South Africa, where the nursing act requires the country's national nursing council to "withdraw or suspend accreditation of a nursing education institution or nursing education programme if the education or training provided does not comply with the prescribed requirements and inform the relevant licensing authority" (Republic of South Africa, 2005).

Once you graduate with your APRN degree, you will likely require a license to practice. *Licensing* is an essential regulatory function carried out by nursing professional regulatory bodies. It is a means to ensure the safety and effectiveness of professional practitioners, as it prohibits those without a license from practicing. In this sense, licensing serves a gatekeeper role by restricting entry into the profession to only those who have demonstrated evidence of competency. Grad (2004) has described the health professional licensing process as it often unfolds in the United States, a process similar to that of many other countries:

> The licensing process begins when the legislature passes a licensing statute to prohibit certain activities unless a license is first obtained. The statute then authorizes the licensing agency, a board of health, a board of regents, or a special professional or occupational board to promulgate rules and regulations relating to license application and to the control of the licensed activity. (p. 120)

This process of broad legislation followed by more detailed regulation is common to lawmaking in several countries. These procedural steps in the United States, which Grad (2004) describes, also occur in Zimbabwe, where legislation requires that a license (or in their words, a "practicing certificate") be obtained prior to nursing practice, while regulations specify procedures and criteria to issue, renew, suspend, and cancel nursing licenses (Zimbabwe, 2004).

In addition to acquiring your APRN degree and your license, you may further be required to register as an APRN with a nursing professional council. *Registration* is a regulatory device to ensure comprehensive information and records on the number, distribution, and other relevant characteristics of professionals in a field, such as nursing. It should be distinguished from licensing, although at times the two terms have been conflated (Grad, 2004).

Now, imagine yourself practicing as an APRN a few years from now. Depending on where you practice, you may also be required to demonstrate continuing competence in order to periodically renew your license or reregister. For example, in Tanzania the law requires that nurses demonstrate proof of completion of continuing professional development with their license renewal application (United Republic of Tanzania, 2010). *Continuing professional development* (CPD) is a means of ensuring quality competent nursing care throughout nurses' careers, and like licensing and registration, is often mandated in national nursing and midwifery legislation or regulations. Requiring CPD and enforcing the requirement are thus further ways in which lawmakers and regulators use the force of law to ensure ongoing professional competence. However, in some countries there is still no formal requirement for nurses to engage in CPD.

In review, accreditation, licensing, registration, and CPD are essential regulatory functions relevant to nursing training and practice. Other essential regulatory functions affecting APRN include the definition of scopes of practice of all nursing cadres, as well as the establishment of codes of ethical conduct or professional responsibility. Hopefully, you now have a greater appreciation for how laws shape your educational path and affect your professional career as an APRN. Such laws and regulations shape advanced practice nursing in your country and throughout the world.

But how might one advance the role of the APRN in disadvantaged, low-income countries through law and regulation? This chapter includes ideas to consider, based on our experience to date with the ARC initiative in 17 countries. First, simply bringing the perspective of a nurse who has been regulated may prove useful. Not all APRNs will have the opportunity to regulate APRN professional training and practice; however, every APN has had to comply with professional regulations and requirements. Whether obtaining the initial license to practice, providing evidence of CPD to renew one's license, or otherwise complying with externally imposed requirements, every

APRN has experienced being the object of professional regulation. This perspective can be a fruitful one to explore when providing advice or technical assistance on how best to regulate. Second, when possible, draw on technical experts who have themselves served on regulatory councils or professional associations that have addressed issues of APRN regulation. Third, consider convening regulators and other nursing professional leaders from within and across countries to facilitate intra- and inter-country learning. For each participant country from sub-Saharan Africa that would like to access technical assistance or a small grant, ARC requires the participation of four nursing leaders, all of whom it considers essential to the functioning of a nursing professional regulatory regime: (a) the Ministry of Health, represented by the Chief Nursing Officer; (b) the Nursing Council, represented by the Registrar; (c) the Nursing Professional Association; and (d) a nursing pre-service training institute. By convening nursing policy makers, regulators, professionals, and academic leaders from within and across countries, ARC fosters a dynamic learning environment to collaboratively advance nursing and midwifery regulation.

In conclusion, advancing APRN globally through laws and regulations is a complex endeavor. Should you choose to dedicate a portion of your career as an APRN to global health, you may want to reflect on these closing pieces of advice. First, try to learn about the nursing legal and regulatory framework in the country you would like to assist. To strengthen or support (or even just comply with) laws or regulations, you must first know what they are. Establishing a legal/regulatory baseline for APRN can therefore be the fundamental first step (McCarthy et al., 2013). Important partners in creating such a baseline may include nursing regulators and legal experts from the country. Publicly available legal research websites may also be of some assistance (WHO International Digest of Health Legislation, GlobaLex). Second, if possible, explore similarities and differences among various national nursing laws and regulations. This comparison provides useful material to inform discussions regarding legal and regulatory reform. Neighboring or similarly situated countries may take dramatically different approaches to resolving the same issues, and these diverse approaches can serve as a learning laboratory. Finally, recognize that what constitutes a "good" nursing professional law may be difficult to discern from an outsider's perspective. What is right for one country's nursing profession and stakeholders may not be right for another's. Furthermore, there is much to be said for a "good" or fair and inclusive process when reforming laws and regulations. Basic procedural safeguards, such as public notice and comment requirements, before finalization of rules and regulations can help ensure that they result from, or at least are informed by, stakeholder input (Gostin, 2008, p. 168). Nevertheless, there are still some objective methods to help determine what constitutes a "good" or "strong" nursing law. International benchmarks exist against which nursing laws may be measured (Verani, 2011). For instance, the ICN has issued several guidance documents on nursing regulation, including a Model Nursing Act. Nursing laws can be compared to guidance issued by the ICN, ICM, and WHO, as countries seek to improve their own nursing legal and regulatory frameworks.

CONCLUSION

With nurses and midwives constituting the largest number of health workers in low-resource settings, health systems and HRH are areas uniquely suitable for research and advanced global nursing practice. Proficiency in this area includes an ability to identify nursing workforce gaps and—in collaboration with local stakeholders—design and evaluate appropriate solutions. Related competencies include prioritizing scarce nursing resources at a macro level and determining whether (or where) further investments are needed. This chapter highlights a regional approach for addressing gaps in nursing regulatory practices and developing an ongoing process for evaluating change. The ARC case study serves as a template for successful APRN engagement within a global context. This chapter also highlighted the importance of assessing national policies and regulatory frameworks and determining the extent to which they harmonize with existing nursing scopes of practice. In conclusion, in order to function as 21st century global nurse practitioners, today's APRNs need analytic skills that enable them to identify nursing needs, design and evaluate proposed interventions, and propose evidence-based policies that ultimately result in improved health care.

(The findings and conclusions in this chapter are those of the authors and do not necessarily represent the decisions, policy, or views of the Centers for Disease Control and Prevention, U.S. Department of Health and Human Services.)

NOTE

1. NIMART is the practice of clinical tasks associated with HIV treatment by nurses, including initiation, prescription, management of follow-up visits, and clinical monitoring, among others.

DISCUSSION QUESTIONS

1. After reviewing the United Nations Development Programme (UNDP) human development index (http://hdr.undp.org/en/statistics), select one country that is categorized as "medium" for human development and another one that is categorized as "low." Then access each country's respective maternal and child health indices, including maternal/infant/ child mortality rates and their respective health service indicators, such as the percentage of the population having access to skilled attended births in a health care facility and percentage of coverage of childhood immunizations. Summarize your findings based on the available published data and compare your results with the available literature regarding each country's health care provider to population ratio. Are your findings consistent with those published by Lincoln Chen and the Joint Learning Initiative? (Refer to full citation in the reference list.)
2. Based on the Institute for Healthcare Improvement (IHI) "breakthrough for change" model, can you identify another global health challenge that might benefit from a similar application? Is adapting this conceptual framework to other situations beneficial? If so, describe how this model can be useful.
3. With regard to the Capability Maturity Model (CMM) that is being used to measure the impact of the ARC initiative, what other kind of global health intervention would be suitable for benchmarking using this evaluation approach?
4. This chapter provides a process for conducting research with regard to nurse-initiated and managed antiretroviral therapy (NIMART). Using this process, identify another research issue of relevance to global APRNs. Then construct a relevant and appropriate research process for the issue that you would investigate.
5. Describe three nursing regulatory functions relevant to APRNs worldwide. How might diverse and legal regulatory environments in the global context affect APRNs?

REFERENCES

Adano, U. (2008).The health worker recruitment and deployment process in Kenya: An emergency hiring program. *Human Resources for Health, 6*, 19.

American Nurses Association. (2009). *Consensus model for APRN regulation: Licensure, accreditation, certification, and education.* Retrieved from http://www.nursecredentialing.org/Certification/APRN Corner

American Public Health Association. (2013). What is public health? Retrieved from www.apha.org /about

The Bill & Melinda Gates Foundation. Retrieved from http://www.gatesfoundation.org

Buchan, J., & Dal Poz, M. R. (2003). Role definitions, skill mix, multi-skilling and "new" workers. In P. Ferrinjho & M. R. Dal Poz (Eds.), *Toward a global health workforce strategy* (pp. 275–300). Antwerp, Belgium: ITG Press.

Callaghan, M., Ford, N., & Schneider, H. (2008). A systematic review of task-shifting for HIV treatment and care in Africa. *Human Resources for Health, 8*, 8. Retrieved from http://www.human-resources -health.com/content/8/1/8

Carnegie Mellon University Software Engineering Institute. (1987). *Characterizing the software process: A maturity framework.* Pittsburgh, PA: W.S. Humphrey.

Chen, L., Evans, T., Anand, S., Boufford, J. L., Brown, H., Chowdhury, M., … Wibulpolprasert, S. (2004). Human resources for health: Overcoming the crises. *Lancet, 364*, 1984–1990.

Dohrn, J., Nzama, B., & Murrman, M. (2009). The impact of HIV scale-up on the role of nurses in South Africa: Time for a new approach. *Journal of Acquired Immune Deficiency Syndrome, 52*(1), S27–S29.

Fairall, L., Bachmann, M. O., Lombard, C., Timmerman, V., Uebel, K., Zwarenstein, M., … Bateman, E. (2012). Task shifting of antiretroviral treatment from doctors to primary–care nurses in South Africa (STRETCH): A pragmatic, parallel, cluster-randomised trial. *Lancet, 380*, 889–898.

Feeley, R., & O'Hanlon, B. (2007). *Why policy matters: Regulatory barriers to better primary care in Africa—Two private sector examples.* Bethesda, MD: United States Agency for International Development.

GlobaLex. Retrieved from www.nyulawglobal.org/Globalex/#

The Global Fund to Fight AIDS, Tuberculosis and Malaria. Retrieved from http://www.theglobalfund .org/en

Gostin, L. O. (2008). *Public health law: Power, duty, restraint.* Berkeley: University of California Press.

Grad, F. P. (2004). *The public health law manual.* Washington, DC: American Public Health Association.

Gross, J. M., Riley, P. L., Kiriinya, R., Rakuom, C., Willy, R., Kamenju, A., … Rogers, M. F. (2010). The impact of an emergency hiring plan on the shortage and distribution of nurses in Kenya: The importance of information systems. *Bulletin of the World Health Organization, 88*, 824–30. doi:10.2471 /BLT.09.072678

Gross, J. M., Rogers, M. F., Teplinsky, I., Oywer, E., Wambua, D., Kamenju, A., … Waudo, A. (2011). The impact of out-migration on the nursing workforce in Kenya. *Health Services Research, 46*(4), 1300–1328. doi:10.1111/j.1475-6773.2011.01251.x

Institute for Health Care Improvement. (2003). *The breakthrough series: IHI's collaborative model for achieving breakthrough improvement.* Boston, MA: IHI. Retrieved from http://www.ihi.org/knowledge /Pages/IHIWhitePapers/TheBreakthroughSeriesIHIsCollaborativeModelforAchievingBreak throughImprovement.aspx

Institute of Medicine. (2010a). *Committee on Envisioning a Strategy for the Long-Term Burden of HIV/AIDS: African needs and U.S. interests.* Retrieved from http://iom.edu/Activities/Global/LongTermAIDS .aspx

Institute of Medicine. (2010b). *Preparing for the future of HIV/AIDS in Africa: A shared responsibility.* Washington, DC: Author. Retrieved from http://books.nap.edu/openbook.php?record_id=12991

International Confederation of Midwives. (2011). Global standards for regulation. The Hague: Author.

International Council of Nurses. (2009). Credentialing. Retrieved from www.icn.ch/publications /regulation

International Council of Nurses. (2009a). *The role and identity of the regulator: An international comparative study* (ICN Regulation Series). Geneva: ICN. Retrieved from http://www.icn.ch/images/stories /documents/publications/free_publications/role_identity regulator.pdf

International Council of Nurses. (2009b). *Model nursing Act* (ICN Regulation Series). Geneva: ICN.

International Council of Nurses. (2010). *Nursing matters: Credentialing* (ICN Fact Sheet Credentialing). Geneva: ICN.

Joint Learning Initiative. (2004). Human resources for health: Overcoming the crisis. Cambridge, MA: Harvard University Press.

Kinfu, Y., Dal Poz, M., Mercer, H., & Evans, D. B. (2009). The health worker shortage in Africa: Are enough physicians and nurses being trained? *Bulletin of the World Health Organization, 87*(3), 225–228. doi:10.2471/BLT.08.051599

McCarthy, C. F., & Riley, P. L. (2012). The African health profession regulatory collaborative. *Human Resources for Health*, 10:26. doi:10.1186/1478-4491-10-26

McCarthy, C. F., Voss, J., Verani, A. R., Vidot, P., Salmon, M. E., & Riley, P. L. (2013). Nursing and midwifery regulation and HIV scale-up: Establishing a baseline in east, central, and southern Africa. *Journal of the International AIDS Society, 16*, 18051. Retrieved from http://www.jiasociety.org/index.php/jias/article/view/18051 doi: 10.7448/IAS.16.1.18051.

Miles, K., Clutterbuck, D. J., Seitio, O., Sebego, M., & Riley, A. (2007). Antiretroviral treatment roll-out in a resource-constrained setting: Capitalizing on nursing resources in Botswana. *Bulletin of the World Health Organization, 85*(7), 555–560.

Miles, K., Seitio, O., & McGilvray, M. (2006). Nurse prescribing in low-resource settings: Professional considerations. *International Nursing Review, 53*(4), 290–296.

Morris, M. B., Chapula, B. T., Chi, B. H., Mwango, A., Chi, H. F., Mwanza, J., ... Reid, S. E. (2009). Use of task-shifting to rapidly scale-up HIV treatment services: Experiences from Lusaka, Zambia. *BMC Health Services Research, 9*(1), 5.

Munjanja, O., Kibuka, S., & Dovlo, D. (2005). The nursing workforce in sub-Saharan Africa. *Global Nursing Review Initiative, 7*. Geneva, International Council of Nurses.

National CNS Competency Task Force. (2010). *Clinical nurse specialist core competencies: Executive summary 2006–2008*. Retrieved from http://nursingcertification.org/pdf/Exec%20Summary%20-%20Core%20CNS%20Competencies.pdf

Pan-American Health Organization/World Health Organization. (2007). The essential public health functions as a strategy for improving overall health systems performance: Trends and challenges since the public health in the Americas initiative, 2000–2007. Retrieved from www.paho.org/english/DPM/SHD/HR/EPHF_2000-2007.pdf

Paulk, M. C., Weber, C. V., Curtis, W., & Chrissis, M. B. (1994). *The capability maturity model: Guidelines for improving the software process*. Reading, MA: Addison Wesley.

PEPFAR Blueprint: Creating an AIDS-free Generation. (2012). Retrieved from www.pepfar.gov/documents/organization/201386.pdf

Philips, M., Zachariah, R., & Venis, S. (2008). Task shifting for antiretroviral treatment delivery in sub-Saharan Africa: Not a panacea. *Lancet, 371*(9613), 682–684.

Plager, K. A., & Razaonandrianina, J. O. (2009). Madagascar nursing needs assessment: Education and development of the profession. *International Nursing Review, 56*(1), 58–64.

President's Emergency Plan for AIDS Relief. Retrieved from www.pepfar.gov

Rajaraman, D., & Palmer, N. (2008). Changing roles and responses of health care workers in HIV treatment and care. *Tropical Medicine and International Health, 13*(11), 1357–1363.

Rakoum, C. (2010). *Nursing human resources in Kenya: Case study*. Geneva: ICN and Florence Nightingale International Foundation.

Reich, M., Takeni, K., Roberts, M., & Hsiao, W. (2008). Global action on health systems: A proposal for the Toyako G8 summit. *Lancet, 371*, 865–869.

Republic of South Africa. (2005). Nursing act. Retrieved from www.denosa.org.za/upload/acts/Nursing_Act.pdf

Riley, P. L., Vindigni, S. M., Arudo, J., Waudo, A. N., Kamenju, A., Ngoya, J., ... Marum, L. H. (2007). Developing a nursing database system in Kenya. *Health Services Research, 42*(3, Pt. 2), 1389–1405.

Samb, B., Celletti, F., Holloway, J., Van Damme, W. V., De Cock, K. M., & Dybul, M. (2007). Rapid expansion of the health workforce in response to the HIV epidemic. *New England Journal of Medicine, 357*(24), 2510–2514.

Sanne, I., Orrell, C., Fox, M. P., Conradie, F., Ive, P., Zeinecker, J., ... Wood, R. (2010). Nurse versus doctor management of HIV-infected patients receiving antiretroviral therapy (CIPRA-SA): A randomised non-inferiority trial. *Lancet, 376*(9734), 33–40.

Seloilwe, E. (2001). *The regulation of nursing in Botswana*. Geneva: International Council of Nurses.

Strutt, J. E., Sharp, J. V., Terry, E., & Miles, R. (2006). Capability maturity models for offshore organizational management. *Environment International, 32*(8), 1094–105.

UNFPA. (2011). *The state of the world's midwifery 2011: Delivering health, saving lives.* Geneva: United Nations Population Fund.

United Republic of Tanzania. (2010). Nursing and midwifery act; Nursing and midwifery training regulations. Retrieved from http://polis.parliament.go.tz/PAMS/docs/12-1997.pdf

USAID. (2010). *Creating an enabling environment for task shifting in HIV and AIDS services: Recommendations based on two African country case studies.* Retrieved from http://www.hciproject.org/communities /chw-central/resources/creating-enabling-environment-task-shifting-hiv-and-aids-services-

Van Damme, W., Kober, K., & Kegels, G. (2008). Scaling-up antiretroviral treatment in Southern African countries with human resource shortage: How will health systems adapt? *Social Science & Medicine, 66*(10), 2108–2121.

Verani, A. R., Shayo, P., & Howse, G. (2011). Using law to strengthen health professions: Frameworks and practice. *African Journal of Midwifery & Women's Health, 5*(4), 181–184.

Walshe, K. (2003). *Regulating healthcare: A prescription for improvement.* Philadelphia, PA: Open University Press.

Willis-Shattuck, M., Bidwell, P., Thomas, S., Wyness, L., Blaauw, D., & Ditlopo, P. (2008). Motivation and retention of health workers in developing countries: A systematic review. *Human Resources for Health, 8,* 274.

WHO. (2005). *Health and the millennium development goals.* Retrieved from www.who.int/hdp /publications/mdg_en.pdf

WHO. (2006). *Taking stock: Health worker shortages and the response to AIDS.* Geneva: WHO Press.

WHO. (2006). *World health report: Working together for health.* Geneva: WHO Press.

WHO. (2007). Task shifting global recommendations and guidelines. Retrieved from http://data.unaids .org/pub/Manual/2007/ttr_taskshifting_en.pdf

WHO. (2008). *International health regulations, 2005* (2nd ed.). Retrieved from http://www.who.int/ihr /publications/9789241596664/en/index.html

WHO. (2009). *Global standards for the initial education of professional nurses and midwives.* Geneva: World Health Organization.

WHO. (2010). *Increasing access to health workers in remote and rural areas through improved retention.* Geneva: WHO Press.

WHO. (2011). *Strengthening midwifery toolkit.* Geneva: WHO Press.

WHO. (2011). *Transformative scale up of health professional education.* Geneva: WHO Press.

WHO-EMRO. (2002). *Nursing and midwifery: A guide to professional regulation.* Cairo, Egypt: World Health Organization Regional Office for the Eastern Mediterranean and Regional Office for Europe.

Zachariah, R., Ford, N., Philips, M., Lynch, S., Massaquoi, M., Janssens, V., & Harries, A. D. (2009). Task shifting in HIV/AIDS: Opportunities, challenges and proposed actions for sub-Saharan Africa. *Transactions of the Royal Society of Tropical Medicine and Hygiene, 103*(6), 549–558.

Zimbabwe. (2004). Health Professions Act. Retrieved from http://apps.who.int/medicinedocs /documents/s18418en/s18418en.pdf

Health Care Policy and Certified Registered Nurse Anesthetists: Past, Present, and Future

Christine S. Zambricki

Certified registered nurse anesthetists (CRNAs) have a proud history of integrating nursing care with specialized knowledge and skill in administering anesthesia and treating pain. The success of the nurse anesthesia profession in the public policy arena over time has not been a matter of chance; it has been a matter of choice. The early leaders of this profession were amazing women who taught so many lessons that resonate today. Nurse anesthetists such as Alice Magaw and Agatha Hodgins had ideas of consequence that predicted and ensured the centrality of CRNAs in contemporary health care delivery.

For a student of the history of nurse anesthesia in America, the most astonishing fact about current challenges is that contemporary health policy issues have roots deeply embedded in the past. Turf wars are not new, nor are battles for reimbursement or attempts to restrict scope of practice. Examining the oldest nursing specialty's saga from its 19th-century beginnings to the present not only brings to light many compelling characters; it also lays to rest numerous myths and allows us to come to grips with the most pressing national health issues of our time. What follows are lessons that we need to learn—but have not—from the history of this storied profession.

BRIEF HISTORICAL BACKGROUND/RELEVANT LITERATURE

Surgery in the early 1800s was a barbaric enterprise, requiring physical force to immobilize the patient only to have many patients die from postoperative surgical infections days later. Nurses in the late 19th century were essential contributors to the two significant advances that paved the way for the "Golden Age of Surgery." Without the ability to prevent surgical infections and the capacity to render a patient insensible to pain, surgery could not progress.

Although the relationship between germs and disease was not completely understood at the time, Florence Nightingale's emphasis on cleanliness, hygiene, and ventilation proved dramatically successful, reducing the death rate in British army hospitals in the 1850s from 40% to 2% (Florence Nightingale International Foundation, accessed 2013). The world took notice when Nightingale began her *Notes on Hospitals* (1863) with the prescient admonition: "It may seem a strange principle to enunciate as the very first requirement in a Hospital that it should do the sick no harm" (Nightingale, 1863, Preface). Florence Nightingale's words still hold true today. If she could see advanced practice nurses now, how proud she would be of their leadership and steadfast commitment to patient care.

With the opening of the first formal school of nursing in New York in 1873, nursing began to achieve recognition in the United States as a respectable profession rooted in the science of Nightingale's work. About the same time, sterile gowns, gloves, and instruments were replacing street clothes, bare hands, and water-rinsed instruments and sponges in the operating room. With the emergence of nursing as a legitimate career choice and the acceptance of asepsis, the foundation for safe surgery was falling into place.

The only barrier remaining to achieve Nightingale's obligation to "do the sick no harm" in surgery was the need for a qualified provider to deliver anesthesia safely and efficiently. Once again, professional nursing fulfilled the need and made possible the advancement of contemporary surgery.

Modern anesthesia began in the 1840s with the introduction of diethyl ether for use as a general anesthetic. Yet it would be decades before the administration of anesthesia became safe and predictable. In the years following the demonstration of the anesthetizing properties of diethyl ether, there were no nurse anesthetists, no anesthesiologists, and it was well recognized that "the life of the patient, no less than the success of the operation, is jeopardized by the careless and ignorant manner in which this important part of the procedure is carried out by a novice just out of medical school" (The Professional Anaesthetizer, 1897). Initially the assignment of anesthesia duties was to the least experienced medical school graduates. These younger interns were more interested in observing the surgery than in monitoring the patient, and the lack of vigilance during administration of anesthesia resulted in significant mortality.

During the Civil War, there were reports of nurse anesthetists using chloroform to anesthetize soldiers in battlefield hospitals, and the demand began to grow for nurse anesthesia services (Sudlow, 2000, p. 9; Thatcher, 1953, pp. 33, 54). After the war, in order to meet the need for dedicated and focused anesthesia providers, surgeons recruited Catholic nursing nuns to train to become nurse anesthetists. The earliest existing records documenting the anesthetic care of patients by nurses were those of Sister Mary Bernard in 1887 at St. Vincent's Hospital in Erie, Pennsylvania (Thatcher, 1953).

In the late 1800s, working with the Mayo brothers in Rochester, Minnesota, nurse anesthetist Alice Magaw, known as the "Mother of Anesthesia," greatly contributed to the fund of knowledge in anesthesia. Magaw perfected techniques for administration of open-drop ether and chloroform, documenting the personal administration of 14,000 surgical anesthetics without a single mortality in 1906 (Koch, 1999). Based on observations of her work, medical leaders turned to nursing as a solution to the need for professional, dedicated anesthetists. Looking at the roots of nurse anesthesia practice, what distinguished nurse anesthetists from the beginning was the "touch" component of the care, coupled with technical excellence and quality patient outcomes. The need for specific training in anesthesia was pressing, and doctors and nurses came from across the globe to learn anesthesia techniques from Magaw and Mayo. Dr. J. M. Baldy, president of the American Gynecologic Society, summed up the current state of affairs in his presidential address in 1908 when he said: "The general administration of anesthetics as it is performed today is the shame of modern surgery, is a disgrace to a learned profession, and if the full unvarnished truth concerning it were known it would be but a short while before it were interfered with by legislative means—and properly so . . . . Many brainy women, fully capable of being trained to this responsible position, have entered the nursing profession and it is from this source that we may look for a solution to our difficulties" (Baldy, 1908).

By World War I, there were four formalized, postgraduate educational programs training nurse anesthetists. In 1915, nurse anesthetist Agatha Hodgins and Dr. George Crile (cofounder of the Cleveland Clinic), having perfected the administration of nitrous oxide/oxygen anesthesia, opened Lakeside (Hospital) School of Anesthesia in Cleveland, Ohio. Through Hodgins's leadership and vision, the alumni association of this program was the nucleus for the formation of the American Association of Nurse Anesthetists (AANA). With the increasing professional recognition of nurse anesthetists, physicians became attracted to the field. A number of legal challenges ensued, the most famous being *Frank v. South* (1917) in the state of Kentucky. In this case, the Jefferson County Medical Society claimed that Margaret Hatfield, a nurse anesthetist, was illegally practicing medicine. The Supreme Court of Kentucky ruled that using discretion and making independent judgments in the process of giving anesthesia was legitimate nursing practice. Approximately 20 years later, *Chalmers-Francis v. Nelson* (1936) was decided in a manner similar to *Frank v. South*, and anesthesia was determined to be both the practice of medicine and the practice of nursing. Thus, the foundation for nurse anesthesia practice was firmly established in U.S. law.

Today, CRNAs are advanced practice registered nurses (APRNs), prepared at the master's or doctoral level, with specialized education in anesthesia and pain management. More than 42,000 CRNAs administer over 32 million anesthetics in the United States each year (AANA, 1999). CRNAs administer anesthesia for all types of surgical cases, from the simplest to the most complex. CRNAs are the predominant anesthesia professionals in rural America; in some states, CRNAs are the sole providers in nearly 100% of the rural hospitals. CRNAs work in all settings in which anesthesia and pain care is delivered: traditional hospital surgical suites and obstetrical delivery rooms; ambulatory surgical centers; in the offices of dentists, podiatrists, and plastic surgeons; and in pain clinics. In 24% of all U.S. counties, CRNAs are the sole anesthesia professionals. Nurse anesthesia predominates in veterans hospitals and in the U.S. Armed Forces. Over 500 full-time CRNAs are employed by the Department of Veterans Affairs health care system.

According to the U.S. Department of Labor, all four types of APRNs, including nurse anesthetists, will be in high demand through the 2010 to 2020 decade, particularly in medically underserved areas such as inner cities and rural areas (U.S. Department of Labor, Bureau of Labor Statistics, 2012–2013). CRNA job growth will occur primarily because of technological advancements permitting a greater number of health problems to be treated through surgery, and the large, aging baby boomer population who will demand more surgical procedures as they live longer, seeking more active lives than previous generations. Health care reform, with its promise of access to services for previously underinsured or uninsured citizens, has also been cited as a predictor of increased surgical procedures. For a multitude of reasons, 21st-century surgical volume continues to increase year after year without sign of abatement.

Over 90% of America's CRNAs are members of the 45,000-member AANA. This is a high percentage of membership by any measure. Since its founding by Agatha Hodgins in 1931, the AANA has placed its responsibilities to the public above or equal to its responsibilities to its membership. The education of nurse anesthetists has been a priority throughout the history of the AANA. The AANA's certification exam was first administered in 1945, nurse anesthesia educational programs were nationally accredited in 1952, a voluntary continuing education program was approved in 1969, and mandatory continuing education became effective in 1978. In 1986, a bachelor's degree in nursing or a related degree was required for admission to nurse anesthesia programs, and by 1998 all programs were required to be at the graduate level, awarding at least a master's degree. Doctoral education for entry into nurse anesthesia practice is required by 2025.

The Council on Accreditation of Nurse Anesthesia Educational Programs (COA) is the accrediting agency for the 113 nurse anesthesia programs in the United States, its territories, and protectorates. The COA's mission is to grant public recognition to nurse anesthesia programs and institutions that award post-master's certificates, master's, and doctoral degrees that meet nationally established standards of academic quality and to assist programs and institutions in improving educational quality (COA, 2013) .

The National Board of Certification and Recertification for Nurse Anesthetists (NBCRNA) is a not-for-profit corporation comprising the Council on Recertification and the Council on Certification of Nurse Anesthetists. The mission of the NBCRNA is to promote patient safety through credentialing programs that support lifelong learning (NBCRNA, 2013).

NBCRNA credentialing provides assurances to the public that certified individuals have met objective, predetermined qualifications for providing nurse anesthesia services. While state licensure provides the legal credential for the practice of professional nursing, private voluntary certification indicates compliance with the professional standards for practice in nurse anesthesia. The certification credential for nurse anesthetists has been institutionalized in health care facilities, and it has been recognized through malpractice litigation, state nurse practice acts, and state rules and regulations.

In order to become a CRNA, a licensed registered nurse must graduate from a nationally accredited nurse anesthesia educational program and pass the national certifying examination administered by the Council on Certification of Nurse Anesthetists. At the time of writing, CRNAs must be recertified every 2 years by the Council on Recertification of Nurse Anesthetists. In 2012, the NBCRNA announced a significant transition from the 40-year-old recertification program to a Continuing Professional Certification (CPC) approach. This new model, when fully implemented, incorporates such changes as continuing education (CE) credits through competency modules and a pass/fail examination (NBCRNA, 2013).

CONCEPTUAL AND THEORETICAL SUPPORT

CRNAs are anesthesia professionals who have been providing anesthesia care and managing pain in the United States for nearly 150 years. The conceptual framework for CRNA practice originates with the scope, standards, guidelines, and position statements set forth by the AANA. As APRNs, the practice of nurse anesthesia is also grounded in the theoretical framework contained within *The Consensus Model for APRN Regulation: Licensure, Accreditation, Certification and Education*, approved in 2008 by the National Council of State Boards of Nursing (NCSBN) along with 44 other nursing organizations including the AANA (NCSBN, 2008).

The AANA Scope of Nurse Anesthesia Practice offers guidance for CRNAs and health care institutions regarding the scope of nurse anesthesia practice, recognizing that scope is continuously evolving based on patient and community needs as well as the development of new science and technology. Contemporary CRNA practice encompasses the responsibilities associated with anesthesia practice as well as pain management. CRNAs, like all health care providers, work as members of interprofessional teams. Every CRNA is individually responsible for the quality of services he or she renders (AANA, 2013). Recognizing the inevitability of overlapping scope of practice with physicians and others, CRNAs' scope of practice is grounded in benefits to the public in terms of quality and access to care within a competency framework.

The practice of anesthesia is a specialty in both nursing and medicine. Anesthesia practice is defined as the art and science of rendering a patient insensible to pain by the administration of anesthetic agents and related drugs and procedures. CRNA scope of practice also includes, but is not limited to, the management of pain associated with obstetrical labor and delivery, management of acute and chronic ventilatory problems, and the management of acute and chronic pain. Education, practice, and research within the specialty are to promote competent anesthesia care encompassing the diversity of patient populations, age, ethnicity, and gender.

The AANA has adopted a Code of Ethics to guide nurse anesthetists in fulfilling their obligations as professionals. CRNAs practice nursing by providing anesthesia and related services such as advanced monitoring and pain management. They accept the responsibility conferred on them by the state, the profession, and society. Each CRNA has a personal responsibility to uphold and adhere to these ethical standards (AANA, 2005). Observance includes responsibility to patients, competence, responsibilities as a professional, responsibilities to society, and ethical behavior in terms of research, business practices, and endorsement of products and services.

The Consensus Model for APRN Regulation: Licensure, Accreditation, Certification and Education (2008) defines APRN practice, describes the APRN regulatory model, identifies the titles to be used, defines each specialty, and describes the emergence of new roles and population foci. APRNs, including CRNAs, are defined as licensed independent practitioners who are expected to practice within standards established or recognized by a licensing body. As such, the CRNA is accountable to patients, the nursing profession, and the licensing board to comply with the requirements of the state nurse practice act and for the quality of advanced nursing care rendered; for recognizing limits of knowledge and experience, and planning for the management of situations beyond the APRN's expertise; and for consulting with or referring patients to other health care providers as appropriate (The Joint Dialogue Group, 2008).

APPLICATION TO APRN PRACTICE

Throughout nurse anesthesia history, key turning points have been marked by nurse anesthetist leaders who were political entrepreneurs. They had visionary ideas, noticed weaknesses in the status quo, and prevailed on decision makers to act to achieve political change.

The major health policy challenges for nurse anesthetists fall into one of two general categories: scope of practice and reimbursement. In general, scope of practice is determined at the state level and reimbursement is driven by decisions at the federal level. The reality is that these two policy issues are inextricably connected because access to reimbursement is essentially a form of economic credentialing. Thus, payment impacts scope. Similarly, scope of practice drives reimbursement with a direct link between what services a professional is authorized to provide and payment under the current fee-for-service system.

The Patient Protection and Affordable Care Act (PPACA) (United States Public Law 111-148, March 23, 2010) proposes significant changes to how health care is paid for in the United States. Alternative delivery and payment models such as accountable care organizations and health insurance exchanges are proposed as innovations to pay for more covered lives. It is incumbent on every nurse anesthetist to understand the value of their services as health care policy evolves. Medicare reimbursement methodology is important to CRNAs because the federal government is the largest health insurance program in the country and also because federal programs are used as a template for private insurers in the states. CRNAs must understand the nuances of anesthesia reimbursement policy beginning with the current system.

Medicare payment policy is set forth in statutes, regulations, and Medicare manuals. Examples of key importance to CRNAs include:

- Omnibus Budget Reconciliation Act of 1986
  - 42 CFR §410.69, 42 CFR §414.60
- Medicare Claims Processing Manual
  - Chapter 12—Physician/Non-physician Practitioners
  - Section 50, Payment for Anesthesiology Services
  - Section 140, CRNA Services

There are four components of Medicare payment. Part A and Part B are of special significance for nurse anesthetist health care policy initiatives.

Part A—Hospital Coverage includes the Conditions of Participation, Conditions for Coverage, and Interpretive Guidelines. Part A also includes the provisions for a reasonable-cost pass-through payment for CRNA services in critical access hospitals. The Conditions of Participation and the Conditions for Coverage outline requirements for hospitals, ambulatory surgery centers, critical access hospitals, and other facilities to participate in the Medicare program. Surveyors use the Interpretive Guidelines to ascertain compliance with the Conditions of Participation and the Conditions for Coverage.

In order for a health care organization to participate in and receive payment from the Medicare or Medicaid programs through Part A, it must be certified as complying with the Conditions of Participation and the Conditions for Coverage. State agencies conduct surveys on behalf of the Centers for Medicare & Medicaid Services (CMS) in order to determine compliance. National accrediting organizations must adopt, at a minimum, these standards that meet the federal requirements if they wish to be recognized by CMS. CMS grants these accrediting organizations "deeming" authority to "deem" a health care organization as meeting the Medicare and Medicaid requirements. If the health care organization has "deemed status" from a national accrediting organization, it is not required to undergo a Medicare survey and certification process. However, Medicare is always free to survey in addition to the national accrediting organization if the CMS wishes. Two national accrediting organizations, the Joint Commission and Det Norske Veritas (DNV) or "The Nordic Truth," have deeming status from CMS.

Part B—Physician Services describes conditions of payment for anesthesia services when provided by CRNAs, anesthesiologists, and anesthesia assistants. Part B also authorizes payment for related services that are medical and surgical in nature rather than anesthesia services. These include such things as pain management, Swan–Ganz catheter insertion, and emergency intubation. In addition, Part B sets forth conditions of payment for medical direction and medical supervision as well as teaching rules.

The remaining Medicare components are less relevant to nurse anesthesia health care policy. Part C refers to Medicare Advantage HMO and Part D describes coverage for the Medicare Drug Benefit.

Policy issues rarely occur in a vacuum. The core competencies of CRNA practice exist within a political context of special interests, cost containment, and partisan politics. The following case examples are illustrative of the intersection among access, quality, and cost within a market framed by politics and timing. In these examples, strategies and tactics are employed to achieve public policy successes which are directly linked to professional practice competencies of the CRNA.

The first case study involves the construct of "physician supervision" as it relates to health care payment policy and state scope of practice. The second example details issues related to the delivery of chronic pain management services by CRNAs and the reimbursement for those services. In both cases, strategy and interventions will be effectively linked with core competencies and outcomes to impact health care policy.

Elimination of Part A Medicare Requirements for Physician Supervision

The concept of "physician supervision" has been misinterpreted, misused, and misunderstood since its inception. In our complex health care world, the reality is that no one, either physician or nurse, practices independently. Particularly in the surgical environment, there must be and will always be interprofessional collaboration and cooperation among members of the operating room team. The concept of supervision for highly trained professionals does not fit the reality of contemporary practice in which each individual brings his or her expertise to the team to provide the very best care for the patient.

The Medicare Part A Conditions of Participation require physician supervision of nurse anesthetists unless an individual state opts out of that requirement. References regarding physician supervision requirements are contained in facility-specific sections within the Conditions of Participation and Conditions for Coverage. This supervision of CRNAs may be by the operating physician or by an anesthesiologist. At the time of writing (Table 32.1), 17 states have opted out of the Medicare physician supervision requirement for CRNAs (Figure 32.1). There is no opt-out mechanism for Anesthesiology Assistants (AAs), who must always be supervised, not just by a physician, but by an anesthesiologist. How did health care policy arrive at this juncture, with physician supervision required and a governor allowed to opt out of the law or opt back in without any requirement for public comment or state legislative oversight?

Organized medicine has long held the belief that the delivery of anesthesia is solely the practice of medicine, despite court decisions to the contrary. After a long hiatus following the *Chalmers-Franci v. Nelson* decision in 1936, the issue of physician supervision became prominent once again in the late 20th century (Blumenreich, 2000). Congress had provided additional financial support for physician education in an attempt to reduce health care costs by increasing the number of doctors. As a result, the number of physicians surged in the last quarter of the century and the number of anesthesiologists tripled. At the same time, the "Captain of the Ship"

TABLE 32.1 Physician Supervision Language in CMS Conditions of Participation

HEALTH CARE FACILITY	CMS CONDITIONS OF PARTICIPATION
Hospitals	42 CFR §482.52(a)(4)
Ambulatory Surgery Centers	42 CFR §416.42(b)(2)
Critical Access Hospitals	42 CFR §485.639(c)(2)

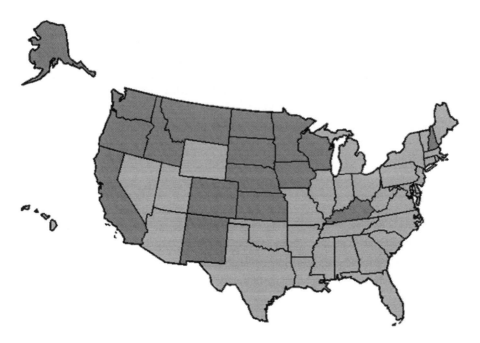

FIGURE 32.1 Opt-out States as of January 2013 (Dark Gray States).

Source: The American Association of Nurse Anesthetists (2013).

doctrine, in which the surgeon is responsible for all damages caused by hospitals and hospital employees, was on the wane. Some anesthesiologists at this time sought to persuade hospitals and surgeons that they were at greater risk when working with nurse anesthetists as compared to anesthesiologists. Fears in this regard were unwarranted, as "the same legal principles that governed the liability of a surgeon for the negligence of a nurse anesthetist also governed the liability of a surgeon for the negligence of an anesthesiologist and had nothing to do with supervision. The issue was whether the surgeon controlled the procedure that gave rise to the injury" (Blumenreich, 2000, p. 407), regardless of whether the procedure was performed by a CRNA or an anesthesiologist.

The CMS Part A reimbursement rules for hospital reimbursement historically required that nurse anesthetists be supervised by either an anesthesiologist or by the procedural physician such as a surgeon or an obstetrician. In December 1997, CMS published a final rule stating that state law would determine which professionals could administer anesthesia and the level of supervision required (United States Health and Human Services, Centers for Medicare and Medicaid Services, 2001, 4674–4687). The agency cited "lack of evidence to support . . . [the] requirement for supervision of Certified Registered Nurse Anesthetists" (United States Health and Human Services, Centers for Medicare and Medicaid Services, 2001, 56762–56769) as the reason for eliminating the physician supervision requirement in Part A Medicare.

Anesthesiologists and organized medicine had vehemently opposed the elimination of physician supervision during the rulemaking period, even though there was no evidence to support the position that supervision adds value in terms of cost or quality. During the comment period, thousands of letters were written, both for and against, and ultimately the agency issued a final rule eliminating the federal requirement for physician supervision of nurse anesthetists.

Some say that making policy is like making sausage: it is not a pretty sight. What happened next is a practical example of the impact of politics and timing. During the interval between publication of the final rule and the effective date of the rule, a new president of the United States took office and immediately pulled back all proposed and final rules of the previous administration if they had not been implemented. The final rule eliminating physician supervision was dead. Months later, after much negotiation and advocacy, the baby was split and the compromise that resulted left both sides unhappy. In November 2001, CMS implemented a rule maintaining physician supervision with the proviso that states may opt out of this federal government requirement.

The process for opt-out is simple. The governor of the state must send a letter to CMS informing Medicare that the state will opt out, that this decision is consistent with state law, and that the governor has consulted with the State Boards of Medicine and Nursing. The governor does not need to obtain the permission of the boards, but merely consult with them. The governor does not need to get approval from CMS to opt out, but only provide notification. When CMS receives the written communication signed by the governor, the opt-out is in effect and the physician supervision requirement for Part A reimbursement no longer applies in that state.

In retrospect, despite the bitter pill of compromise, the benefit of the final rule was that it created a unique opportunity to conduct a retrospective study comparing the difference in patient outcomes between states that had opted out with states that had not. This study was executed, and the results of this research demonstrated conclusively that there is no harm found when nurse anesthetists work without supervision by physicians (Dulisse & Cromwell, 2010).

Repealing the federal Medicare requirement for physician supervision remains a strategic goal. This rule is an example of unnecessary government regulation that is not evidence based. Scope of practice and supervision requirements are best determined at the state level, and in today's challenging environment, health care facilities need the flexibility to innovate in determining the best anesthesia care delivery model. Contemporary anesthesia practice is extremely safe (Li, Warner, & Lang, 2009) and of the highest quality; therefore, communities may look at factors such as cost and access when seeking to meet the unique needs of their patient population.

As mentioned, physician supervision is a requirement for Medicare Part A payment to hospitals outlined in the Conditions of Participation. It is important to recognize the distinction between physician supervision as a condition of health care facility reimbursement in Part A and the payment methodology for medical direction and physician supervision in Medicare Part B payment to providers. This distinction is critical, as recent findings relative to provider payment practices raise questions about the federal requirement for supervision in Part A. Physician supervision is a Part A requirement for hospital reimbursement and it refers to general supervision by either an anesthesiologist or by the procedural physician such as a surgeon. Part B provider reimbursement includes the construct of medical direction and also a different construct of medical supervision. These refer only to anesthesiologists and describe two different ways that anesthesiologists get paid when they work with CRNAs.

There are three options for CRNA practice relative to the Medicare Part A supervision requirement. CRNAs may personally provide anesthesia care without physician supervision if a state has opted out of the federal supervision requirement. The operating physician may supervise the CRNA or the CRNA may be supervised by an anesthesiologist. The Part A requirement for supervision of anesthesiologist assistants is different from that of CRNAs. Anesthesiology assistants must always be supervised by an anesthesiologist.

Professional reimbursement for anesthesia providers is governed by Part B of Medicare. In 1987, through the strong legislative advocacy of the AANA and others, CRNAs became the first nursing group to be paid directly by Medicare reimbursement when the Omnibus Reconciliation Act became law (AANA, 2013). Part B describes the payment methodology for two types of services—anesthesia services and related services (medical and surgical)—when provided by CRNAs, anesthesiologists, and anesthesia assistants. Part B also defines teaching rules for situations where anesthesiologists or CRNAs are being paid for supervising residents or nurse anesthesia students.

There are three options for Medicare CRNA reimbursement in Medicare Part B. CRNAs are paid 100% of the allowable physician Medicare fee when providing anesthesia services if there is no anesthesiologist billing medical direction or medical supervision for the same patient. In this case, the CRNA may also be paid 100% for each of two patients if the CRNA is supervising two students. The nurse anesthetist receives only 50% of the payment when an anesthesiologist is billing either medical direction or medical supervision for that same case.

Payment for an anesthesia service performed by a CRNA may be made to the CRNA or to the individual or entity that the CRNA has an employment or contract relationship with if the CRNA signs over his or her billing rights. This is commonly a CRNA group, an anesthesiologist group, or a health care facility. The conditions for a CRNA to be paid require that the CRNA accept assignment; that is, the CRNA must accept the Medicare payment as payment in full for the service and not bill the balance to the patient. CRNAs must personally provide the service, or they may supervise nurse anesthesia students.

In contrast, there are four options by which Medicare pays an anesthesiologist for anesthesia services through Part B reimbursement. They may be paid for personally providing anesthesia services (100% payment), for medically directing CRNAs (50% payment), for medically supervising CRNAs (three base units plus one additional base unit if present for induction), and for supervising residents (100% payment for each of two residents).

An anesthesiologist may meet the requirement for Part A supervision of the CRNA and yet not bill medical supervision or medical direction in Part B. By law, the operating physician is never eligible to be paid for anesthesia services in Part B even if he or she is serving as the supervising physician for Part A requirements. In other words, either an operating physician or an anesthesiologist may be designated the supervising physician of the CRNA to meet Part A supervision requirements, but only the anesthesiologist may bill for medical direction or medical supervision for Part B. If an anesthesiologist provides Part A physician supervision but does not bill for medical direction or for medical supervision for a given patient, then the CRNA may bill for 100% of the fee or personally provided anesthesia care. Whenever the anesthesiologist bills Part B for medical direction or medical supervision, then the CRNA must revert to the 50% billing.

Anesthesiologists are permitted to bill for medical direction of up to four concurrent cases. In order to be compliant with Medicare requirements, when billing Part B medical direction, the anesthesiologist is required to fulfill seven steps (Table 32.2) for each case. At the time of enactment, the Medicare agency emphasized that these seven steps were payment requirements and not quality of care standards (United States Health and Human Services, Health Care Financing Administration, 1998).

Anesthesiologists are also allowed to bill for Part B medical supervision for more than four procedures concurrently. This is called Part B medical supervision. When billing medical supervision, the anesthesiologist is paid three base units per case. If the anesthesiologist documents presence at induction, one additional unit is allowed per case for a maximum of four base units.

Regardless of whether or not a state has opted out of Part A physician supervision requirements, CRNAs in all states can bill for personally provided anesthesia care in Medicare in Part B. In order to properly bill for services, anesthesiologists and CRNAs must use "modifiers" or codes that describe how the providers are involved in the patient's care (Table 32.3).

To make things even more complex, the anesthesia payment calculation is based on a formula that includes base units, known as relative value units, a taxonomy adopted by Medicare that is related to the complexity of the case and time units that are calculated by dividing actual time by 15-minute intervals. For example, an appendectomy is 6 base units and coronary bypass surgery is 20 base units. The total units are multiplied by a Medicare conversion factor set annually that varies with state and often with location within the state in order to arrive at a total charge. Generally Medicare pays 80% of this total charge and either the patient's Medicare gap insurance policy or the patient is responsible for the remaining 20%. The formula for calculating payment is

$$\text{Total units (Base units + Time units)} \times \text{Conversion Factor}$$
$$= \text{Total anesthesia professional Part B charge}$$

The following is an example of how Medicare pays for anesthesia services in the case of a 90-minute appendectomy when a CRNA and/or anesthesiologist is involved in the case. There are six relative value units for an appendectomy. It is also important to note that anesthesia time is paid in increments of 15 minutes. Medicare determines an amount paid per billing unit annually. This amount varies with state and with region within a state, and is known as the conversion factor. After computing the fee for the case, Medicare pays 80% of the total. Reimbursement for the appendectomy will be

$$6 \text{ (base units)} + 6 \text{ (15-minute time units)} = 12 \text{ (total units)}$$
$$12 \text{ (total units)} \times \$21.00 \text{ (sample conversion factor)} = \$252.00 \times 0.8$$
$$\text{(Medicare pays 80\%)} = \$201.60$$

TABLE 32.2 Tax Equity and Financial Responsibility Act (TEFRA). Seven Required Steps for Anesthesiologists to Legally Bill for Medical Direction of Up to Four Cases

ANESTHESIOLOGISTS BILLING MEDICAL DIRECTION ARE REQUIRED TO MEET 7 STEPS
Perform a pre-anesthetic examination and evaluation
Prescribe the anesthesia plan
Personally participate in the most demanding aspects of the anesthesia plan including, if applicable, induction and emergence
Ensure that any procedures in the anesthesia plan that he or she does not perform are performed by a qualified individual as defined in operating instructions
Monitor the course of anesthesia administration at frequent intervals
Remain physically present and available for immediate diagnosis and treatment of emergencies
Provide indicated post-anesthesia care

Source: 42 CFR §415.110.

TABLE 32.3 CMS Modifiers for CRNAs and Anesthesiologists

ANESTHESIA PROVIDER	ANESTHESIA SERVICE	MODIFIER	PAYMENT
CRNA	Personally performed	QZ	100%
	CRNA providing service when anesthesiologist bills for medical direction	QX	50%
	CRNA providing service when anesthesiologist bills for medical supervision	QX	50%
	CRNA personally performed service with 2 students	QZ	100% for each for up to 2 cases
	CRNA providing supervision of 2 students when anesthesiologist bills for medical direction	QX	50% base units + discontinuous time units
Anesthesiologist	Personally performed	AA	100%
	Medical supervision of > 4 concurrent cases	AD	3 base units per case plus 1 unit if documented presence at induction
	Medical direction of 1 CRNA	QY	50%
	Medical direction of 2, 3, or 4 concurrent procedures while meeting the 7 steps for all cases	QK	50% for each case
	Supervision of a resident	GC	100% for each of up to 2 cases
	Medical direction of 2 CRNAs supervising 2 students each	QK	50% for each case

The anesthesiologist is deemed to have met the Medicare requirement to be reimbursed for medical direction if he or she has performed and documented all 7 criteria for each concurrent case.

See *Medicare Claims Processing Manual*, Chapter 12, Section 50 for other modifiers; available at http://www.cms .gov/Regulations-and-Guidance/Guidance/Manuals/downloads/clm104c12.pdf.

An anesthesiologist may medically direct up to four rooms. In order to be paid for medical direction, the anesthesiologist must comply with the seven steps described in the Tax Equity and Financial Responsibility Act (TEFRA). If the anesthesiologist bills for Part B medical direction, then the anesthesiologist and the CRNA will each receive 50% of the payment for the case. The anesthesiologist will receive $100.80 and the CRNA will receive $100.80. If the anesthesiologist is medically directing four concurrent cases, then he or she will receive a total compensation that is the sum of 50% of the payment for each of the four concurrent cases. Although it is more likely that a medically directing anesthesiologist in the real world would be medically directing four different types of cases, for the sake of this example, if the anesthesiologist were to medically direct four concurrent appendectomies, he or she would receive $403.20. At the same time, each CRNA would receive 50% of the total amount paid for their individual case.

An anesthesiologist may medically supervise five or more rooms, according to Part B payment rules. In the case of Part B medical supervision, the anesthesiologist does not need to comply with the seven TEFRA steps in order to be paid. The anesthesiologist who is medically supervising will be paid three base units for

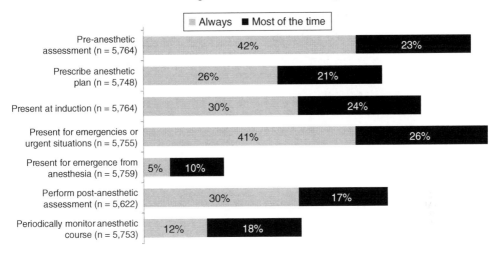

FIGURE 32.2 AANA Membership Data on Compliance With the 7 Steps

Source: AANA 2011 member survey, Unpublished.

each case. If they document that they were present on induction, they will be paid one additional base unit for that case. When an anesthesiologist bills Part B medical supervision, each CRNA receives 50% of the payment for that case. In the appendectomy example, the CRNA will receive $100.80. The anesthesiologist will be paid 3 (base units) × $21.00 (conversion factor) = $63.00 per case. For concurrent medically supervised cases where the anesthesiologist documents presence at induction, the anesthesiologist will receive $84.00 (an additional base unit of $21).

An anesthesiologist or a CRNA may personally provide the anesthetic care without involvement of medical direction or medical supervision. In this case, the CRNA or the anesthesiologist who is personally providing the appendectomy anesthetic will receive the full Medicare payment of $201.60.

For years, nurse anesthesia annual survey responses reported that anesthesiologists do not comply with the seven steps for medical direction in the majority of cases (Figure 32.2). The concept of medical direction as a measure of anesthesiologist work effort was further undermined when *Anesthesiology*, the official publication of the American Society of Anesthesiologists, published a review of one year of data from a tertiary hospital showing that lapses in compliance commonly occurred during first-case-of-the-day starts even with a 1:2 medical direction ratio (Epstein & Dexter, 2012). According to the study, anesthesiologists' failure to comply with the steps required to qualify for payment is substantial (Figure 32.3).

Medical direction adds unnecessary cost to the health care system. Without evidence to support the value proposition of medical direction for every case, having two anesthesia providers when one is sufficient is not consistent with best use of resources, particularly in light of health workforce shortages. The "one size fits all" approach does not take into account the individual needs of a patient based on health status, anesthetic plan, or type of procedure. Whether the cases are cataract procedures or open heart surgery, one anesthesiologist may be paid for medically directing

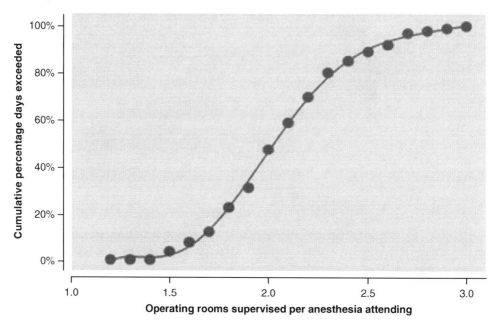

FIGURE 32.3 Lapses in Anesthesiologist Compliance With Requirements for Medical Direction Payment.

Source: Epstein and Dexter (2012).

up to four cases. Compliance with the seven steps required for reimbursement results in operating room delays while patients, surgeons, and staff in the operating room wait for the anesthesiologist to finish in one room. Many hospitals stagger starts by 15 minutes to accommodate this revolving anesthesiologist model, but do not stagger employee start times, with shifts generally beginning at the top of the hour. The cost of this staffing inefficiency is multiplied by the number of operating room team members impacted: at a minimum, a CRNA, an operating room nurse, and a surgical tech for each operating room. At an estimated cost of $20 per minute, the operating room is considered the most expensive real estate in the hospital (Marshall, Steele, & Associates, 2013). Recognizing that the cost of operating room time is variable based on many factors (Macario, 2010), all organizations, including hospitals, have compelling reasons to reduce costs.

Administrative costs associated with an anesthesia team care model are greater than with personally provided anesthesia. Medical direction incurs a greater administrative burden because two anesthesia bills must be generated rather than one. Unfortunately, in too many cases this results in denials, two appeals, and two appeal decisions, multiplying the administrative burden of providing care.

In addition, hospital administrators are often incorrectly led to believe that they must have an anesthesiologist to supervise the CRNAs. It is not uncommon for anesthesiologist groups to require the hospital to pay a subsidy to make up for the income shortfall that the anesthesiologist group perceives will result from direct reimbursement for the case volume that is available. Subsidies to anesthesiologist groups represent a significant cost to health care facilities. The 2012 Subsidy Study by HealthCare Performance Strategies reports that subsidies have risen substantially over the past 5 years to approximately $160,090 per anesthetizing location. Extrapolating based on the previous 2008 study, it is estimated that U.S. hospitals with over 25 beds pay well over $158 billion in anesthesiology subsidies annually (Health Performance Strategies, 2012).

From the 20,000 foot view, scrutiny of the cost of various anesthesia delivery models suggests that CRNA-only anesthesia is the most economically viable under the widest range of conditions and case volumes. Analysis of claims data to compare the cost of providing anesthesia by provider type and by delivery model demonstrates that CRNAs deliver quality care in the most cost-effective manner when compared with medically directed or anesthesiologist-only services. CRNAs are also the most cost-effective providers in terms of the cost to educate. The total estimated expense of pre-anesthetic and anesthetic graduate education for a CRNA is $161,809, whereas for an anesthesiologist it is $1,063,795 (Hogan, Seifer, & Moore, 2010).

Complete transparency of anesthesia workforce practices and billing is necessary to capture the anesthesia care experience at a granular level. Often what happens in the operating room stays behind closed doors and policy makers do not realize the reality of how the operating room actually functions. Systematic monitoring of the safety and quality of care, measured against prices, costs, and work effort of various providers, will reduce waste and reward high-value care while eliminating duplication of services.

CHRONIC PAIN MANAGEMENT

Contemporary challenges to CRNA practice are neither new nor unexpected. For nearly a decade, organized medicine has attempted to restrict CRNA scope of practice, control the anesthesia market through supervision and other requirements, and limit reimbursement for CRNA services. Facing health policy problems head on has profound effects, with long-lasting impact beyond present-day concerns. Surgery and pain management are inflection points where patients can emerge healthier than before and CRNAs are facilitators of that process. For the greatest good of the public, it is critical to ensure that patients continue to have access to CRNA pain care that is known to be of high quality, to cost less than alternatives, and is offered in their home community. This second case study speaks to strategies and interventions in health care policy advocacy relative to CRNAs' role in chronic pain management.

Chronic pain management is an evolving field that deals with the treatment of intractable pain, generally of duration beyond what is expected based on the patient's condition. On January 1, 2013, Medicare implemented a final rule that reinforced, and in some cases restored, the long-standing policy of directly reimbursing CRNAs for chronic pain management services. The story of this recent challenge to CRNA scope of practice and reimbursement, including the historical context, policy foundation, and political strategy, provides a captivating example of the effective use of timing, data, and coalition building to accomplish health policy goals. In this case, the goal of nurse anesthesia is the goal of advanced practice nurses as articulated by the Institute of Medicine (IOM): nurses should practice to the full extent of their education/training (Institute of Medicine, 2010).

On March 17, 2011, Noridian Administrative Services (Noridian) issued a bulletin entitled "CRNA Practice and Chronic Pain Management" notifying providers and the public that as a Medicare Administrative Contractor (MAC), Noridian would cease the practice of reimbursing CRNAs for chronic pain management services. Noridian's policy would have the effect of reducing or eliminating access to treatment for unrelenting chronic pain experienced by many Medicare beneficiaries, particularly in rural areas and in frontier states. Under the direction of a new Noridian Medical Director for Part B reimbursement, the bulletin took the position that CRNAs were not adequately trained to provide chronic pain management services, thus making an unfounded distinction between other related services such as acute pain management and the delivery of chronic pain care. Within months, a second MAC, Wisconsin Physician Services, Inc. (WPS), issued a similar bulletin borrowing heavily from language used in the Noridian statement.

A Local Coverage Determination (LCD) is a decision about whether a contractor will cover a particular service; it delineates the circumstances under which the service is considered reasonable and necessary (United States Department of Health and Human Services, Centers for Medicare and Medicaid Services, 2012b, Ch. 13, §13.1.3). From a policy perspective, the Noridian notices had the same impact as an LCD, yet there was no opportunity for comment as is required when an LCD is released. CMS directs that LCDs "shall be based on the strongest evidence available" (United States Department of Health and Human Services, Centers for Medicare and Medicaid Services, 2012b, Ch. 12, §13.7.1), yet Noridian and WPS issued denials of payment without any evidence base for these decisions in terms of quality, outcomes, access, or cost.

For more than two decades, Medicare law had supported reimbursement of chronic pain management services administered by CRNAs as permitted by state law. The Social Security Act recognizes CRNAs, nurse practitioners, and clinical nurse specialists as providers of "medical and other health services" (42 U.S.C § 1395x(s)). The Omnibus Reconciliation Act of 1986 (Public Law 99-509) called for direct payment for the services of a CRNA under Medicare Part B, beginning in 1989. The Medicare regulation implementing the law states, "Medicare Part B pays for anesthesia services and related care furnished by a certified registered nurse anesthetist who is legally authorized to perform the services by the State in which the services are furnished" (42 CFR § 410.69(a)).

The *Medicare Claims Processing Manual* provides further guidance on what is meant by "related care," stating that "[p]ayment can be made for medical or surgical services furnished by non-medically directed CRNAs if they are allowed to furnish those services under State law. These services may include … pain management . . . . Payment is determined under the physician fee schedule" (United States Department of Health and Human Services, CMS, 2012a, at Ch. 12, 140.4.3). Medicare does not make a distinction between "chronic pain management" and "acute pain management" when referring to "related services" or "medical and surgical services" that CRNAs are authorized to provide and be paid for. "Pain management" is an intentionally broad term, encompassing all pain management services that CRNAs are permitted to furnish under state law. The term "pain management" is not defined anywhere in statutes, regulations, or regulatory guidance.

Through these citations, it is clear that Medicare policy provided for coverage of pain management services provided by CRNAs without physician supervision. "Anesthesia service furnished by CRNAs can be medically directed or non-medically directed, but related care services are medical or surgical services, not anesthesia procedures, and are therefore not subject to the general medical direction rules." "Payment for related care services furnished by CRNAs on or after January 1, 1992 will be consistent with payment for physicians." "We will recognize separate payment for the same related care services furnished by anesthesiologists or CRNAs" (Part B and Other Services Payment, 1992).

At various points Medicare states that payment for related care services furnished by a CRNA will be consistent with payment for a physician and that separate payment is recognized for the same related care services whether furnished by anesthesiologists or CRNAs. As previously mentioned, the hospital Conditions of Participation for anesthesia services under Part A require physician supervision of CRNAs for "anesthesia services" (unless a state has opted out). There is no Part A or

Part B requirement for physician supervision of CRNAs providing "medical or surgical" services such as pain management, insertion of Swan–Ganz catheters, central venous pressure lines, emergency intubation, or the pre-anesthetic examination and evaluation of a nonsurgical patient.

When Noridian and WPS ceased payment for CRNA pain services, they questioned aspects of pain care relative to the scope of practice of CRNAs. The question of scope is rightfully within the authority of each state, not the authority of an insurance company or Medicare. Federal statute is clear on the role of state law in determining CRNA scope of practice. "The term 'services of a certified registered nurse anesthetist' means anesthesia and related care furnished by a certified nurse anesthetist . . . which the nurse anesthetist is authorized to perform as such by the State in which the services are furnished" (United States Code, 2011, 42 U.S.C. §1395x(bb)(1)). States define scope of practice in general terms in order to allow for the evolution of patient needs, health care technology, and professional education over time. The states in these jurisdictions permitted and in some cases required a CRNA to perform a thorough diagnostic assessment and develop a treatment plan—the very things that the MAC said CRNAs were not qualified to do. Medicare law makes clear that CRNAs may be reimbursed for pain management services if they are allowed to furnish those services under state law.

The linkage between pain practice and core competencies is delineated in the national standards set forth by the AANA, the COA, and the NBCRNA. CRNAs' specialized training in pain management is recognized in nurse anesthesia program accreditation standards (COA, 2009), scope of practice (AANA, 2013), position statements (AANA, 2010), and guidelines for core clinical privileges (AANA, 2010).

To be certified, a CRNA must have graduated from a nationally accredited program whose curriculum includes training to develop pain management skills. This rigorous graduate-level curriculum includes content in pain management, anatomy, pharmacology, chemistry, biochemistry, physics, patient assessment, and advanced principles of anesthesia practice. Student nurse anesthetists complete a minimum of 550 clinical cases, including the full scope of procedures, techniques, and specialty practice caring for patients with all comorbidities and levels of risk. The average student graduates with over 100 clinical cases in regional anesthesia (NBCRNA, 2011).

The NCSBN considers CRNAs, nurse practitioners, and clinical nurse specialists all to be APRNs, "licensed independent practitioners who are expected to practice within standards established or recognized by a licensing body," but only the CRNA is recognized for pain management and anesthesia-related skills (NBCRNA, 2011). The American Nurses Association supports CRNA pain practice, stating that "through extensive approved continuing education programs, CRNAs further advance and refine their skills in all areas of practice including pain management. CRNAs' authority to make independent professional judgments and utilize multiple anesthetic techniques including all forms of regional techniques . . . is critical to meeting a vast array of chronic pain management and surgical needs at a reasonable cost" (*Spine Diagnostics Center of Baton Rouge v. Louisiana State Board of Nurse et al.*, 2008).

Pain medicine is an evolving field with rapid advances in technology, pharmacology, and imaging propelling the specialty forward at lightning speed. The education and skills required to administer many chronic pain management procedures are based on the same foundation as those that CRNAs use every day as they perform various blocks for surgical and labor analgesia. With the advent of high-tech imaging and new approaches, advances in the pain specialty are happening at increasing speed. Contemporary pain practice was unknown as recently as 20 years ago, a reality that requires every pain practitioner to keep up through workshops, fellowships, hands-on coursework, and wet-lab experiences. CRNAs who specialize in pain management are held to the same standard of professional accountability as any CRNA; that is, to maintain competency relative to their practice specialization.

ACCESS, COST, AND QUALITY IMPERATIVES

There are compelling policy considerations in favor of CRNA-provided chronic pain care. Chief among these are access to care in rural and frontier communities, and cost and quality of care. These issues were addressed in the 2011 IOM report to Congress, which the Patient Protection and Affordable Care Act required in recognition of chronic pain's growing impact on Americans and on the economy. This report estimates that 100 million American adults suffer from chronic pain at a cost of over $650 billion per year. The report notes that "a number of barriers . . . including regulatory, legal, institutional, financial and geographic . . . limit the availability of pain care" (Institute of Medicine, 2011). According to survey data, 3,360 CRNAs indicated that they specialize in pain management and in the same year, the American Board of Anesthesiology (ABA) recognized 3,900 physicians as pain subspecialists. Clearly the number of pain management specialists is inadequate to meet this public health challenge.

In many rural and frontier areas, Medicare beneficiaries must travel hundreds of miles to access alternative care, and CRNAs often are the only health care professionals trained in pain management in these communities. In these cases, referring practitioners choose to refer their patients to CRNAs for high-quality pain care, and patients choose to receive their care from a CRNA in their local community rather than travel long distances. This practice is the essence of patient-centered care: providing services where and by whom the patient selects. Without CRNAs to administer chronic pain management services, Medicare beneficiaries in vast rural and frontier areas would lose access to vital treatment, which could result in poor health care outcomes, lower quality of life, and unnecessary costs to patients, Medicare, and the health care system. According to a case study analysis by the Lewin Group (2012), using real-life situations of four individuals living in rural communities representing different geographic locations throughout the United States, the direct medical costs of alternatives such as surgery or nursing home care range from 2.3 times to more than 150 times the cost of a CRNA providing these services in the community. By choosing not to reimburse CRNAs for pain care, Noridian and WPS were limiting or eliminating access to legitimate pain specialists and requiring beneficiaries to seek other more costly, more inconvenient, and in some cases, more dangerous alternatives.

Another important health care policy consideration is the economics of chronic pain management provided by CRNAs. At a time when there is national concern about the cost of federal health care spending (Figure 32.4), the economics of reimbursement for CRNA-provided services versus more expensive physician-provided services cannot be overlooked. It is more economical for a facility to employ a CRNA rather than a physician when both possess the requisite training and skills. CRNAs typically provide anesthesia services at the lowest economic cost and generally do not require subsidization from the health care facility (Hogan, 2010).

This case study is an excellent example of why advanced practice nurses such as CRNAs must become involved in policy development. The rationale for such sponsorship lies beyond protecting reimbursement and scope of practice. Advanced

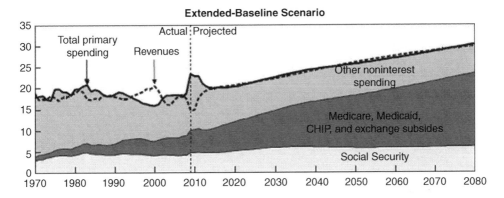

FIGURE 32.4 Federal Health Care Spending Impact on Federal Budget Projections.

practice nursing advocacy is essential to ensuring access to quality care for patients and reducing health disparities.

What accounts for the fact that nurse anesthetists are recognized as leaders in health care advocacy and influence? Much of the explanation can be found in the growing power of public opinion, brought about by the spread of education, communication technology, mass media, and professional organizations—all of which have heightened recognition of the benefits of CRNA care in terms of cost, quality, and access. For APRNs, outcomes and core competencies are linked to professional practice at a level that is significantly distinguishable from registered nurse practice even at the expert level. As a result, APRNs must invest heavily in health policy development at a personal and a professional association level.

The AANA adopted a two-pronged approach to support access to CRNA pain care. Coined Protect My Pain Care, this initiative was built on a foundation of a tactical team and a strategic group. The strategic group met monthly to provide the 30,000-foot view, evaluating results of efforts to date, changing direction or cadence when needed, and staying focused on progress toward meeting goals and objectives. The tactical team met weekly to update operational activities, including grassroots action; grass tops activity (large organizations), public relations and communication, state support, research, legislative impact, and regulatory influence.

Through essential work of the tactical team, Protect My Pain Care employed devices such as the establishment of an online micro-site for patients and providers. The group enlisted the support of the community of interest such as AARP, the National Rural Health Association, and many state boards of nursing and state hospital associations. The tactical team oversaw a grassroots campaign of CRNAs, referring physicians, patients, and their families who wrote over 4,000 letters in support of CRNA-provided pain care. The Lewin Group published case studies showing the high cost of alternative pain care without CRNAs. Democratic and Republican groups participated in focus sessions that provided insights into the importance of having the right to choose one's health care provider. Through the tactical team advocacy work, legislators and their staff reached out to CMS and others to support continued payment for CRNA pain services in order to protect their home state citizens.

At the request of this network of stakeholders, including professional organizations, patients, hospitals, and physicians, access to pain care by CRNAs was protected. The Medicare agency published a final rule on November 1, 2012, stating that "Anesthesia and related care means those services that a certified registered nurse anesthetist is legally authorized to perform in the state in which the services are furnished." The agency noted in its descriptive preamble, "we agree with commenters that the primary responsibility for establishing the scope of services CRNAs are sufficiently trained and thus should be authorized to furnish, resides with the states."

In doing so, the Medicare agency maintained a consistent national policy authorizing direct reimbursement of chronic pain management services provided by CRNAs, as well as adjunct imaging, and evaluation and management services that nurse anesthetists are allowed to furnish under state law. CMS removed regulatory barriers to access for CRNA pain care and deferred to states for scope of practice decisions. Noridian's and WPS's decision to withhold payment for CRNA chronic pain management services was overturned.

EVALUATION

While health care costs continue to grow at an unsustainable rate, Congress and health care policy makers continue to seek ways to make health care work better, cost less, be more accessible to patients, and of higher quality. Landmark research and advisory papers published over time underscore the value of CRNAs in promoting crucial societal goals. This scientific evidence base has been a powerful foundation for actions, interventions, and strategies aimed at developing robust health care policy. Key studies and papers are summarized below.

Numerous research studies have found no significant differences among nurse anesthetists in mortality or anesthesia complications (Needleman & Minnick, 2008; Pine, Holt, & Lou, 2003; Simonson, Ahern, & Hendryx, 2007; Hoffman, 2002). The quality of care by all anesthesia providers is excellent, resulting in a very low incidence of anesthesia-related morbidity or mortality. Though these previous studies have demonstrated the high quality of nurse anesthesia care, the results of a 2010 study published in *Health Affairs* (Dullise & Cromwell, 2010) led researchers to recommend that costly and duplicative supervision requirements for CRNAs should be eliminated. The study analyzed outcome by type of professional and found that there are no differences in patient outcomes based on whether the anesthesia was delivered by a CRNA without physician supervision, an anesthesiologist, or by a CRNA supervised by an anesthesiologist. The study compared anesthesia patient outcomes (mortality and complications) in 14 states that opted out of the Medicare physician supervision requirement for CRNAs from 2001 to 2005 with those that did not opt out. As of 2013, 17 states have opted out. From a population health perspective, the researchers found that anesthesia has continued to grow more safe in opt-out and non-opt-out states alike. There was no difference in outcomes in the states that had opted out when compared to the states that had not. Based on the evidence contained in this study, the authors concluded that "we recommend that CMS allow certified registered nurse anesthetists in every state to work without the supervision of a surgeon or anesthesiologist" (Dulisse & Cromwell, 2010, p. 1469). Reviewing the study, the *New York Times* stated, "In the long run, there could also be savings to the health care system if nurses delivered more of the care" (New York Times Editorial, 2010).

Among all anesthesia delivery models, nurse anesthesia care is 25% more cost-effective than the next least costly model, according to a Lewin Group study published in *Nursing Economic$* (Hogan et al., 2010). Based on claims data, researchers determined that CRNAs practicing independently were the lowest cost to the private payer. Because CRNAs safely provide the full range of anesthesia services, the use of additional duplicative supervision represents additional health care cost that can be saved or allocated elsewhere in the health system, while maintaining a high standard of quality and patient safety. The authors also compared the marginal cost of pre-anesthesia and anesthesia graduate education between nurse anesthetists and anesthesiologists. The total estimated direct costs of education and clinical experience prior to anesthesia education and during anesthesia graduate education were found to be $161,809 for a CRNA and $1,083,795 for an anesthesiologist (Hogan et al., 2010, p. 168). Because both CRNAs and anesthesiologists provide high-quality care using the same skill set and techniques for all types of surgical procedures and all categories of patients, the contrasting cost to society of training these two categories of anesthetists gives pause during times of fiscal uncertainty.

To ensure patient access to high-quality care, a 2010 IOM report, *The Future of Nursing*, recommended that APRNs should be able to practice to the full extent of their education and training (Institute of Medicine, 2010). By eliminating regulatory and other policy barriers to the use of APRNs, including CRNAs, the health care system makes the most efficient use of the available workforce of health care professionals. This ensures patient access to high-quality care, and promotes local control of health care delivery.

ETHICAL CONSIDERATIONS

At this point, it is helpful to explore the relationship between the economics of health care and ethical practices within the health care system. Why do policies continue over time even though they are wasteful and there are better alternatives? A practical recommendation to reduce the unsustainably rising health care costs is to incorporate evidence-based decision making when creating health care policy. A case in point includes requirements for physician supervision that have no evidence base or the promulgation of regulations that make it more difficult for lower-cost providers to give needed pain care.

The standard response to health care needs in the United States is more: more highly trained physician specialists and more access to top technology. After more than a century of progress in education, pharmaceuticals, and technology resulting in huge gains in patient safety, as a country we have failed to articulate a health care delivery system that is efficient and cost-effective.

Health care coverage must be affordable and sustainable for society. Health care policy should promote access to high-quality care that is effective, efficient, safe, timely, patient centered, and equitable (Institute of Medicine, 2004). These societal needs support the premise that all health care providers should practice at the top of their education, training, and license.

In the conceptual framework of bioethics, questions concerning access to health care are directly related to principles of justice. Justice within this context relates to whether people who require services receive them. Concepts of fairness, health care services as a "right," and availability of these resources to those who need them come into play. Case in point, pain in America is a compelling health care challenge. Disparities in access to care, severity of suffering, and the cost to society are just a few of the contributing factors. There are substantial differences in pain prevalence and rates of undertreatment in vulnerable populations. Access to pain care is far from equitable. Race and ethnicity, geographic variation, and education and income impact availability of pain care. Attempts to prevent qualified pain care providers, such as nurse anesthetists, from delivering needed care to vulnerable populations legitimately raise the question of justice.

Do nurse anesthetists have any obligation to improve the health care system? The Code of Ethics for the CRNA requires that nurse anesthetists fulfill an individual, professional responsibility to society in "promoting community and national efforts to meet the health needs of the public" (AANA, 2005). CRNAs have an obligation to try to change the system as a part of their duty to patients. Despite the explosion in knowledge, innovation, and capacity to manage catastrophic conditions, the U.S. health care system "falls short on such fundamentals as quality, outcomes, cost, and equity" (Institute of Medicine, 2012).

FUTURE OF NURSE ANESTHESIA

Despite the many accomplishments of the profession of nurse anesthesia to date, there is much more to be done in the future. The need still exists within the profession to transform practice. CRNAs should practice to the full extent of their education and training. Obstacles to accomplishing this goal remain at the federal and state levels in the form of outdated statutes, rules, and regulations that are based on historical politics rather than a base of evidence. On the reimbursement front, barriers still exist to CRNA practice, particularly at the state and local health care plan levels. In 2013, the AANA began a program of state reimbursement advocacy with the establishment of the State Reimbursement Specialist (SRS) program. The SRS serves as a coordinator of contacts with state reimbursement decision makers and is the clearinghouse for all information regarding state health plan reimbursement, including private plans, federal and state exchanges, Medicaid plans, and the MACs. Over the coming years, this program will develop to be a powerful strategic tool as more reimbursement battles shift from the federal to the state level.

In the future, the nurse anesthesia profession must continue to evolve in transforming education of CRNAs. Nurse anesthetists must achieve high levels of education and training, evolving to the minimal standard of a doctoral degree by the year 2025. There has been strong movement in this direction, and efforts must not get sidetracked along the way. In order to successfully accomplish this goal, current faculty must return to obtain their doctoral degrees in large numbers and educational programs must design flexible curricula that accommodate the needs of working professionals using advanced technology and innovative teaching approaches. Lifelong learning is moving to a continuing competency model that will include competency-based modular offerings as well as interval testing. The area of pain management holds tremendous promise for the nurse anesthesia profession to take a leading role in designing comprehensive pain care education that follows the holistic model put forth by the IOM in the 2012 report *Pain in America* (IOM, 2012). Through these efforts and others, the profession of nurse anesthesia can remain at the forefront of advancing nursing education for the future.

There is great opportunity for nurse anesthetists to become full partners with physicians and other health professionals in redesigning health care and the health care system. With their advanced education and expert clinical knowledge, nurse anesthetists are prime candidates to assume leadership roles in health care systems and in the university setting. The profession needs to accelerate efforts to advance the placement of CRNAs on decision-making boards and regulatory bodies in order to contribute the special expertise of nurse anesthetists to the advancement of an imaginative and successful future for our country's health care system.

In order to accomplish this future vision, the profession of nurse anesthesia, in collaboration with the accrediting body and the certification/recertification board, must seek to strengthen data integrity relative to the CRNA workforce, anesthesia and pain care quality outcomes, and the best educational approaches. Effective workforce planning and policy making require an improved information infrastructure.

Although there is strong evidence demonstrating the quality of nurse anesthesia practice, the cost advantage of nurse anesthesia care, and the reach of nurse anesthetists in providing access to disparate populations, it is not enough. There are many questions that remain to be answered and the profession must step up to the plate in a leadership role to contribute to this essential body of knowledge.

There are still many opportunities for nurse anesthesia leadership in addressing these pressing challenges and contributing to the betterment of society. CRNAs, working through the professional association, can facilitate the use of evidence-based clinical practice guidelines in anesthesia and pain management practice. Nurse anesthetists must engage in lifelong learning, accessing, managing, and applying new evidence to deliver safe care. CRNAs must find ways to fully involve patients for a truly patient- and family-centered approach to anesthesia and pain care. As payment models shift to reward desired care outcomes, payment models will change, and CRNAs must be ready for plan designs that support high-quality, team-based care. The profession of nurse anesthesia must increase the availability of information about the quality, cost, and outcomes of nurse anesthesia care, with full transparency for payers and decision makers. Nurse anesthetists have always been leaders in nursing and in the health professions as a whole. Concepts of continuous learning and quality improvement must be incorporated into professional education, certification, and accreditation requirements. The imperatives are clear, but the roadmap has yet to be drawn.

CONCLUSION

CRNAs, and all advanced practice nurses, have a key role to play in the development of our nation's health care policy. CRNA's superior knowledge and skill in anesthesia and pain care, makes them uniquely qualified to improve the health care system for their patients and society. With greater education comes greater responsibility, and nurse anesthetists are well positioned to use their significant talents for the greater good of society's health care delivery system.

As clinical experts, as educators, as administrators, and as researchers, CRNAs must use their experience at the leading edge of patient care to drive change that is needed. Throughout their history to the present, nurse anesthetists have been defined by providing access to excellent quality care at less cost than alternative providers. The success of the nurse anesthesia profession during times of crisis is well documented, and the contributions during times of war well recognized.

Every nurse anesthetist must become involved, at some level, in influencing health care reform. Advocacy may involve writing a letter or sending an e-mail to a member of Congress, making an appointment in the district to meet with a legislator, or attending a town hall meeting in the community. CRNAs may become involved in lobbying days in their state or in Washington, DC. They may attend conferences to stay current on key issues for the profession or make a contribution to the political candidate of their choice. State nurse anesthesia associations welcome volunteers with an interest in government relations. At the national level, the AANA offers many opportunities for leadership, including becoming a Federal Political Director or a State Reimbursement Director, or joining the CRNA-PAC Committee. With over 92% of nurse anesthetists belonging to the professional association, CRNAs have a high level of engagement and a high level of responsibility. Beneficial change to the anesthesia delivery system will require attention by CRNAs through focused advocacy, education, and research. Nurse anesthetists must be willing to challenge the system when it is in patients' best interests to do so, while understanding that health care spending competes with other important needs of society, and efforts to reduce costs will mean better access to care for all. The future is bright for this storied profession as health policy incentives align to reward the value that CRNAs bring to the patient experience.

DISCUSSION QUESTIONS

1. The Affordable Care Act (Sec. 1206) contains a "Non-discrimination" provision that prohibits health plans from discriminating against qualified health care providers by licensure. Where are the likely sources of opposition to the language? What arguments could be made against the nondiscrimination provision? What bullet points would you make if asked to provide written comment during the notice-and-comment rulemaking process by CMS?
2. Anesthesia care is safer than ever in the history of the specialty. In the advent of new anesthesia techniques, drugs, and enhanced training, anesthesia mortality risk has declined 100 fold to less than 1 in 100,000, according to recent studies. What are the implications of this improvement in outcomes for health care policy relative to nurse anesthetists? How does the increase in safety relate to advocacy efforts?
3. A bill has just been introduced that will allow payment for telemedicine supervision of nurse anesthetists in rural hospitals. Discuss this proposal in terms of the ethical considerations for health care sustainability. Develop a strategy for advocacy to address this proposal and describe the following: community of interest, opponents and supporters, key talking points, and elements of a media plan.

REFERENCES

American Association of Nurse Anesthetists. (2005). Code of ethics for the certified registered nurse anesthetist. Retrieved from http://www.aana.com/resources2/professionalpractice/Documents/PPM%20Code%20of%20Ethics.pdf

American Association of Nurse Anesthetists. (2010a). Guidelines for core clinical privileges for certified registered nurse anesthetists. Retrieved from http://www.aana.com/resources2/professional practice/Pages/Guidelines-for-Core-Clinical-Privileges.aspx

American Association of Nurse Anesthetists. (2010b). Position statement no. 2.11: Pain management. American Association of Nurse Anesthetists. Retrieved from http://www.aana.com/resources2/professionalpractice/Pages/Pain-Management.aspx

American Association of Nurse Anesthetists. (2013a). Certified registered nurse anesthetists at a glance. Retrieved from http://www.aana.com/ceandeducation/becomeacrna/Pages/Nurse-Anesthetists-at-a-Glance.aspx

American Association of Nurse Anesthetists. (2013b). Qualifications and capabilities of the certified registered nurse anesthetist. Retrieved from http://www.aana.com/ceandeducation/become acrna/Pages/Qualifications-and-Capabilities-of-the-Certified-Registered-Nurse-Anesthetist-.aspx

American Association of Nurse Anesthetists. (2013c). Scope of nurse anesthesia practice. Retrieved from http://www.aana.com/resources2/professionalpractice/Documents/PPM%20Scope%20and%20Standards.pdf

Baldy, J. M. (1908). The nurse as an anesthetist. Taken from the address of the President of the American Gynecological Society in May, Philadelphia. *American Journal of Nursing, 8*, 979–982.

Blumenreich, G. A. (2000). Supervision. *AANA Journal, 68*(3), 404–408.

Chalmers-Francis v. Nelson, 6 Cal. 2d 402 (1936).

Council on Accreditation of Nurse Anesthesia Educational Programs. (2009). Standards for accreditation of nurse anesthesia educational programs. Retrieved from http://home.coa.us.com/accreditation /Documents/Standards%20for%20Accreditation%20of%20Nurse%20Anesthesia%20Education %20Programs_January%202013.pdf

Council on Accreditation of Nurse Anesthesia Programs. (2013). Retrieved from http://home.coa.us .com/about/Pages/default.aspx

Dulisse, B., & Cromwell, J. (2010). No harm found when nurse anesthetists work without supervision by physicians. *Health Affairs, 29*(8), 1469–1475.

Epstein, R., & Dexter, F. (2012). Influence of supervision ratios by anesthesiologists on first-case starts and critical portions of anesthetics. *Anesthesiology, 116*, 683–691.

Florence Nightingale International Foundation. The Florence Nightingale legacy. Retrieved from http: //www.fnif.org/nightingale.htm

Frank v. South, 175 Ky. 416, 194 S.W. 375 (1917).

Health Performance Strategies. (2012). *Anesthesia subsidy surveys* (pp. 1–8). Ft. Lauderdale, FL: Author.

Hoffman, K., Thompson, G., Burke, B., & Derkay, C. (2002). Anesthetic complications of tympanostomy tube placement in children. *Archives of Otolaryngology Head & Neck Surgery, 128*(9), 1040–1043.

Hogan, P., Seifer, R., & Moore, C. (2010). Cost effectiveness analysis of anesthesia providers. *Nursing Economic$, 28*(3), 159–169.

Institute of Medicine. (2010). The future of nursing: Leading change, advancing health. Washington, DC: National Academy Press.

Institute of Medicine. (2011). Relieving pain in America: A blueprint for transforming prevention, care, education, and research. Washington, DC: National Academies Press.

Institute of Medicine. (2012). Best care at lower cost: The path to continuously learning health care in America. Washington, DC: National Academies Press.

Institute of Medicine, Committee on Consequences of Uninsurance. (2004). Insuring American's health: Principles and recommendations. Retrieved from www.iom.edu/uninsured

Joint Dialogue Group. (2008). The consensus model for APRN regulation: Licensure, accreditation, certification and education. Retrieved from https://www.ncsbn.org/aprn.htm

Koch, E. (1999). Alice Magaw and the great secret of open drop anesthesia. *AANA Journal, 67*(1), 33–38. [Includes a reprint of Magaw's article "A review of over fourteen thousand surgical anaesthesias."]

The Lewin Group. (2012). Cases: Costs of alternative pain management paths. Retrieved from http:// www.lewin.com/s~/media/Lewin/Site_Sections/Publications/CRNAPainMgtCaseStudies.pdf

Li, G., Warner, B., & Lang, B., (2009). Epidemiology of anesthesia-related mortality in the United States, 1999–2005. *Anesthesiology, 110*(4), 759–765.

Marshall, Steele & Associates. (2013). Operating room efficiency program. Retrieved from http://www .marshallsteele.com/OREfficiencyProgramOverview.pdf

National Board of Certification and Recertification of Nurse Anesthetists. (2011). Annual report.

National Board of Certification and Recertification of Nurse Anesthetists. (2013). Retrieved from http: //www.nbcrna.com/about-us/Pages/Mission-and-Vision.aspx

National Board of Certification and Recertification of Nurse Anesthetists. (2013). Retrieved from http: //www.nbcrna.com/cpc/Pages/default.aspx

National Council of State Boards of Nursing. (2008). The consensus report. Retrieved from https://www .ncsbn.org/FINAL_Consensus_Report_070708_w._Ends_013009.pdf

Needleman, J., & Minnick, A. (2008). Anesthesia provider model, hospital resources and maternal outcomes. *Health Services Research, 44*, 464–482.

Omnibus Budget Reconciliation Act of 1986, Pub. L. No. 99–509.

Part B and Other Services Payment (57 Fed. Reg. 33878 et seq., July 31, 1992).

Patient Protection and Affordable Care Act. (2010). Pub. L. No. 111–148, §2702, 124 Stat. 119, 318–319. Retrieved from http://www.gpo.gov/fdsys/pkg/BILLS-111hr3590enr/pdf/BILLS-111hr3590enr .pdf

Pine, M., Holt, K., & Lou, Y. (2003). Surgical mortality and type of anesthesia provider. *AANA Journal, 71*(2), 109–116.

The professional anaesthetizer. (Editorial). (1897). *Medical Record (NYC), 51,* 522. 18.

Simonson, D., Ahern, M., & Hendryx, M. (2007). Anesthesia staffing and anesthetic complications during cesarean delivery: A retrospective analysis. *Nursing Research, 56*(1), 9–17.

Spine Diagnostics Center of Baton Rouge v. Louisiana State Board of Nurses (2008). Docket No. 09 C 1444, Supreme Court of Louisiana, Brief of Amici Curiae by the American Nurses Association, Louisiana State Nurses Association, Louisiana Alliance of Nursing Organizations in Support of the Application for Writ of Certiorari Filed by the Louisiana State Board of Nursing through the Louisiana Department of Health and Hospitals and the Louisiana Association of Nurse Anesthetists.

Sudlow, L. L. (2000). *A vast army of women: Maine's unaccounted forces in the American Civil War.* Gettysburg, PA: Thomas Publications.

Thatcher, V. S. (1953). *History of anesthesia with emphasis on the nurse specialist.* Philadelphia, PA: J.B. Lippincott.

United States Code. (2011). 42 U.S.C §1395x(s)(11).

United States Code. (2011). 42 U.S.C. §1395x(bb)(1).

United States Code of Federal Regulations. (2011). 42 CFR 410.69 – Services of a certified registered nurse anesthetist or an anesthesiologist's assistant: Basic rule and definitions.

United States Department of Labor, Bureau of Labor Statistics. (2012-2013). *Occupational outlook handbook.* Retrieved from http://www.bls.gov/ooh/healthcare/registered-nurses.htm

United States Department of Health and Human Services, Centers for Medicare and Medicaid Services. (2001a). Medicare and Medicaid programs: Hospital conditions of participation; anesthesia services. *Federal Register, 66*(12), 4674–4687.

United States Department of Health and Human Services, Centers for Medicare and Medicaid Services. (2001b). Medicare and Medicaid programs: Hospital conditions of participation; anesthesia services. *Federal Register, 66*(219), 56762–56769.

United States Department of Health and Human Services, Centers for Medicare and Medicaid Services. (2012a). *Medicare claims processing manual,* Chapter 12: Physicians/Nonphysician practitioners. Pub. 100-04.

United States Department of Health and Human Services, Centers for Medicare and Medicaid Services. (2012b). *Medicare program integrity manual.* Pub. 100-08.

United States Department of Health and Human Services, Health Care Financing Administration. (1998). Medicare program; Revisions to payment policies and adjustments to the relative value units under the physician fee schedule for calendar year 1999. 63 *Fed. Reg.* 58843, Nov. 2, 1998.

Who should provide anesthesia care? (2010, September 6, Opinion Section). *New York Times.* Retrieved from http://www.nytimes.com/2010/09/07/opinion/07tue3.html?_r=0

Index

AACN. *See* American Association of Colleges of Nursing
AANA. *See* American Association of Nurse Anesthetists
AARP
  Center to Champion Nursing in America, 96–97
  definition, 95–96
  Future of Nursing: Campaign for Action, 98
  Graduate Nurse Education (GNE)
    Demonstration Program, 99
  IOM report recommendations, 97–98
  on nursing, 99–100
  Policy Book 2010 Revision, 97
  Public Policy Institute publications, 99
  strategic initiatives, 100
Accountable Care Organizations (ACOs), 91, 376
  ACO model
    features, 276
    vs. HMO and MCO, 276
  APRNs
  attribution of ACO beneficiaries, 279–280
  Medicare beneficiaries, attaining and
    maintaining, 280
  meeting quality and cost-efficiency
    measures, 282
  patient activation and engagement, 280–282
  Medicare Shared Savings Program
    ACO providers, 277–278
    MedPAC recommendation, 277
    payments and treatment, 278–279
    requirements, 278
  non-Medicare shared savings programs,
    282–283
  PPACA, programs and demonstration projects
    Center for Medicare and Medicaid
      Innovation, 275–276
    health home, 275
    home demonstration project, 274–275
    National Pilot Program on Payment
      Bundling, 274

    pediatric ACO demonstration project, 275
    quality of health care, 379–378
accreditation, consensus model, 60–62
ACOs. *See* Accountable Care Organizations
advanced practice registered nurses (APRNs)
    Alma Ata Declaration, 340–341
barriers to practice, 202–205, 346
  clinical nurse specialist, 345–346
  CNSs and APNs, 387
    competencies, 340
    educational preparation, 340
  family nurse practitioner, 344–345
    Global Advisory Group, 341
  global perspectives, 346
    nurse midwives, 339
  OECD countries, 343–344
  oncology care and, 245–246
  Patient Protection and Affordable Care Act, 92
    professional support, 339
    scope of practice, 339
advocacy
  competencies, 136–137
  definition, 3
  strategy tools and resources, 140–142
Affordable Care Act (ACA), 5, 379
African Health Professions Regulatory
    Collaborative (ARC) for Nurses and
    Midwives
  baseline survey, 401–402
  Capability Maturity Model, 403–406
  collaborative regulatory improvement, 399, 400
  core objectives, 398
  evaluation, 401
  law and regulation, 409–411
  nurse-initiated and managed antiretroviral
    therapy
    data collection and analysis, 408
    dissemination of findings, 408–409
    domains of inquiry, 407
    literature review, 407

African Health Professions Regulatory
Collaborative (ARC) for Nurses and
Midwives (*cont.*)
   research collaboration, 407
   study design and implementation, 408
   regulatory improvement grants, 400
   technical assistance, 400–401
aging population
   Consensus Model, 194
   health care needs of, 189–191
   new opportunities, 191–192
   outcomes, 192–194
   scope of practice, reimbursement, and
      prescriptive authority, 186–189
American Association of Colleges of Nursing
   (AACN), 25
American Association of Nurse Anesthetists
   (AANA), 419, 420–421, 433, 435
American Nurses Association (ANA)
   advanced education and licensure, 314–315
   American Nurses Credentialing Center,
      312–313
   APRN movement, 311–312
   clinical nurse specialists
      certification, 312–313
      councils, 314
   collaboration, 316–317
   constituent and state nurses associations
      CAPNAP, 317
      Georgia Nurses Association, 319
      Iowa Nurses Association, 319
      Maryland Nurses Association, 318
      Missouri Nurses Association, 318
      Oregon Nurses Association, 317–318
      Rhode Island Nurses Association, 318
      South Carolina Nurses Association, 318
      Vermont State Nurses Association, 318
      WV Nurses Association, 318
   federal work, 315–316
   nurse practitioner
      certification, 312–313
      councils, 313
      national alliance of, 315
   organizational affiliates, 319
   policy priorities, 319–320
American Nurses Credentialing Center (ANCC),
   312–313, 350
American Organization of Nurse Executives
   (AONE), 26
American Society of Clinical Oncology
   (ASCO), 244
ANA. *See* American Nurses Association
ANCC. *See* American Nurses Credentialing
   Center
AONE. *See* American Organization of Nurse
   Executives
ASCO. *See* American Society of Clinical Oncology

California Association of Psychiatric Mental
   Health Nurses in Advanced Practice
   (CAPNAP), 317

Campaign for Action: Future of Nursing, 77–79
   AARP, 98
   challenges, 80
   dashboard indicators, 81–82
   evaluation, 80–81
   future plans, 81–84
   National Summit, 79
cancer burden, United States, 240
Cancer Care Continuum
   cancer as chronic condition, 239–240
   palliative care, 243–245
   prevention, 240–241
   risk assessment and counseling, 241–242
   survivorship, 243–245
   treatment, 243
cancer genetic and genomic testing, 241–243
Capability Maturity Model (CMM)
   components, 403
   nursing and midwifery regulation, 403–404
   Regulatory Function Framework, 405–406
   software design, 403
   stages, 403
   validation and pilot testing, 404–405
CAPNAP. *See* California Association of
   Psychiatric Mental Health Nurses in
   Advanced Practice
care coordination
   clinical nurse specialist, 388
   PMH nursing practice, 168, 171
CCNA. *See* Center to Champion Nursing in
   America
Center for Medicare and Medicaid Innovation
   (CMMI), 43
   PPACA initiatives, 275–276
Centers for Medicare and Medicaid Services
   (CMS), 330
Center to Champion Nursing in America
   (CCNA), 96–97
certifications
   clinical nurse specialists, 312–313
   Consensus Model, 63
   oncology advanced practice registered
      nurse, 238
certified nurse midwives (CNMs)
   collegial barriers, 202–204
   core competencies, 200–201
   financial barriers, 204–205
   midwifery domination, 200
   outcome measures, 206
   PPACA, 206–208
   regulatory barriers, 201–202
   therapeutic alliance, 200
certified registered nurse anesthetists (CRNAs)
   Medicare reimbursement methodology, 422
   Patient Protection and Affordable Care Act,
      421–422
   physician services, 422–423
   scope of practice and reimbursement, 421
   chronic pain management, 431–436
   core competencies, 423
   ethical considerations, 437–438

evaluation, 436–437
future aspects, 438–439
historical background, 418–420
physician supervision, 424–429
   Tax Equity and Financial Responsibility
      Act, 426–428
Champion Nursing Coalition, 96
clinical nurse specialist (CNS)
   care quality and safety, 383–385
   care transitions, 382–383
   challenges, 380
   chronic illness, 387–388
   community-based care, 386–387
   health policy, 380–381
   QSEN competencies, 385–386
   wellness and preventive care, 389
CMM. *See* Capability Maturity Model (CMM)
CMMI. *See* Center for Medicare and Medicaid
   Innovation
CMS. *See* Centers for Medicare and Medicaid
   Services
CNMs. *See* certified nurse midwives
CNS. *See* clinical nurse specialist
COA. *See* Council on Accreditation of Nurse
   Anesthesia Educational Programs
Coalition for Patients' Rights (CPR), 69
   advanced practice registered nurses and,
      71–72
   advantages, 68–69
   description, 67–68
   and Scope of Practice Partnership, 69–71
Conditions of Participation (CoPs), 218
Consensus Model
   aging population, 194
   applications to APRNs, 60–64
   evaluation of, 64
   as health policy, 64–65
   older adults, 194
   oncology advanced practice registered nurse,
      237–238
Continuing Professional Certification (CPC)
   approach, 420
Continuing Professional Development (CPD), 410
CoPs. *See* Conditions of Participation
Council on Accreditation of Nurse Anesthesia
   Educational Programs (COA), 420, 433
CPD. *See* Continuing Professional Development
CPR. *See* Coalition for Patients' Rights
credentialing
   advanced practice vs. specialization, 355–356
   American Nurses Credentialing Center, 350
   Australia's health care system, 353–354
   global processes and procedures, 354–355
   internal regulation, 356–357
   International Council of Nurses (ICN),
      349–350
   New Zealand mental health nurse, 351–353
     Te Ao Maramatanga, 352–353
   professional specialist, 351
   Royal College of Nursing, 350–351
CRNAs. *See* certified registered nurse anesthetists

direct-to-consumer (DTC) genetic testing, 242
Diversity Steering Committee, 52–53
dying patient's bill of rights, 221

education
   Consensus Model, 63–64
   interprofessional workforce, 36–37
   oncology advanced practice registered nurse,
      237–238
EGAPP. *See* Evaluation of Genomic Applications
   in Practice and Prevention
EHPs. *See* emergency hire programs (EHPs)
emergency hire programs (EHPs), 397–398
end-of-life care
   conceptual and theoretical framework, 222–223
   ethics, 230–231
   health policy, 223
   history, 218–220
   Measure Applications Partnership, 229
   outcome measures, 229
   palliative care, 220–222
   policy changes, 217–218
   practice implications, 229–230
ethical issues
   advanced practice registered nurse, 18–19
   end-of-life care, 230–231
   PMH nursing practice, 175
   White House Joining Forces initiative, 129
Evaluation of Genomic Applications in Practice
   and Prevention (EGAPP), 242

Federal Employees Health Benefits Program
   (FEHBP), 291
federally qualified health centers (FQHCs), 31, 47
Federal Trade Commission (FTC), 332
fee-for-service payment, 288
FEHBP. *See* Federal Employees Health Benefits
   Program
fiscal transparency, 9
5As model, 107
5Rs model, 107
FQHCs. *See* federally qualified health centers
FTC. *See* Federal Trade Commission
Future of Nursing
   Campaign for Action
     AARP, 98
     challenges, 80
     dashboard indicators, 81–82
     evaluation, 80–81
     future plans, 81–84
     National Summit, 79
   IOM report
     Diversity Steering Committee, 52–53
     recommendations, 48–52

Genetic Information Nondiscrimination Act
   (GINA), 242
Georgia Nurses Association (GNA), 319
GINA. *See* Genetic Information
   Nondiscrimination Act

GNA. *See* Georgia Nurses Association
Graduate Nurse Education (GNE)
    Demonstration, 99, 155–158

Health and Human Services (HHS)
    Accountable Care Organizations, 379–380
    National Quality Strategy, 379
health care reform, 163–164
health care services, result-oriented
        reimbursement, 8–9
health care spending
    administrative systems, 290
    competitive bidding, 289–290
    defensive medicine, 291–292
    exchanges and state employee plans, 289
    fee-for-service payment, 288
    nonphysician providers, 291
    payment rates, 288
    physician self-referrals, 291
    transparency of prices, 290
health care system models, quality and safety
    health literate organizations, 262
    high-reliability organizations, 261
    just culture, 261
    learning health care systems, 263–264
    patient engagement, 263
    person-centered care, 262
health care workforce, in APRNs
    chronic care, 33
    disease management, 33
    health information technology, 34
    medical homes, 34
    medical resident care, 32–33
    primary care, 32
    retail clinics, 34
    telehealth, 34
    vulnerable populations, 33
health information technology (HIT)
    health care workforce, 34
    PMH nursing practice, 168–169, 171–172
health literate organizations, 262
Health Maintenance Organization (HMO), 276
health promotion, 92
Henderson's theory, 124–125
HHS. *See* Health and Human Services (HHS)
high-reliability organizations (HROs), 261
HIT. *See* health information technology
HMO. *See* Health Maintenance Organization
home care nursing services, 376–377
home demonstration project, 274–275
Hospice and Palliative Nurses Association
        (HPNA) 2010 Public Policy Guiding
        Principles, 225
HROs. *See* high-reliability organizations
human resources for health
    educational investments, 396–397
    emergency hire initiatives, 397–398
    Joint Learning Initiative, 394–395
    Nurse Education Partnership Initiative, 396
    task sharing, 397

ICN. *See* International Council of Nurses
illness prevention, nursing theorists, 7–8
Institute of Medicine (IOM)
    Future of Nursing report, 42–48
        Diversity Steering Committee, 52–53
        recommendations, 48–52
        services by NMHCs, 46–47
    integrated workforce, 34–37
    and Robert Wood Johnson Foundation, 41–42
integrated health care, 166–167, 169–170
integrated workforce
    data improvement, 37
    interprofessional education, 36–37
    outcome-driven policy, 35
    patient-centered care, 35
    professional protectionism, 36
    quality gaps, 36
    reform provider reimbursement, 37
International Council of Nurses (ICN), 362
    APN scope of practice, 339
    credentialing, 349–350
    educational preparation of the APN, 340
    INP/APNN, 338
    nurse midwives, 339
    professional support, 339
    RN competencies, 340
international perspectives
    advanced practice nursing, 361–362
    APN education requirements
        Ireland, 367
        Israel, 367–368
        Republic of South Africa, 366–367
    APN role and responsibilities
        Netherlands, 368–369
        New Zealand, 369–370
        Republic of South Africa, 368
        United Kingdom, 369
    authorization, APN roles
        Australia, 364
        France, 363
        Ireland, 364
        Israel, 365–366
        Oman, 363
        policy-driven support, 362–363
        Republic of South Africa, 365
        Saudi Arabia, 365
        Singapore, 364
    International Council of Nurses, 362
    United States, 361
interprofessional workforce education, 36–37
IOM. *See* Institute of Medicine
Iowa Nurses Association, 319

JLI. *See* Joint Learning Initiative
Johnson & Johnson *Campaign for Nursing's
        Future*
    description, 23–24
    local, regional scholarships and fundraisers, 25
    NLN partnership, 25–28
    nurse educator initiatives, 25

Joint Learning Initiative (JLI), 394–395
just culture principles, 261

legislatures, 138
licensing boards, 139
licensure, Consensus Model, 59–60
Local Coverage Determination (LCD), 432
long-term skilled nursing care, 376–377
low-income countries
    ARC
        baseline survey, 401–402
        Capability Maturity Model, 403–406
        collaborative regulatory improvement,
            399, 400
        core objectives, 398
        evaluation, 401
        law and regulation, 409–411
        NIMART, 407–409
        regulatory improvement grants, 400
        technical assistance, 400–401
    health systems, 394–395
    human resources for health
        educational investments, 396–397
        emergency hire initiatives, 397–398
        Joint Learning Initiative, 394–395
        Nurse Education Partnership Initiative, 396
        task sharing, 397
    system-level changes, 406

MAC. *See* Medicare Administrative Contractor
Managed Care Organization (MCO), 276
Maryland Nurses Association (MNA), 318
MCO. *See* Managed Care Organization
Measure Applications Partnership measures, 229
Medical Home Model, 376
medical homes
    health care workforce, 34
    Patient Protection and Affordable Care Act, 91
medical marijuana, 246
Medicare Administrative Contractor (MAC),
    431–432
Medicare Modernization Act (MMA), 87
Medicare Payment Advisory Commission
    (MedPAC), 277
Medicare Shared Savings Program
    ACO providers, 277–278
    general requirements, 278
    MedPAC recommendation, 277
    payments and treatment, 278–279
    quality and reporting requirements, 278
MedPAC. *See* Medicare Payment Advisory
    Commission (MedPAC)
mental health care. *See* psychiatric mental health
    (PMH) nursing practice
mental health nurse credentialing
    Australia's health care system, 353–354
    New Zealand
        credentialed status, 353
        evidence-based record (EBR), 352
        mental health issues, 351

periodic recredentialing, 352
        registered nurses skills, 351–352
        responsibility, 352
        Te Ao Maramatanga, 352–353
mental illness, prevalence, 165
midwifery domination, 200
midwifery guardianship, 200
military service members, 125
Million Hearts® initiative, 103–116
Million Hearts® Pledge, 106
Missouri Nurses Association (MONA), 318
MMA. *See* Medicare Modernization Act
MNA. *See* Maryland Nurses Association
MONA. *See* Missouri Nurses Association

NACNS. *See* National Association for Clinical
    Nurse Specialists
National Association for Clinical Nurse
    Specialists (NACNS), 329–300
National Board for Certification of Hospice and
    Palliative Nurses (NBCHPN®), 218,
    226–228
National Board of Certification and
    Recertification for Nurse Anesthetists
    (NBCRNA), 420, 433
National Consensus Project (NCP) for Quality
    Palliative Care, 244
National Council of State Boards of Nursing
    (NCSBN), 57–58
National Healthcare Quality Report 2011, 36
National Institute of Nursing Research (NINR),
    223–224
National League for Nursing's (NLN) Faculty
    Leadership and Mentoring Program,
    25–28
National Pilot Program on Payment Bundling,
    274
National Quality Strategy (NQS), 106
National Summit, *Future of Nursing: Campaign for
    Action*, 79
NBCHPN®. *See* National Board for Certification
    of Hospice and Palliative Nurses
NBCRNA. *See* National Board of Certification
    and Recertification for Nurse
    Anesthetists
NCSBN. *See* National Council of State Boards of
    Nursing
NEPI. *See* Nurse Education Partnership Initiative
NIMART. *See* nurse-initiated and managed
    antiretroviral therapy
NINR. *See* National Institute of Nursing Research
NMHCs. *See* nurse-managed health clinics
NQS. *See* National Quality Strategy
NTA. *See* Nurse Training Act
Nurse Education Partnership Initiative
    (NEPI), 396
nurse-initiated and managed antiretroviral
    therapy (NIMART), 397
    data collection and analysis, 408
    dissemination of findings, 408–409

nurse-initiated and managed antiretroviral
    therapy (NIMART) *(cont.)*
  domains of inquiry, 407
  literature review, 407
  research collaboration, 407
  study design and implementation, 408
nurse-managed health clinics (NMHCs), 46, 159
Nurse Practice Act, 138
nurse practitioners
  current situation, 374–375
  future aspects
    Accountable Care Organizations, 376
    home care nursing services, 376–377
    long-term skilled nursing care, 376–377
    Medical Home Model, 376
    transitional and coordinated care, 376
  history, 373–374
Nurse Training Act (NTA), 147–149
nursing education funding
  Congressional action, 147–150
  federal funding, 150–152
  GNE Demonstration, 155–158
  Patient Protection and Affordable Care Act,
    152–155
  public health nursing, 145
  Public Health Service, 145–146
Nursing Need Theory, 124
Nursing Pledge, 128
nursing theorists, illness prevention, 7

older adults
  Consensus Model, 194
  health care needs of, 189–191
  outcomes, 192–194
  scope of practice, reimbursement, and
    prescriptive authority, 186–189
ONA. *See* Oregon Nurses Association (ONA)
ONCC. *See* Oncology Nurse Certification
  Corporation
oncology advanced practice registered nurse
  in Accountable Care Organizations, 238
  Cancer Care Continuum
    cancer as chronic condition, 239–240
    palliative care, 243–245
    prevention, 240–241
    risk assessment and counseling, 241–242
    survivorship, 243–245
    treatment, 243
  in collaborative oncology care, 238–239
  competencies, 235–237
  Consensus Model, 237–238
  prescriptive authority
    barriers to practice, 245–246
    medical marijuana, 246
  specialty nursing practice, 235
Oncology Nurse Certification Corporation
  (ONCC), 238
Oncology Nursing Society (ONS), 235–237
ONS. *See* Oncology Nursing Society
Oregon Nurses Association (ONA), 317

organizational policy, definition, 14
Organization for Economic Co-operation and
  Development (OECD) countries, 343–344

palliative care
  advanced practice registered nurse, 225–228
  Cancer Care Continuum, 243–245
  end-of-life care, 220–222
patient-centered care
  clinical nurse specialist, 387
  integrated workforce, 35
  PMH nursing practice, 169, 172
Patient Centered Outcomes Research Institute
  (PCORI)
  chronic disease care, 388
  quality and safety, 266–267
Patient Protection and Affordable Care Act
  (PPACA), 421–422
  Accountable Care Organization, 91
  American Nurses Association, 316
  disease prevention, 92
  health promotion, 92
  insurance exchanges, 91
  Medicaid expansion, 92
  medical homes, 91
  nurse practitioners, 90–91
  nursing education funding, 152–155
  obstacles/barriers, 92
  programs and demonstration projects
    Center for Medicare and Medicaid
     Innovation, 275–276
    health home, 275
    home demonstration project, 274–275
    National Pilot Program on Payment
     Bundling, 274
    pediatric ACO demonstration project, 275
  protection and provisions, 88–89
  psychiatric mental health nursing practice,
    165–166
  transitional care and care coordination, 91–92
PCORI. *See* Patient-Centered Outcomes Research
  Institute
pediatric ACO demonstration project, 275
person-centered care, health care system
  models, 262
PGP. *See* Physician Group Practice
PHS. *See* Public Health Service
Physician Group Practice (PGP), 277
policy
  competencies, 136–137
  definition, 3
  drivers of, 5
  organizational, 14
  professional, 14
  public, 14
policy making
  development stages of, 4–5
  in government bodies, 137–139
  illness prevention, 7–8
  new delivery models, 10

with nursing process, 5
result-oriented reimbursement, 8–9
scope of practice, 8
well-being promotion, 4–7
PPACA. *See* Patient Protection and Affordable
        Care Act
prescriptive authority, oncology APRNs,
        245–246
President's Emergency Fund for AIDS Relief
        (PEPFAR) initiative, 396
professional nursing organizations
    APRN organizations, 301–302
    health policy issues, 302–305
    IOM quality reports, 305–307
    leadership, 307–309
    nursing's social policy statement, 299–300
    and policy process, 297–298
professional policy, definition, 14
professional protectionism, 36
psychiatric mental health (PMH) nursing practice
    ethical issues, 175
    evaluation initiatives, 172–173
    health care reform, 163–164
    impact of
        care coordination, 168, 171
        health information technology, 168–169,
            171–172
        integrated health care, 166–167, 169–170
        patient-centered care, 169, 172
        wellness, 167, 170–171
    outcomes and core competencies, 174
    PPACA, 165–166
public health nursing, 145
Public Health Service (PHS), 145–146
public policy, definition, 14, 135–136
Public Policy Institute (PPI) publications, 99

QIOs. *See* quality improvement organizations
Quad Council's Competencies for Public Health
        Nurses, 329
quality and safety
    data collection and reporting challenges,
        265–266
    driving forces, 255–256
    evidence-based practice, 264–265
    health care delivery, 255
    health care system models
        health literate organizations, 262
        high-reliability organizations, 261
        just culture, 261
        learning health care systems, 263–264
        patient engagement, 263
        person-centered care, 262
    nursing alliance, 256–258
    Patient-Centered Outcomes Research Institute,
        266–267
    policy vs. quality, 254–255
    strategies, 267–268
    strengthening competencies, 268–269
    transparency, 259–260

Quality and Safety Education for Nurses (QSEN)
        competencies, 385–386
quality improvement organizations (QIOs), 10

RCN. *See* Royal College of Nursing
residency programs, in APRNs, 158–159
retail clinics, health care workforce, 34
Rhode Island Nurses Association, 318
Robert Wood Johnson Foundation (RWJF), 41–42,
        75–76
Royal College of Nursing (RCN), 350–351
RWJF. *See* Robert Wood Johnson Foundation

Scope of Practice Partnership (SOPP), 69–71
social identity theory
    controversies, 325–326
    geographic identity, 326
    LACE institution, 325
    uniqueness, 325
SOPP. *See* Scope of Practice Partnership
South Carolina Nurses Association, 318
SRS program. *See* State Reimbursement Specialist
        (SRS) program
stakeholders, speaking for APRNs, 139
Stark law, 291
State-Based Coalition (SBC) Program, 69
state-based regulatory implementation,
        Consensus Model
    definition, 323–324
    evaluation and application, 332
    vs. model act and rules, 324
    policy concepts
        constraints, 324
        incrementalism, 326–327
        social construction and policy design, 325
        social identity theory, 325–326
    social construction and social identity, 327–330
    successful strategies, 331–332
state board of nursing, 138
state regulatory boards, speaking for APRNs, 139
State Reimbursement Specialist (SRS)
        program, 438
"Sunshine laws," 139

Tax Equity and Financial Responsibility Act
        (TEFRA), 426–427
TEFRA. *See* Tax Equity and Financial
        Responsibility Act (TEFRA)
telehealth, health care workforce, 34
therapeutic alliance, 200
transparency, quality and safety, 259–260

United Nations Millennium Development Goals
        (MDGs), 394
U.S. Preventive Services Task Force (USPSTF),
        109–110
USPSTF. *See* U.S. Preventive Services Task Force

Vermont State Nurses Association, 318

wellness, PMH nursing practice, 167, 170–171
West Virginia Nurses Association (WVNA), 318
White House Joining Forces initiative
    application to APRNs, 125–126
    ethical issues, 129
    evaluation concepts, 126
    Nursing Pledge, 128

WHO. *See* World Health Organization
World Health Organization (WHO)
    Alma Ata Declaration, 340–341
    Global Advisory Group, 341
    primary health care, 341
WVNA. *See* West Virginia Nurses Association
    (WVNA)

Made in the USA
Middletown, DE
10 August 2016